NCLEX-RN® Review Guide

Top Ten Questions for Quick Review

Cynthia Chernecky, PhD, RN, AOCN, FAAN
Professor
Department of Physiological and Technological Nursing
School of Nursing
Medical College of Georgia
Augusta, GA

Nancy Stark, RN, MSN, CNAA, BC
Instructor
Department of Physiological and Technological Nursing
School of Nursing
Medical College of Georgia
Augusta, GA

Lori Schumacher, PhD, RN, CCRN
Associate Professor and Interim Chair
Department of Physiological and Technological Nursing
School of Nursing
Medical College of Georgia
Augusta, GA

JONES AND BARTLETT PUBLISHERS
Sudbury, Massachusetts
BOSTON   TORONTO   LONDON   SINGAPORE

World Headquarters

Jones and Bartlett Publishers
40 Tall Pine Drive
Sudbury, MA 01776
978-443-5000
info@jbpub.com
www.jbpub.com

Jones and Bartlett Publishers Canada
6339 Ormindale Way
Mississauga, Ontario L5V 1J2
Canada

Jones and Bartlett Publishers International
Barb House, Barb Mews
London W6 7PA
United Kingdom

Jones and Bartlett's books and products are available through most bookstores and online booksellers. To contact Jones and Bartlett Publishers directly, call 800-832-0034, fax 978-443-8000, or visit our website www.jbpub.com.

Substantial discounts on bulk quantities of Jones and Bartlett's publications are available to corporations, professional associations, and other qualified organizations. For details and specific discount information, contact the special sales department at Jones and Bartlett via the above contact information or send an email to specialsales@jbpub.com.

The authors, editor, and publisher have made every effort to provide accurate information. However, they are not responsible for errors, omissions, or for any outcomes related to the use of the contents of this book and take no responsibility for the use of the products and procedures described. Treatments and side effects described in this book may not be applicable to all people; likewise, some people may require a dose or experience a side effect that is not described herein. Drugs and medical devices are discussed that may have limited availability controlled by the Food and Drug Administration (FDA) for use only in a research study or clinical trial. Research, clinical practice, and government regulations often change the accepted standard in this field. When consideration is being given to use of any drug in the clinical setting, the health care provider or reader is responsible for determining FDA status of the drug, reading the package insert, and reviewing prescribing information for the most up-to-date recommendations on dose, precautions, and contraindications, and determining the appropriate usage for the product. This is especially important in the case of drugs that are new or seldom used.

Additional credits appear on page xiv, which constitutes a continuation of the copyright page.

Production Credits

Executive Editor: Kevin Sullivan
Acquisitions Editor: Emily Ekle
Associate Editor: Amy Sibley
Editorial Assistant: Patricia Donnelly
Production Director: Amy Rose
Production Editor: Carolyn F. Rogers
Senior Marketing Manager: Katrina Gosek
Associate Marketing Manager: Rebecca Wasley

Senior Photo Researcher and Photographer: Kimberly Potvin
Associate Photo Researcher and Photographer: Christine McKeen
Interactive Technology Manager: Dawn Mahon Priest
Manufacturing and Inventory Coordinator: Amy Bacus
Compositor: Publishers' Design and Production Services, Inc.
Cover Design: Kristin E. Ohlin
Cover Image: © ErikN/ShutterStock, Inc.
Printing and Binding: Malloy, Inc.
Cover Printing: Malloy, Inc.

Library of Congress Cataloging-in-Publication Data

Chernecky, Cynthia C.
    NCLEX-RN review guide : top ten questions for quick review / Cynthia Chernecky, Nancy Stark, and Lori Schumacher.
        p. ; cm.
    Includes bibliographical references.
    ISBN-13: 978-0-7637-4039-9
    ISBN-10: 0-7637-4039-X
    1. Nurses—Licenses—Study guides. 2. Nursing—Examinations, questions, etc. I. Stark, Nancy, 1956–
II. Schumacher, Lori. III. Title.
    [DNLM: 1. Nursing—Examination Questions. WY 18.2 C521n 2007]
    RT55.N7458 2007
    610.73076—dc22

                                                                                    2007000618

6048

Printed in the United States of America
11 10 09 08 07   10 9 8 7 6 5 4 3 2 1

CONTENTS

WHAT IS THE NCLEX EXAMINATION?

Entry into the practice of nursing in the United States and its territories is regulated by the licensing authorities within each jurisdiction. To ensure public protection, each jurisdiction requires candidates for licensure to pass an examination that measures the competencies needed to perform safely and effectively as a newly licensed, entry-level registered nurse. The National Council of State Boards of Nursing, Inc. (NCSBN), has developed a licensure examination, called the National Council Licensure Examination for Registered Nurses (NCLEX-RN), which is used by state, commonwealth, and territorial boards of nursing to assist in making licensure decisions.

Information regarding how and where to take the NCLEX-RN examination is available at the NCSBN Web site at www.ncsbn.org. There you will find complete information on the following subjects surrounding the NCLEX exam:

- Scheduling an appointment to take the NCLEX
- What to expect on the day of the examination
- Results reporting

ADDITIONAL INFORMATION ABOUT THE NCLEX EXAMINATION

Examination Length

The NCLEX-RN is a variable-length adaptive test. The exam is taken electronically via a computer and is not offered in paper-and-pencil or oral examination formats. More information on the adaptive format of the NCLEX is available at the NCSBN Web site at www.ncsbn.org.

Reviewing the Answers and Guessing

Two questions that many students have about the NCLEX exam are:

How much time should I spend on each question?

and

Should I guess on a question if I don't know the answer and am I penalized for guessing?

There are important things to note when considering how to answer questions on the

NCLEX exam. First, you must answer every item even if you are not sure of the right answer. The computer will not allow you to go on to the next item without answering the one on the screen. If you are unsure of the correct answer, make your best guess and move on to the next item. After you select an answer to an item, you will have a chance to think about your answer and change it as many times as you like. However, once you confirm your answer and go on to the next item, you will not be allowed to return to any previous item on the examination. Second, rapid guessing can drastically lower your score. On any adaptive test, this strategy can be disastrous! Additional information about how to approach the questions in the NCLEX-RN exam is provided at the NCSBN Web site (www.ncsbn.org).

THE *NCLEX-RN®* TEST PLAN

Introduction

The *NCLEX-RN® Test Plan* is the outline that the creators of the exam follow to determine which questions will be included on the exam. The *NCLEX-RN® Test Plan* was most recently updated in April of 2007. This book follows this latest version of the test plan.

The content of the *NCLEX-RN® Test Plan* is organized into four major categories based on patient needs. Two of the four categories are further divided as follows:

Safe and Effective Care Environment
- Management of Care
- Safety and Infection Control
Health Promotion and Maintenance
Psychosocial Integrity
Physiological Integrity
- Basic Care and Comfort
- Pharmacological and Parenteral Therapies
- Reduction of Risk Potential
- Physiological Adaptation

Distribution of Content

The percentage of test questions assigned to each patient needs category and subcategory of the *NCLEX-RN® Test Plan* is based on the results of the *Report of Findings from the 2005 RN Practice Analysis: Linking the NCLEX-RN® Examination to Practice*

(NCSBN, 2006), and expert judgment provided by members of the NCSBN Examination Committee.

Patient Needs	Percentage of Items from Each Category/Subcategory
Safe and Effective Care Environment	
Management of Care	13–10%
Safety and Infection Control	8–14%
Health Promotion and Maintenance	6–12%
Psychosocial Integrity	6–12%
Physiological Integrity	
Basic Care and Comfort	6–12%
Pharmacological and Parenteral Therapies	13–19%
Reduction of Risk Potential	13–19%
Physiological Adaptation	11–17%

Again, the book you hold in your hands, *NCLEX-RN® Review Guide: Top Ten Questions for Quick Review*, follows the current *NCLEX-RN® Test Plan*. It also follows the percentage breakdown of the various patient needs areas shown above. Visit the NCSBN's Web site at www.ncsbn.org to find more information about each of the patient needs categories. There, you will find the latest information about computerized adaptive testing (CAT) and everything you might need to know about taking the NCLEX-RN exam.

TOP TEN NCLEX-RN REVIEW: HOW THIS BOOK WORKS

Top Ten

The first section of this review guide presents 10 questions from each of the major categories from the *NCLEX-RN® Test Plan*:

- Care of the Childbearing Family and the Neonate
- Care of Children
- Care of Adults
- Care of Patients with Psychiatric and Mental Health Problems
- Trends and Current Issues in Nursing
- Math, Dosage Calculations, and Related Problems
- Care of Patients with Diabetes
- Care of Patients with Hypertension and Cardiac Problems

These "top ten" questions represent the most essential concepts from each topic. If you can correctly answer these questions, you are well on your way to proficiency in that subject area. Designed specifically to help you gauge your competency level, these questions will help you develop a thorough study plan for the NCLEX.

Did you answer all of the top 10 questions for math correctly, but miss 4 of the cardiac questions? You'll know to spend your valuable study time brushing up on cardiology and you can feel a little more self-assured about your math skills.

Sections II–X

Once you have completed the top 10 questions for each section, it is time to move on to the major content areas. Sections II through X cover the previously mentioned topics with percentages of questions (per the *NCLEX-RN® Test Plan*) in the following categories and subcategories:

Safe and Effective Care Environment
- Management of Care
- Safety and Infection Control
Health Promotion and Maintenance
Psychosocial Integrity
Physiological Integrity
- Basic Care and Comfort
- Pharmacological and Parenteral Therapies
- Reduction of Risk Potential
- Physiological Adaptation

Each section contains 222 questions, the majority of which are standard multiple choice. Scattered throughout each section, in proportions according to the test plan, are a number of alternative-format questions (discussed later).

After you have completed Sections II through X, it is often helpful to return to Section I (the top 10 questions) to see the progress you have made. We hope you can now answer all of the top 10 questions correctly and with confidence!

Alternative Item Formats

An alternative item format is an examination item, or question, that uses a format other than standard, four-option, multiple-choice questions to assess candidate ability. Alternative item formats may include

- Multiple-response items that require a candidate to select one or more than one response
- Fill-in-the-blank items that require a candidate to type in terms or numbers in a calculation item
- Hot-spot items that ask a candidate to identify an area on a picture or a graphic
- Chart/exhibit-format items in which candidates are presented with a problem and need to read the information in the chart or exhibit to solve the problem
- Drag-and-drop items that require a candidate to rank-order or move options to provide the correct answer

Alternative-format items allow candidates to demonstrate their entry-level nursing competence in ways that are different from the standard multiple-choice items. In addition, some nursing content areas can be assessed more readily and authentically with alternative-format items. As with standard multiple-choice items, alternative-format items are scored as either right or wrong; there is no use of partial credit in the scoring of these items.

Interactive CD-ROM

Inside this book, you'll find a CD-ROM. This CD contains all of the questions from the book itself, but using the CD lets you do the following:

- Sort the questions by subject area
- Sort the questions by patient need category as described in the *NCLEX-RN® Test Plan*
- Randomize the questions
- Grade yourself! The "grade-yourself" feature allows you to review the questions you answered incorrectly. This feature will also indicate which subject areas are your strongest and which might require additional time and attention.
- Practice taking exams electronically

TEST-TAKING SKILLS

Nothing is more important to successful test taking than studying. A thorough understanding of the test material is essential to your success. While test-taking strategies are not a substitute for good study habits, these skills will enhance your overall performance on a test as long as you have a good grasp of the knowledge being measured. Follow the study plan guidelines discussed previously and use the hints provided here to increase your probability of choosing the correct answer. Remember—the right answer is right there in front of you. Have confidence in yourself.

Plan Ahead

The night before the test is not the time for cramming. Review the test-taking strategies discussed next, and then put your books away. Relax and get a good night's sleep. Plan to wear comfortable clothes. It is difficult to predict the climate variations of most testing sites, so dress in layers and bring a sweater. Avoid confusion on the day of the test by being well prepared. Bring your admission ticket, your photo identification, and a watch. Make sure you are familiar with the route to the testing site and allow yourself plenty of time

to get there. Arrive early and choose a seat where you feel comfortable. A little bit of anxiety is a positive force and planning ahead will help keep your anxiety at this positive level. Relaxation techniques such as controlled breathing will help you feel calm and unhurried when the test begins.

Read Each Question Carefully

Read each question all the way through. Pay attention to detail; every word counts. Be alert for key words. Words such as "only," "never," "first," "last," "always," "except," or "never" are strong words that limit the choice of the correct answer. Ask yourself, "What is this question asking?" Consider the question as it is written. At the same time, do not read anything into it—no one is trying to trick you. If it helps, try to rephrase and answer the question in your own words.

Read Each Answer Choice Carefully

Even if the first or second answer choice looks good to you, it is a mistake to think that you don't need to read the other options. Sometimes another choice provides a more precise answer or makes you realize that you misunderstood the question. Under the stress of taking a test, you might be tempted to select the first answer choice that looks right. Resist this temptation! Careful examination may reveal that your first choice does not answer the question at all.

Eliminate the obviously incorrect options quickly and compare the plausible options for similarities or conflicts. Given that there is only one correct answer to each of the standard multiple-choice questions, options that are similar must both be wrong. If two options are polar opposites, one of them is frequently correct. Eliminate the wrong answer choices one by one. This process of elimination will be completed quickly for simple recall questions, but may take longer for more complex questions.

Although this method sounds time-consuming, it will assist you in clarifying the question and selecting more correct answers. Practicing this method of eliminating answers on the sample tests included in this book will help you to develop the speed you need in the real exam.

Reread the Question and the Answer Choices

Choose your answer from your remaining choices based on your rereading of the question. Spend time considering the plausible choices. Have confidence in your selection, but if you are unable to answer the question after eliminating the obviously wrong choices, move on to the next question. Remember, in an NCLEX exam, you must provide an answer to the current question before you can move on to the next question. Don't get bogged down on any single question. Spending too much time on a difficult question could compromise your final test score.

Stay Focused

Keep yourself focused. Think only about the question in front of you. If stray thoughts distract you, or you find your mind wandering back to a previous question, bring your focus back to the question at hand. Congratulate yourself for being in control of the situation.

Pace Yourself

On the one hand, don't puzzle too long over any question. On the other hand, don't race through the test so fast that you make careless errors. Pace yourself. Plan your timing strategy in advance. Use the practice questions in this book to practice pacing yourself. Rushing to finish a test will not benefit your score. Do not be distracted by other students who leave the testing room before you do. Everyone works at a different pace, and paying attention to what others are doing takes time away from your test.

TOP TEN NCLEX-RN REVIEW: THIS BOOK WILL HELP YOU PASS

Begin the task of studying for the NCLEX—one of the most important tests you'll ever take—by concentrating on those subject areas where you need the most help. Section 1, on the top 10 questions, will help you do just that. No other NCLEX-RN review guide offers such a precise measurement of your true ability. The more than 1,500 practice questions will help you hone your skills and zero in on your areas of weakness. By the time you're done, you'll feel confident and prepared to take the next step—taking the exam!

Unless otherwise indicated, photographs and art are owned by Jones and Bartlett Publishers.

SECTION I

Page 8: © Elena Kalistratora/ShutterStock, Inc.
Page 17: © Elena Kalistratora/ShutterStock, Inc.

SECTION III

Page 73: Courtesy of Kristen Rogers.
Page 77: © Johanna Goodyear/ShutterStock, Inc.
Page 92: Courtesy of Kristen Rogers.
Page 95 (left): © Johanna Goodyear/ShutterStock, Inc.

SECTION VI

Page 186–187: From *Arrhythmia Recognition: The Art of Interpretation*, courtesy of Tomas B. Garcia, MD.
Page 188: Courtesy of Kristen Rogers.

SECTION VII

Pages 231, 234, 245, and 247: Courtesy of Kristen Rogers.

SECTION VIII

Pages 258, 262, 274, 275, and 276: Courtesy of Kristen Rogers.

SECTION IX

Page 295: Adapted from Phipps, W. J., Long, B. C., & Woods, N. F. (1995). *Medical-surgical nursing: Concepts and clinical practice* (5th ed.). St. Louis, MO: Mosby.
Page 307: Adapted from Lewis, S. M., Heitkemper, M. M., & Dirksen, S. R. (2000). *Medical-surgical nursing: Assessment and management of clinical problems* (5th ed.). St. Louis, MO: Mosby-Yearbook.
Page 308 (top): Adapted from Caremark. (2004). *Health A to Z: Traction*. Retrieved May 15, 2007, from http://healthresources.caremark.com/topic/topic100587587
Page 308 (middle): Adapted from Lewis, S. M., Heitkemper, M. M., & Dirksen, S. R. (2000). *Medical-surgical nursing: Assessment and management of clinical problems* (5th ed.). St. Louis, MO: Mosby-Yearbook.
Page 319–320: Adapted from Phipps, W. J., Long, B. C., & Woods, N. F. (1995). *Medical-surgical nursing: Concepts and clinical practice* (5th ed.). St. Louis, MO: Mosby.

SECTION X

Pages 332, 334–336, 351–353, 360: From *Arrhythmia Recognition: The Art of Interpretation*, courtesy of Tomas B. Garcia, MD.
Page 339: Adapted from Weight-Control Information Network (WIN). An information service of the National Institute of Diabetes and Digestive and Kidney Diseases (NIDDK). *Weight and waist measurements: Tools for adults*. Retrieved May 4, 2007, from: http://win.niddk.nih.gov/publications/tools.htm#bodymassindex

Top Ten Review

CARE OF THE CHILDBEARING FAMILY AND THE NEONATE

Multiple Choice

1. A nurse is caring for a patient in labor having a Pitocin (oxytocin) induction. The nurse notes that the contractions are occurring every 2 minutes, last 90 seconds, and have +3 palpated intensity. The baseline fetal heart rate is 150, with uniformed decelerations that begin at the peak of the contraction and return to baseline after the contraction is over. What should the nurse do?

1. Increase the primary IV rate, as these are signs of dehydration.
2. Discontinue the Pitocin drip, as these are signs of hyperstimulation.
3. Increase the Pitocin, as this is a dysfunctional labor pattern.
4. Give oxygen per face mask and increase the IVF to perform intrauterine resuscitation.

2. The grandmother of an infant, born 1 hour ago via c-section, wants to take the baby to the mother's room. The mother had an emergency c-section and is still in recovery although her room has been assigned. What should the nursery nurse do?

1. Allow the grandmother to escort the baby to the room.
2. Obtain permission from the mother for the grandmother to take the baby from the nursery.
3. Not allow the grandmother to have the baby unless hospital staff can obtain permission from a family member.
4. Verify that the infant's mother is a patient and that her room is ready.

3. The nurse is coming on to her shift at 7 A.M. She has the following patients assigned to her care:

- Gravida 4 term 3 patient who is being induced and is 8 cm dilated
- Gravida 1 term 0 patient who is 4–5 cm dilated with an epidural and Pitocin
- Gravida 2 term 3 patient who has pregnancy-induced hypertension with a cervidil in place that is due to be removed within the hour

Which patient should the nurse see first?

1. Induction patient.
2. Patient who is 4–5 cm dilated.
3. Patient with hypertension.
4. None of these patients—complain that this is a heavy load.

4. A nurse on the postpartum unit is faced with several patient needs—three of her patients have called out in the last 5 minutes. The nursing assistant offers to conduct the vital sign recheck on a hypertensive patient. What should the nurse do?

1. Send the nursing assistant to give a sitz bath to a patient with a fourth-degree laceration.

2. Thank the nursing assistant for the offer and have her complete the task.

3. Thank the nursing assistant but say that she cannot help the nurse with any of her patients at the moment.

4. Send the nursing assistant to give Colace (docusate sodium) to the 2-day postoperative c-section patient.

5. A postpartum nurse is caring for a 16-year-old patient who is giving her baby up for adoption. Which of the following statements is most applicable in this situation?

1. This decision requires communication between a social services worker and the patient.

2. The patient's parents need to be present.

3. A cophysician must be present at the time of patient discharge.

4. The patient should not be allowed to see the infant after birth.

6. A patient who is a gravida 2 term 1 comes to labor and delivery with a birth plan reflecting her desire to have an unmedicated vaginal delivery. Her first delivery was via c-section for a breech presentation. When the patient's provider comes to perform an initial pelvic exam, she states, "You are going to have a repeat c-section, correct? I mean, why go through all that pain when we can just do a c-section?" How should the nurse respond to the patient?

1. "She is right—there is no need for you to go through the pain of labor."

2. "This is your birth, and I will support your decision."

3. "It is not recommended that you try to have a vaginal birth after a c-section."

4. "I had my babies vaginally—it is no big deal."

7. A patient delivered 30 minutes ago and has an IV of lactated Ringer's with 25 units of Pitocin infusing. The nurse evaluates her lochia and finds it to be excessive. The patient's vital signs are blood pressure 150/98, pulse 80, respirations 18, and temperature 98°F. The nurse notifies the provider and the following order is received: Methergine (methylergonovine) 0.2 mg IM now. What should the nurse do?

1. Question the order, as the medication is contraindicated in this patient.

2. Do not give the medication but increase the IV fluids.

3. Request to give the medication intravenously—this is an emergency.

4. Give the medication and reevaluate the bleeding.

8. An infant was just admitted to the nursery after an emergency c-section. The nurse's initial assessment is that the infant's skin has a slightly yellow tint. She looks in the maternal history for

1. Maternal Rh factor.

2. The presence of recreational drug use.

3. Thyroid disease.

4. ABO incompatibility.

9. A nurse performs an assessment on an infant who is 4 hours old. She notes a change in his color from an initial overall pink color except for acrocyanosis to a current central pallor. His vital signs are as follows: heart rate 125; respirations 60; temperature 98.6°F. The nurse knows the following lab work will need to be drawn:

1. Hematocrit, indirect Combs.

2. Kleinhaure-Betke, hematocrit.

3. Indirect Combs, Kleinhaure-Betke.

4. None—this is a normal physiologic adaptation.

10. The provider just performed an amniotomy on a patient who is 6 cm dilated. Following the procedure, the contractions are 3 minutes apart, last 60–70 seconds, and are +2 palpated intensity. The baseline fetal heart rate was originally 135 with good variability, but is now 95–100 for approximately 45 seconds. What is the nurse's first action?

1. Take a full set of vital signs.

2. Perform a vaginal exam.

3. Prepare for a delivery.

4. Dry the perineum, and provide clean pads.

CARE OF CHILDREN

Multiple Choice

1. A 15-month-old child is scheduled for measles, mumps, and rubella (MMR) immunization. Identify the observation that indicates the nurse should withhold the immunization.

1. The child's temperature is 100.5°F.

2. The child's temperature after the last immunization was 103.5°F.

3. The child is currently receiving antibiotics for otitis media with effusion.

4. The child has a congenital immunodeficiency.

2. A 9-year-old child has been taking Ritalin (methylphenidate hydrochloride) for 2 months to assist with symptoms of attention-deficit hyperactivity disorder. During a follow-up visit to the clinic, which statement indicates the medication is achieving a positive outcome?

1. The child is easily distracted and finds homework difficult to complete.

2. The child completes homework in 15 minutes with multiple errors.

3. The child completes household chores with only one reminder.

4. The child is agitated and complains of frequent headaches.

3. The parents of a 2½-year-old child are frustrated with their child's behavior, which includes constantly saying "no." They are also concerned that the child is becoming a picky eater, saying "no" to foods and juices. What is the best response by the nurse?

1. "You should try to offer choices; this behavior is common as children become more independent."

2. "This is not a common behavior. We need to be concerned about malnourishment and growth."

3. "You will need to see a counselor and nutritionist to best deal with the situation and plan meals the child will eat."

4. "You will need to be firm with your child and set limits and rewards for the behavior displayed."

4. What nursing observation indicates a major complication in a child receiving a blood transfusion?

1. Difficulty breathing.

2. Brisk capillary refill.

3. Temperature of 98.3°F.

4. Sleeping soundly.

5. An 8-year-old child has fallen out of a tree and sustained a closed head injury. At the time of admission, the child was unconscious, with decorticate posturing to noxious stimuli. The nurse assesses the child 1 hour later. Which observation indicates the child is deteriorating neurologically?

1. The child is lethargic, with clear fluid draining from the nose.

2. The child exhibits bilateral flexion of the upper extremities to noxious stimuli.

3. The child is confused and reports diminished visual acuity.

4. The child exhibits bilateral extension of the upper extremities to noxious stimuli.

6. An 11-year-old child with a thoracic spinal cord injury is admitted to the unit. Vital signs and laboratory results are as follows:

Blood pressure = 106/60

Pulse = 62

Respiratory rate = 12

Arterial pH = 7.28

Arterial pCO_2 = 64 mm Hg

Arterial pO_2 = 89 mm Hg

Arterial HCO_3 = 32 mm Hg

Based on the preceding information, which nursing action would be the best to implement?

1. Notify the physician to request an order for a sedative, and reevaluate in 20 minutes.

2. Notify the physician about metabolic acidosis, and anticipate increasing the oxygen concentration.

3. Evaluate airway patency, and administer pain medication to ensure effective coughing and deep breathing exercises.

4. Evaluate airway patency, and elevate the head of the bed while implementing coughing and deep breathing exercises.

7. A 9-year-old with hemophilia complains of increased bruising when playing with siblings. Which lab value would provide an explanation for the finding?

1. White blood cell count = 8,000/μL.

2. Platelet count = 120,000/μL.

3. Red blood cell count = 4.2 million/mm³.

4. Hemoglobin = 13 g/dL.

8. The nurse is assessing a young mother's understanding of injury prevention for her 6-month-old child. Which statement by the mother would indicate a need for further teaching?

1. "The car seat is an infant model and is securely anchored."

SECTION I
SECTION II
SECTION III
SECTION IV
SECTION V
SECTION VI
SECTION VII
SECTION VIII
SECTION IX
SECTION X

2. "The car seat is rear-facing in the back passenger seat."

3. "The car seat is securely anchored and the harness fastens snugly."

4. "The car seat is front-facing in the back passenger seat."

9. A 10-year-old is admitted to the unit with metastatic osteosarcoma. The child's parents inform the nurse that the child's grandfather died 3 weeks ago. The nurse walks into the room and observes the child crying; the child asks the nurse if she is going to die. What is the best response by the nurse?

1. "Yes, everyone dies sometime."

2. "You will need to ask your parents when they come and visit."

3. "Let's talk about it. What do you think?"

4. "You do not need to focus on that; you need to put your energy into getting better."

10. The nurse is caring for an infant who has just returned to the unit from surgery. Which observation would indicate the infant is experiencing pain?

1. A rating of 5 on the faces pain rating scale.

2. Crying and pointing to the area producing pain.

3. Increased heart rate and sleeping soundly.

4. Crying steadily and kicking.

CARE OF ADULTS

Multiple Choice

1. A patient returns to the unit from the recovery room after surgery. Identify the correct sequence of care for this patient.

1. Administer pain medication, assess vital signs, assess dressing.

2. Assess urinary output, change gown, attain warm blanket.

3. Assess vital signs, administer pain medication, assess dressing.

4. Assess vital signs, assess dressing, assess presence of pain.

2. The nurse is caring for a patient who has had a right total hip replacement. The patient informs the nurse that he would be more comfortable without the pillow between his legs and wants the pillow

removed. Identify the statement that explains a possible reason for keeping the pillow in place.

1. "The pillow is to prevent the inadvertent movement of your right leg too far away from the body."

2. "The pillow is to prevent you from getting up during the night, as you might awake confused."

3. "The pillow is to prevent the inadvertent movement of your right leg crossing over to the left side."

4. "The pillow is to prevent you from touching your knees together and to avoid the formation of bed sores."

3. A patient is being discharged from the hospital and will need to perform dressing changes at home. Which statement by the patient indicates understanding of aseptic technique?

1. "I should wash my hands prior to removing the old dressing and again before placing the new dressing over the wound."

2. "I need to take a pain pill 30 minutes before changing the dressing."

3. "I should use sterile gloves to apply the new dressing, and wash my hands before and after the dressing change."

4. "I should wash my hands and use an over-the-counter antimicrobial ointment to speed the healing process."

4. A postoperative patient refuses to use the incentive spirometer and states that it hurts too much when she deep-breathes and coughs. What is the best intervention for the nurse to implement?

1. Explain the importance of the activity.

2. Respect the patient's wishes.

3. Inform the patient that she will definitely catch pneumonia.

4. Notify the physician.

5. A patient is admitted to the unit with episodes of bradycardia. Currently, the patient's vital signs are as follows: blood pressure 82/36; heart rate 42. An epinephrine infusion is initiated at 2 µg/min. What effect on cardiac output would be expected from the epinephrine infusion?

1. Cardiac output will diminish.

2. Cardiac output will improve.

3. Cardiac output will remain unchanged.

4. The patient will progress to cardiac arrest.

6. A patient is admitted to the unit and is confused, disoriented, and combative. Based on this information, which nursing action would be the best to implement to prevent the patient from harming himself?

    1. Place the bed in a low position, and administer a sedative and antipsychotic.

    2. Place all four side rails in the up position, and encourage the family to stay with the patient.

    3. Activate the bed alarm, and encourage the family to stay with the patient.

    4. Place the patient in a vest restraint and administer a sedative.

7. A patient is admitted with a closed head injury. On admission, vital signs were as follows: temperature 99.2°F; blood pressure 120/72; heart rate 104; respirations 24. Thirty minutes later, the nurse observes the patient exhibiting Cushing's triad signs. Which assessment findings are abnormal and should be immediately reported to the physician?

    1. Blood pressure 136/72; heart rate 94; respirations 22.

    2. Blood pressure 154/78; heart rate 68; respirations 14.

    3. Blood pressure 110/70; heart rate 124; respirations 30.

    4. Blood pressure 152/88; heart rate 128; respirations 16.

8. The nurse is caring for a patient who is in left-sided heart failure and is receiving continuous venonenous hemofiltration for anuria and acute renal failure. Identify the items pertinent to document regarding the care of this patient.

    1. Daily weight, lab values, and urinary output.

    2. Type of dialysate, amount of dwell time, and characteristics of the fluid drained.

    3. Appearance of peritoneal site and amount of fluid removed.

    4. Daily weight, blood pressure, type of dialysate used, and amount of fluid removed.

9. The probable occurrence of alcohol withdrawal symptoms in a patient is assessed by determining

    1. Blood alcohol level, drinking history, and type of alcoholic beverage last consumed.

    2. Past alcohol withdrawal episodes, blood alcohol level, and time last alcoholic beverage consumed.

    3. Drinking history, and time and amount of alcoholic beverage last consumed.

    4. Blood alcohol level, and type and amount of alcoholic beverage last consumed.

10. The nurse caring for a patient with chronic obstructive pulmonary disease encourages the patient to quit smoking. Identify the statement that explains a possible reason supporting the cessation of smoking for this patient.

    1. Smoking decreases the amount of mucus production within the respiratory tract.

    2. Smoking allows hemoglobin to become highly oxygenated.

    3. Smoking shrinks the alveoli in the lungs.

    4. Smoking damages the ciliary cleansing mechanism of the respiratory tract.

CARE OF PATIENTS WITH PSYCHIATRIC AND MENTAL HEALTH PROBLEMS

Multiple Choice

1. Gerald is a 56-year-old male who was first diagnosed with bipolar disorder at age 24. He is an English professor at the local university. Gerald stayed up all night writing a novel and tells his wife the next morning that he has racing thoughts. He paces the floor, writes two words, paces the floor again, and repeats this process. Gerald is currently dressed in orange-colored shorts, no shirt, and a purple pullover hat; he is barefoot. He has not taken his lithium in more than 3 months as it interferes with his ability "to be the next great novelist of the world." What is an appropriate patient outcome once Gerald is admitted to the inpatient mental health unit?

    1. Gerald will adhere to established limits and expectations of fluid ingestion.

    2. Gerald will dress himself appropriately for his age and status.

    3. Gerald will maintain a positive sodium and potassium electrolyte balance.

    4. Gerald will express the desire to leave the hospital, go home, and meet his goal of being the greatest novelist in the world.

2. Robin is a 38-year-old mother of two children. She has just learned that her mother has been diagnosed with lung cancer. Yesterday, her husband divorced her and married his secretary. Robin has a 15-year history of manic behavior. She calls her ex-husband at his office and tells him she wants to die. Her ex-husband calls an ambulance, and Robin is admitted to the hospital. She admits that she has

not been taking her lithium for "5 weeks or so." What is the priority nursing diagnosis for Robin?

1. Impaired social interaction.
2. Ineffective coping related to low self-esteem.
3. Self-care deficit.
4. Risk for self-directed violence.

3. Barry is a 48-year-old male who came to the Emergency Department complaining of chest pain and shortness of breath. The standard cardiac workup was within normal limits. Barry stated to the staff that his son committed suicide 3 months ago after a long history of alcohol abuse and that his wife is having a long-term extramarital affair and recently asked him for a separation. Barry is concerned about financial matters as well. The Clinical Nurse Specialist in psychiatric mental health nursing interviews Barry. Based on the preceding information, what is the primary nursing diagnosis?

1. Decreased decision and conflict resolution behaviors.
2. Sexual dysfunction.
3. Anxiety.
4. Altered sleep patterns.

4. Maria Gonzalez is a 50-year-old Hispanic woman whose husband died 6 months ago in a car accident. She comes to your clinic complaining of dizziness. Upon taking a history, you note that Mrs. Gonzalez is a practicing Catholic, is dressed in black, and answers questions briefly but accurately. The nursing assistant states that Mrs. Gonzalez's vital signs are blood pressure 154/92, pulse 96, respirations 22, and temperature 99.6°F orally. Based on this information, which nursing diagnosis or problem is *not* likely to be one associated with Mrs. Gonzalez?

1. Delayed bereavement.
2. Anxiety.
3. Hypertension.
4. Potential for infection.

5. You are a 38-year-old nurse caring for a 22-year-old patient with depression. You are considering a sexual relationship with the patient. You know that preventing harm should be a major consideration in your nursing role. Which ethical issue applies in this situation?

1. Autonomy.
2. Paternalism.

3. Distributive justice.
4. Beneficence.

6. For the last 8 months, Monique has displayed the following symptoms: delusions, hallucinations, frequent incoherent speech, grossly disorganized and flat affect. Based on this information, Monique displays the symptoms of

1. Obsessive-compulsive disorder.
2. Schizophrenia.
3. Detoxification.
4. Anxiety.

7. Which of the following conditions could be 100% preventable?

1. Schizophrenia.
2. Obsessive-compulsive disorder.
3. Chronic depression.
4. Fetal alcohol syndrome.

8. Which of the following measures would be appropriate to use if you wanted to assess for dementia?

1. Mini-Mental Status Examination (MMSE).
2. World Health Organization Analgesic Tool (WHO-AT).
3. Caregiver Status Scale.
4. State, Trait Anxiety Scale.

9. Which of the following is a physical symptom associated with anorexia nervosa?

1. Tachycardia.
2. Constipation.
3. Menstrual cramps.
4. Weight that is 20% above the ideal weight.

10. William is a 32-year-old black male who has been drinking alcohol excessively since the age of 14. He has recently started a new job after being unemployed for the last 7 months. Three days after starting his new job, William's apartment was flooded and he lost all his possessions. He also states that he finds riding public transportation back and forth to work each day somewhat frustrating. Which of the following physiologic stressors would you, as a nurse, be concerned about because it can potentially be a cause of illness?

1. Common daily frustrations.
2. Job change.

Trends and Current Issues in Nursing 7

SECTION
I

SECTION
II

SECTION
III

SECTION
IV

SECTION
V

SECTION
VI

SECTION
VII

SECTION
VIII

SECTION
IX

SECTION
X

3. Excessive alcohol intake.

4. Disaster due to flooding.

TRENDS AND CURRENT ISSUES IN NURSING

Multiple Choice

1. Which of the following tasks is appropriate for a registered nurse to delegate?

   1. Vital signs to a certified nursing assistant who has documented competency in the skill.

   2. Diabetic discharge teaching to a nursing assistant who also has diabetes.

   3. Admission assessment of an unstable patient to an LPN in orientation.

   4. Evaluation of a patient's response to treatment of a surgical wound.

2. Which of the following is an example of a health disparity?

   1. The complication rate for all patients undergoing bronchoscopy is 2%.

   2. Women with cardiovascular disease are underdiagnosed and undertreated as compared to men.

   3. The screening rates for prostate cancer in outpatient primary care facilities are consistent for African Americans and Asian Americans.

   4. Ability to pay is not considered a criterion for treatment in outpatient clinics.

3. A nurse is teaching a class on interventions that decrease the risk of cervical cancer to a group of young adults. What intervention would be appropriate to include?

   1. Administer human papillomavirus (HPV) vaccination to prevent cervical cancer.

   2. Avoid the use of tampons on a routine basis.

   3. Take daily doses of echinacea to prevent cervical cancer.

   4. Practive daily vaginal douching to prevent yeast infections.

4. Which health risks are commonly associated with obesity?

   1. Hypertension, insulin resistance, cardiovascular disease.

   2. Liver disease, decreased insulin production, skin cancer.

   3. Chronic obstructive pulmonary disease, type 1 diabetes, colon cancer.

   4. Cardiomyopathy, type 2 diabetes, hypolipidemia.

5. A patient has been administered the wrong oral medication. Which action should the nurse take first?

   1. Complete a medication error report.

   2. Notify the prescribing physician.

   3. Assess the patient.

   4. Contact the pharmacist.

6. A male patient with a diagnosis of acute lymphocytic leukemia is admitted to the hospital with complaints of fever, chills, fatigue, and pallor over the past week. Labs are drawn and the results reported. Which lab data will provide the most likely explanation for the fatigue and pallor?

   1. Magnesium = 2.0 mEq/L.

   2. Hemoglobin = 6.5g/dL.

   3. White blood cells = 12.6×10^3/μL.

   4. Creatinine = 2.5 mg/dL.

7. A patient with type 2 diabetes has glycated hemoglobin (HbA_{1C}) of 15%. What is the best interpretation of the laboratory value by the nurse?

   1. The value is normal and the patient has established glycemic control.

   2. The value is abnormal and the patient should increase the medication dosage.

   3. The value is high and the patient has not achieved glycemic control.

   4. The value is low and the patient needs to have adjustments made in medications.

8. A patient is being taught about the validity of health information available on the Internet. Which site description would *decrease* the likelihood of obtaining valid health information from an online source?

   1. A government information site on health promotion activities that is dated and revised every 6 months.

   2. An herbal supplement site that is sponsored by the company selling the product.

   3. A peer-reviewed site that identifies clinical manifestations of a disease.

4. A site that identifies treatment modalities for depression that can be cross-referenced with print or electronic resources.

9. The nurse is working at a flu shot clinic. Four patients are waiting for vaccinations, but there is enough vaccine for only one patient. Which of the following patients is at highest risk for influenza and should receive the available vaccine?

   1. An adolescent who attends a crowded high school.
   2. A middle-aged healthcare worker who is employed in an acute care hospital.
   3. An elderly female with an acute, febrile illness.
   4. A child who is 10 years old and attends an after-school day-care program.

10. The charge nurse working in an emergency room is notified that a massive explosion has occurred at a local industrial plant. More than 30 victims and casualties from the explosion are expected. What action should the nurse take first?

   1. Activate the emergency response plan.
   2. Call in available personnel.
   3. Obtain additional supplies.
   4. Move existing patients to rooms in the hospital.

MATH, DOSAGE CALCULATIONS, AND RELATED PROBLEMS

1. Clinically you often mix insulins in one syringe, such as regular insulin and NPH insulin, always drawing up the regular insulin first into a syringe (clear drawn up before cloudy). On the figure below, draw an arrow corresponding to the dose of *regular* insulin if you have a total insulin dose of 65 units of which 38 units consists of NPH insulin.

Short Answer

2. Determine the total units of insulin based on glucose levels and carbohydrates consumed. Administer 1 unit of regular insulin for every 30 mg/dL increase in blood glucose above 150 mg/dL, and administer 2 units regular insulin for every 25 g of carbohydrates consumed.

   Blood glucose = 210 mg/dL

   Carbohydrates consumed = 25 g + 35 g + 15 g + 50 g

What is the total number of units of regular insulin you should administer?

Multiple Choice

3. Your patient is prescribed ampicillin by piggyback. You receive the mini-bag labeled as follows:

   Normal saline 50 mL

   500 mg ampicillin

   Total infusion time of 30 minutes

What is the rate at which the ampicillin should infuse?

   1. 30 mL/h.
   2. 100 mL/h.
   3. 50 mL/h.
   4. 10 mL/h.

4. Using the following IV prescriptions, determine the flow rate that you will program into the electronic infusion pump. **Prescription:** Rocephin (ceftriaxone sodium) 1 g IVPB (intravenous piggyback) prior to surgery (pharmacy label D_5W 100 mL infuse in 30 minutes). What is the flow rate in mL/h?

   1. 100 mL/h.
   2. 10 mL/h.
   3. 33 mL/h.
   4. 200 mL/h.

Care of Patients with Diabetes **9**

SECTION
I

SECTION
II

SECTION
III

SECTION
IV

SECTION
V

SECTION
VI

SECTION
VII

SECTION
VIII

SECTION
IX

SECTION
X

5. Determine the bolus dose of heparin (in units) and adjust the dose of heparin IV bolus (units) based on the PTT results using the weight-based heparin protocol as follows:

Bolus heparin at 80 units/kg.

For PTT results:

PTT < 35: Give 80 units/kg bolus.

PTT 35–45: Give 40 units/kg bolus.

PTT 46–70: No change.

PTT > 70: Call physician immediately.

Patient's weight = 62 kg. PTT = 34.

1. Bolus dose of heparin is 4,800 units; adjust the dose of heparin based on PTT results by administering 4,800 units heparin.
2. Bolus dose of heparin is 4,960 units; adjust the dose of heparin based on PTT results by administering 4,960 units heparin.
3. Bolus dose of heparin is 6,400 units; adjust the dose of heparin based on PTT results by administering 6,400 units heparin.
4. Bolus dose of heparin is 1,364 units; adjust the dose of heparin based on PTT results by administering 80 units heparin.

6. Your patient is prescribed digoxin (Lanoxin) 250 μg (micrograms) PO daily. The pharmacy sends up digoxin 0.125 mg (milligram) tablets. The patient's vital signs are blood pressure 120/80, heart rate 58, respirations 18, temperature 98.6°F, and pain score 1. It is time for you to administer morning medications. What action should you take?

1. Administer 1 tablet of digoxin.
2. Administer 2 tablets of digoxin.
3. Administer no digoxin because the pain score is too low.
4. Administer no digoxin because the pulse rate is too low.

7. Prescription: Nitrostat 1/150 grain (0.4 mg) sublingually 5 minutes apart for angina. Do not take more than 3 tablets in 15 minutes. The patient reports that he has taken 3 tablets. How many total milligrams has he taken?

1. 3/150 mg.
2. 120/150 mg.
3. 0.4 mg.
4. 1.2 mg.

8. Your patient is prescribed the liquid medication Pepcid (famotidine), and the pharmacy sends up a multidose bottle. You know the prescription calls for your patient to receive 200 mg daily. The strength/volume ratio is 40 mg/5 mL, and the total strength is 400 mg in a total volume of 50 mL. How much medication do you give the patient daily?

1. 50 mL.
2. 25 mL.
3. 20 mL.
4. 40 mL.

9. Mr. Goldstein has a fungal infection of the mouth and is prescribed Nystatin (mycostatin) oral suspension 300,000 units by mouth every 6 hours. The Nystatin is provided as 100,000 units per mL. How much volume do you pour for each dose every 6 hours?

1. 3.33 mL.
2. 0.3 mL.
3. 2 mL.
4. 3 mL.

Short Answer

10. The physician has prescribed penicillin V potassium 2 g for a patient who needs pretreatment with an antibiotic prior to a surgical procedure. The transporters have come for the patient. You determine that you have penicillin V potassium in stock as three capsules of 500 mg/capsule and six capsules of 250 mg/capsule. What is the best way to administer the 2-g dose that will require the patient to swallow the fewest capsules?

CARE OF PATIENTS WITH DIABETES

1. Mr. Woldon is an insulin-dependent diabetic. His wife called 911 because her husband was "acting funny." Mr. Woldon comes into the Emergency Department via ambulance stretcher. His workup reveals a blood sugar of 800 mg/dL, ketones are absent in his urine, and he is dehydrated and has altered mental status. Based on these data, what is your evaluation of Mr. Woldon?

1. He has diabetic ketoacidosis (DKA).
2. He is in hyperosmolar nonketotic coma (HNKC).
3. He has acute renal failure.
4. He has diabetic retinopathy.

2. Mrs. Kirkland comes into the clinic and states she might be having trouble with her diabetes management. She says that she often feels nauseated, is restless, perspires, is fatigued, and is hungry. Her pulse is about 90 beats per minute. What do these signs indicate?

1. Hypoglycemia.
2. Hyperglycemia.
3. Diabetic nephropathy.
4. Diabetic retinopathy.

3. Mrs. Smolinski comes to the clinic for monitoring of her diabetes. Upon talking to her, you discover she has carbuncles, vulvovaginitis, cellulitis of the right ankle, nasal congestion, periodontal disease, and a urinary tract infection. Of these discoveries, which one could you *not* contribute to poorly controlled diabetes mellitus?

1. Cellulitis.
2. Vulvovaginitis.
3. Urinary tract infection.
4. Nasal congestion.

4. Ms. Effington works out of her home from her computer about 10 hours per day, 6 days per week. She is 48 years old, is 5 feet 3 inches tall, weighs 232 pounds, and has little time to exercise. Based on these data, which of the following conditions is she most at risk of developing?

1. Pancreatic cancer.
2. Duodenal ulcer.
3. Insulin-dependent diabetes mellitus (type 1).
4. Non-insulin-dependent diabetes mellitus (type 2).

5. To maintain normalized blood sugars, Mr. Hernandez has the following sliding-scale insulin prescription: Give 1 unit of regular insulin for every 20 g of carbohydrates eaten plus if the blood glucose is

< 130 mg/dL, administer 0 units of insulin.

130–160 mg/dL, administer 2 units of regular insulin.

161–190 mg/dL, administer 4 units of regular insulin.

191–220 mg/dL, administer 6 units of regular insulin.

221–250 mg/dL, administer 8 units of regular insulin.

> 250 mg/dl, administer 10 units of regular insulin and contact the physician immediately.

Mr. Hernandez has eaten 40 g of carbohydrates and his blood sugar is 204. What is the total amount of regular insulin you should administer?

1. 2 units.
2. 6 units.
3. 8 units.
4. 10 units.

6. To reduce the risk of hyperglycemia, Mrs. Murphy is to inject herself with 1 unit of regular insulin for every 8 g of carbohydrates consumed at mealtime and 1 unit of regular insulin for every 30 mg/dL increase in blood sugar above 130 mg/dL. For lunch, she has eaten a hamburger bun (20 g carbohydrates), a 3-ounce hamburger (10 g), 6 ounces of french fries (45 g), one cup of baked beans (45 g), and a 12-ounce diet soda (0 g). Her blood sugar is now 190 mg/dL. How much total insulin should Mrs. Murphy inject?

1. 6 units.
2. 12 units.
3. 17 units.
4. 19 units.

7. Mrs. Gill has been an insulin-dependent diabetic since age 13. When she came into your clinic for a follow-up visit, you noticed she had many scratches on her right ankle and a resulting infection and cellulitis. When you question her about this problem, Mrs. Gill states, "Oh, my cat Hercules must have been using my leg as a scratching post again and I did not even feel it." Which diabetic complication does Mrs. Gill have?

1. Nephropathy.
2. Neuropathy.
3. Macroangiopathy.
4. Retinopathy.

8. Because of the lack of insulin in diabetics, the body cannot use carbohydrates for energy and instead uses proteins and fats. Which sign of diabetes does this metabolism cause?

1. Polydipsia.
2. Overhydration.
3. Weight loss.
4. Paresthesia.

Care of Patients with Orthopedic Problems **11**

SECTION
I

SECTION
II

SECTION
III

SECTION
IV

SECTION
V

SECTION
VI

SECTION
VII

SECTION
VIII

SECTION
IX

SECTION
X

9. Nursing assessment of diabetic patients includes the assessment of which body system if you are assessing for hypertension and peripheral vascular disease?

1. Sensory/neurological.
2. Musculoskeletal.
3. Metabolic.
4. Cardiovascular.

Short Answer

10. Your hospital provides you with three types of insulin syringes: 30 units, 50 units, and 100 units per syringe. If your patient is to receive 20 units of regular insulin plus 28 units of NPH insulin in one syringe, which syringe should you choose based on total dose of insulin and best readability of the syringe?

CARE OF PATIENTS WITH ORTHOPEDIC PROBLEMS

Multiple Choice

1. Identify the statement that differentiates osteoarthritis from rheumatoid arthritis.

1. Osteoarthritis is a degenerative joint disease caused by an autoimmune response.
2. Swan neck and boutonniere deformities are associated with osteoarthritis.
3. Osteoarthritis is a systemic disease that has local joint manifestations.
4. Osteophyte formation occurs as a result of destruction of subchondral bone in osteoarthritis.

2. A patient has been taking aspirin 650 mg four times a day for the last 9 months to relieve the symptoms of arthritis. During a follow-up visit to the clinic, the patient tells the healthcare provider that he has had increasing fatigue and his stools have been black and tarry for the past 3 to 4 weeks. Identify the statement that explains a possible reason for the finding.

1. Production of cylooxygenase-1 is inhibited, which can result in gastric erosion and ulceration.
2. Production of cyclooxygenase-2 is increased, which can result in a decrease in platelet aggregation.
3. The clinical manifestations are normal findings associated with long-term administration of aspirin.

4. Prostaglandin synthesis and gastrointestinal mucosa production are increased.

3. A patient is taking a disease-modifying antirheumatic drug (DMARD), methotrexate (Rheumatrex), for rheumatoid arthritis. Which patient statement would indicate a need for further teaching?

1. "I will begin to see an effect of the drug in 3 to 6 weeks."
2. "I will need to take a nonsteroidal anti-inflammatory drug to relieve my symptoms until the methotrexate becomes effective."
3. "I will be cured once I complete the full course of the prescribed medication."
4. "I should not become pregnant while taking the drug and for as long as 6 months after stopping the medicine."

4. Which two hormones regulate calcium and phosphate levels in the blood and stimulate (or inhibit) bone cell activity?

1. Parathyroid hormone and calcitonin.
2. Vitamin D and erythropoietin.
3. Serotonin and acetylcholine.
4. Thyroid hormone and cortisol.

5. A 50-year-old patient with newly diagnosed osteoporosis asks the nurse why bone mass is being lost. What is the nurse's best response?

1. The rate of bone resorption exceeds the rate of bone formation.
2. A diet high in calcium and vitamin D promotes osteoclastic activity.
3. An increase in the blood estrogen levels promotes the loss of bone mass.
4. The parathyroid gland is unable to respond to decreasing levels of calcium.

6. A patient experienced a lower extremity fracture. The injury was immobilized with a cast for 6 weeks to promote healing. Upon removal of the cast, the patient notices a decrease in the size of the muscle. What is the best explanation for the change?

1. Aging has produced a change in muscle cells during the period the cast was applied.
2. Cellular ischemia and muscle cell damage caused the formation of scar tissue.
3. Muscle dysplasia developed in response to the abnormal accumulation of muscle tissue proteins.

4. Atrophy of the muscle cells developed as a result of disuse.

7. After radiographic examination, a patient with a hand fracture was diagnosed with malunion. What is one reason why malunion might occur?

1. Bleeding at the fracture site.
2. Inadequate reduction or alignment of the fracture.
3. Significant displacement of bone at the time of injury.
4. Nerve injury in association with the fracture.

8. A patient complains of numbness and tingling of the fingers, muscle cramps, and tetany. Which lab value would provide an explanation for the findings?

1. Serum calcium = 6 mg/dL.
2. Serum potassium = 3.5 mg/dL.
3. Serum sodium = 145 mEq/L.
4. Serum magnesium = 2.7 mg/dL.

9. A patient experienced fractures of the radius and the ulna. The nurse assesses the extremity immediately after the fractures are reduced. Which neurovascular assessment findings are abnormal and should be immediately reported to the physician?

1. Pallor, paresthesia, capillary refill > 5 seconds, nonpalpable radial pulse.
2. Pink, weak pulse, normal sensation, palpable popliteal pulse.
3. Warm, dry, capillary refill < 2 seconds, palpable radial pulse.
4. Rubor, echymosis, edema, palpable dorsalis pedis pulse.

10. A patient with a transverse, midshaft fracture of the femur is scheduled for an open reduction and internal fixation. The patient asks the nurse, "Why can't they just put my leg in a cast?" What is the nurse's best response?

1. Reduction of bone fragments is best achieved by application of a cast, but immobilization is prolonged.
2. A cast would not provide for sufficient immobilization of the bone fragments to promote healing and prevent complications.
3. A long leg cast is used only when a closed reduction and immobilization of less than 3 weeks are needed.

4. The length of time during which the femur would need to be immobilized is increased when a short leg cast is used.

CARE OF PATIENTS WITH HYPERTENSION AND CARDIAC PROBLEMS

Multiple Choice

1. What is the first-line treatment for hypercholesteremia?

1. Smoking cessation and bile acid-binding resins.
2. Niacin and a low-fat diet.
3. Weight loss and an exercise regimen.
4. A 1,800-calorie diet and insulin.

2. A neighbor with a history of angina calls a nurse to report that her chest pain has not been relieved after taking three nitroglycerin tablets 5 minutes apart. Which action should the nurse take next?

1. Offer to contact the neighbor's cardiologist.
2. Advise the neighbor to take two aspirins and go to bed.
3. Drive the neighbor to the nearest emergency room.
4. Contact the local emergency management system (911).

3. A patient with peripheral vascular disease presents with symptoms of intermittent claudication. Which of the following statements best describes the pathophysiology of the symptom?

1. Oxygen demand exceeds supply, resulting in ischemic pain.
2. Oxygen supply exceeds demand, resulting in peripheral edema.
3. Thrombus formation occurs, resulting in decreased blood flow.
4. Vasodilation occurs, resulting in decreased preload.

4. According to the Joint National Committee on Detection, Evaluation, and Treatment of Hypertension (JNC 7), which systolic blood pressure (SBP) and diastolic blood pressure (DBP) values are diagnostic for stage 1 hypertension?

1. SBP > 140 mm Hg and DBP > 90 mm Hg.
2. SBP > 140 mm Hg or DBP > 80 mm Hg.
3. SBP > 160 mm Hg and DBP >100 mm Hg.
4. SBP > 160 mm Hg or DBP > 90 mm Hg.

Care of Patients with Hypertension and Cardiac Problems   **13**

SECTION
I

SECTION
II

SECTION
III

SECTION
IV

SECTION
V

SECTION
VI

SECTION
VII

SECTION
VIII

SECTION
IX

SECTION
X

5. A patient is admitted to the Emergency Department with chest pressure, pain radiating down the left arm, nausea, and diaphoresis after shoveling snow. Which initial general treatment priorities should the nurse anticipate for the patient?

1. Oxygen, nitroglycerin, aspirin, morphine.
2. Aspirin, thrombolytics, heparin, oxygen.
3. Beta blockers, morphine, nitroglycerin, glycoprotein inhibitors.
4. Heparin, glycoprotein inhibitors, ace inhibitors, beta blockers.

6. The home care plan for a patient with congestive heart failure includes rest, oxygen therapy, and diuretics. What is the expected outcome of the care plan?

1. Increased afterload.
2. Increased preload.
3. Decreased myocardial contractility.
4. Decreased workload of the heart.

7. The nurse is assessing a patient who has been admitted for observation after undergoing coronary angioplasty via the right femoral artery. Upon assessment, the nurse notes that the right leg is cool and has a decreased pulse and that an orange-size hard area is palpable in the right groin. Which intervention would be the first priority for the nurse to implement?

1. Instruct the patient to notify the nurse if there is any bleeding from the site.
2. Apply pressure immediately to the groin site.
3. Monitor the patient for possible deep vein thrombosis.
4. Observe the site again in 15 minutes for any changes.

8. Which of the following statements accurately describes the pathophysiology of the clinical manifestations associated with acute myocardial infarction?

1. Chest pain is related to the release of catecholamines from the ventricle.
2. Cool, clammy skin is related to the vasoconstriction that occurs due to the stimulation of the sympathetic nervous system.
3. Bradycardia occurs secondary to the stimulation of the sympathetic portion of the autonomic nervous system.
4. Accumulation of myoglobin in the gastrointestinal tract results in nausea and vomiting.

9. A patient who has been diagnosed with hypertension asks, "Why do I need to take expensive blood pressure medication when I don't feel bad?" What is the most appropriate response by the nurse?

1. Hypertension is a chronic condition that can have serious complications if you do not comply with the treatment plan.
2. Tell me what you know about hypertension and the treatment of the disease.
3. You will need to take the medication only until your blood pressure is within the recommended parameters.
4. I will ask the social worker to discuss financial support for medication expenses with you.

10. A patient is taking prescribed medications for congestive heart failure. The lab reports a serum potassium level of 2.4 mg/dL. Which of the prescribed drugs is the most likely cause of the potassium level?

1. Furosemide (Lasix).
2. Nitroglycerin (Nitrobid).
3. Metoprolol (Lopressor).
4. Spironolactone (Aldactone).

ANSWERS AND RATIONALES

CARE OF THE CHILDBEARING FAMILY AND THE NEONATE

1. Correct Answer: <u>2</u>

   Rationale: This situation involves hyperstimulation as a result of the Pitocin; the infant is having late decelerations. It is imperative that the Pitocin be stopped immediately and that intrauterine resuscitation measures follow.

2. Correct Answer: <u>2</u>

   Rationale: The infant should not be released to anyone who does not have authority to take the child as designated by the mother.

3. Correct Answer: <u>1</u>

   Rationale: The most active patient is the one who is 8 cm dilated; she should be evaluated first. Because she has had three other children, her second stage could happen very quickly.

4. Correct Answer: <u>1</u>

   Rationale: The nursing assistant cannot perform a vital signs assessment on a patient who needs those vital signs taken as part of a diagnostic assessment, as is the case with a known hypertensive patient having a reevaluation. A nursing assistant can help administer comfort measures.

5. Correct Answer: <u>1</u>

   Rationale: This complex situation falls outside the skill set of registered nurses and cannot be handled by the nurse alone. It will require the activation of other resources.

6. Correct Answer: <u>2</u>

   Rationale: The nurse's role is to advocate for the patient and to support her plans as long as they are not contraindicated by an evidence-based standard of nursing practice.

7. Correct Answer: <u>1</u>

   Rationale: Methergine (methylergonovine) is contraindicated in a patient with a blood pressure greater than 140/90.

8. Correct Answer: <u>1</u>

   Rationale: Pathologic jaundice can be caused by Rh incompatibility in a mother not treated with RhoGAM prenatally.

9. Correct Answer: <u>2</u>

   Rationale: This color change could be a sign of anemia. The hematocrit needs to be evaluated and a maternal blood smear (Kleinhaure-Betke) obtained to evaluate for fetal erythrocytes that would indicate hemolysis as a result of Rh incompatibility.

10. Correct Answer: <u>2</u>

    Rationale: After the amniotic sac is ruptured either spontaneously or artificially, there is a risk for a cord prolapse. This condition will be manifested in the fetal heart rate as a sudden and sustained bradycardia. A pelvic exam will rule out cord prolapse and should be done immediately.

CARE OF CHILDREN

1. Correct Answer: <u>4</u>

   Rationale: A known altered immunodeficiency is a true contraindication for withholding the MMR immunization.

2. Correct Answer: <u>3</u>

   Rationale: Achieving a positive outcome for a patient on Ritalin would decrease the symptoms and allow the child to reach accomplishments.

3. Correct Answer: <u>1</u>

   Rationale: During toddlerhood, a child develops autonomy. Refusal is expected behavior at this stage of development.

4. Correct Answer: <u>1</u>

   Rationale: Difficulty breathing could indicate an air embolism, which is a complication that can occur during blood transfusion.

5. Correct Answer: <u>4</u>

   Rationale: Extension of upper extremities to noxious stimuli is decerebrate posturing and signals further neurological deterioration.

6. Correct Answer: **4**

   Rationale: The first priority is to evaluate airway patency. The child is retaining excess CO_2 and breathing must be stimulated.

7. Correct Answer: **2**

   Rationale: The platelet count is low and could contribute to the increased bruising.

8. Correct Answer: **4**

   Rationale: Car seat safety for an infant includes using a car seat that is sized for infants. The car seat is placed rear-facing in the back passenger seat and should be securely anchored with a harness that fits snugly.

9. Correct Answer: **3**

   Rationale: The best intervention by the nurse is to facilitate open communication.

10. Correct Answer: **4**

    Rationale: Observations of pain in an infant would include crying, increased heart rate, increased blood pressure, and restlessness.

CARE OF ADULTS

1. Correct Answer: **4**

   Rationale: Vital signs should be the first item assessed for a patient returning from surgery, followed by the dressing and the presence of pain (which would be included in the head-to-toe assessment).

2. Correct Answer: **3**

   Rationale: The pillow prevents adduction beyond the midline, which could dislodge the implanted prosthesis.

3. Correct Answer: **1**

   Rationale: Hand washing is the most important aspect of aseptic technique.

4. Correct Answer: **1**

   Rationale: Communication is essential. Explaining the importance and reason for the activity will help the patient understand why it is necessary.

5. Correct Answer: **2**

   Rationale: The cardiac output equals the stroke volume multiplied by the heart rate. Epinephrine increases heart rate and increases afterload, thereby increasing cardiac output.

6. Correct Answer: **3**

   Rationale: Initially, the nurse should implement measures that would not be considered restraints.

7. Correct Answer: **2**

   Rationale: Late increased intracranial pressure is manifested by Cushing's triad, which includes severe hypertension, widened pulse pressure, bradycardia, and slowed, irregular respirations.

8. Correct Answer: **4**

   Rationale: Continuous hemofiltration through the patient's venous system is dependent on blood pressure. Weight and blood pressure must be documented along with the type of dialysate solution used.

9. Correct Answer: **3**

   Rationale: The probable occurrence of alcohol withdrawal is best determined by obtaining the drinking history and noting the time and quantity of the last alcoholic beverage consumed.

10. Correct Answer: **4**

    Rationale: Ciliary movement in the respiratory tract is a protective mechanism that is damaged by smoking.

CARE OF PATIENTS WITH PSYCHIATRIC AND MENTAL HEALTH PROBLEMS

1. Correct Answer: **2**

   Rationale: He will preserve his self-esteem and avoid embarrassment by dressing appropriately.

2. Correct Answer: **4**

   Rationale: She is at risk for self-directed violence due to suicidal ideation.

3. Correct Answer: **3**

   Rationale: His anxiety is related to the loss of his son and the threats to his social and economic status.

4. Correct Answer: **1**

   Rationale: This patient's cultural expression of grief includes wearing black for one year or longer.

5. Correct Answer: **4**

   Rationale: This term refers to bringing about good and the imperative of primum no nocere ("First do no harm").

6. Correct Answer: **2**

Rationale: According to the *DSM-IV* classification, these symptoms match those for schizophrenia. To warrant this diagnosis, the patient must have the symptoms for at least 6 months, with symptoms lasting at least 1 month in the active phase.

7. Correct Answer: **4**

Rationale: Fetal alcohol syndrome is 100% preventable if the pregnant woman abstains from alcohol use throughout her pregnancy.

8. Correct Answer: **1**

Rationale: The MMSE measures cognitive impairment that is part of dementia.

9. Correct Answer: **2**

Rationale: Constipation is a common side effect of overuse of laxatives and lack of food intake.

10. Correct Answer: **3**

Rationale: Ingestion of chemical substances such as alcohol is a physiological stressor, not a psychosocial stressor.

TRENDS AND CURRENT ISSUES IN NURSING

1. Correct Answer: **1**

Rationale: According to the National Council of State Boards of Nursing, delegation is the transferring of authority to perform a selected nursing task, in a certain situation, to a competent individual. Factors for successful delegation include the right task, in the right circumstances, to the right person, under the right direction/communication and right supervision/evaluation. Registered nurses may delegate the task of taking vital signs to unlicensed assistive personnel who have documented competency in the skill.

2. Correct Answer: **2**

Rationale: Health disparities are differences that occur based on gender, race or ethnicity, education or income, disability, geographic location, or sexual orientation. The underdiagnosis and undertreatment of cardiovascular disease in women is an example of a health disparity.

3. Correct Answer: **1**

Rationale: HPV is the leading cause of cervical cancer in women. A vaccine has been developed to protect women against this virus. The Centers for Disease Control and Prevention's Advisory Committee on Immunization

Practices recommendation calls for the routine vaccination of girls at 11–12 years of age. The recommendations also allows for vaccination of girls beginning at 9 years old as well as vaccination of girls and women 13–26 years old.

4. Correct Answer: **1**

Rationale: Obesity is excess body fat that results from an imbalance between energy intake and energy consumption. Health risks associated with obesity include hypertension, insulin resistance, and cardiovascular disease. Other conditions associated with obesity include hyperlipidemia; type 2 diabetes; infertility; endometrial, breast, colon, and prostate cancers; and gallbladder disease.

5. Correct Answer: **3**

Rationale: The first responsibility of the nurse when a medication error is discovered is to assess the patient. The assessment should focus on the current health status of the patient and identify whether there are any adverse effects from the medication administered in error. The assessment also serves as a baseline for further monitoring for adverse effects.

6. Correct Answer: **2**

Rationale: The hemoglobin content of the blood is normally 14–16.5 g/dL in a male patient . A patient with a hemoglobin level of 6.5 g/dL is experiencing severe anemia. Red blood cells contain hemoglobin, which transports oxygen to the cells. Because of decreased levels of hemoglobin and an associated decrease in oxygen-carrying capacity, the patient would be expected to exhibit the clinical manifestations of fatigue and pallor.

7. Correct Answer: **3**

Rationale: A glycated HbA_{1C} reading provides an index of average glucose levels over a period of 3 to 6 months. The goal for a diabetic patient is to maintain an HbA_{1C} level of less than 7%. An HbA_{1C} level of 15% is high. The finding indicates the patient has not achieved glycemic control and suggests the medical treatment plan and the patient's compliance with the treatment plan should be assessed.

8. Correct Answer: **2**

Rationale: An Internet site that provides information for the purpose of selling a product should generate concerns regarding the validity of information available from the site.

Answers and Rationales **17**

SECTION

I

SECTION

II

SECTION

III

SECTION

IV

SECTION

V

SECTION

VI

SECTION

VII

SECTION

VIII

SECTION

IX

SECTION

X

9. Correct Answer: **2**

Rationale: A healthcare worker should be immunized, owing to the risk of complications for patients who come in contact with the worker and are at high risk for transmission.

10. Correct Answer: **1**

Rationale: Activation of an emergency response plan would be the first action that the charge nurse should take. Moving existing emergency room patients to hospital beds, calling in available personnel, and obtaining additional supplies would all be components of an emergency response plan.

MATH, DOSAGE CALCULATIONS, AND RELATED PROBLEMS

1. Correct Answer:

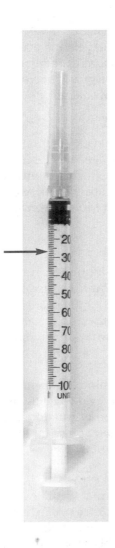

2. Correct Answer: **7 units.**

Rationale: $210 - 150 = 60$; $60/30 = 2$ units. $25 + 35 + 15 + 50 = 125$; $125/25 = 5$ units. Therefore, 2 units + 5 units = 7 units.

3. Correct Answer: **2**

Rationale: 50 mL/30 min = x mL/60 min; $x = 100$ mL/h.

4. Correct Answer: **4**

Rationale: Proportion is 100 mL/30 min = x mL/60 min; $x = 200$ mL/h.

5. Correct Answer: **2**

Rationale: $80 \times 62 = 4{,}960$; bolus is 80×62 or 4,960 units.

6. Correct Answer: **4**

Rationale: The pulse rate is less than 60 beats per minute, which necessitates that you hold the digoxin.

7. Correct Answer: **4**

Rationale: 0.4 mg $= x/3$; $x = 1.2$ mg.

8. Correct Answer: **2**

Rationale: Proportion is $40:5 = 200:x$; $40x = 1{,}000$; $x = 25$.

9. Correct Answer: **4**

Rationale: $300{,}000/100{,}000 = 3$.

10. Correct Answer: **Administer three 500-mg capsules and two 250-mg capsules.**

CARE OF PATIENTS WITH DIABETES

1. Correct Answer: **2**

Rationale: HNKC includes absent ketones, increased blood sugar, altered mental status, and dehydration.

2. Correct Answer: **1**

Rationale: These are classic signs of hypoglycemia.

3. Correct Answer: **4**

Rationale: Nasal congestion is not due to poorly controlled diabetes.

4. Correct Answer: **4**

Rationale: Sedation, overweight, lack of exercise, and age are risk factors for non-insulin-dependent diabetes mellitus (type 2 diabetes).

5. Correct Answer: **3**

   Rationale: 40/20 = 2 units for carbohydrate intake and 6 units for sliding scale = 2 + 6 = 8.

6. Correct Answer: **3**

   Rationale: 20 + 10 + 45 + 45 = 120; 120/8 = 15 units for food. 190 − 130 = 60; 60/30 = 2 units; 2 × 1 = 2 units for blood sugar. Thus 15 food + 2 blood sugar = 17 units.

7. Correct Answer: **2**

   Rationale: Neuropathy is loss of sensation, nephropathy is kidney dysfunction, macroangiopathy is arteriosclerosis, and retinopathy is an eye complication.

8. Correct Answer: **3**

   Rationale: Weight loss is due to using up proteins and fats, which results in acidosis and the buildup of ketones.

9. Correct Answer: **4**

   Rationale: Cardiovascular assessment includes assessing for hypertension, PVD, and coronary artery disease.

10. Correct Answer: **50-unit syringe.**

CARE OF PATIENTS WITH ORTHOPEDIC PROBLEMS

1. Correct Answer: **4**

   Rationale: Osteoarthritis is a degenerative joint disease caused by synovitis and the chronic loss of articular cartilage. Healthy articular cartilage in combination with synovial fluid promotes joint movement. As articular cartilage is worn away and damaged, synovial fluid enters cracks in the cartilage, leading to destruction of the subchondral bone and formation of osteophytes.

2. Correct Answer: **1**

   Rationale: Cyclooxygenase (COX) is a substance that converts arachidonic acid into prostaglandins. Prostaglandins protect the stomach by decreasing gastric acid secretion and increasing bicarbonate secretion, mucosal blood flow, and mucus production. Aspirin inhibits the production of COX-1 and its protective actions in the stomach. The result can be gastric ulceration. Clinical manifestations of gastric ulceration can include fatigue from chronic blood loss and the presence of blood in the GI tract as evidenced by black, tarry stools.

3. Correct Answer: **3**

   Rationale: Rheumatrex disrupts cellular metabolic processes (such as DNA synthesis) and produces immunosuppression. Because rheumatoid arthritis is an inflammatory disease that results from an immune response, the use of Rheumatrex can slow disease progression, but does not cure the disease.

4. Correct Answer: **1**

   Rationale: Parathyroid hormone is released in response to a negative feedback mechanism that is triggered by an abnormally low serum calcium level. The secretion of parathyroid hormone results in the release of calcium from bones (stimulation of bone cell activity), conservation of calcium by the kidney, and increased intestinal absorption of calcium. Calcitonin is released in response to increased blood calcium levels and acts to inhibit the release of calcium from bones (inhibition of bone cell activity) and decrease renal reabsorption of calcium.

5. Correct Answer: **1**

   Rationale: The development of osteoporosis is influenced by age, gender, nutrition, and genetics. The underlying pathophysiology of the disease is an imbalance between bone resorption and formation, which results in bone loss.

6. Correct Answer: **4**

   Rationale: With immobilization of the extremity, the workload for the muscle tissue decreases. The cells adapt to the change in workload by decreasing in size and metabolic functioning. The muscle tissues can be restored with use.

7. Correct Answer: **2**

   Rationale: Malunion is a complication of fracture healing that is evidenced by healing with deformity angulation or rotation. Inadequate reduction or alignment of the fracture can be a cause of malunion.

8. Correct Answer: **1**

   Rationale: A normal serum calcium is in the range of 8.5–10.5 mg/dL. This electrolyte plays an important role in neuromuscular and cardiac excitability. A serum calcium level of

6 mg/dL indicates hypocalcemia, and clinical symptoms may include numbness, tingling, muscle spasms or cramping, and tetany. Additional symptoms may include cardiac dysrhythmias, hypotension, and seizures.

9. Correct Answer: <u>1</u>

Rationale: Assessment of the neurovascular status of an extremity is an important nursing intervention for a patient who has suffered a musculoskeletal injury. The affected extremity should be assessed for color, temperature, capillary refill, presence of pulses, edema, numbness, sensation, motor function, and pain. Abnormal findings could indicate a neurological or vascular injury and should be reported promptly to prevent further complications. A vascular problem would be indicated by the findings of pallor, prolonged capillary refill, and a nonpalpable pulse. Paresthesia is an abnormal neurological finding indicating nerve injury. Prompt reporting of the findings can result in more timely interventions and preservation of function.

10. Correct Answer: <u>2</u>

Rationale: Once a fracture has occurred, the injury must be reduced and immobilized to promote healing. The goals of fracture treatment include anatomical realignment of the bone fragments (reduction), immobilization to maintain realignment, and restoration of normal function. Fracture reduction can be accomplished by manipulation, closed and open reduction, and traction. Immobilization is accomplished by casting, traction, and internal or external fixation. A transverse femur fracture is treated by open reduction; immobilization in this case is accomplished either by internal fixation (e.g., use of pins, plates, and rods) at the time of realignment or by the use of traction. A femur fracture cannot be effectively reduced or immobilized by a cast.

CARE OF PATIENTS WITH HYPERTENSION AND CARDIAC PROBLEMS

1. Correct Answer: <u>3</u>

Rationale: The preferred method for reducing LDL cholesterol levels is therapeutic lifestyle changes to include weight control, exercise, and smoking cessation. If treatment of the hypercholesteremia with therapeutic lifestyle changes is not successful, pharmacologic treatments may be added.

2. Correct Answer: <u>4</u>

Rationale: The standard dosing regimen for nitroglycerin is one tablet sublingually repeated every 5 minutes, up to three doses. If anginal pain is not relieved after three sublingual nitroglycerin tablets, the patient should be advised to immediately seek emergency medical care by contacting the local emergency management system (911).

3. Correct Answer: <u>1</u>

Rationale: Intermittent claudication is ischemic pain that is precipitated by exercise, resolves with rest, and is reproducible. The pain associated with claudication arises when cellular oxygen demand exceeds supply. Increased demand results in anaerobic cellular metabolism to meet the cellular energy needs. Anaerobic by-products such as lactic acid accumulate and result in the stimulation of nerve fibers, which produces pain. With rest, the metabolic by-products are cleared from the system and pain diminishes.

4. Correct Answer: <u>1</u>

Rationale: JNC 7 defines stage 1 hypertension as a systolic blood pressure greater than 140 mm Hg or a diastolic blood pressure greater than 90 mm Hg.

5. Correct Answer: <u>1</u>

Rationale: The patient's clinical symptoms are suggestive of cardiac ischemia—that is, pain associated with decreased blood flow to the myocardium. There are four general treatment priorities in such cases: oxygen, aspirin, morphine, and nitroglycerin. Oxygen is used to increase delivery of O_2 to the myocardium. Aspirin is given for its antiplatelet effect. Morphine is used to treat the ischemic pain. Morphine and nitroglycerin act by decreasing preload and afterload, thereby reducing the myocardial workload.

6. Correct Answer: <u>4</u>

Rationale: The desired outcome for a patient with congestive heart failure is to decrease the workload of the heart. Interventions that decrease preload and afterload and balance myocardial oxygen demands with cellular needs are used to achieve the goal.

SECTION I

SECTION II

SECTION III

SECTION IV

SECTION V

SECTION VI

SECTION VII

SECTION VIII

SECTION IX

SECTION X

7. Correct Answer: **2**

Rationale: The assessment findings of a cool leg with a decreased pulse and an orange-size, hard, palpable area in the right groin are indicative of inadequate hemostasis of the right femoral artery following coronary angioplasty. The nurse should immediately apply pressure to the groin site to control bleeding and achieve hemostasis of the artery.

8. Correct Answer: **2**

Rationale: Sympathetic nervous system stimulation during a myocardial infarction results in vasoconstriction of the peripheral blood vessels. Its development is associated with skin that is cool to the touch and diaphoresis.

9. Correct Answer: **2**

Rationale: Hypertension is a chronic disease that progresses slowly and often has few overt symptoms. The lack of symptoms makes it difficult for patients to maintain adherence to treatment regimens that include lifestyle modifications and medications, all of which have adverse effects and are costly. With treatment, essential hypertension can be controlled and complications decreased. Without treatment, hypertension may lead to heart and kidney disease and stroke. By asking an open-ended question to assess what the patient knows about the disease and its treatment, the nurse can begin to work with the patient on strategies to promote adherence to the treatment plan.

10. Correct Answer: **1**

Rationale: Furosemide is a loop (high-ceiling) diuretic that inhibits the reabsorption of sodium and chloride and results in diuresis. Potassium is lost through excretion in the distal nephrons when the patient receives the drug. The lab result is interpreted as hypokalemia, which is an adverse effect associated with the administration of furosemide (Lasix).

Care of the Childbearing Family and the Neonate

MANAGEMENT OF CARE

Multiple Choice

1. A physician determines that a primigravida who has labored for 14 hours and has had no dilation for 3 hours should have a cesarean section for cephalopelvic disproportion. He informs the patient of the possible risks associated with the procedure. When the nurse asks the patient to sign the consent form, the patient's husband says, "I'll sign it for her. She's too upset by what is happening to make this decision." What should the nurse do?

1. Ask the patient if this is acceptable to her.
2. Have the patient and her husband both sign the consent form.
3. Ask the patient to sign the consent form.
4. Ask the doctor to witness the consent form.

2. While caring for a 33-week preterm infant, you note that he is having an apneic episode. What should your first course of action be?

1. Notify the doctor.
2. Increase the amount of oxygen that the infant is receiving through his nasal cannula.
3. Begin giving rescue breaths.
4. Use tactile stimulation.

3. Which of the following actions would you take first if you found an infant to be severely hypothermic?

1. Place the infant in passive skin-to-skin contact with the parent.
2. Place the infant under a warmer with a skin probe attached to the chest.
3. Perform tactile stimulation to see if more movement will raise the temperature.
4. Check the parents' room for adequate temperature.

4. A nurse is caring for a patient in labor having a Pitocin (oxytocin) induction. The nurse notes that her contractions are every 2 minutes and last 90 seconds; there have been three consecutive late decelerations. What is the nurse's *first* action?

1. Increase the primary IV rate.
2. Discontinue the Pitocin drip.
3. Turn the patient to the opposite side.
4. Give oxygen per face mask.

5. A 36-year-old patient has been admitted with a diagnosis of eclampsia. The nurse observes that the patient is experiencing a seizure. What is the nurse's primary goal?

1. Roll the patient to her side.
2. Start an IV.
3. Record the activity.
4. Call for help.

6. When should a woman who is Rh-negative receive RhoGAM (Rho D immune globulin)?

1. After an amniocentesis.
2. After a car accident.
3. After a miscarriage.
4. All of the above.

7. A patient is pregnant and has been identified as Rh-negative. When should she receive RhoGAM (Rho D immune globulin)?

1. 14 weeks gestation.
2. 36 weeks gestation.
3. Prior to delivery.
4. 28 weeks gestation.

True/False

8. True or False: Eye prophylaxis is required by law in all states in the United States.

9. True or False: Once informed consent is given for human immunodeficiency virus (HIV) testing, patients may refuse to have the test.

Multiple Choice

10. A neonatologist is present in the operating room after a cesarean delivery. The nurse explains to the patient that the neonatologist is there because neonates born by cesarean delivery have a higher incidence of

1. Congenital abnormalities.
2. Respiratory distress syndrome.
3. Meconium aspiration syndrome.
4. Pulmonary hypertension.

11. The *first* nursing responsibility after artificial rupture of membranes (AROM) or spontaneous rupture of membranes (SROM) is to

1. Take a full set of maternal vital signs.
2. Observe for changes in the fetal heart rate.
3. Place the patient in knee-chest position.
4. Dry the perineum, and provide clean pads.

12. Your postpartum patient's blood type is O-negative. She tells you that she received RhoGAM (Rho D immune globulin) at 28 weeks gestation and wonders if she needs another dose now. What is your first action?

1. Call the doctor for an order.
2. Call the blood bank to see if the medication is ready.
3. Ascertain the baby's blood type.
4. Order an antibody test for the patient.

13. A male infant born at 41 weeks gestation is scheduled for circumcision. Prior to the procedure, the nurse needs to verify that

1. The parents want pain medication for the procedure.

2. The infant has had a bowel movement.
3. A consent form has been signed and is on the chart.
4. The table and instruments are ready.

14. A nurse received a phone call on the labor and delivery unit from her patient's mother. Her daughter is in labor, and the mother wants to check to see how she is progressing. What should the nurse do?

1. Tell the mother how her daughter is doing.
2. Do not tell her any information.
3. Pretend she does not have that patient.
4. Ask the charge nurse to speak with the mother.

15. A postpartum patient who delivered 30 minutes ago has an increase in lochia. What should the nurse do?

1. Notify the doctor and request medication orders.
2. Give the patient Pitocin (oxytocin).
3. Evaluate the patient's vital signs.
4. Evaluate the patient's bladder and fundus.

16. A nurse prepares to conduct an assessment of a mother 15 minutes after her delivery of a normal healthy infant. The mother is breastfeeding and requests that the exam be delayed for at least 30 minutes. What should the nurse do?

1. Honor the patient's request.
2. Perform the exam without interrupting breastfeeding.
3. Stop the breastfeeding for 5 minutes to do a quick exam.
4. Ask the certified nursing assistant to complete the assessment.

17. A patient is 2 days post vaginal delivery and has done very little to provide hands-on care to her infant even though she reacts very positively to the baby. What should the nurse do?

1. Encourage the mother to change the diaper under the supervision of the nurse.
2. Call for a social work consult.
3. Ask the family what is wrong with the patient.
4. Make a note in the chart.

18. A 16-year-old patient delivers her first baby and is on the postpartum unit. She has done very little to care for the infant and does not maintain eye contact with the infant. What should the nurse do?

1. Make a referral to the social worker.

2. Notify the provider.

3. Make a referral to the lactation consultant.

4. Notify the charge nurse.

19. A 30-year-old patient is breastfeeding her 1-day-old infant who is not latching on correctly to the breast. What should the nurse do?

   1. After an attempt to help without success, make an appointment for a lactation consultation.

   2. After an attempt to help, ask an experienced nurse to help.

   3. After an attempt to help, ask another patient for some help.

   4. Suggest the mother should use formula, as it is easier and just as nutritious as breast milk.

20. A patient is at the clinic for her 36-week checkup. She is 18 years old and wants to have her tubes tied after her baby is born. What should the nurse do?

   1. Tell the patient she will probably want more children and should rethink her decision.

   2. Tell the patient it is a good decision, as she already has three other children.

   3. Encourage the patient to discuss all of her options for birth control with the provider.

   4. Obtain the consent form and have the patient sign it before she leaves.

21. An 18-year-old postpartum patient is interested in getting a bilateral tubal ligation after her delivery. The nurse understands her role in the process is to

   1. Explain the patient's options for different surgical procedures.

   2. Document information provided as well as the patient's comprehension of informed consent.

   3. Contact the ethics committee because the patient is younger than 20 years of age.

   4. Physically prepare the patient for surgery.

22. A labor and delivery nurse who works in a facility that receives federal funding understands that her role in advanced directives is

   1. Nothing—women don't usually die while delivering a baby.

   2. To ask all patients if they have knowledge of advanced directives.

   3. Nothing—this is done when the patient is admitted.

   4. To give all patients a brochure when they are admitted to their rooms.

23. A patient is 18 weeks pregnant, and the nurse is assisting the provider during her prenatal visit. She overhears the provider tell the patient that the alpha-fetoprotein (AFP) level is a required prenatal test. The nurse knows that this test

   1. Is not required, and the patient has a right to refuse it.

   2. Is required, because the patient is high risk because of her age.

   3. Is a simple blood test, and all women get it between 15 and 18 weeks gestation.

   4. Is not required, but is often associated with false-negative results.

24. A labor patient at 42 weeks gestation is having labor induction for post dates. The patient is on Pitocin (oxytocin), and the fetal heart rate begins to show late decelerations. What should the nurse do?

   1. Call the physician immediately.

   2. Give the patient oxygen.

   3. Increase the Pitocin (oxytocin) and deliver the patient quickly.

   4. Stop the Pitocin (oxytocin) and begin fetal resuscitative efforts.

25. A postpartum nurse gives a pain medication to the wrong patient. What should the nurse do?

   1. Nothing—the patient is not allergic and has not experienced any side effects.

   2. Notify the pharmacist.

   3. Complete an incident report and notify the physician.

   4. Notify the physician.

26. The nurse is coming on to her shift at 7 A.M. She has the following patients assigned to her care:

   - An induction for pregnancy-induced hypertension
   - A patient who is 2 cm dilated with an epidural and Pitocin
   - A patient who is 6 cm dilated

Which patient should she see first?

   1. The patient who is 6 cm dilated.

   2. The patient who is undergoing induction.

   3. The patient who is 2 cm dilated.

   4. None of them—complain that this is a heavy load.

27. The nurse is coming on to her shift at 7 A.M. on a postpartum unit. Her patients include a patient who is 2 days postoperative cesarean section, a patient who underwent a vaginal delivery 2 hours ago, and a patient who is dressed and waiting for discharge. Which patient should the nurse assess first?

1. The patient who underwent a vaginal delivery 2 hours ago, because she is at risk for bleeding.
2. The patient who is ready to go home, because she is waiting.
3. The 2-day postoperative patient, because she is at risk for bleeding.
4. The patient who underwent a vaginal delivery 2 hours ago, and have the nursing assistant discharge the waiting patient.

28. A nurse in the newborn nursery has several patient needs. Indicate all activities that can be delegated to a nursing assistant:

1. Changing a baby's diaper.
2. Feeding an infant of a diabetic mother.
3. Performing an initial admission assessment.
4. Giving an antibiotic.

29. A nurse on the postpartum unit has several patient needs. Indicate all activities that can be delegated to a nursing assistant:

1. Giving a sitz bath to a patient with a fourth-degree laceration.
2. Checking vital signs on a new admission to the unit.
3. Checking the fundus of a newly delivered mother.
4. Giving Colace (docusate sodium) to a patient who is 2 days postoperative c-section.

30. A nurse on the labor and delivery unit has several patient needs. Indicate all activities that can be delegated to a nursing assistant:

1. Giving a patient an enema.
2. Assisting with an epidural insertion.
3. Taking the blood pressure of a hypertensive patient.
4. None of the above.

31. A nurse on a high-risk pregnancy unit is caring for a patient with type 1 diabetes who was admitted for poor insulin control. The nurse has cared for this patient for the past 3 days, during which time the patient had not received her correct diet. The nurse knows that

1. This problem always happens with the dietary department.
2. This problem is a quality assurance issue that needs to be addressed.
3. Her diet alterations are minimal and would not affect the patient.
4. This problem should be reported to the physician.

32. A 21-year-old patient is admitted for incompetent cervix. Her 18 weeks gestation can not be salvaged. The nurse recognizes a knowledge deficit when the patient says:

1. "My baby will be fine—he can just go to the neonatal intensive care unit."
2. "I do hope a cerclage will help with my next pregnancy."
3. "I am so sad I am losing this baby—it is my third loss."
4. "What medication will I receive after the baby is born?"

33. A patient admitted for hyperemesis will need a referral to which of the following?

1. Radiology department for an ultrasound.
2. Maternal fetal medicine.
3. Nutritionist.
4. Pharmacist.

34. A nurse is precepting a new graduate on the labor and delivery unit. Today, the graduate nurse needs to insert an intravenous line (IV) in a labor patient. The patient is hurting and wants pain medication. What must the new graduate do first?

1. Place a towel under the patient to catch the blood.
2. Put on her gloves.
3. Prep the patient's arm with iodine.
4. Get the pain medication and have it waiting.

35. A postpartum nurse is caring for a patient who plans to give her baby up for adoption. The nurse knows

1. This decision requires communication between social services and the patient.
2. This decision is not uncommon and can be handled without incident.
3. The physician must be present at the time of patient discharge.

4. The charge nurse needs to coordinate the patient's care.

36. A new admission to the labor and delivery unit is HIV-positive. The charge nurse assigns the patient to a nurse who says, "I can't take that patient; I am pregnant and will get HIV." The charge nurse

1. Knows this is true and reassigns the patient.

2. Is aware that the nurse won't get HIV if she only wears goggles during the delivery.

3. Realizes there is a potential need for staff education on HIV transmission.

4. Knows this could be true depending on the nurse's gestational age.

37. A 40-year-old patient refuses an amniocentesis after having a positive alpha-fetoprotein test. How should the nurse counsel the patient?

1. She is making a mistake, as she is at high risk for delivering a child with Down syndrome.

2. She should do whatever her provider suggests.

3. The decision to accept or reject testing is hers.

4. She will need to get consent from the baby's father before she can make that decision.

38. The grandmother of an infant in the nursery wants to take the baby to the mother's room. What should the nurse do?

1. Allow the grandmother to escort the baby to the room.

2. Obtain permission from the mother for the grandmother to take the baby from the nursery.

3. Do not allow the grandmother to have the baby.

4. Call the charge nurse.

39. A nurse who is working in the genetics clinic understands that she must be able to

1. Obtain an accurate family history.

2. Provide a supportive environment.

3. Understand and communicate the basics of genetic disease.

4. All of the above.

40. A 16-year-old patient in a family planning clinic asks the nurse which form of birth control the nurse would recommend. When advising this patient, the nurse must first

1. Be aware of her own beliefs regarding family planning and sexuality.

2. Discourage the patient from using birth control, as she is too young to engage in sexual intercourse.

3. Be aware of all birth control options.

4. Involve the patient's boyfriend in the decision-making process.

41. A gravida 6 para 5 patient who is Group B *Streptococcus* (GBS)-positive comes to labor and delivery. She is 9 cm dilated and ready to push. The nurse knows the patient needs to receive intravenous antibiotics for the GBS. What should the nurse do?

1. Give the patient an epidural to eliminate her urge to push.

2. Attempt to start the antibiotic administration but notify the nursery of inadequate coverage.

3. Ignore the fact that the patient is GBS-positive and encourage her to push.

4. Call the pharmacist.

42. A nurse on the labor and delivery unit overhears another nurse talking about her patient at the nurses' station. The patient came in with a lengthy, detailed birth plan, and her nurse says she is sure the patient will end up with a cesarean section because of it. This attitude demonstrates a lack of

1. Advocacy.

2. Continuity of care.

3. Delegation.

4. Ethics.

43. A patient comes to the labor and delivery unit with a birth plan that does not include an epidural. When the patient's provider comes to perform a pelvic exam, she states, "You are going to get an epidural, correct? I mean, why go through all that pain when we have medication that can take it all away?" How should the nurse respond to the patient?

1. "She is right—there is no need for you to have any pain in labor."

2. "This is your birth and I will support your decisions."

3. "Labor won't hurt, so you really won't need anything for pain."

4. "I had my babies with an epidural—it is no big deal."

44. A patient has stated that she wishes to not have an episiotomy. During the delivery of the infant and while the head is crowning, the nurse sees the provider pick up the scissors to cut an episiotomy. What should the nurse do?

1. Nothing—the provider is the ultimate decision maker in terms of patient care.
2. Tell the patient she is about to have an episiotomy.
3. Notify the provider that the patient does not want an episiotomy.
4. Turn away and finish charting.

SAFETY AND INFECTION CONTROL

Multiple Choice

45. A patient's husband accompanies her to all her prenatal visits. You suspect spousal abuse when you note the following:

1. The patient seems withdrawn at each visit.
2. The husband answers questions that are directed to him.
3. The patient has a list of discomforts that she wishes to discuss.
4. The husband excuses himself during invasive procedures.

46. Which of the following is *not* associated with postpartum risk for infection?

1. Anemia.
2. Surgical procedures.
3. Multiple pelvic examinations.
4. Preterm labor.

47. Daily umbilical cord care to prevent infection should include which one of the following measures?

1. Bathe daily with warm water and pat dry.
2. Apply oil to the cord.
3. Apply lotion to the area just next to the cord.
4. Keep the cord and area directly surrounding it clean and dry.

48. A postpartum patient has not been immunized against rubella. The nurse understands the patient needs rubella immunization prior to her discharge. What instruction will the nurse give the patient regarding this injection?

1. She can get the injection at her postpartum visit.
2. She should not become pregnant in the next 3 months.

3. She should not take her prenatal vitamins once she receives the injection.
4. She cannot take birth control pills after receiving the injection.

49. A postpartum nurse notices that two medications with identical packaging and similar names are stored next to one another in the floor's medication administration machine. What should the nurse do?

1. Announce this fact in the staff meeting.
2. Tell the charge nurse.
3. Notify the pharmacy.
4. Tell her colleagues working that shift.

50. A nurse is transcribing medication orders from the chart of a new admission. She has trouble reading the dose of a common medication used on the postpartum unit. What should the nurse do?

1. Call the provider for order clarification.
2. Call the pharmacist to see how the pharmacist read the order.
3. Ask the charge nurse.
4. Assume it is the common medication dose routinely used by this provider.

51. A nurse is caring for an infant of a mother who is infected with herpes simplex virus. The nurse uses gloves with all contact and knows that

1. This measure is required with universal precautions.
2. She will still need to wash her hands between patients.
3. This measure is all that is needed with this particular diagnosis.
4. The infant does not have the disease—only the mother—so nothing else needs to be done.

52. A nurse is precepting a new graduate with inserting an intravenous line (IV) in a labor patient. The patient is hurting and wants pain medication. The new graduate uses perfect technique in starting the IV and gets it on the first try but did not use gloves. What should the nurse do?

1. Congratulates the new graduate on her technique and speed.
2. Tell the new graduate she needs to wear gloves with all IV starts.
3. Get the pain medication to the patient quickly.
4. Question the new graduate on her technique of IV insertion.

True/False

53. True or False: Wearing protective gear during deliveries is not necessary as it is not an invasive procedure.

Multiple Choice

54. A newly pregnant patient comes to the clinic because her boyfriend has tested positive for *Chlamydia*. The nurse knows

1. This infection cannot be transmitted through intercourse.
2. This infection cannot be treated with antibiotics.
3. The patient needs to be tested for the infection.
4. The patient just needs to use condoms from now on.

55. A 32 weeks pregnant patient is positive for *Chlamydia*. The nurse knows

1. The patient is at risk for a postpartum infection.
2. The infant is at risk for ophthalmia neonatorum.
3. The infant will be born with red lesions.
4. *Chlamydia* can cause brain damage in infants.

56. A gynecology patient has tested positive for *Chlamydia*. The nurse knows that, if she is not treated, the patient is at risk for

1. Ectopic pregnancy.
2. Pelvic inflammatory disease.
3. Tubal factor infertility.
4. All of the above.

57. What is (are) the risk(s) associated with amniocentesis?

1. Infection.
2. Hemorrhage.
3. Miscarriage.
4. All of the above.

58. A patient is tested for Group B *Streptococcus* at 36 weeks of gestation. The patient asks, "Is this infection a sexually transmitted disease?" How should the nurse respond?

1. "No, this infection involves bacteria normally found in your intestinal tract."
2. "No, this infection involves bacteria normally found in your bladder."

3. "Yes, you will need to use condoms."
4. "Yes, you will need to receive an antibiotic."

59. A patient is tested for Group B *Streptococcus* at 36 weeks of gestation and is found to be positive. The patient asks, "How do we treat this?" How should the nurse respond?

1. "There is no need to treat you—only the baby will receive treatment."
2. "We will give you a prescription for an antibiotic."
3. "You will be treated in labor with intravenous antibiotics."
4. "There is no need to treat this infection, as it involves bacteria normally found in the vagina."

60. A patient is tested for Group B *Streptococcus* at 36 weeks of gestation and is found to be positive. The patient asks, "Is this dangerous for me and the baby?" How should the nurse respond?

1. "Yes, it can kill you and your baby."
2. "No, it is a normal finding and we won't do anything about it."
3. "I am not sure; ask the provider when you see him."
4. "It is not harmful to you, but it could make your baby very sick once it is born."

61. A nurse is counseling a newly pregnant patient about handling her cat's litter box. The nurse does so in an effort to prevent maternal infection with

1. Trichomoniasis.
2. Toxoplasmosis.
3. *Chlamydia*.
4. Bacterial vaginosis.

True/False

62. True or False: Wearing protective gear in the postpartum unit is not necessary, as no invasive procedures take place in this unit; it is more like respite care.

Multiple Choice

63. Pelvic inflammatory disease (PID) can

1. Be cured.
2. Can cause infertility.
3. Can cause ectopic pregnancies.
4. All of the above.

64. The following symptoms may signify the past or current presence of sexual abuse in a patient:

1. Postpartum blues.

2. Low self-esteem, insomnia, extreme anger.

3. Waking every few hours in the last weeks of pregnancy.

4. Shortness of breath during pregnancy.

65. It is important to educate a pregnant patient about the following:

1. Headaches and blurred vision after 28 weeks of pregnancy.

2. Nausea and vomiting before 12 weeks of pregnancy.

3. Clear or white nipple discharge during pregnancy.

4. Frequent urination after the second trimester.

66. A nurse is assessing the fundal height of a patient at 32 weeks gestation. It is noted to be 28 cm. The nurse knows

1. This reflects the fact that the patient just moved her bowels and caused the baby to shift.

2. This reflects the fact that the baby is in a breech position.

3. This may indicate a lack of fetal growth.

4. This is a normal finding in this gestation.

HEALTH PROMOTION AND MAINTENANCE

67. A pregnant patient comes to the clinic with her boyfriend for a prenatal visit. The nurse suspects physical abuse. How should the nurse address her concern?

1. Ask the patient if she being abused.

2. Ask the boyfriend to leave and then ask about safety issues.

3. Do nothing, as her suspicions are unlikely to be borne out.

4. Make a note in the chart about her suspicions.

68. According to the American Academy of Pediatrics, what is the *best* form of infant nutrition?

1. Exclusive breastfeeding until 2 months of age.

2. Exclusive breastfeeding until 6 months of age.

3. Commercially prepared infant formula for 1 year.

4. Commercially prepared infant formula until 4–6 months of age.

69. A 26-week, G1P0 patient confides to the nurse that her husband refuses to have intercourse because he is afraid he will hurt the baby by introducing germs. What information would be helpful to this couple?

1. A mucous substance called leukorrhea will clear the vagina of any unfriendly bacteria.

2. Douching with warm saline solution after intercourse will protect the baby from bacteria.

3. The mucous plug that seals the cervix acts as a barrier against bacterial invasion during pregnancy.

4. Couples having sexual problems during pregnancy should consider making an appointment with a marriage counselor.

70. During a late-pregnancy visit, a patient is distraught about the dark red "stretch marks" that have just appeared on both sides of her lower abdomen. She wants to know what to do to ensure they will disappear after she delivers. What is the nurse's *best* response?

1. "There is no treatment for stretch marks, but after birth they usually fade to a lighter pink."

2. "Stretch marks seem to be familial, so you might want to see who had them in your family and what they used to make them fade."

3. "Many women get these stretch marks, and yours seem less severe than many I've seen."

4. "Stretch marks are from hormone-induced pigmentation changes during pregnancy, and they disappear after delivery."

71. A patient presents today for her first new obstetric visit. The nurse takes her history. Here is what the patient says about her past pregnancies:

1991: ectopic pregnancy

1992: spontaneous miscarriage at 5 weeks

1998: cesarean section at 41 weeks gestation

1999: normal spontaneous vaginal delivery at 38 weeks

2002: intrauterine fetal death at 18 weeks

Which of the following represents her GTPAL?

1. 62032.

2. 45232.

3. 52122.

4. 42132.

Health Promotion and Maintenance **29**

SECTION
I

SECTION
II

SECTION
III

SECTION
IV

SECTION
V

SECTION
VI

SECTION
VII

SECTION
VIII

SECTION
IX

SECTION
X

72. A G1 patient is 20 weeks pregnant. She presents to the office today for her routine prenatal visit. The patient complains of palpitations. What is the nurse's best response?

1. "Palpitations are normal and are often related to the normal increase in your blood volume and pulse in pregnancy."
2. "This issue needs further investigation now."
3. "Palpitations are normal and are related to the normal increase in your respiratory rate during pregnancy."
4. "You need to keep a record of when these episodes occur and bring it to your next visit."

73. A nurse is giving nutrition counseling to a patient who is 18 weeks pregnant. The nurse tells her that the ideal pregnancy weight gain is around 35 pounds. The patient says, "Don't babies weigh just 6 or 7 pounds?" What is the nurse's best response?

1. "That's true, but let me explain where the additional weight is distributed."
2. "Please don't worry about that now. We want you to concentrate on eating well."
3. "It may sound like a lot of weight, but it is important for your baby's health."
4. "Are you concerned about your body image?"

74. Second-trimester teaching includes all *except*:

1. Safe use of seat belts.
2. Pelvic rock exercises.
3. Signs of potential problems.
4. Restriction of tub bathing.

75. A patient who is 26 weeks pregnant complains of sharp, stabbing, unilateral lower abdominal pain, which occurs intermittently while she is walking or getting up from sitting. What is the most likely cause of this pain?

1. Appendicitis.
2. Preterm labor.
3. Round ligament pain.
4. Increased intestinal motility.

76. A postpartum patient's husband asks, "When can my wife and I resume intercourse?" What is the nurse's best response?

1. "Anytime your wife feels like she wants to."
2. "In 6 months."
3. "When her birth control method starts to work."

4. "It is advised to wait until after her 6-week checkup."

77. Lack of immunity to rubella identified in the prenatal period requires:

1. Monitoring of antibody titers during the second trimester.
2. Administration of the vaccine once the lab result is received.
3. Administration of the vaccine during the postpartum period.
4. Testing of the newborn's antibody levels within 24 hours of birth.

78. In a mother who chooses not to breastfeed, what breast changes can she expect during the postpartum period?

1. The breasts will return to the prepregnant state in 48 hours.
2. Engorgement may occur for 24 to 36 hours.
3. Engorgement occurs only with breastfeeding.
4. The breasts will return to the prepregnant state in about 6 weeks.

79. A mother desires to exclusively breastfeed her full-term infant. On admission to the mother/baby unit, the nurse discusses the ideal situation to enhance early and exclusive breastfeeding, which includes all of the following *except*:

1. Keeping the baby in the mother's room 24 hours (day and night).
2. Letting the baby spend the first night in the nursery so the mother can sleep.
3. Performing skin-to-skin contact when possible.
4. Feeding the infant with proper latch-on when hunger cues are present.

80. Which point about breast milk production is the best basis for counseling breastfeeding mothers?

1. It is hormone driven.
2. It is infant driven by quantity and quality of infant suckling.
3. Human placental lactogen, glucocorticoids, and thyroid-stimulating hormone are major factors in milk production.
4. It depends on the size of the ducts and ductules.

81. A patient confides in the nurse that she eats dirt. The nurse knows this practice, which is called pica, is of concern because:

1. It is not normal and the patient needs a psychiatric consult.

2. It involves the consumption of low-nutritional-value products.

3. It is reflective of the patient's normal dietary pattern when not pregnant.

4. It will influence the eating habits of her baby.

82. A 16-year-old patient comes to the clinic for a new obstetric appointment and is accompanied by her mother. Prior to taking the patient's history, the nurse should:

1. Have the patient go to the bathroom as the interview process may take a while.

2. Ask the patient's mother to wait in the waiting room during the interview.

3. Have the patient don a gown so the provider can conduct the physical immediately after the interview.

4. Have the patient get her lab work done first.

83. The nurse counsels a postpartum patient on the frequency and timing of breast self-exams. When should the exams be conducted in this patient?

1. Weekly and mid-cycle.

2. Monthly mid-cycle.

3. Monthly during the menstrual cycle.

4. Every day during the menstrual cycle.

84. A 20-year-old patient comes to the clinic for preconceptual counseling. She reports that her past gynecology history is positive for cervical dysphasia. The nurse understands that all of the following are risk factors for this condition:

1. Later age for first sexual intercourse.

2. Cigarette smoking.

3. Herpes.

4. Monogamy.

85. A patient comes to the clinic for her 6-week checkup after having her second baby. She asks when she can get pregnant again, because she wants a large family. How should the nurse respond?

1. "Any time—it is better to have children when you are young."

2. "Once you stop breastfeeding."

3. "It is advised to wait at least 1 year between pregnancies."

4. "Two years between children is a good idea."

86. A patient comes to the clinic because she is trying to conceive and has been unsuccessful. The nurse looks at her chart and identifies the following as a risk factor:

1. Smoker.

2. Exercise 4 times per week.

3. Age 25.

4. History of two past sexual partners.

PSYCHOSOCIAL INTEGRITY

Multiple Choice

87. The patient has a toddler who is 2 years old and a child who is 7 years old. What is appropriate sibling preparation for this family?

1. Arrange for the children to stay with their grandparents out of state during labor and the early postpartum period.

2. Move the 2-year-old from the crib to a larger bed during the last month of pregnancy.

3. Tell the children that you know they will love this baby.

4. Let the children listen to the fetal heartbeat and feel the baby move.

88. A patient is taken for an emergency c-section for fetal distress. When she awakes she states "I really wanted to have a vaginal delivery. I am a failure." The nurse's best response is:

1. "I am sure the epidural you got caused the fetal distress. It is not your fault."

2. "At least your baby is healthy. How it is delivered really doesn't matter."

3. "Tell me why you feel like like having a c-section represents failure?"

4. "Once you see your baby, you will forget all about the c-section."

89. Which nursing diagnosis would be most likely in a patient who is G4P0 1 week after a spontaneous abortion?

1. Ineffective family coping.

2. Situational low self-esteem.

3. Social isolation.

4. Loss of intimacy.

90. A multigravida woman is admitted to the hospital for a trial of labor and a vaginal birth after cesarean (VBAC). She had her first cesarean section for fetal distress. The current fetus has severe repetitive late decelerations and fetal distress, and an emergency cesarean section is performed under general anesthesia. After the delivery, the patient tells the nurse, "I feel terrible. This is exactly what happened during my first delivery." What is a priority nursing diagnosis for this patient?

1. High risk for hemorrhage related to previous cesarean section.

2. Anxiety related to neonatal outcome.

3. Pain related to surgical incision and uterine cramping.

4. Low self-esteem related to inability to deliver vaginally.

91. Your patient has been moved to an intensive care unit (ICU) after developing severe anemia and DIC related to a bleeding episode. Her baby remains in the regular nursery for full-term infants. Which nursing intervention would be *most* helpful for this family during the first 24 hours?

1. Bring the baby for regular visits to the mother's bedside as her condition allows.

2. Allow only the father to feed the baby in the nursery.

3. Discharge the baby to relatives as soon as possible.

4. Assign the baby to one nurse in the nursery to provide total care.

92. Your postpartum patient does not speak any English, and she resists your beckoning to her to take a shower. What should your next step be?

1. Offer her a bed bath instead.

2. Assume that showering is a taboo in her culture.

3. Call for an interpreter.

4. Wait for her family to arrive to provide her care.

93. You are having a conversation with a pregnant woman in the park where her children are playing. Of the following information that she shares with you, which issue places her at high risk for postpartum depression?

1. She is excited about having another baby.

2. She has lived in the same city all of her life.

3. Her children playing on the swings are 4, 6, and 8 years of age.

4. Her husband cannot find work since he lost his job.

94. A mother of a 6-week-old baby begins yelling at you because you woke her baby to take vital signs. What is your best response?

1. "The doctor has ordered vital signs to be done every 4 hours on your baby."

2. "I understand that you are tired and frustrated, but I want to be sure that your baby is doing okay."

3. "Would you like to leave the hospital for a while to take a break?"

4. "I'm sorry that I disturbed you. Let me know when I can come back to get these vital signs."

95. Your patient has just been brought to your postpartum unit after delivering a stillborn baby girl. She is crying as you help her into bed. What is the nurse's *best* response?

1. "I feel very sad for you. What can I do for you?"

2. "God had a purpose for her."

3. "Even though you are hurting now, it is better for this to happen now than after you had time to really get to know her."

4. "Now you have an angel in heaven."

96. A patient who is 15 weeks pregnant comes to her routine prenatal visit with her husband. The husband says, "My wife acts strangely lately. One minute she is happy, and the next minute she is crying." How should the nurse respond?

1. "The physical stress of pregnancy is hard. Your wife can speak with our social worker today."

2. "Emotional highs and lows are a sign of psychiatric issues. Does your wife have a history of any such disorders?"

3. "We don't know why this happens, but it may be related to hormone changes in pregnancy. It is normal to experience this."

4. "Be sure to tell the midwife when she comes in to see you. This behavior is not normal and may be a problem she needs to address."

97. A patient at 28 weeks gestation is admitted in preterm labor. She says to her nurse, "I just knew I should have quit jogging when I discovered I was pregnant." Which response by the nurse would be most helpful?

1. "The doctor will be able to tell you the reason for your preterm labor as soon as your test results are back."

SECTION II

SECTION III

SECTION IV

SECTION V

SECTION VI

SECTION VII

SECTION VIII

SECTION IX

SECTION X

2. "What other risky activities did you do that might possibly contribute to your preterm labor?"

3. "Most women wonder what causes preterm labor, but we don't always know the answer."

4. "Try not to worry. Stress can make contractions worse and they are bad now."

98. A nurse is caring for a patient who has just delivered a 20-week gestation born dead. The nurse encourages the patient to give the baby a name. Why?

1. It is required for the death certificate.

2. The name that is chosen will not be given to a future child.

3. Naming the baby will distract her from her grief.

4. It will make the loss become real to her and her family.

99. In counseling a husband and wife who have experienced a perinatal loss, an important concept to emphasize is

1. The couple can get pregnant again.

2. Men and women grieve in different ways.

3. They should avoid talking about the baby to minimize their pain.

4. A funeral is the best way to resolve grief.

100. Which of the following remarks is helpful to say to bereaved parents following a stillbirth?

1. "The living must go on."

2. "God had a purpose for her."

3. "I am so sorry."

4. "You can still have other children.

101. Which of the following women needs the *most* careful follow-up for postpartum depression after discharge home with a newborn?

1. G2P1 married with a 2-year-old child and whose neighbor has promised to help.

2. G1P0 single with an older sister with a child coming to help.

3. G4P3 married with a husband who is away at work during the day.

4. G4P3 single who is living with parents and grandparents.

102. A patient comes in for a new obstetric visit after having experienced a voluntary interruption of pregnancy 2 months prior because of early diagnosis of Down syndrome. The patient asks the

nurse, "What should I do to prevent this baby from having the same problem?" How should the nurse respond?

1. "Make sure you take your prenatal vitamins."

2. "Make sure you see a genetic counselor."

3. "You did nothing to cause this."

4. "Nothing—it is likely to happen again."

103. A first-time mother begins to breastfeed for the first time. The infant attempts to latch and then continually pulls off the nipple. The patient says, "She doesn't like me or my breast milk." The nurse understands

1. Incorrect latch-on can contribute to infants pulling off the breast.

2. The mother is correct and will need to formula feed.

3. This is an unusual finding, and the nurse will need to get the lactation specialist.

4. She should stop trying and start again the next day.

104. The postpartum nurse is giving instructions regarding prevention of postpartum depression. What information should those instructions include?

1. Postpartum depression is very rare and unlikely to occur.

2. Share your feelings with someone; avoid isolation.

3. Reconnect into all your previous activities as soon as possible.

4. You will not need any help when you get home.

105. Which characteristics describe the postpartum blues?:

1. Postpartum blues occur 3–5 days after delivery and are short-lived.

2. Postpartum blues can last up to 6 weeks.

3. The mother may feel like hurting her baby.

4. The mother will have insomnia.

106. A 20-year-old patient comes to the reproductive health clinic for an abortion at 8 weeks gestation. What is the nurse's role in this process?

1. To have the patient give informed consent.

2. To provide unconditional support through the process.

3. To refer the patient to a family who wants to adopt.

4. To help the patient see how she can keep the baby.

BASIC CARE AND COMFORT

Multiple Choice

107. On the second postpartum day, your patient with a cesarean delivery complains of gas pains. You should instruct the patient to

1. Ask her provider for a prescription for Colace (docusate sodium).
2. Chew on some ice chips.
3. Maintain bed rest.
4. Ambulate more often.

108. Which interventions for shortness of breath—a common complaint during the last trimester of pregnancy—should the nurse suggest?

1. Consume 16 ounces of water four times per day.
2. Get a back massage.
3. Keep the bladder empty.
4. Sleep with extra pillows under the head.

109. Care for pregnant women that almost all cultures emphasize includes

1. Working until the due date to prevent boredom.
2. Refraining from raising arms above the head to prevent knots in the umbilical cord.
3. Prohibiting sexual activity during the second half of pregnancy.
4. Maintaining a harmonious and agreeable environment.

110. Following the vaginal delivery of an 11-pound baby, the nurse encourages the mother to breastfeed her newborn. What is the *primary* purpose of this action?

1. To facilitate maternal–newborn interaction.
2. To initiate the secretion of colostrum.
3. To stimulate the uterus to contract.
4. To prevent neonatal hyperglycemia.

111. Your patient has been 7 cm dilated for the past 3 hours. You decide to try some nonpharmacologic methods to speed the progress of her labor. Which of the following can result in prolonged labor?

1. Restricting a woman's position during labor.
2. A previous history of precipitous deliveries.
3. Fluid overload during this labor.
4. A low platelet count.

112. A patient who is having her second baby complains of round ligament pain. The nurse suggests

1. Nothing—this is a normal finding.
2. Use of a prenatal belt.
3. Taking tub baths three times a day.
4. Walking daily to facilitate the stretching for labor.

113. A patient who is 20 weeks pregnant tells the nurse that her prenatal vitamin makes her feel sick. Which is the best suggestion?

1. Take the vitamin with breakfast.
2. Stop taking the vitamin for a few days and then resume.
3. Take the vitamin at bedtime.
4. Take the vitamin with milk between meals.

114. A postpartum patient complains of abdominal cramping with breastfeeding. The nurse knows

1. This reaction is normal; the nurse explains this to the patient and suggests she take Motrin (ibuprofen).
2. This reaction is normal; the nurse suggests placing a heating pad on her abdomen right away.
3. This reaction is not normal; the nurse evaluates the patient's blood loss by taking vital signs and making peripad assessments.
4. This reaction is not normal; the nurse notifies the physician.

115. A patient phones the office on postpartum day 4 with a complaint of breast engorgement; she is not breastfeeding. The nurse suggests all of the following measures *except*

1. Take a warm shower while rubbing the breasts.
2. Apply cold compresses.
3. Wear a tight-fitting bra.
4. Take anti-inflammatory medications as needed.

116. A woman is experiencing back labor and complains of intense pain in her lower back. Which of the following would be the most effective relief measure?

1. Effleurage.
2. Breathing techniques (slow-paced).
3. Counterpressure against the sacrum.
4. Guided imagery.

SECTION I

SECTION II

SECTION III

SECTION IV

SECTION V

SECTION VI

SECTION VII

SECTION VIII

SECTION IX

SECTION X

117. The most effective nursing intervention for perineal discomfort in the first 12 hours after delivery is

  1. Application of an ice pack.
  2. Administration of oral estrogen.
  3. Application of local anesthetic cream.
  4. Administration of a warm sitz bath.

118. A patient who is 9 weeks pregnant calls the office complaining of morning sickness. What should the nurse suggest?

  1. Eat small frequent meals.
  2. Morning sickness is normal and will pass.
  3. Eat only three meals per day.
  4. Add more fat in the diet, as it aids with digestion.

119. A patient who is 36 weeks pregnant calls the office complaining of epigastric discomfort. What should the nurse suggest?

  1. Eat small frequent meals.
  2. Eat only fruits and vegetables until the discomfort resolves.
  3. Avoid foods with lactose.
  4. Not to worry—epigastric discomfort is normal.

120. A Hispanic patient at 36 weeks gestation complains about heartburn. The nurse knows this is

  1. A good reason for the patient to change from her cultural diet.
  2. Abnormal and requires provider notification.
  3. Normal but can be relieved with antacids.
  4. A sign of preterm labor.

True/False

121. True or False: A woman who is breastfeeding can no longer eat her native food if it is very spicy.

Multiple Choice

122. A woman comes to the clinic for her 6-week checkup. She complains of urinary incontinence. What should the nurse suggest?

  1. The patient stop drinking any caffeinated beverages.
  2. The patient stop drinking so much water.
  3. The patient tell the provider.
  4. The patient do Kegel exercises.

123. A woman in her first trimester complains of nausea and vomiting, especially when she brushes her teeth. What should the nurse suggest?

  1. Not to worry about it—the patient's teeth will be fine if she does not brush them.
  2. It is still important to brush, because cavities can form.
  3. This problem probably will last throughout the entire pregnancy.
  4. Call the dentist.

124. A patient who is 28 weeks pregnant complains of lower back pain. What should the nurse suggest?

  1. The patient pay close attention to her body posture and mechanics, as these are the cause of back pain in pregnancy.
  2. The patient tell her provider immediately, because she is in preterm labor.
  3. Lower back pain is part of being pregnant, and there is nothing the patient can do about the pain.
  4. The patient take Motrin as needed.

125. It is recommended that a pregnant woman rest

  1. Four times per day.
  2. In the side-lying position.
  3. Minimally.
  4. On her back.

126. As women progress in their pregnancy, it is recommended that their seat belts should

  1. Not be worn.
  2. Be a lap belt.
  3. Fit across the pelvic bone and above the uterus.
  4. Have padding across the shoulder harness to prevent chaffing.

127. A patient at 30 weeks gestation tells the nurse that she will be traveling cross-country by car to visit family. She asks the nurse's advice for traveling while pregnant. The nurse makes a recommendation based on the knowledge that pregnant women who are traveling should

  1. Take advantage of the time and sleep the entire trip.
  2. Do nothing special.
  3. Travel only 2 hours per day.
  4. Schedule periods of activity and rest.

PHARMACOLOGICAL AND PARENTERAL THERAPIES

Multiple Choice

128. The nurse is recommending how to prevent iron-deficiency anemia in a healthy, full-term, exclusively breastfed infant. What should the nurse suggest?

1. Iron drops after 1 month of age.
2. Iron-fortified commercial formula by 4–6 months of age.
3. Iron-fortified infant cereal by 2 months of age.
4. Iron-fortified infant cereal by 4–6 months of age.

129. You are to administer surfactant to a 10-day-old infant with respiratory distress syndrome who has been admitted to the neonatal intensive care unit (NICU). What is the benefit of surfactant for this baby?

1. It increases surface tension in the lungs.
2. It acts as a bronchodilator in the lungs.
3. It is a steroid that is used to decrease edema in the airway.
4. It decreases surface tension in the lungs.

130. A drug commonly used to manage postpartum hemorrhage is

1. Betamethasone.
2. Factor VIII.
3. Methergine (methylergonovine).
4. Magnesium sulfate.

131. Your patient has been admitted in preterm labor and is receiving magnesium sulfate as a tocolytic. You prepare her for the common side effects of this medication, which include drowsiness, lethargy, feeling warm, and

1. Tremulousness.
2. Tachycardia.
3. Muscular weakness.
4. Palpitations.

132. The newborn whose mother has received a large amount of magnesium sulfate will show which of the following signs?

1. Hypertonia.
2. Hypotonia.
3. Tachypnea.
4. Polycythemia.

133. You are caring for a 22-day-old neonate in the NICU. She has been placed on theophylline for management of apneic episodes. Which of the following would be a sign of theophylline toxicity?

1. Bradycardia.
2. Hyperthermia.
3. Irritability.
4. Listlessness.

134. The medication orders for a postpartum patient indicate that she is to receive Percocet (Endocet, Roxicet, Tylox) for pain. The patient is allergic to Tylenol. The nurse knows

1. The patient will be allergic to Percocet.
2. It is safe for the patient to take the medication.
3. She needs to get a new order from pharmacy.
4. She can just give the patient Motrin (ibuprofen).

135. A patient arrives at the office today for her annual gynecology appointment. She tells the nurse that she and her husband are actively trying to get pregnant. What preconceptual counseling, with regard to vitamin supplementation, would the nurse give her?

1. Suggest she take a vitamin that contains 400 milligrams of folic acid.
2. Suggest she take a vitamin that contains 400 micrograms of folic acid.
3. Suggest she take a vitamin that contains 2 grams of folic acid.
4. Suggest she take a vitamin that contains 4 grams of folic acid.

136. A patient has a subcutaneous terbutaline (Brethine) pump for treatment of preterm labor. Which of the following findings warrants a call to the physician?

1. The patient feels nervous and jittery.
2. The patient's pulse is 124 beats per minute.
3. Fetal movements are more than 12 per hour.
4. Fetal movements are fewer than 12 per hour.

137. A patient in labor has pregnancy-induced hypertension. Her blood pressure is elevated, and the physician orders labetalol hydrochloride (Normodyne). The nurse knows

1. This medication may cause maternal headache and flushing.
2. It is important to get the blood pressure down quickly.

3. The fetus will not be affected by the medication.

4. One dose of the medication will alleviate the elevated blood pressure.

138. A patient delivered 30 minutes ago and has an IV of lactated Ringer's with 25 units of Pitocin infusing. The nurse evaluates her lochia and finds it to be excessive. The patient's vital signs are as follows: blood pressure 150/98, pulse 80, respirations 18, temperature 98°F. The nurse notifies the provider, and the following order is received: Methergine (methylergonovine) 0.2 mg IM now. What should the nurse do?

1. Give the medication and reevaluate the bleeding.

2. Question the order, as this medication is contraindicated in the patient.

3. Do not give the medication but increase the IV fluids.

4. Request to give the medication IV as this is an emergency.

139. In a postpartum hemorrhage, the nurse understands all of the following medications may be given but knows that the first-line treatment is

1. Pitocin (oxytocin).

2. Hemabate (prostaglandin).

3. Methergine (methylergonovine).

4. Methyldopa.

True/False

140. True or False: Hemabate (prostaglandin) can be given intramyometrially and intra-abdominally as needed.

Multiple Choice

141. Which of the following medications is used to treat some ectopic pregnancies?

1. Pitocin (oxytocin).

2. Hemabate (prostaglandin).

3. Methergine (methylergonovine).

4. Methotrexate.

142. Indicated use of magnesium sulfate in pregnancy is

1. To trigger breast milk letdown.

2. To prohibit preterm labor.

3. To prevent seizures.

4. Both to prohibit preterm labor and to prevent seizures.

143. The physician orders a loading dose of magnesium sulfate of 10 grams over 20 minutes. What is the nurse's response?

1. Calculate the dose in milliliters to infuse on a pump.

2. Call the pharmacy to get assistance with the calculation.

3. Verify the order—this is an incorrect dose.

4. Verify patient's allergies prior to infusion.

144. Which of the following medications is considered a tocolytic?

1. Brethine (terbutaline).

2. Magnesium sulfate.

3. Procardia (nifedipine).

4. All of the above.

145. What is the recommended route of administration for terbutaline (Brethine) for preterm labor?

1. Subcutaneous.

2. Intravenous.

3. Oral.

4. Rectal.

146. What is the recommended route of administration for nifedipine (Procardia) for preterm labor?

1. Subcutaneous.

2. Intravenous.

3. Sublingual.

4. Rectal.

147. Indomethacin is given as a treatment for preterm labor. What is a potentially significant fetal side effect of this drug?

1. Premature closure of the ductus arteriosus.

2. Premature closer of the ductus venosus.

3. Bradycardia.

4. Decreased fetal movement.

148. Which of the following tests might be ordered for a patient in preterm labor who is being treated with indomethacin?

1. Amniotic fluid index.

2. Amniocentesis.

3. Chorionic villus sampling.

4. Alpha-fetoprotein.

149. A postpartum patient is Rh-negative; her infant is Rh-positive. What medication does the mother need to receive prior to discharge?

1. RhoGAM.
2. Rubella vaccine.
3. Ritodrin (Yutopar).
4. Raloxifene.

150. A woman who is 8 weeks pregnant is status post chorionic villus sampling and is Rh-negative. What dose of RhoGAM should she receive?

1. 300 micrograms.
2. 500 micrograms.
3. 50 micrograms.
4. 30 micrograms.

151. A postpartum patient is Rh-negative; her infant is Rh-positive. What dose of RhoGAM should she receive?

1. 300 micrograms.
2. 500 micrograms.
3. 50 micrograms.
4. 30 micrograms.

152. A postpartum patient is not immune to rubella. The nurse understands that this patient needs rubella immunization prior to her discharge. By which of the following routes is the vaccine given?

1. Intramuscular.
2. Sublingual.
3. Subcutaneous.
4. Oral.

153. Erythromycin ophthalmic ointment 0.5% is given immediately after an infant is born to provide prophylaxis against

1. *Neisseria gonorrhoea.*
2. *Chlamydia trachomatis.*
3. Syphilis.
4. Both *Neisseria gonorrhoea* and *Chlamydia trachomatis.*

154. Vitamin K is given to newborn infants after birth to

1. Help their guts digest the first feeding.
2. Prevent hemorrhagic disorders.
3. Provide vitamin supplementation for a month.
4. Protect against genetic blood disorders.

155. The nurse is drawing up a vitamin K injection for a newborn. What should the dose be?

1. 0.5–1 milligrams.
2. 10–50 micrograms.
3. 12 milliliters.
4. 1–2 milligrams.

156. A nurse is administering Pitocin (oxytocin) to a laboring patient as a means of augmenting her inadequate labor pattern. Which of the following is a common side effect of this medication?

1. Maternal tachycardia.
2. Uterine hyperstimulation.
3. Maternal fever.
4. Fetal arrhythmias.

157. A patient is admitted in active labor. The nurse reviews her prenatal history and sees that the patient tested positive for group B *Streptococcus* at her 36-week checkup. Which medication should the patient receive as first-line treatment?

1. Penicillin G.
2. Clindamycin.
3. Flagyl (metronidazole).
4. Ciproflaxin (Cipro).

158. A nurse takes over care of a laboring patient and assesses that she is currently receiving 40 milliunits of Pitocin per minute. What should the nurse do?

1. Document the dose and continue the assessment.
2. Stop the medication, as this dose is higher than recommended.
3. Notify the provider, as this is not a therapeutic dose.
4. Evaluate the contraction pattern.

159. A patient who is postpartum cesarean section received keterolac (Toradol) for pain. The patient's orders also state that she should begin Motrin (ibuprofen) when she can tolerate fluids and foods by mouth. What should the nurse do?

1. Follow this order and evaluate the patient's oral intake.
2. Clarify the orders with the provider, as Motrin is also a nonsteroidal anti-inflammatory agent.
3. Give the patient morphine instead of keterolac.
4. Check the patient's allergies.

SECTION I
SECTION II
SECTION III
SECTION IV
SECTION V
SECTION VI
SECTION VII
SECTION VIII
SECTION IX
SECTION X

160. Docusate sodium (Colace) is often prescribed in the postpartum period. What is its purpose?

1. To dry up milk production in non-breastfeeding women.
2. To prevent perineal pain after an episiotomy.
3. To soften stool.
4. To help women sleep.

REDUCTION OF RISK POTENTIAL

Multiple Choice

161. While caring for her 1-month-old infant, a mother asks the nurse to "get some milk for my baby, please." What action should the nurse take based on the knowledge she has regarding infant nutrition?

1. Ask the mother if she prefers whole milk or 2%.
2. Warm the milk in the microwave before presenting it to the baby.
3. Ask the mother what type of formula the baby drinks.
4. Place the whole milk in a sippy cup for the baby.

162. Your patient expresses concern about preventing sore nipples during early breastfeeding. Which of the following should the nurse stress in her teaching?

1. Limit feedings to 5 minutes on each breast at each feeding.
2. Check for correct positioning and latching.
3. Alternate supplemental bottles with each breastfeeding.
4. Wash the nipples with warm water before each feeding.

163. Education of a woman in the postpartum period with deep vein thrombosis includes all of the following *except*

1. Continue bed rest until it has resolved.
2. Frequent massage of the affected area is encouraged.
3. Medication will be given to thin the blood.
4. Lab work will be drawn on a frequent basis.

164. A G1P0 30-year-old patient at 38 weeks gestation is admitted with heavy, bright red bleeding. The initial nursing assessment should include all of the following *except*

1. Asking about pain.

2. Taking vital signs.
3. A vaginal examination.
4. Fetal monitoring.

165. An Rh-positive infant is born to an Rh-negative mother. What test should be carried out on the cord blood?

1. Kleinhauer-Betke test.
2. Indirect Coombs test.
3. Direct Coombs test.
4. RhoGAM.

166. On the first postpartum day, a patient with a cesarean delivery is ordered a full liquid diet to advance as tolerated. Before providing the tray, the nurse should assess the patient's

1. Thirst.
2. Desire to eat.
3. Bowel sounds.
4. Degree of discomfort.

167. A patient asks, "If I get pregnant again, will I need to have another cesarean section?" The nurse should explain to the patient that a vaginal birth after cesarean (VBAC) is

1. Possible if the patient did not have a classic uterine incision.
2. Possible if the patient has a history of rapid labor.
3. Not possible because the patient is a multipara.
4. Not possible because the patient had a low transverse abdominal and uterine incision.

168. The nurse makes all of the following observations of a 12-hour-old African-American newborn. Which of these observations requires further assessment?

1. Bilateral yellow-tinged sclera.
2. Blue-black patches on sacral area and buttocks.
3. Silky hair covering occipital and parietal areas.
4. Fingertip pigmentation darker than that of the fingers.

169. Nursing care in the first 30 minutes after a cesarean section includes

1. Ambulation.
2. Oral hydration and nutrition.
3. Fundal and lochia assessments.
4. Vital signs every hour.

Reduction of Risk Potential **39**

SECTION I

SECTION II

SECTION III

SECTION IV

SECTION V

SECTION VI

SECTION VII

SECTION VIII

SECTION IX

SECTION X

170. A 40-year-old patient who is 8 weeks pregnant and desires fetal testing is able to have the following tests at this time:

1. Biophysical profile.
2. Chorionic villus sampling.
3. Amniocentesis.
4. Alpha-fetoprotein test.

171. For a patient who lost 1,500 mL of blood at delivery and has a hemoglobin level of 8, what discharge teaching is important?

1. Increase her dietary iron and protein intake.
2. Walk at least 5,000 steps per day.
3. Increase the number of sitz baths to four per day.
4. Decrease contact with the baby.

172. A biophysical profile consists of all of the following measures *except*

1. Fetal breathing.
2. Femur length.
3. Nonstress test.
4. Amniotic fluid index.

173. Fetal lung maturity is confirmed by phosphatidylglycerol (PG) and lecithin/sphingomyelin (L/S) ratio. Patient education regarding this test is

1. Take nothing by mouth after midnight in preparation for an early-morning blood draw.
2. An amniocentesis will be done to test the amniotic fluid.
3. Remember to eat a meal before testing, as a mother's low blood sugar can alter the test results.
4. An amniocentesis will be done to test the cord blood.

174. What is the primary reason an ultrasound is done in the *first trimester*?

1. Evaluate fetal structure.
2. Measure amniotic fluid.
3. Determine sex.
4. Determine gestational age.

175. Which of the following does the alpha-fetoprotein (AFP) test screen for?

1. Inborn errors of metabolism.
2. Neural tube defects.
3. Cystic fibrosis.
4. Diabetes.

176. What lab work is ordered on a pregnant patient suspected of having HELLP syndrome?

1. Glucose screen and CBC.
2. Liver biopsy and liver enzymes.
3. CBC, platelet count, and liver enzymes.
4. Nonstress test and a biophysical profile.

177. A urine pregnancy test measures which of the following?

1. Human chorionic gonadotropin.
2. Estradiol.
3. Alpha-fetoprotein.
4. Estrogen/progesterone ratio.

178. Variable decelerations are caused by

1. Maternal infection.
2. Umbilical cord compression.
3. Prolonged labor.
4. Utero-placental insufficiency.

179. A laboring patient expresses a desire to receive an epidural. The nurse is aware that the epidural would be contraindicated if the patient had

1. Recently been on antibiotic therapy.
2. Experienced a previous spontaneous abortion.
3. A history of pelvic inflammatory disease.
4. Abnormal coagulation studies.

180. What is the cause of late decelerations?

1. Utero-placental insufficiency.
2. Umbilical cord compression.
3. Prolonged labor.
4. Head compression.

181. The nurse is taking care of a patient whose fetus is having late decelerations. The nurse looks at the mother's history and realizes the late decelerations are most likely caused by

1. Previous miscarriage.
2. Breech presentation.
3. Pregnancy-induced hypertension.
4. An Rh-negative mother.

182. During labor, late decelerations occur after the mother receives an epidural. The nurse understands

1. The late decelerations were caused by the position the mother assumed for the epidural insertions.

2. The late decelerations can be related to hypotension that occurs in the mother after receiving an epidural.

3. Late decelerations are normal and do not require any action.

4. The late decelerations are related to the medication used in the epidural.

183. Early decelerations

1. Require immediate physician notification.

2. Are a sign of fetal compromise.

3. Are an indication for a cesarean section.

4. Are a sign of fetal head compression.

Fill in the Blank

184. A risk associated with amniocentesis is _____.

Multiple Choice

185. The test used to screen for gestational diabetes is given

1. At a preconceptual counseling appointment.

2. At 26–28 weeks gestation.

3. In the first trimester.

4. Postpartum.

186. The tests that may be used to screen for diabetes include

1. Urine test.

2. One-hour oral glucose tolerance test.

3. Three-hour oral glucose tolerance test.

4. All of the above.

187. The nurse taking care of a woman who has gestational diabetes and is in labor knows the patient and fetus are at risk for

1. Shoulder dystocia.

2. Late decelerations.

3. Hypoglycemia.

4. All of the above.

Fill in the Blank

188. The primary risk when the amniotic sac is ruptured is _____.

Multiple Choice

189. A patient being induced for post dates with the use of Pitocin has a maternal habitus that is very large, making external fetal monitoring difficult. The nurse requests that the provider

1. Perform a cesarean section, as it will be safer than vaginal delivery.

2. Place an internal uterine pressure catheter so that the fetal heart rate can be adequately monitored.

3. Use a vacuum extractor for the delivery.

4. Use an internal scalp electrode so that the fetal heart rate can be monitored.

190. The passage of meconium in utero can be

1. Caused by fetal distress.

2. A result of post dates status.

3. Spontaneous.

4. All of the above.

191. In which of the following cases should the last-trimester patient notify her provider?

1. Excessive fetal movements.

2. Light spotting after intercourse.

3. Irregular contractions.

4. Bright red bleeding.

192. A patient who is 36 weeks gestation phones the clinic to report no fetal movement in the past 2 hours. What should the nurse advise the patient to do?

1. Come to the clinic immediately.

2. Go to the labor and delivery unit immediately.

3. Eat and drink something, rest for 2 hours, and count the movements; call back if no movement is felt at that point.

4. Continue your day as usual; if you do not feel any movement in 24 hours, call back.

193. A patient just delivered an 8-pound infant 30 minutes ago. The nurse assesses her vital signs and finds the following: blood pressure 120/60, respirations 18, pulse 120, temperature 98°F. What should the nurse do?

1. Nothing—these are normal findings.

2. Assess the patient's current and past blood loss, as her pulse is elevated.

3. Notify the physician, as these are not normal findings.

4. Encourage the patient to drink more fluids, as her blood pressure is lower than usual.

PHYSIOLOGICAL ADAPTATION

Multiple Choice

194. As blood flows through the heart of a child with an atrial septal defect, it flows

1. From the right atrium to the left atrium.
2. From the right atrium to the pulmonary artery.
3. From the left atrium to the right ventricle.
4. From the left atrium to the pulmonary vein.

195. When does jaundice typically appear in the newborn with hemolytic disease?

1. In the first 24 hours of life.
2. Between the second and fourth days of life.
3. After the tenth day of life.
4. After the first month of life.

196. Baby Joanna has a congenital heart defect called patent ductus arteriosus. How will you explain this defect to her mother?

1. "Joanna has a persistent connection between the pulmonary artery and the aorta."
2. "Joanna has a hole in her heart between the two ventricles."
3. "Joanna has a hole in her heart between the two atria."
4. "Joanna has one vessel that forms both the aorta and the pulmonary artery."

197. A patient 24 hours postpartum asks you to feel her baby's head. You note there is swelling over the entire right parietal skull bone. You explain to the mother that the swelling is called _____; it means _____; and it should resolve _____.

1. Caput succedaneum; there was birth trauma; in a few days.
2. Hydrocephalus; there is pressure inside the skull; after a shunt is placed.
3. Cephalhematoma; there was birth trauma; in weeks to months.
4. Cephalhematoma; there was birth trauma; in about 1 week.

198. Which of the following, seen in a patient's history, is a risk factor for placenta previa?

1. A previous baby weighing more than 9 pounds.
2. Previous low cervical cesarean birth.
3. Low weight gain during this pregnancy.
4. A first pregnancy.

199. When caring for a woman in labor, which finding might be a sign of an abrupted placenta?

1. Bright red bleeding from the vagina.
2. A baby in a persistent transverse lie.
3. A woman having her first baby.
4. A uterus that does not relax between contractions.

200. After cesarean section for placenta previa, which of the following signs would be an expected clinical finding?

1. Moderate lochia rubra.
2. A small trickle of bright red blood.
3. Urine output of less than 30 cc/h.
4. A soft, relaxed, nontender uterus.

201. Which of the following refers to an infant born before completion of 37 weeks gestation, regardless of birth weight?

1. Post-term (post date).
2. Preterm or premature.
3. Low birth weight.
4. Small for gestational age.

202. Which one of the following injuries due to birth trauma may contribute to hyperbilirubinemia?

1. Caput succedaneum.
2. Subconjunctival hemorrhage.
3. Petechiae.
4. Cephalhematoma.

203. A mother is upset because her newborn has erythema toxicum neonatorum. The nurse should reassure the mother that this condition is

1. Easily treated.
2. Benign and transient.
3. Usually not contagious.
4. Usually not disfiguring.

204. A multipara has delivered a neonate at 24 weeks gestation. What is the major threat to the neonate's survival?

1. Hyperbilirubinemia.
2. Rh sensitization.
3. Reactions to blood transfusions.
4. Respiratory distress syndrome.

SECTION I

SECTION II

SECTION III

SECTION IV

SECTION V

SECTION VI

SECTION VII

SECTION VIII

SECTION IX

SECTION X

205. The nurse is caring for a primipara who delivered a neonate with myelomeningocele. The physician has discussed the treatment with the patient. The nurse determines that the patient needs further instructions when she says,

1. "If the baby has the surgery, the baby probably will be able to walk normally."
2. "The sac will be covered with a sterile pad."
3. "The baby will be positioned on its side to prevent pressure."
4. "The baby may suffer from incontinence, even with surgical correction."

206. Which of the following are parts of the fetal circulation?

1. Ductus arteriosis, foramen ovale, ductus venosus.
2. Ductus arteriosis, choanal atresia, foramen ovale.
3. Foramen ovale, tricuspid atresia, subaortic stenosis.
4. Foramen ovale, ductus venosus, tricuspid atresia.

207. What is the major anemia found in pregnancy?

1. Sickle cell anemia.
2. Megaloblastic anemia.
3. Iron-deficiency anemia.
4. Cooley's anemia.

208. Your patient in labor has just received an epidural block. What is the *most* important nursing intervention?

1. Limit oral fluids.
2. Encourage the woman to lie on her back.
3. Monitor maternal pulse for possible bradycardia.
4. Monitor blood pressure for possible hypotension.

209. A patient is hospitalized for severe pregnancy-induced hypertension (PIH). Her hematocrit has increased two points since the previous day. What is the probable cause of this increase?

1. Increased hematopoiesis in the red bone marrow.
2. Decreased red blood cell destruction by the spleen.
3. A shift of red blood cells from the fetus.

4. A shift of fluid from the vascular compartment.

210. A G2P1 patient at 28 weeks gestation is admitted for a bleeding episode. Ultrasound examination reveals a low-lying placenta. After the patient is stabilized (i.e., bleeding stops), what is the preferred management for her?

1. Pelvic examination with immediate cesarean section if another bleeding episode occurs.
2. Expectant management (observation and bed rest) in the hospital.
3. Home management with frequent testing and readily available transportation.
4. Either expectant management in the hospital or home management with frequent testing and readily available transportation.

211. The nurse might suspect von Willebrand's disease in a postpartum patient if which of the following was present?

1. Bleeding that does not respond to the usual measures.
2. No family history of the disease.
3. Complaint of pain in both lower extremities.
4. Foul-smelling lochia.

212. A patient with eclampsia begins to seize. What is the nurse's primary goal?

1. Roll the patient to her side.
2. Start an IV.
3. Record the activity.
4. Call for help.

213. Why is maintaining a thermoneutral environment essential for the neonate?

1. Metabolism slows dramatically in the neonate who experiences cold stress.
2. The neonate produces heat by increasing activity and shivering.
3. A thermoneutral environment permits the neonate to maintain a normal core temperature with minimum oxygen consumption.
4. A thermoneutral environment permits the neonate to maintain a normal core temperature with increased caloric consumption.

214. The part of the fetus that enters the pelvic inlet first and leads through the birth canal is referred to as the fetal

1. Presentation.
2. Attitude.
3. Station.
4. Molding.

215. Which of the following physiologic findings is expected during labor?

1. Decreased white blood cell count.
2. Decreased blood pressure.
3. Increased cardiac output.
4. Increased blood glucose level.

216. The nurse has received a report that a laboring woman's last vaginal exam was recorded as 4 cm, 80%, and –1. How does the nurse interpret this assessment?

1. The cervix is effaced 4 cm and dilated 80%; the presenting part is 1 cm below the ischial spines.
2. The cervix is dilated 4 cm and effaced 80%; the presenting part is 1 cm above the ischial spines.
3. The cervix is effaced 4 cm and dilated 80%; the presenting part is 1 cm above the ischial spines.
4. The cervix is dilated 4 cm and effaced 80%; the presenting part is 1 cm below the ischial spines.

217. A patient who is at 14 weeks gestation comes to the office for an appointment. She tells the nurse that her nephew has German measles and spent the weekend at her house. She wonders if that might be harmful to her and her baby. The nurse knows

1. The patient will need to see a genetic counselor to have her question answered.
2. If the patient has had a rubella vaccine, she will be immune.
3. The nurse will need to check the patient's rubella immunity status from her prenatal lab work.
4. Because the patient is early in the second trimester, any potential teratogenic effects are minimal.

218. A patient is in the emergency room with a positive pregnancy test, bleeding, and severe abdominal pain. The suspected diagnosis is ectopic pregnancy. The nurse's primary concern is the patient's alteration in

1. Comfort.

2. Emotional status.
3. Hemodynamics.
4. Fertility.

219. Your patient delivered her third child by vaginal delivery 6 hours ago. She plans to breast-feed. You explain to her that the "afterbirth" pains she may experience are caused by

1. Hormone imbalances.
2. Blood collecting in the uterus.
3. Contractility of the uterus.
4. Bladder spasms.

220. A patient in active labor has not changed her cervix in 2 hours. Which of the following factors will *not* affect the process of labor in this patient?

1. Her contraction pattern.
2. The shape of her pelvis.
3. Her anxiety as it relates to pain in labor.
4. The time at which her water broke.

221. A patient in active labor is 6 cm dilated and wants an epidural. The nurse knows

1. The patient is too far dilated to receive an epidural.
2. An epidural is not an intervention indicated for this stage in labor.
3. The patient will need to have labs drawn.
4. An epidural is not an invasive procedure.

222. A patient in active labor is 8 cm dilated, 90% effaced, and –3 station when her water breaks. Immediately thereafter, the fetal heart rate decelerates into the 60s. The nurse knows

1. This is a normal response when the membranes rupture.
2. This is a normal fetal heart rate pattern.
3. This could be a sign of uterine rupture.
4. This could be a sign of cord prolapse.

223. What is the most likely cause of a slight temperature elevation (99.6°F) in a new mother at 12 hours after delivery?

1. Infection.
2. Hemorrhage.
3. Exhaustion.
4. Dehydration.

MANAGEMENT OF CARE

1. Correct Answer: **3**

   Rationale: The patient is the only person who can give consent for procedures if she is cognitively intact.

2. Correct Answer: **4**

   Rationale: Often stimulation is all that is needed to correct an apneic episode.

3. Correct Answer: **2**

   Rationale: Severe hypothermia can lead to cold stress and requires immediate action.

4. Correct Answer: **2**

   Rationale: Pitocin can cause hyperstimulation and fetal distress.

5. Correct Answer: **1**

   Rationale: Even though all of these are reasonable concerns, maintaining a clear airway is of the utmost importance. The leading cause of mortality with seizures is aspiration.

6. Correct Answer: **4**

   Rationale: RhoGAM should be administered after any episode that could precipitate fetal–maternal blood transfusion.

7. Correct Answer: **4**

   Rationale: Around 28 weeks gestation, Rh-negative women are assessed for maternal sensitization. If this test is negative, patients will receive RhoGAM.

8. Correct Answer: **True**

9. Correct Answer: **True**

   Rationale: The patient has the right to refuse any test. Nevertheless, it should be stressed that early detection leads to better outcomes for both mother and infant.

10. Correct Answer: **2**

    Rationale: Because babies delivered by cesarean section do not experience the vaginal squeeze that helps clear fluid from their lungs, these newborns often have transient tachypnea that can cause respiratory difficulties after birth.

11. Correct Answer: **2**

    Rationale: Observing the fetal heart rate pattern is important to evaluate how the infant tolerated the intervention. Once the amniotic sac ruptures, the cord could prolapse through the cervix. Cord prolapse is a medical emergency requiring an immediate cesarean section.

12. Correct Answer: **3**

    Rationale: If the baby has an O-negative blood type, there is no need for RhoGAM.

13. Correct Answer: **3**

    Rationale: It is the nurse's ultimate responsibility to ensure that informed consent has been given by the parents and that they have signed the form prior to beginning the procedure.

14. Correct Answer: **2**

    Rationale: Patient information is confidential unless the patient indicates in writing who can be informed of his or her status.

15. Correct Answer: **4**

    Rationale: The most common cause of uterine atony is a full bladder. After verifying the bladder is empty, fundal massage remedies most episodes of bleeding.

16. Correct Answer: **2**

    Rationale: The exam cannot be delayed because the greatest risk of postpartum hemorrhage occurs within the first hour after delivery. A viable compromise is to perform the exam without interrupting breastfeeding if at all possible.

17. Correct Answer: **1**

    Rationale: The patient has reacted positively to the infant, but her lack of initiative toward infant care may be a reflection of her insecurities. Offering to supervise a skill such as changing a diaper may give the patient the confidence and reassurance she needs.

18. Correct Answer: **1**

Rationale: These signs could represent bonding issues and need to be explored by a professional with counseling skills.

19. Correct Answer: **1**

Rationale: Once a floor nurse has offered assistance, it is best to make a referral to a professional who has the necessary skill set to resolve the difficulties efficiently and effectively.

20. Correct Answer: **3**

Rationale: This patient needs informed consent regarding the permanence of the procedure as well as other options of birth control methods available to her.

21. Correct Answer: **2**

Rationale: The nurse's role is to document when informed consent is given, what information was delivered, and how well the patient understands the information received.

22. Correct Answer: **2**

Rationale: In federally funded facilities, the nurse is required to ask patients about their knowledge of advanced directives and to provide them with information about these directives if necessary.

23. Correct Answer: **1**

Rationale: Any patient has the right to refuse any tests.

24. Correct Answer: **4**

Rationale: Pitocin can cause utero-placental insufficiency and lead to a fetal heart rate response in the form of late decelerations. It is imperative to stop the Pitocin and allow for fetal resuscitation.

25. Correct Answer: **3**

Rationale: It is important for patient safety initiatives to provide a written report of the incident; you must also notify the physician and ask for further orders. Systems are the cause of most errors, but they cannot be modified if problems are not identified.

26. Correct Answer: **1**

Rationale: The most active patient is the one who is 6 cm dilated. She should be evaluated first.

27. Correct Answer: **1**

Rationale: The patient that delivered 2 hours ago has the most urgent assessment need. Her risk for hemorrhage outweighs the risks associated with the other patient situations.

28. Correct Answers: **1 and 2**

Rationale: These activities can be handled within the skill set of a nursing assistant.

29. Correct Answers: **1 and 2**

Rationale: The registered nurse can delegate both of these activities to a nursing assistant.

30. Correct Answer: **1**

Rationale: A nursing assistant can help with the administration of an enema.

31. Correct Answer: **2**

Rationale: Diet adherence can significantly alter blood glucose levels in patients and can lead to increased length of stay if diets consumed are not congruent with what is ordered. This discrepancy has quality assurance implications, so this deficit needs to be addressed.

32. Correct Answer: **1**

Rationale: An 18 weeks gestation is not suitable for treatment in a NICU; the NICU is not an option for this infant.

33. Correct Answer: **3**

Rationale: It will be essential for this patient to receive nutritional counseling for when she returns home.

34. Correct Answer: **2**

Rationale: All potential contact with body fluids requires the use of gloves.

35. Correct Answer: **1**

Rationale: Dealing with an adoption requires a multidisciplinary team collaboration that will involve both nursing and social services.

36. Correct Answer: **3**

Rationale: Nurses should use universal precautions with all patients. It should be assumed that all patients have the potential to transmit infections regardless of a known diagnosis. The nurses response indicates the need for education related to standard use of protective wear and a lack of knowledge related to HIV transmission to health workers.

SECTION I

SECTION II

SECTION III

SECTION IV

SECTION V

SECTION VI

SECTION VII

SECTION VIII

SECTION IX

SECTION X

37. Correct Answer: 3

Rationale: The patient has the right to refuse any tests. Nevertheless, it is the job of the nurse to ensure that proper information regarding all tests has been given and is understood by the patient.

38. Correct Answer: 2

Rationale: The nurse obtains permission from the baby's mother regarding who can have contact with her infant.

39. Correct Answer: 4

Rationale: All of these skills are necessary for a nurse who works with patients regarding genetic issues.

40. Correct Answer: 1

Rationale: It is of primary importance for the nurse to understand her own beliefs regarding sexuality and birth control options before she can provide unbiased and nonjudgmental information to her patients.

41. Correct Answer: 2

Rationale: Even though the patient should receive the antibiotic, it is unlikely that any step the nurse can take will stop a multiparous woman from pushing in transition. The nurse should notify the pediatrician and nursery that there was inadequate antibiotic coverage due to precipitous delivery.

42. Correct Answer: 1

Rationale: This behavior represents a lack of advocacy on the part of the nurse. She has destined the patient for a c-section based on a written birth plan. By doing so, the nurse becomes unable to effectively advocate for this patient.

43. Correct Answer: 2

Rationale: The patient's wishes must be respected. When a patient presents with a written plan, it is the nurse's role to advocate for the patient and support her plans as long as they are safe for both mother and baby.

44. Correct Answer: 3

Rationale: The nurse is responsible for advocating for the patient when she is unable to do so for herself. The nurse has information she is compelled to pass along when she sees something that directly conflicts with the patient's wishes.

SAFETY AND INFECTION CONTROL

45. Correct Answer: 1

Rationale: A withdrawn attitude may be a sign of abuse and needs to be explored further.

46. Correct Answer: 4

Rationale: Preterm labor is not a source of postpartum infection.

47. Correct Answer: 4

Rationale: All that is needed to promote healing and prevent infection is to keep the cord area dry and clean.

48. Correct Answer: 2

Rationale: The rubella vaccine is a live vaccine. Women need to avoid conceiving within 3 months of receiving this injection, as it can cause birth defects.

49. Correct Answer: 3

Rationale: This setup is a potential source of errors and should be brought to the attention of pharmacy, which stocks and orders the medications. It is important that system errors such as those related to similar packaging and storage practices be mitigated before the wrong medications or doses inadvertently reach patients.

50. Correct Answer: 1

Rationale: All unreadable orders need to have provider clarification.

51. Correct Answer: 2

Rationale: Regardless of the situation, hand washing between patients is the best method of infection control.

52. Correct Answer: 2

Rationale: All potential contact with body fluids requires the use of gloves.

53. Correct Answer: False

Rationale: Standard precautions are recommended when any exposure to body fluids can occur, which is certainly the case in a delivery.

54. Correct Answer: 3

Rationale: *Chlamydia* infection is a sexually transmitted disease and requires a test, treatment, and a test of cure.

55. Correct Answer: **2**

    Rationale: *Chlamydia* infections are the cause of ophthalmia neonatorum.

56. Correct Answer: **4**

    Rationale: All of these are risk factors for untreated *Chlamydia* infection.

57. Correct Answer: **4**

    Rationale: All of these are risks associated with amniocentesis.

58. Correct Answer: **1**

    Rationale: Group B *Streptococcus* is a bacterium that is normally found in varying degrees of colonization in some women. Its presence does not affect the mother but can negatively affect an infant after delivery.

59. Correct Answer: **3**

    Rationale: The treatment for Group B *Streptococcus* is intravenous antibiotics given during labor.

60. Correct Answer: **4**

    Rationale: This bacterium does not harm the mother and, in fact, is normally found in the gastrointestinal tract. However, Group B *Streptococcus* can make some infants very sick if they are infected as they pass through the birth canal.

61. Correct Answer: **2**

    Rationale: Toxoplasmosis is a protozoan infection associated with the consumption of infested raw or undercooked meat and with poor hand washing after handling infected cat litter.

62. Correct Answer: **False**

    Rationale: Standard precautions are required whenever there is a risk of body fluid contact.

63. Correct Answer: **4**

    Rationale: PID is a result of an infectious agent such as *Chlamydia* entering the genital tract and infecting the reproductive organs. If left untreated or if treatment is delayed, it can cause infertility and ectopic pregnancies. PID can be treated with antibiotics.

64. Correct Answer: **2**

    Rationale: These and other signs such as mood swings, suicidal thoughts, and memory lapse may indicate a history of sexual abuse and require further evaluation.

65. Correct Answer: **1**

    Rationale: These are signs of high blood pressure and need further evaluation.

66. Correct Answer: **3**

    Rationale: The weeks of gestation should correspond to the number of centimeters when measuring fundal height by ±2 cm. A difference of more than 2 cm could indicate a lack of fetal growth and needs further evaluation.

HEALTH PROMOTION AND MAINTENANCE

67. Correct Answer: **2**

    Rationale: The nurse should ask anyone accompanying the patient to leave prior to asking personal questions such as those dealing with abuse.

68. Correct Answer: **2**

    Rationale: Exclusive breastfeeding provides adequate nutrition for infants during the first 6 months of life.

69. Correct Answer: **3**

    Rationale: Men are often afraid they will harm the baby by having intercourse with their pregnant wives. It is important to educate the couple about anatomy and physiology to help them understand what is harmful and what is not.

70. Correct Answer: **1**

    Rationale: Stretch marks are a fact of pregnancy and will fade in the postpartum period.

71. Correct Answer: **1**

    Rationale: GTPAL: G = number of pregnancies, 6 (all previous including present); T = number of term pregnancies, 2 (all that have completed the 37th week of gestation) ; P = number of preterm pregnancies, 0 (all pregnancies born prior to the completion of the 37th week of gestation and after the completion of the 20th week); A = number of abortions, either voluntary or spontaneous, 3; L = number of living children, 2.

72. Correct Answer: **1**

    Rationale: Physiologic changes occur in the cardiovascular system, such as heart enlargement, displacement of the heart upward, and rotation of the heart to the left. There is also an increase in cardiac output

SECTION I

SECTION II

SECTION III

SECTION IV

SECTION V

SECTION VI

SECTION VII

SECTION VIII

SECTION IX

SECTION X

induced by blood volume changes. At 14–20 weeks gestation, the pulse increases 10–15 beats/min, which can cause palpitations.

73. Correct Answer: **1**

Rationale: It is important for women to understand how the weight is distributed so they will not be concerned about an overall weight gain of 35–40 pounds.

74. Correct Answer: **4**

Rationale: Tub baths are permitted in women who are pregnant.

75. Correct Answer: **3**

Rationale: It is important to rule out pathological causes of abdominal pain but this description is highly indicative of round ligament discomfort, which is common at this gestational age.

76. Correct Answer: **4**

Rationale: It is recommended that a patient wait until the 6-week checkup to ensure that her stitches have healed correctly if she had an episiotomy and for her uterus to return to normal size. This rest period also protects against the inadvertent introduction of germs into the uterus as the placental site is healing.

77. Correct Answer: **3**

Rationale: The postpartum period is a good time to administer the rubella vaccine if the woman is non-immune because you know the patient is not pregnant and the vaccine is a live virus. It is important to give instructions regarding the need for birth control measures during the following 3 months after the injection.

78. Correct Answer: **2**

Rationale: Engorgement occurs 24–36 hours after childbirth regardless of whether the mother is breastfeeding.

79. Correct Answer: **2**

Rationale: Keeping the baby and the mother separated does not facilitate exclusive breastfeeding.

80. Correct Answer: **2**

Rationale: Understanding that breastfeeding is solely based on the "supply and demand" principle is pivotal for successful breast milk establishment and maintenance.

81. Correct Answer: **2**

Rationale: The excessive consumption of low-nutritional products associated with pica is of concern with regard to maternal/fetal nutrition.

82. Correct Answer: **2**

Rationale: The patient may not reveal pertinent health history if her mother is in the room. It is wise to take health histories when only the patient is present.

83. Correct Answer: **3**

Rationale: Breast exams should be done monthly during the menstrual cycle when hormone levels are low and are least likely to influence breast changes.

84. Correct Answer: **2**

Rationale: Cigarette smoking, infection with human papilloma virus, multiple sex partners, and early age of first sexual intercourse are all risk factors.

85. Correct Answer: **3**

Rationale: It is recommended to wait a year between pregnancies to allow the woman's body to restore its levels of needed nutrients, which are often depleted with pregnancies.

86. Correct Answer: **1**

Rationale: Smoking is a risk factor for infertility. Women should be counseled regarding this risk factor.

PSYCHOSOCIAL INTEGRITY

87. Correct Answer: **4**

Rationale: It is important to make siblings part of the process when possible.

88. Correct Answer: **3**

Rationale: All the other responses do not acknowledge the patients feelings. It is important to help patients explore the origins of their feelings.

89. Correct Answer: **2**

Rationale: Women often blame themselves after a miscarriage, which could lead to situational low self-esteem.

90. Correct Answer: **4**

Rationale: Women may perceive having a cesarean section as a failure, leading them to feel guilty or at fault for the surgical outcome.

91. Correct Answer: **1**

Rationale: It is important to connect the baby with the mother as soon as possible.

92. Correct Answer: 3

Rationale: It is important to relay information to patients in their spoken language to avoid misunderstandings and miscommunication.

93. Correct Answer: 4

Rationale: Job loss is a family stressor that could put this woman at risk for postpartum depression.

94. Correct Answer: 2

Rationale: Acknowledge that she is probably tired and wants her infant to sleep. At the same time, letting her know these assessments are necessary for infant well-being is essential for the patient to understand your actions.

95. Correct Answer: 1

Rationale: Honestly admitting your feelings and offering to help is the therapeutic answer. All of the other choices are clichés that should be avoided.

96. Correct Answer: 3

Rationale: Helping patients and their family understand that changes in physical and emotional status will happen with pregnancy is essential to normalizing their experience.

97. Correct Answer: 3

Rationale: Women often blame themselves when problems arise in pregnancy. It is important to validate this guilt as a normal feeling and to confirm we do not always know why these things happen.

98. Correct Answer: 4

Rationale: Ignoring a loss does not make it go away. The experience should be embraced and the grief process facilitated.

99. Correct Answer: 2

Rationale: It is important to prepare men and women for the likelihood that they will grieve differently and that their behaviors will be different in this process.

100. Correct Answer: 3

Rationale: Acknowledges the sorrow you both feel. The other answers are not therapeutic.

101. Correct Answer: 3

Rationale: This woman already has three children and will be home alone without any support.

102. Correct Answer: 3

Rationale: Patients often feel responsible for any poor outcome, even when it is out of their control. It is important to clarify any misconception about how things happen, particularly with genetic abnormalities, and to reassure patients that they were not to blame.

103. Correct Answer: 1

Rationale: Incorrect positioning and latch-on are reasons that infants might appear not to want the breast. It is important to communicate this fact to the patient, as she is taking the infant's response personally.

104. Correct Answer: 2

Rationale: It is important to share feelings with someone close and to not isolate oneself. It will take time to resume previous activities, and it is important to have help when returning home so that the patient can obtain adequate rest.

105. Correct Answer: 1

Rationale: Postpartum blues occur within a specific time frame and are not chronic.

106. Correct Answer: 2

Rationale: It is important that patients receive nonjudgmental support through the process. Allowing patients to have an opportunity to explore their feelings about the procedure in an accepting environment is a critical role for the nurse.

BASIC CARE AND COMFORT

107. Correct Answer: 4

Rationale: Ambulation increases intestinal motility and improves the passing of intestinal gas.

108. Correct Answer: 4

Rationale: Shortness of breath is common in women when they sleep. Elevating the head helps alleviate this discomfort.

109. Correct Answer: 4

Rationale: Stress has been shown to be a factor in precipitating preterm labor, so decreasing stressors is important.

110. Correct Answer: 3

Rationale: A woman who delivers an 11-pound baby is at risk for postpartum hemorrhage. Breastfeeding releases oxytocin in the body,

SECTION I

SECTION II

SECTION III

SECTION IV

SECTION V

SECTION VI

SECTION VII

SECTION VIII

SECTION IX

SECTION X

which stimulates uterine contractions and helps prevent excessive blood loss.

111. Correct Answer: **1**

Rationale: Encouraging mobility in labor helps labor progress.

112. Correct Answer: **2**

Rationale: Prenatal belts can relieve some of the fetal weight that contributes to round ligament pain, especially in women having a subsequent pregnancy.

113. Correct Answer: **3**

Rationale: When prenatal vitamins cause a bit of nausea, it is suggested that patients take the medication at bedtime so they may experience less nausea while they sleep.

114. Correct Answer: **1**

Rationale: These normal afterbirth pains are stimulated by the release of oxytocin associated with breastfeeding. They can best be treated with NSAIDs such as ibuprofen (Motrin).

115. Correct Answer: **1**

Rationale: Warm water and stimulation will merely increase engorgement and, therefore, should be restricted.

116. Correct Answer: **3**

Rationale: Lower back pain in labor is usually a result of the occiput pressing on the sacrum. Counter-pressure helps relieve this discomfort.

117. Correct Answer: **1**

Rationale: Applying ice immediately after delivery and in the first 12 hours postpartum decreases swelling and provides comfort.

118. Correct Answer: **1**

Rationale: Eating small, frequent meals does not overload the digestive system and maintains adequate blood glucose levels.

119. Correct Answer: **1**

Rationale: Eating small, frequent meals is encouraged to maintain adequate blood glucose levels. As the pregnancy progresses and the uterus grows, the GI tract will be displaced upward, leading to a decrease in holding capacity and making consumption of large meals more difficult. Gastric reflux will occur.

120. Correct Answer: **3**

Rationale: It is normal for women to get more indigestion as the uterus enlarges. The growing fetus displaces the GI tract upward, causing gastric reflux. This discomfort is particularly common in patients late in pregnancy.

121. Correct Answer: **False**

Rationale: The consumption of spicy foods by mothers does not affect infants who consume their breast milk.

122. Correct Answer: **4**

Rationale: Kegel exercises will help strengthen the pelvic floor muscles and improve muscle tone.

123. Correct Answer: **2**

Rationale: It is not uncommon for women to avoid brushing their teeth because of the nausea and vomiting. Nevertheless, it is important for them to continue this health practice.

124. Correct Answer: **1**

Rationale: Changes in the woman's center of gravity plus softening and relaxing of the pelvic joint place stress on the abdominal musculature as the pregnancy progresses and can add undue strain to the lower back. It is important for pregnant women to pay close attention to their body mechanics and posture.

125. Correct Answer: **2**

Rationale: It is important for pregnant women to rest throughout the day when possible. They should lie on their sides, as this position increases profusion to the uterus and thus to the infant, minimizes back strain, and minimizes orthostatic hypotension.

126. Correct Answer: **3**

Rationale: The lower belt should be placed over the pelvic bone. The shoulder harness should be placed above the gravid uterus and below the neck.

127. Correct Answer: **4**

Rationale: It is important to alternate periods of activity and rest to avoid becoming fatigued or developing venous stasis.

PHARMACOLOGY AND PARENTERAL THERAPIES

128. Correct Answer: <u>4</u>

Rationale: If the infant is weaned by 6 months of age, then commercial formula is recommended. However, this baby is exclusively breastfed and, therefore, will have adequate hemoglobin for the first 6 months. After then, iron-fortified cereals should be added to the child's diet.

129. Correct Answer: <u>4</u>

Rationale: Surfactant lowers surface tension, requiring less pressure to keep the lungs' alveoli open and to maintain alveolar stability by changing surface tension as the size of the alveoli changes.

130. Correct Answer: <u>3</u>

Rationale: Methergine (methylergonovine) is given intramuscularly to produce sustained uterine contractions.

131. Correct Answer: <u>3</u>

Rationale: Magnesium sulfate is a smooth muscle relaxant and central nervous system depressant. It competes with calcium entry into muscles leading to a decrease in the intensity of uterine contractions and overall muscle weakness.

132. Correct Answer: <u>2</u>

Rationale: Magnesium sulfate is a smooth muscle relaxant and central nervous system depressant. It competes with calcium entry into muscles and caused muscle weakness

133. Correct Answer: <u>3</u>

Rationale: This respiratory and myocardial stimulant is metabolized by the liver into caffeine.

134. Correct Answer: <u>1</u>

Rationale: Percocet is a combination of acetaminophen and oxycodone hydrochloride. Thus an allergy to Tylenol (acetaminophen) would make Percocet contraindicated in this patient.

135. Correct Answer: <u>2</u>

Rationale: The correct dose is 400 micrograms.

136. Correct Answer: <u>2</u>

Rationale: A side effect of terbutaline (Brethine) is tachycardia. Women should be monitored for elevation of the heart rate over 120 beats/min, and dosing adjusted accordingly.

137. Correct Answer: <u>1</u>

Rationale: These are known side effects of this medication. A rapid decrease in blood pressure can cause maternal/fetal complications.

138. Correct Answer: <u>2</u>

Rationale: Methergine (methylergonovine) is contraindicated in a patient with a blood pressure greater than 140/90.

139. Correct Answer: <u>1</u>

Rationale: Pitocin is first followed by Methergine and then by Hemobate.

140. Correct Answer: **True**

Rationale: This medication can be given directly into the uterus if bleeding is excessive and does not respond to Pitocin (oxytocin) or Methergine (methylergonovine).

141. Correct Answer: <u>4</u>

Rationale: All other medications listed are treatments for postpartum hemorrhage.

142. Correct Answer: <u>4</u>

Rationale: Magnesium sulfate is used to mitigate preterm labor and in women with pregnancy-induced hypertension, as it is a smooth muscle relaxant and central nervous system depressant. It competes with calcium entry into muscles and decreases the intensity of uterine contraction.

143. Correct Answer: <u>3</u>

Rationale: The standard loading dose is 4–6 grams given over 20 minutes. The ordered dose of 10 grams over 20 minutes should not be given.

144. Correct Answer: <u>4</u>

Rationale: All of the medications listed are used to stop preterm labor.

145. Correct Answer: <u>1</u>

Rationale: Although terbutaline (Brethine) can be given by mouth, it is most efficacious when given subcutaneously.

146. Correct Answer: <u>3</u>

Rationale: This is the only route of administration.

SECTION I

SECTION II

SECTION III

SECTION IV

SECTION V

SECTION VI

SECTION VII

SECTION VIII

SECTION IX

SECTION X

147. Correct Answer: **1**

Rationale: If given in excess, this medication could potentially cause premature closure of ductus arteriosus.

148. Correct Answer: **1**

Rationale: This medication can cause oligohydramnious. Thus careful monitoring of the amniotic fluid is required.

149. Correct Answer: **1**

Rationale: RhoGAM is given to all postpartum women who are Rh-negative and have Rh-positive infants. This medication destroys any fetal red blood cells that are in the maternal circulation before the woman's immune system is activated to produce antibodies that might endanger future pregnancies.

150. Correct Answer: **3**

Rationale: The standard dose is 300 micrograms for postpartum or intrapartum routine injections. A smaller dose is given at 8 weeks because the dose is titrated based on potential fetal/maternal red blood cell exposure.

151. Correct Answer: **1**

Rationale: The expected postpartum dose of RhoGAM is 300 micrograms.

152. Correct Answer: **3**

Rationale: The medication is administered in a subcutaneous injection.

153. Correct Answer: **4**

Rationale: The ointment is used to prevent against ophthalmia neonatorum in newborns whose mothers have gonorrhea and against conjunctivitis in newborns whose mothers are infected with *Chlamydia*.

154. Correct Answer: **2**

Rationale: Vitamin K is produced in the gastrointestinal tract starting around day 8. This initial injection bridges the gap between the birth and day 8 of life.

155. Correct Answer: **1**

Rationale: The recommended does is 0.5–1 milligram.

156. Correct Answer: **2**

Rationale: This medication induces contractions and, if not properly monitored, can cause excessive contractions.

157. Correct Answer: **1**

Rationale: Penicillin G is the drug of choice provided the patient does not have an allergy to penicillin.

158. Correct Answer: **2**

Rationale: Maximum dosing is 20 milliunits/min. The medication should be discontinued at this rate and an appropriate dose obtained.

159. Correct Answer: **2**

Rationale: Both Toradol and Motrin are NSAIDs. Giving both would be redundant and might increase the risk of gastrointestinal bleeding.

160. Correct Answer: **3**

Rationale: Ducosate sodium (Colace) helps to prevent constipation by incorporating water into the stool so that it will be softer when passed.

REDUCTION OF RISK POTENTIAL

161. Correct Answer: **3**

Rationale: At this age, an infant should consume only breast milk or infant formula. Neither should ever be warmed in a microwave oven.

162. Correct Answer: **2**

Rationale: The key to successful breastfeeding begins with correct positioning and latch-on.

163. Correct Answer: **2**

Rationale: It is contraindicated to rub the affected area, as this action may dislodge the blood clot.

164. Correct Answer: **3**

Rationale: A vaginal exam is contraindicated in a woman with bright red bleeding.

165. Correct Answer: **3**

Rationale: A <u>direct</u> Coombs test is done on the infant postpartum; cord blood is obtained, and the test looks for maternal cells in the fetal system. An indirect Coombs test is done on the mother prenatally.

166. Correct Answer: **3**

Rationale: The presence of bowel sounds indicates that the bowel has recovered from anesthesia and is able to digest food.

167. Correct Answer: **1**

Rationale: The only contraindication to a VBAC is a vertical scar called a classical incision.

168. Correct Answer: <u>1</u>

Rationale: Yellow sclera is not a normal finding and should be evaluated further.

169. Correct Answer: <u>3</u>

Rationale: Evaluation of the fundus and lochia give reassurance against the possibility of hemorrhage related to uterine atony.

170. Correct Answer: <u>2</u>

Rationale: Chorionic villus sampling (CVS) is the only genetic test that can be done at this early stage of gestation.

171. Correct Answer: <u>1</u>

Rationale: The patient is most likely anemic and will need to increase her iron consumption by taking supplements.

172. Correct Answer: <u>2</u>

Rationale: Femur length is not part of a biophysical profile.

173. Correct Answer: <u>2</u>

Rationale: An amniocentesis obtains amniotic fluid, which contains PG. It, along with the L/S rate, indicates fetal lung maturity.

174. Correct Answer: <u>4</u>

Rationale: Sonography in the first trimester is best used for determining the fetus's gestational age.

175. Correct Answer: <u>2</u>

Rationale: This screening determines the level of AFP in the maternal bloodstream. High levels indicate an opening in the fetal spine that has allowed the fetus's spinal fluid to escape into the maternal system.

176. Correct Answer: <u>3</u>

Rationale: Hemolysis, elevated liver enzymes, and low platelets are the hallmark lab results of HELLP syndrome, which is a variant of pregnancy-induced hypertension.

177. Correct Answer: <u>1</u>

Rationale: The direct measure of pregnancy is the presence of HCG in the urine and blood of women.

178. Correct Answer: <u>2</u>

Rationale: Umbilical cord compression is the most common cause of variable decelerations.

179. Correct Answer: <u>4</u>

Rationale: Inability of the patient's blood to clot correctly is a contraindication to receiving an epidural.

180. Correct Answer: <u>1</u>

Rationale: The lack of blood flow from the mother to the fetus via the placenta is the cause of late decelerations.

181. Correct Answer: <u>3</u>

Rationale: Pregnancy-induced hypertension causes vascular constriction in the mother and placenta, leading to compromised blood flow.

182. Correct Answer: <u>2</u>

Rationale: A common side effect of an epidural is maternal hypotension. This decrease in blood flow can cause late decelerations in the fetal tracing.

183. Correct Answer: <u>4</u>

Rationale: Early decelerations are normal and are a sign of fetal head compression, which usually happens when a patient is dilated to 4 cm or is almost completely dilated and ready to push.

184. Correct Answers: <u>**Infection, fetal trauma, puncture of the umbilical cord, bleeding, miscarriage, fetal death.**</u>

185. Correct Answer: <u>2</u>

Rationale: The most appropriate time to screen for gestational diabetes, if a patient does not have risk factors that would otherwise warrant early testing, is between 26 and 28 weeks gestation.

186. Correct Answer: <u>4</u>

Rationale: During pregnancy, the urine is screened at each visit. The 1-hour and 3-hour tests are used sequentially—that is, if the 1-hour test is positive, the 3-hour test is then conducted.

187. Correct Answer: <u>4</u>

Rationale: Shoulder dystocia often occurs because women with gestational diabetes typically have larger babies. Diabetes is a vascular disease and may affect placental profusion. If the mother's diabetes has not been well controlled, the infant may be born with excess insulin in his or her system, which could lead to hypoglycemia once the infant's food supply has ended through the placenta.

188. Correct Answer: <u>**infection**</u>

189. Correct Answer: <u>**4**</u>

Rationale: Internal monitoring is the best solution when obtaining the fetal heart rate or contraction patterns is necessary for the safety of the mother and infant and such monitoring cannot be done externally.

190. Correct Answer: <u>**4**</u>

Rationale: All of the listed items are causes of early passage of meconium in utero. Often this problem occurs without any identifiable cause.

191. Correct Answer: <u>**4**</u>

Rationale: Bright red bleeding is not normal in pregnancy and should be evaluated immediately.

192. Correct Answer: <u>**3**</u>

Rationale: Often fetal movement is occurring, yet the mother does not feel it. It is important to make sure that the pregnant woman is properly hydrated and nourished. Once this occurs, encouraging rest with the sole purpose of fetal movement counting is recommended, with a return call being place if no movement is felt in that 2-hour time frame.

193. Correct Answer: <u>**2**</u>

Rationale: The elevated pulse is the first indication of excessive blood loss and should be evaluated.

PHYSIOLOGICAL ADAPTATION

194. Correct Answer: <u>**1**</u>

Rationale: The defect causes the blood to flow from the right to left atrium.

195. Correct Answer: <u>**1**</u>

Rationale: A common cause of hemolytic disease of the newborn is Rh incompatibility. This disease is manifested by jaundice in the first 24 hours of life.

196. Correct Answer: <u>**1**</u>

Rationale: The fetal circulation—that is, is the connection between the pulmonary artery and the aorta—does not close at birth.

197. Correct Answer: <u>**4**</u>

Rationale: Cephalhematoma does not cross the suture lines and is a result of birth trauma. It

will resolve spontaneously in a week after the child's birth.

198. Correct Answer: <u>**2**</u>

Rationale: Previous uterine scars put women at increased risk for placenta previa.

199. Correct Answer: <u>**4**</u>

Rationale: Although bleeding can be a sign, a more consistent sign is abdominal findings such as a tetanic contraction.

200. Correct Answer: <u>**1**</u>

Rationale: This is the expected description of normal postpartum bleeding.

201. Correct Answer: <u>**2**</u>

Rationale: Until a pregnant woman has completed the 37th week of gestation, the fetus is considered a preterm infant. Preterm classification is based on gestational age, not weight.

202. Correct Answer: <u>**4**</u>

Rationale: Cephalhematoma is a bleed between the skull and scalp that does not cross the suture lines. Extra blood will create more bilirubin as it breaks down.

203. Correct Answer: <u>**2**</u>

Rationale: This normal skin change in newborns does not require any intervention and will go away in time.

204. Correct Answer: <u>**4**</u>

Rationale: Preterm infants do not have fully developed lungs, so respiratory issues tend to be their main problems.

205. Correct Answer: <u>**1**</u>

Rationale: The ability to walk normally is not a guaranteed result of surgery. The mother needs further education regarding the infant's condition and diagnosis.

206. Correct Answer: <u>**1**</u>

Rationale: These three in utero adaptations occur as the body adjusts to maintain the fetal circulation and adequate oxygenation.

207. Correct Answer: <u>**3**</u>

Rationale: Iron-deficiency anemia is the most common anemia in women and is caused by poor iron nutrition.

208. Correct Answer: **4**

Rationale: Epidural anesthesia causes maternal hypotension, which can lead to fetal bradycardia.

209. Correct Answer: **4**

Rationale: The pathology behind PIH is a fluid shift that occurs from the vasculature to the tissues, which causes edema and leads to an increase in hematocrit.

210. Correct Answer: **4**

Rationale: Depending on the clinical picture, the patient can be managed either in the hospital or at home.

211. Correct Answer: **1**

Rationale: Von Willebrand's disease—a type of hemophilia resulting from a factor VIII deficiency—is the most common hereditary bleeding disorder.

212. Correct Answer: **1**

Rationale: Even though all of these are reasonable concerns, maintaining a clear airway is of the utmost importance, as the leading cause of mortality with seizures is aspiration.

213. Correct Answer: **3**

Rationale: Thermoregulation is a very important and sensitive state in any newborn, because these infants cannot use mechanisms such as shivering to generate heat.

214. Correct Answer: **1**

Rationale: Presentation can be vertex, breech, footling, brow, and so on.

215. Correct Answer: **3**

Rationale: During labor, cardiac output, vital signs, and respirations all increase.

216. Correct Answer: **3**

Rationale: 4 cm refers to the cervical dilation, 80% refers to the cervical effacement (how

thinned out the cervix is), and −1 indicates the relationship of the fetal head to the ischial spines.

217. Correct Answer: **3**

Rationale: Verifying immune status via prenatal lab work can definitively determine the patient's risk from exposure to German measles. Receiving the vaccine does not guarantee immunity.

218. Correct Answer: **3**

Rationale: While all of these are valid nursing concerns, of primary importance with an ectopic pregnancy is the potential for rupture and hemorrhagic shock.

219. Correct Answer: **3**

Rationale: The release of oxytocin with breastfeeding causes the uterus to contract, increasing patient discomfort.

220. Correct Answer: **4**

Rationale: All of the other items affect the delivery: passenger, passageway, powers, and emotional status. Membrane status does not necessarily affect cervical change directly.

221. Correct Answer: **3**

Rationale: The patient must have a normal platelet count before the epidural can be given.

222. Correct Answer: **4**

Rationale: A cervical exam finding of 8/90% and −3 indicates that the fetal head is not engaged in the pelvis. This puts the patient at risk for cord prolapse, particularly in light of her ruptured membranes.

223. Correct Answer: **4**

Rationale: Dehydration is a common cause of maternal temperature elevation in the postpartum period.

SECTION
I

SECTION
II

SECTION
III

SECTION
IV

SECTION
V

SECTION
VI

SECTION
VII

SECTION
VIII

SECTION
IX

SECTION

SECTION
X

Care of Children

MANAGEMENT OF CARE

Multiple Choice

1. A 2-month-old infant is to receive required immunizations during a clinic visit. What would that immunization include?

   1. MMR and varicella.

   2. MMR only.

   3. DTP and IPV.

   4. Hepatitis A and DTP.

2. Which of these interventions would be most appropriate when teaching the parents of a 6-month-old client how to administer medications through a gastrostomy tube? (Select all that apply.)

   1. Clamp the tube after flushing.

   2. Cut the tablet in half and push it through the tube.

   3. Mix the medication with enteral formula in a medication cup.

   4. Warm the medication in a microwave.

   5. It is appropriate to crush an enteric-coated aspirin.

   6. Pour the medication into a syringe.

3. Implementing which client's plan of care first would indicate that the nurse has an appropriate understanding of how the workload should be prioritized?

   1. A 13-year-old admitted with acute appendicitis.

   2. A 9-year-old in sickle cell crisis.

   3. An 11-year-old admitted with chronic renal failure.

   4. A 5-year-old with cerebral palsy.

4. A 4-week-old infant is brought to the Emergency Department. The child is lethargic and minimally cries when stimulated. Upon assessment, the fontanel is bulging and bruising is found on the arms and legs. Shaken baby syndrome is suspected. What action should the nurse take based on this assessment?

   1. Document the assessment findings and provide education to the parents.

   2. Discharge the infant to home with no follow-up necessary.

   3. Document the assessment findings and report them to local authorities.

   4. Discharge the infant and assign a case worker to the case.

Fill in the Blank

5. A 14-year-old boy was involved in a motor vehicle crash and sustained a traumatic amputation of his left leg. The client has been in the hospital for 2 weeks. His parents are actively involved in the care of their son. A Child Life Specialist has been working with the client to provide schooling and diversional activities. The pastor from the church has been visiting routinely. Mobility is an issue that needs to be addressed and the client wants to begin exercising. Which healthcare team member should the nurse expect a consultation from?

_____

Multiple Choice

6. Which nursing action is a priority for a child admitted with suspected bacterial meningitis?

1. Place the child in isolation.
2. Prepare for a lumbar puncture procedure.
3. Administer the prescribed antibiotic.
4. Initiate intravenous fluids.

7. Which assignment would be most appropriate to assign a certified nursing assistant (CNA) to perform?

1. Changing a peripherally inserted central catheter (PICC) dressing on a 14-year-old client.
2. Administering acetaminophen syrup to a 3-year-old client with a temperature of 102.5°F.
3. Bathing a 6-year-old child who has been incontinent of urine and feces and is in a halo brace.
4. Delivering a lab specimen collected from a 4-year-old client after performing a venipuncture to collect the blood.

8. The nurse presents the informed consent form for the insertion of a Port-a-Cath to the parents of a 6-year-old child with cancer. The parents tell the nurse that they are confused about what the surgeon told them. Which nursing action is most appropriate?

1. Have the parents sign the form and tell them that you will call the surgeon.
2. Explain the procedure to the parents and have them sign the form.
3. Notify the surgeon that the parents have questions and the form is not signed.
4. Have the parents sign the form so not to delay surgery and treatment of their child.

9. The philosophy of family-centered care is an integral aspect of delivering health care to children. Which nursing action best corresponds to family-centered care?

1. Information is shared openly between the parents and the healthcare team.
2. Strict adherence to visiting hours is enforced.
3. The family and child should be viewed as separate entities.
4. Family spiritual beliefs should not be incorporated into the child's care.

10. An 18-year-old client has an intravenous infusion initiated for continuous IV fluids and antibiotic therapy. To administer the first IV piggyback, select the steps that would be needed to infuse the antibiotic.

1. Hang the IV antibiotic bag lower than the continuous IV fluid bag.
2. Connect the antibiotic IV tubing to the closest port to the continuous fluid IV bag.
3. Detach the primary IV fluid bag and insert the antibiotic IV tubing.
4. Connect the antibiotic IV tubing to the closest port to the patient.
5. Hang the IV antibiotic bag higher than the continuous IV fluid bag.

11. Before administering a subcutaneous injection of NPH insulin to a 9-year-old client with type 1 diabetes mellitus at 10 A.M., the nurse should

1. Test the urine for ketones.
2. Document the client's vital signs.
3. Check the client's glycosated hemoglobin value.
4. Instruct the client to eat lunch and dinner.

12. Which of these clients would be the most appropriate assignment for an LPN?

1. An 8-year-old who is newly admitted to the unit with non-Hodgkin's lymphoma.
2. A 6-year-old with nephroblastoma who is receiving chemotherapy.
3. A 2-year-old with a right dislocated hip who is in Buck extension traction.
4. A 9-year-old with newly diagnosed diabetes who is being discharged and needs teaching.

13. A nurse is assigned several pediatric clients. Which would be first to receive care at the start of the shift?

1. A child infected with human immuno-deficiency virus (HIV).
2. A child with asthma exacerbation.
3. A child with a recent cleft palate repair.
4. An infant infected with rotavirus.

14. Which of these interventions would be most appropriate when performing central line site care on a 10-year-old with a Groshong catheter? (Select all that apply.)

1. Put on gloves and remove the dressing, and then discard the dressing and gloves.
2. Inspect the skin and insertion site.
3. Wash your hands.
4. Put on gloves and remove the dressing, and then discard the dressing.

5. No dressing change is needed—this device is implanted.

6. Use a circular motion with each antiseptic swab.

15. An RN assigns the care of a 7–year-old client with a wound requiring sterile dressing changes every 8 hours to an LPN. As the nurse walks into the room, the LPN is observed using clean gloves to perform the dressing change. How should the RN handle the situation?

1. Inform the LPN that the LPN is doing the procedure incorrectly and that a report will be placed in the personnel file after the RN has finished the dressing change.

2. Inform the LPN that they need to talk after the dressing change has been completed.

3. Use the situation to teach the LPN how to perform the procedure correctly and, upon exiting the client's room, counsel the LPN.

4. Document the LPN's actions in a report to be placed in the personnel file.

16. Which observation indicates that the nurse should withhold a scheduled immunization for measles, mumps, and rubella (MMR) for a 15-month-old child?

1. The client has a congenital immunodeficiency.

2. The client is receiving antibiotics for otitis media with effusion.

3. The client had a temperature of 103.5°F after the last immunization.

4. The client's current temperature is 100.5°F.

17. In caring for a 15-year-old client in the terminal stages of cancer who is refusing any more treatment, the nurse should provide ethical care that

1. Ensures a cure and benefits the client's parents.

2. Allows the client to determine his or her care.

3. Requires treatment to be continued.

4. Promotes equity and prevents litigation.

18. The charge nurse is making assignments for the next shift. In a semi-private room, Client A, who is 6 years old, has idiopathic thrombocytopenic pupura. Client B is 8 years old and has possible viral pneumonia. Which assignment is the most appropriate?

1. Place client A is a private room. Assign different nurses to care for client A and client B.

2. Assign the same nurse to care for client A and client B in the same room.

3. Place client B in another room with a 3-year-old client. Assign the same nurse to care for client A and client B.

4. Assign one nurse to client A and another nurse to client B in the same room.

19. A client is returning from surgery for repair of a patent ductus arteriosus (PDA). A chest tube is in place. To care for this patient postoperatively, select all the equipment that should be at the bedside.

1. Sterile gloves.

2. Wall suction.

3. Sterile petroleum-covered gauze.

4. Thoracotomy tray.

5. Sterile gauze.

6. Endotracheal tube.

7. Sterile glass bottles.

20. During the planning phase of the nursing process for a 5-year-old client who was admitted for a tonsillectomy, the nurse

1. Collects information about past medical problems.

2. Determines if the goal of care has been met.

3. Establishes outcomes.

4. Identifies the problem and nursing diagnosis.

21. A 5-year-old client is admitted with deep partial-thickness and full-thickness burns of the chest from a firecracker explosion. Multiple dressing changes to the chest will be performed, and the expected patient outcome while hospitalized is the absence of a wound infection. Which intervention is most appropriate in meeting this outcome?

1. Administer prophylactic antibiotics to prevent an infection and colonization of wounds.

2. Gloves, gowns, masks, and caps must be worn during the care of this client and sterile gloves must be worn for the dressing changes.

3. Intubation and aggressive ventilatory management are needed to reverse the effects of an inhalation burn injury.

4. The use of good hand washing technique is adequate and is the only intervention that is needed.

22. A nurse is preparing to administer oral Dilantin (phenytoin) to a 13-year-old client with a seizure disorder. Before administering the medication, which action is the most important for the nurse to perform?

1. Initiate an IV with normal saline infusing.
2. Document that the medication was administered.
3. Check the medication dose and the client's identification.
4. Count the available medication available and sign for the medication.

23. A staff nurse has been caring for a 5-year-old patient in respiratory and chronic renal failure. The client has a tracheostomy, is on a ventilator, and is receiving gastric tube feedings. Which information is critical to communicate to the next nurse caring for this client? (Select all that apply.)

1. Room temperature.
2. Amount, color, and consistency of tracheal secretions.
3. Ventilator settings.
4. Vital signs.
5. PO intake.
6. Arterial blood gas results.
7. New orders.

24. The nurse is providing care to an 8-year-old client who has undergone a surgical procedure and has just been received from the recovery room. Which sequence of care is correct for caring for this client?

1. Administer pain medication, check vital signs, and assess the dressing.
2. Check vital signs, administer pain medication, and assess the dressing.
3. Check vital signs, and assess the dressing and presence of pain.
4. Assess urinary output, change the client's gown, and obtain a warm blanket.

25. A 3-year-old child from a prominent family is admitted to the hospital. A reporter for the local newspaper telephones the nursing unit and asks for an update on the client's status. What should the nurse do before providing any information?

1. Verify the reporter's identity.
2. Nothing—provide detailed information now.
3. Obtain signed parental authorization.
4. File a complaint with the newspaper.

26. When the Clinical Nurse Specialist (CNS) gives information that is pertinent to a current performance improvement project on reducing the number of nosocomial urinary tract infections and urinary catheter utilization rates, the CNS may

1. Display the information on the bulletin board in the unit's locker room and bathroom.
2. Share the information at a monthly unit staff meeting.
3. Only share the information with the unit's performance improvement committee.
4. Share the information with the multidisciplinary team that provides care on the unit.

27. A 3-year-old client is scheduled to have blood drawn and the client's father is in the room. Which positioning techniques would assist in obtaining the specimen? (Select all that apply.)

1. Have client's father leave and go to the waiting room.
2. Place the child in the father's lap and use a straddling sitting position.
3. Place the child in arm restraints.
4. Have the client's father stay and assist.
5. Place the child in a mummy restraint.

28. In performing a chart audit, the nurse is evaluating the nursing documentation. Which should be present in the chart for a 7-year-old client who is anuric and receiving peritoneal dialysis?

1. Client weight, lab values, and urine output.
2. Fistula site location, appearance, and presence of thrills and bruits.
3. Client weight, dialysate dwell time, and description of fluid drained.
4. Dialysate, amount of blood dialyzed, and fluid removed.

29. A 10-year-old client is admitted to the hospital with a brain tumor. The client is covered by the parents' insurance, which consists of an HMO. After the initial treatment, the client's ongoing and specific needs for care would be coordinated by

1. The neurosurgeon.
2. The case manager.
3. The charge nurse.
4. Home healthcare nurses.

30. Home healthcare nurses are visiting a family with a 5-year-old child with cystic fibrosis to assist in reinforcing the teaching of chest physiotherapy (CPT). Evaluation and outcome management for this client and family would include

1. A reduction in hospitalizations for pneumonia.
2. Physical activity and the intake of a well-balanced diet.

3. The satisfaction survey on the home health nurses.

4. The ability to use an inhaler to deliver a bronchodilator.

31. A nurse is demonstrating colostomy care to the mother of a child with a new colostomy. Which actions would the nurse teach the mother to perform? (Select all that apply.)

1. Wash hands.
2. Apply sterile gloves.
3. Observe for any irritation.
4. Apply talcum powder.
5. Cut the skin barrier to size.
6. Use an antimicrobial ointment on the skin.

32. During a preoperative assessment of a 2-year-old client undergoing a myringotomy, the nurse identifies a risk for latex allergy when the mother of the client reports an allergy to

1. Milk.
2. Tomatoes.
3. Bananas.
4. Apples.

33. A 3-year-old client needs dressing changes at home. Which statement made by the mother of the client indicates a correct understanding of aseptic technique?

1. "I should use sterile gloves to apply the new dressing."
2. "I should wash my hands prior to removing the old dressing and again before redressing the wound."
3. "I need to give my child pain medication 30 minutes before changing the dressing."
4. "I should wash my hands and use an over-the-counter antimicrobial ointment to help the healing process."

34. Select the blood products that would require use of a microaggregate filter to infuse them in a child needing multiple types of blood products. (Select all that apply.)

1. Packed red blood cells.
2. Platelets.
3. Clotting factors (VIII, IX).
4. Fresh frozen plasma.
5. Whole blood.

35. A 6-year-old client was admitted yesterday and has been placed in a room with a child with cancer who receives chemotherapy. Now the 6-year-old presents with a rash that itches. Varicella-zoster infection is suspected. Which measure should the nurse take to prevent the spread of virus?

1. No isolation precautions are necessary; just place the child in a private room.
2. This child can be left in the semi-private room with the child with cancer.
3. Place the child in a private room and adhere to strict isolation precautions.
4. Observe good hand washing technique and move the child with cancer.

36. Which nursing observation would indicate a major complication in a 5-year-old client who is receiving a blood transfusion?

1. Temperature of 98.3°F.
2. Difficulty breathing.
3. Sleeping soundly.
4. Brisk capillary refill.

37. Which nursing action has the highest priority for a 14-month-old client admitted with burns to 40% of the body and smoke inhalation?

1. Maintain strict fluid restriction.
2. Encourage play.
3. Monitor respiratory status.
4. Administer antibiotics.

38. The charge nurse is making shift assignments. Which client assignment to an LPN indicates that the charge nurse demonstrates an understanding of appropriate delegation?

1. A 13-month-old with inflammatory bowel disease.
2. A 14-year-old receiving a bone marrow transplant.
3. A 15-month-old just admitted with multiple fractures.
4. An 11-year-old receiving conscious sedation.

39. A 3-year-old client is crying and points to the IV in the arm; the client also screams when touched. Which symptom would a nurse become concerned with for possible IV infiltration?

1. Slight swelling.
2. Softness at the insertion site and the surrounding tissue.

3. No redness around the insertion site.

4. Cool skin.

40. When performing an eye irrigation procedure on a 4-year-old client, which sequence would be the most appropriate for the nurse to follow?

1. Wash hands, don gloves, tilt the head toward the unaffected eye, irrigate until clear.

2. Wash hands, tilt the head toward the affected eye, don gloves, irrigate until clear.

3. Don gloves, tilt the head toward the un-affected eye, irrigate until clear, wash hands.

4. Prepare a sterile field, wash hands, don sterile gloves, irrigate until clear.

41. During the insertion of a urinary catheter in a 3-year-old client, the tip of the catheter brushes against the arm of the nurse when the child squirms and kicks. Which nursing action is most appropriate?

1. Continue with the catheter insertion and have the parent restrain the child.

2. Wipe the catheter with betadine and continue the catheter insertion.

3. Obtain a new catheter and seek assistance to hold and comfort the child.

4. Soak the catheter in sterile saline and reattempt insertion in 15 minutes.

42. The nurse on a pediatric unit observes smoke billowing from a room next to a room that holds a 7-year-old client whose parents have left for the evening. Which action should first be taken by the nurse?

1. Yell, "Fire."

2. Close the client's door.

3. Grab the fire extinguisher.

4. Evacuate the 7-year-old client.

43. A mother of an 8-month-old client states that the infant has received all required immunizations. These would include

1. Two doses of DPT and two doses of IPV.

2. Three doses of DPT and two doses of IPV.

3. One dose of DPT and IPV.

4. Three doses of DPT and MMR.

44. Which technique is correct when administering eardrops to a 20-month-old client?

1. Pull the earlobe down and back.

2. Pull the earlobe down and forward.

3. Pull the earlobe up and back.

4. Pull the earlobe up and forward.

SAFETY AND INFECTION CONTROL

Multiple Choice

45. Which client would be the highest risk for poisoning?

1. A 2-week-old infant.

2. A 6-week-old infant.

3. A 3-month-old infant.

4. A 6-month-old infant.

46. A 9-month-old infant is brought to the Emergency Department to be evaluated for injuries after a bookcase fell on top of her. The parents report that the infant was pulling herself up by using the bookcase when it fell over on top of the infant. Which clinical findings would confirm the suspicion of potential maltreatment of the infant?

1. Crying.

2. Hugging the mother tightly.

3. Spiral fracture of the leg.

4. Bend fracture of the fibula.

47. A 9-year-old client is admitted with suspected meningitis. A lumbar puncture is to be performed by the physician. To promote safety, which safety measure would the nurse implement while a cerebrospinal fluid specimen is obtained?

1. Place the child in a sitting position with the head extended.

2. Place the child in a side-lying position with the front closest to the edge of bed.

3. Do not wear gloves because the physician is collecting the specimen.

4. Place one arm behind the child' neck and the other behind the knees.

48. Select the "rights" that pertain to administering medications to a child. (Select all that apply.)

1. Right time.

2. Right physician.

3. Right medication.

4. Right dose.

5. Right client.

6. Right route.

49. Which statement made by a young mother indicates she understands child-proofing her home and preventing injuries for her 3-year-old son?

    1. "The only way I can get my child to take his medicine is to pretend that it is candy."
    2. "All medications have child-resistant caps and are stored in the medicine cabinet above the sink."
    3. "My child is allowed to play in the backyard with a friend while I watch from the window and care for my newborn."
    4. "The electrical outlets are covered with protective devices and our front door is only locked and chained at night for our protection."

50. A 17-year-old client is admitted after a motor vehicle crash, and use of methamphetamine is suspected. Which assessment findings would indicate this client has a possible overdose of methamphetamine?

    1. Hypertension, tachycardia, diarrhea.
    2. Hypotension, tachycardia, papillary constriction.
    3. Hypertension, tachycardia, cardiac arrhythmias.
    4. Hypotension, bradycardia, cardiac arrhythmias.

51. A mother and her 6-month-old infant are in the clinic for a routine visit. Which statement by the mother indicates a knowledge deficit and need for more teaching?

    1. "The car seat is securely anchored and the harness fastens snugly."
    2. "The car seat is an infant model and is securely anchored."
    3. "The car seat is front-facing in the back passenger seat."
    4. "The car seat is rear-facing in the back passenger seat."

52. A child is admitted with a history of seizures. To promote safety, what equipment should be in use or available at the bedside? (Select all that apply.)

    1. Tongue depressor.
    2. Suction.
    3. Restraints.
    4. Padded side rails.
    5. Pulse oximeter.
    6. Code cart.

53. Which instruction should be given to the parents of a 6-month-old child regarding injury prevention?

    1. "Balloons make wonderful toys and keep children entertained."
    2. "Keep sharp objects out of reach."
    3. "You may give hard candy to help with teething."
    4. "Remove all crib toys strung across the top of the crib."

54. Which foods should parents be taught to avoid giving their 6-month-old child?

    1. Scrambled eggs.
    2. Milk.
    3. Iron-fortified rice cereal.
    4. Applesauce.

55. Which statement made by a mother of a 7-year-old child indicates she understands strategies to prevent accidents?

    1. "A helmet is not necessary now that my child has learned how to ride a bicycle."
    2. "My child has taken swimming lessons and swims unsupervised in our pool."
    3. "My child wears a helmet, wrist guards, and knee and elbow pads when skateboarding."
    4. "My child wears a helmet while being the sole operator of an all-terrain vehicle."

56. A staff nurse has been caring for a 4-year-old client with poisoning. In preparing to be discharged, which information is critical to communicate regarding all types of injury prevention? (Select all that apply.)

    1. Never leave the child unattended in a shopping cart.
    2. Assure that medications have child-resistant caps.
    3. Restrain the child when in a high chair.
    4. Store medications in a locked cabinet.
    5. The child may in-line skate while wearing a helmet.
    6. Keep the laundry chute door locked.

57. Multiple documentation entries have been made in the nurses' notes from previous shifts. An error is made in these notes. Which method would be the most accurate way to correct the documentation error?

    1. Use a black marker to cover up the entry and continue to chart.
    2. Draw a single line through the entry and write "error" and your initials above or beside the entry.

3. Use correction fluid to cover the entry and write over the entry.

4. Discard the page on which the error occurred and begin documentation on a new page by hand-copying the previous entries.

58. Which statement concerning the transmission of tinea capitis (*Trichophyton tonsurans, Microsporum canis*) would be the most important teaching delivered by the nurse?

1. This viral infection rarely results in permanent hair loss.

2. This viral infection is spread by skin-to-skin contact.

3. This fungal infection is spread from animal to person.

4. This fungal infection disappears spontaneously.

59. To promote safety in the environment of a 6-year-old client with hemophilia, the nurse would

1. Provide oral care using a soft-bristle toothbrush.

2. Administer aspirin for a temperature of 102.5°F.

3. Change all medication so that it is delivered IM once a day.

4. Administer vitamin K daily.

60. While teaching the parents of a 3-year-old client with pediculosis capitis, the nurse should stress which information?

1. Only children of low socioeconomic status are susceptible to this condition.

2. Machine-wash everything washable and dry in the sun on a clothesline.

3. Nonwashable items should be placed in plastic bags for 14 days.

4. Allow the child to share cookies and play beauty parlor with other children.

61. Which of these interventions would be most appropriate when caring for an 8-year-old client in Buck traction? (Select all that apply.)

1. Apply the ordered traction weight plus 5 pounds to prevent sliding.

2. Maintain the correct body alignment.

3. Check the pin sites frequently.

4. Check the pulses in the affected area.

5. Apply the correct amount of traction weight.

6. Apply antibiotic ointment to the pin sites.

62. A 14-year-old client is scheduled for a sterile dressing change of an open chest wound. Which action is necessary to maintain asepsis?

1. While pouring the sterile wound solution into the dressing tray, if some splashes on the sterile field, you should start the procedure over.

2. If the new dressing is ready to be applied and a piece is dropped on the outer aspect of the sterile field, it may be left there until the dressing change is completed.

3. After removing the old dressing, it is appropriate to set it on the outermost portion of the sterile field and then discard it along with all the materials from the procedure.

4. After washing the hands, sterile gloves are applied to begin the dressing change.

63. Which nursing approach would be most appropriate for following airborne precautions with a 2-year-old client?

1. Wear gloves and a mask when entering the room.

2. Place the client in a semi-private room and wear a gown when in the room.

3. Place the client in a private room and wear gloves, a mask, and a gown when in the room.

4. Place the client in a private room and wear gloves and a gown when in the room.

64. The nurse is changing a dressing of a 22-month-old client with impetigo. What is the best way for the nurse to perform this procedure?

1. Soften and then gently remove crusts and debris.

2. Cleanse the wound with soap and water.

3. Apply a topical antibiotic to the lesions.

4. Administer oral antibiotics and apply hot, moist compresses.

65. A nurse is caring for a 7-week-old infant with dehydration. The physician's order reads "1,000 cc lactated Ringer's to infuse in 2 hours." What is the nurse's first action?

1. Assess breath sounds.

2. Call and verify the order with the physician.

3. Call and verify the order with the pharmacist.

4. Initiate a second IV line.

66. Which action indicates that the nurse has an understanding of safe medication administration for a 5-month-old client?

1. Add the medication to the child's formula to ensure the total dose is administered.

2. Confirm the order with the medication package and chart after the medication has been administered.

3. Prior to administering the medication at the bedside, confirm the client's identity by looking at the arm band.

4. Contact the physician to clarify possible adverse reactions prior to administering any medications.

HEALTH PROMOTION AND MAINTENANCE

Multiple Choice

67. Which instructions should be given to a mother of a 6-month-old-infant regarding the introduction of solid foods?

1. The order of introducing foods begins with cereal and meats, followed by fruits and vegetables.

2. Introduce one food at a time, at intervals of 4 to 7 days.

3. Chopped table food or commercially prepared junior foods are appropriate.

4. The quantity of formula will stay the same as the amount of solid food increases.

68. Which observation made during a school screening would indicate suspected scoliosis in an 11-year-old child?

1. Shoulder symmetry.

2. Presence of lordosis.

3. Positive Adam's test.

4. Presence of kyphosis.

69. The nurse should teach the mother of a 14-month-old child which concept regarding dental hygiene?

1. Brushing and flossing are not necessary until permanent teeth have come in.

2. Taking a bottle of milk to bed strengthens the enamel on the teeth.

3. A trip to the dentist and the use of fluorinated mouthwash is encouraged.

4. Six to eight strokes of a toothbrush should be used for effective brushing.

70. In the initial presentation of type 1 diabetes mellitus in a 9-year-old child, which symptoms would the nurse expect to assess?

1. Blurred vision and weight gain.

2. Weight loss and hypotonic reflexes.

3. Short attention span and hyperactivity.

4. Polydipsia and polyphagia.

71. In which circumstance would a nurse be concerned about the language development of a 3-year-old child?

1. Conversation with the child is 50% intelligible.

2. The child uses pronouns and prepositions when talking.

3. The child has a vocabulary of about 900 words.

4. The child is inquisitive and asks "why" a majority of the time.

72. The parents of a 20-month-old child are ready to begin toilet training with their child. Toilet training can be frustrating. Which signs would indicate this child was ready to begin toilet training? (Select all that apply.)

1. Regular bowel movements.

2. Appropriate age.

3. Expresses desire to use toilet.

4. Increased number of wet diapers.

5. Wakes up from nap dry.

6. Able to dress and undress himself or herself.

73. Which information is most important to teach a 17-year-old client about contraception and safe sexual practices?

1. Taking an oral contraceptive is the safest method to prevent pregnancy and sexually transmitted diseases.

2. Teenagers who are sexually active need to worry about only genital herpes and trichomoniasis.

3. Peer pressure makes it difficult to make choices about sexual activity, and it is important to role-play situations.

4. There is no need to demonstrate how to use contraceptive products because the directions are included in the package.

74. The parents of a 2-year-old child state that they are frustrated with the child always saying "no" to food and juices and becoming a picky eater. Which response from the nurse would be most appropriate?

1. "This is not a common behavior, and we need to worry about malnourishment and development."
2. "You will need to see a counselor and nutritionist to best deal with this situation."
3. "You need to be firm with the child and set limits and rewards."
4. "You should try to offer choices; this behavior is common as children become more independent."

75. A 3-year-old child has an imaginary friend. While the child is undergoing a check-up, the child's mother states that she is worried because her child speaks about the imaginary friend incessantly. What should the nurse emphasize when guiding the parents of this child?

1. Enroll the child in daycare or preschool 3 days a week.
2. Imaginary friends usually disappear when the child is older.
3. The parents need to take a class and join a support group.
4. The child is emotionally scarred and will need a psychiatrist soon.

76. A child with Duchene muscular dystrophy is undergoing a routine check-up. Which statement indicates that the mother understands the cause of this disorder in the child?

1. "Both my husband and I carry a recessive trait for this disease."
2. "The disease is inherited through the X chromosome and came from my side of the family."
3. "The trait for the disease is on chromosome 21 and came from my side of the family."
4. "The disease came from my husband's side of the family and is inherited on the Y chromosome."

77. During a routine physical, a 13-year-old girl reports that she believes she is overweight and wants to lose 20 pounds. Her current height is 5 feet 4 inches and her weight is 106 pounds. Which response by the nurse would be best?

1. "I understand your concern because you desire to have a slim figure and not become fat."
2. "I would not worry about your weight; you are growing and need to eat."
3. "The best thing you can do is talk with your parents about this issue and cut down on the amount of food you eat."

4. "I understand your concern about becoming fat, and I do think it best that you exercise more and eat less."

78. A 6-month-old child is undergoing a routine check-up. Select all findings the nurse would expect to find during an assessment of this child.

1. Doll's eyes.
2. Presence of the anterior fontanel.
3. Extrusion of the tongue when receiving cereal.
4. Weight has doubled since birth.
5. Sits with support.
6. Grabs for rattle.

79. A parent is asking questions related to immunizations for a 5-year-old child who is scheduled to start school. Which statement made by the nurse indicates an appropriate understanding of immunizations?

1. "A tetanus and first MMR vaccination will be needed before the child can enter school."
2. "A DPT, IPV, and second booster for MMR vaccination will be needed prior to the child beginning school."
3. "A DPT, second IPV, and Hib vaccinations will be needed sometime during the first year the child attends school."
4. "No immunizations are needed until the child begins the third grade."

80. What should the nurse emphasize when guiding parents about teething of their 6-month-old infant?

1. Drooling is not normal and indicates that something is wrong.
2. Most infants will have a high fever and will be irritable and refuse to eat.
3. The use of teething powders and hard candy is encouraged.
4. Providing a frozen teething ring helps relieve the inflammation.

81. Which assessment finding indicates an 8-day-old client treated for an infection is fully recovered?

1. Respiratory rate of 50.
2. Heart rate of 204.
3. Axillary temperature of 99°F.
4. Easily takes bottle every 2 hours.

82. Which action by a 7-year-old child indicates further instruction regarding management of asthma is needed?

SECTION I

SECTION II

SECTION III

SECTION IV

SECTION V

SECTION VI

SECTION VII

SECTION VIII

SECTION IX

SECTION X

1. The child lies down when using a peak expiratory flow meter.
2. The child holds his or her breath for 5 seconds upon inhaling the inhaler mist.
3. The child waits 1 minute between metered-dose inhaler puffs.
4. The child uses breathing exercises to promote chest wall mobility.

83. Which assessment finding would be abnormal in a 6-week-old infant?

1. Presence of hip movement toward the side of the spine touched.
2. Presence of a rooting reflex.
3. Presence of a positive Babinski reflex.
4. Presence of tongue extrusion when feeding.

84. A 4-year-old client is in skeletal traction. Which activity would be appropriate to offer the child? (Select all that apply.)

1. Crayons and coloring books.
2. Riding in a wagon.
3. Finger painting.
4. Stringing beads.
5. Watching television.
6. Squeaky animals and toys.

85. A 23-month-old child is hospitalized for a repair of a hernia. The child clings to a worn, tattered teddy bear and screams if anyone attempts to take the bear away. Which plan would be most appropriate?

1. Replace the teddy bear with a new, clean stuffed toy.
2. Allow the child to keep the teddy bear and place it on the night stand.
3. Replace the teddy bear with a clean hospital blanket.
4. Allow the child to keep the worn, tattered teddy bear.

86. During assessment of a newborn, the nurse is evaluating the rooting reflex. Which assessment techniques and findings would indicate the presence of this reflex? (Select all that apply.)

1. The cheek is stroked.
2. The tongue is depressed.
3. The outer sole of the foot is stroked.
4. The infant flexes the hands and toes.
5. The infant coughs.
6. The infant begins to suck.

PSYCHOSOCIAL INTEGRITY

Multiple Choice

87. Which approach should be included in the plan of care for a 14-year-old client who is admitted following a sexual abuse incident?

1. Medicate the client with Ativan (lorazepam).
2. Limit communication with the client's parents and reinforce the secrets.
3. Encourage communication and listen attentively.
4. Encourage the client to immediately engage in normal routines and social activities.

88. An 8-year-old child is hospitalized for a conduct disorder of uncontrolled aggression and to begin a behavior modification program. Which initial assessment is necessary in establishing a successful program?

1. Monitor the therapeutic effectiveness of antianxiety medications prescribed.
2. Collect the history, and identify aggressive behaviors and their frequency.
3. Ask why the child behaves this way.
4. Discharge the child and observe the child in the home and school settings for accuracy.

89. A 6-year-old child has moderate mental retardation. In planning for school activities for this child and his or her family, which nursing action would be most appropriate?

1. Prepare the family to isolate the child to protect him or her from teasing.
2. Assist the family in determining the child's readiness to learn and setting realistic goals.
3. Encourage the family to place the child in an institution.
4. Encourage the family to enroll the child in a traditional school setting.

90. An 11-year-old client with metastatic osteosarcoma is admitted to the unit. The child's grandfather died 2 months ago. The nurse walks into the room and finds the child crying. The child asks the nurse if he is going to die. Which response by the nurse would be the most appropriate?

1. "You don't need to focus on that; you need to put your energy into getting better."
2. "You will need to ask the doctor when he comes to check you."
3. "Let's talk about it. What do you think?"
4. "Yes, everyone dies sometime."

91. Which clinical finding would indicate an attention-deficit/hyperactivity disorder in a 6-year-old child? (Select all that apply.)

   1. The child is impulsive and has difficulty waiting for his or her turn.
   2. The child talks little and pays close attention to directions.
   3. The child has difficulty organizing and is forgetful.
   4. The child listens attentively and follows directions carefully.
   5. The child frequently squirms and fidgets in class.
   6. The child is easily distracted.

92. A 7-year-old client is in the terminal stages of cancer. Which nursing action will provide the most support to the child and family during this time?

   1. Promote open communication about what to expect.
   2. Promote rest by limiting visitation.
   3. Prevent information overload by communicating once a week.
   4. Begin decreasing the current treatment regimen.

93. Which plan is most appropriate for meeting the dietary practices of a 9-year-old Muslim client while hospitalized?

   1. Breakfast foods would include eggs, sausage, and toast.
   2. Lunch would consist of a hamburger, an apple, and macaroni and cheese.
   3. Lunch would include cheese and pepperoni pizza and a soft drink.
   4. Dinner would include a slice of ham, green beans, and fruit cocktail.

94. A 13-year-old girl is admitted to an inpatient psychiatric unit after attempting suicide. What is the initial nursing priority?

   1. Increase the client's self-esteem and promote her sense of identity.
   2. Establish a therapeutic play session.
   3. Ensure the client's safety.
   4. Establish recreational therapy.

95. The physician has ordered Ritalin (methylphenidate hydrochloride) for a 9-year-old client with attention-deficit/hyperactivity disorder. After 2 months, which evaluation indicates that the medication is having a positive outcome?

   1. The child is agitated and complains of headaches.
   2. The child is easily distracted and finds homework difficult.
   3. The child completes household chores with only one reminder.
   4. The child completes homework in 10 minutes with multiple errors.

96. Which evaluation indicates that a 15-year-old girl with anorexia nervosa has made a positive accomplishment toward the plan of care outlined for her?

   1. Eating small portions followed by 1 hour of strenuous exercise.
   2. Attending group therapy and weight loss of 2 pounds in a week.
   3. Eating small portions of high-caloric food and weight gain of 0.5 pound.
   4. Eating large portions and weight loss of 3 pounds in a week.

97. The parents of a 4-year-old child state that they are having difficulty controlling their child. They indicate that the child is always defiant and hostile toward adults and is totally resistant to direction or bargaining. In designing a behavior modification program for this child, which interventions would be appropriate? (Select all that apply.)

   1. Use of a colored chart with goals listed.
   2. Establishment of a behavioral contract.
   3. Use of a reward system for accomplishments.
   4. Allowing small outbursts.
   5. Enrollment in vocational training.
   6. Establishment of limits and consequences.

98. Which behavior is associated with the protest phase of separation anxiety for a 2½-year-old child who is hospitalized?

   1. Clings to the parent.
   2. Sucks thumb.
   3. Withdraws to a corner of the room.
   4. Interacts with caregivers.

99. Which nursing action is most appropriate when caring for a 6-year-old child who is hospitalized with depression?

   1. Promote solitary play.
   2. Promote continued dependency and reliance on others.
   3. Promote therapeutic play activities.
   4. Assess frequently for suicidal ideation.

SECTION I

SECTION II

SECTION III

SECTION IV

SECTION V

SECTION VI

SECTION VII

SECTION VIII

SECTION IX

SECTIO X

100. In a 16-year-old client, which observation is indicative of cocaine use?

1. Constricted pupils and bradycardia.
2. Nasal mucosal swelling and irritability.
3. Intense craving for sweets and salt.
4. Sleepiness and hypertension.

101. A trusting relationship is crucial in providing care. Which behavior indicates that a 14-year-old male client with schizophrenia is developing this trusting relationship?

1. The client mimics the same behavior and follows the nurse around the unit.
2. During group therapy, the client describes vividly the hallucinations he experiences.
3. The client openly describes his feelings to the nurse during a therapeutic session.
4. During group therapy, the client states that he is feeling normal and wants to go home.

Fill in the Blank

102. The nurse is assessing a 6-year-old boy. The client shares that he is embarrassed to spend the night at a friend's house because he wets the bed 3 to 4 times a week. By what name does the nurse refer to this disorder?

_____

Multiple Choice

103. A newborn is born with Down syndrome. The parents are devastated at the thought of not having a perfect child. After 2 days of grieving and minimal contact with the baby, which comments would be considered a sign that the parents are making progress in their emotional state?

1. "Was this caused by something that we did during the pregnancy?"
2. "We would rather you took care of our baby."
3. "When are we scheduled to take our baby home?"
4. "Is it safe for us to hold and feed our baby?"

104. The mother of a newborn is exhibiting signs of heroin withdrawal. Her newborn is suspected to have neonatal abstinence syndrome. In planning activities for the newborn, which nursing action would be appropriate?

1. Rock and wrap the baby snugly.
2. Increase the baby's external stimulation.
3. Place the baby in a car seat for feedings.
4. Place a mobile above the crib that plays music.

105. Which finding in an 8-week-old infant with a non-organic failure to thrive indicates that the client is responding positively to the plan of care? (Select all that apply.)

1. The infant avoids eye contact.
2. The infant's weight is currently within the 15th percentile.
3. The infant is apathetic and withdrawn.
4. The infant smiles and coos.
5. The infant screams at strangers.
6. The infant takes 3–4 ounces of formula every 3 hours.

106. Sudden infant death syndrome is suspected to be the cause of death for a 6-month-old child who was admitted to the Emergency Department. The nurse who cared for the infant brings the parents to the room. The parents are grief stricken and want to hold their baby. Which nursing action would be most appropriate in helping the parents at this time?

1. Kindly ask the parents to leave the room and say good-bye to their child, and then accompany them to the waiting room.
2. Allow the parents to say goodbye and to hold and rock the child.
3. Discourage the parents from touching the child.
4. Encourage the parents to say good-bye to the child, accompany them to the waiting room, and call the chaplain.

BASIC CARE AND COMFORT

Multiple Choice

107. Which instruction would be included in the teaching plan of a 5-year-old child with self-perpetuating constipation?

1. Administer an enema twice a week.
2. Provide snacks such as raisins and popcorn.
3. Hold the urge to have a bowel movement until at home.
4. Increase the amount of milk and juice, but discourage intake of broccoli.

108. In planning care for a 7-year-old client with Graves' disease, what should the nurse do?

1. Encourage strenuous physical activity.
2. Encourage a decreased caloric intake.
3. Encourage frequent rest periods.
4. Administer thyroid hormone replacement daily.

109. A 6-month-old infant has returned to the unit from surgery. Which assessment finding would indicate that the infant was experiencing pain?

1. The child sleeps soundly, with an increased pulse rate and decreased blood pressure.
2. The child has a rating of 6 on the Faces Pain Rating Scale.
3. The child cries steadily and kicks.
4. The child points to the area producing the pain.

110. A 4-week-old infant is diagnosed with acute congestive heart failure and hypoplastic left heart syndrome. The nurse observes that the infant develops cyanosis, has increased difficulty breathing, and tires easily during activities. In caring for this infant, which would be the most appropriate nursing action?

1. Put the child in the prone position with the head slightly elevated.
2. Feed the child small volumes every 2 to 3 hours.
3. Feed the child normal volumes every 4 hours.
4. Give the child a bath and a diaper change prior to feeding.

111. A 5-year-old child is diagnosed with right lower lobe pneumonia. In which position should the child be placed to maximize oxygenation?

1. High Fowler's.
2. Supine.
3. Right side-lying.
4. Left side-lying.

112. The nursing evaluation of the respiratory status of a 3-year-old client who is newly admitted with acute epiglottitis would include the following findings:

1. Irritability, coarse crackles bilaterally, and low-grade fever.
2. Drooling, decreased pulse, and stridor.
3. Croupy cough, high fever, and hoarseness.
4. Irritability, drooling, and absence of spontaneous cough.

113. An 8-year-old child has fallen out of a tree and sustained a closed head injury. At the time of admission, the child is unconscious and exhibits decorticate posturing with noxious stimulation. One hour later, the nurse assesses the client. Which findings should the nurse report to the physician? (Select all that apply.)

1. Lethargic state.
2. Bilateral flexion of the upper extremities to noxious stimuli.
3. Bilateral extension of the upper extremities to noxious stimuli.
4. Small, reactive pupils.
5. Clear fluid draining from the nostrils.
6. Slight drainage from facial lacerations.
7. Diminished visual acuity.

114. A 5-month-old child is admitted with suspected shaken baby syndrome and possible increased intracranial pressure (ICP). Which assessment finding would be most indicative of increased ICP in this client?

1. Bulging anterior fontanel.
2. Bulging posterior fontanel.
3. Unchanged occipitofrontal circumference.
4. Weak, soft cry.

115. A 2-month-old infant is diagnosed with failure to thrive. Consumption of which item would indicate compliance with the plan to increase the child's caloric intake?

1. Evaporated milk with iron and vitamin C supplements.
2. Rice cereal with every feeding.
3. Similac formula.
4. Whole milk.

116. A 15-year-old client sustained a thoracic spine injury and is confined to a wheelchair. Which nursing assessment indicates the need for intervention?

1. Voiding 300 mL/day.
2. Consumption of 4 glasses of milk a day.
3. Weight gain of 2 pounds.
4. Nonproductive cough.

117. During the initial assessment of a 3-month-old client with aortic stenosis, the nurse would carefully observe for which symptoms?

1. Hypotension.
2. Bradycardia.
3. Strong, bounding pulses.
4. Clubbing.

118. A 4-year-old client is admitted for a series of tests to verify the diagnosis of pheochromocytoma. Which assessment findings would support this diagnosis?

1. Anuria.
2. Weight gain.
3. Hypertension.
4. Diarrhea.

119. A 7-year-old client is to have a nasogastric tube placed. Organize the following steps in chronological order for this procedure.

1. Measure the tube for approximate placement length.
2. Insert the tube along the base of the nose.
3. Place the client supine in a sniffing position.
4. Check the position of the tube placement and secure the tube.
5. Lubricate the tube.
6. Advance the tube straight back toward the occiput.

120. A 9-year-old client is admitted to the unit for treatment of hypoparathyroidism. Current lab results are as follows: WBC 6,000/μL, hemoglobin 13.0 g/dL, hematocrit 41%, calcium 6.8 mg/dL, and phosphorus 10.4 mg/dL. Which potential diagnosis would be the nursing priority?

1. Infection related to an elevated white cell count.
2. Seizures due to elevated calcium levels.
3. Fluid volume deficit related to decreased hematocrit levels.
4. Ineffective airway clearance due to laryngospasm.

121. A 10-year-old child was admitted after a motor vehicle crash with multiple fractures, including an open compound left femur fracture. The client is in skeletal traction. During an assessment, the nurse finds the client's right foot to be warmer than the left foot. What should the nurse do?

1. Encourage active range of motion of both legs but particularly the left.
2. Assess bilateral foot color, sensation, capillary refill, and toe wiggle.
3. Recognize that the traction weight is too heavy and remove some weight.
4. Recognize that vascular compromise is taking place and notify the physician.

122. An 11-year-old child is admitted for radio-frequency ablation. When providing post-procedure care for this client, which intervention should the nurse implement?

1. Assess the sternal dressing every hour for bleeding.
2. Assess the drainage of the chest tube.
3. Observe the insertion site for hematoma.
4. Ambulate the client an hour after arrival on the unit.

Fill in the Blank

123. A 4-year-old child is admitted to the Emergency Department with an acute asthmatic attack. An audible wheeze is heard on auscultation, and substernal retractions are noted. In which position should the nurse place this client to maximize oxygenation?

_____

Multiple Choice

124. An infant is born with spina bifida and is scheduled for surgery the next day. Which nursing action has the greatest priority?

1. Preventing rupture of the meningocele sac.
2. Preventing infection by supine positioning.
3. Encouraging the parents to hold, cuddle, and feed the infant.
4. Promoting range-of-motion exercises.

125. A 3-year-old client with leukemia is admitted to receive a chemotherapy treatment. The child has a white blood cell count of 4,000/μL. Which nursing intervention is most important?

1. Restrict fluids.
2. Administer an antiemetic.
3. Restrict visitors.
4. Monitor the client's temperature.

126. A 12-year-old client has a right tibia fracture that is casted. This client needs instruction regarding how to walk on crutches using a three-point gait prior to being discharged from the Emergency Department. Which instructions would be included? (Select all that apply.)

1. Weight bearing is permitted on the left foot.
2. The hands and arms support the body's weight.
3. Weight bearing is permitted on the right foot.
4. The axillary area supports the body's weight.
5. Advance both crutches and swing both feet forward.
6. The right foot acts like a balance.
7. The body swings through and beyond the crutches.

PHARMACOLOGICAL AND PARENTERAL THERAPIES

Multiple Choice

127. A 4-year-old child has been admitted with second-degree burns and is undergoing debridement of the wounds. Morphine 1 mg IV push has been administered. Following administration of this medication, the nurse makes the following observations:

- Pulse: 96
- Respirations: 28
- Blood pressure: 84/62
- Child sleeping quietly

Which nursing action is most appropriate?

1. Administer 100% oxygen.
2. Keep the code cart at the bedside.
3. Allow the child to sleep quietly.
4. Administer naloxone (Narcan).

128. While initiating a blood transfusion for a child with a hemoglobin 8.5 g/dL, what would be the priority of care for this client?

1. Administer the first 50 mL of blood slowly and infuse the rest over 30 minutes.
2. Allow the blood to warm at room temperature for 2 hours.
3. Administer prophylactic epinephrine.
4. Administer the first 50 mL of blood slowly and monitor the child closely.

129. A 7-year-old child has an order for IV fluid of normal saline, 250 cc, to run from 12 midnight to 6 A.M. At what rate should the nurse set the infusion pump?

1. 21 mL/h.
2. 42 mL/h.
3. 50 mL/h.
4. 84 mL/h.

130. Which statement made by a 9-year-old client who is newly diagnosed with diabetes indicates an understanding of the daily diabetes management?

1. "I might need to eat a snack before playing ball."
2. "I need to prick my finger once a week."
3. "Every time I need insulin, I should give myself a shot in my left arm."
4. "I can eat anything I want."

Fill in the Blank

131. An order reads as follows: "Heparin 12,500 U in 250 mL of D_5W intravenously. Infuse at 20 U/kg/hr." The child is 10 years old and weighs 66 pounds. What is the flow rate in milliliters per hour?

_____

Multiple Choice

132. After administering Amoxcil oral suspension to their 2-year-old child with an ear infection, the parents inform that nurse that the child developed a chest rash. What is the most appropriate action for the nurse to take?

1. Tell the parents to adhere to the schedule for giving the Amoxcil.
2. Tell the parents to decrease the dose by half for the next dose.
3. Tell the parents to administer syrup of ipecac.
4. Inform the physician and tell the parents to stop the medication.

133. In addition to the dosage of the drug, what needs to be discussed with the parents of a 6-year-old child with Crohn's disease fibrosis in the teaching session for taking sulfasalazine?

1. Possibility of weight gain.
2. Need to take a folic acid supplement.
3. Taking the sulfasalazine prior to meals for better absorption.
4. Limiting water and beverage intake.

134. Which parameter should the nurse check before administering oral digoxin to a 1-year-old client?

1. Blood pressure.
2. Weight.
3. Heart rate.
4. Potassium level.

135. Which action would be appropriate to minimize pain and local reactions when administering immunizations to a 6-month-old client?

1. Select a 2-inch needle to deposit the antigen deep into the muscle mass.
2. Administer the injection into the deltoid muscle.
3. Apply a topical anesthetic to the injection site 1 hour before the injection.
4. Give an oral syrup of pain medicine on arrival to the clinic.

SECTION I

SECTION II

SECTION III

SECTION IV

SECTION V

SECTION VI

SECTION VII

SECTION VIII

SECTION IX

SECTIO X

136. Which technique should be used in the administration of the measles, mumps, and rubella (MMR) vaccine to a 12-month-old client? (Select all that apply.)

1. Hold the skin tight around the injection site.
2. Insert the needle into the injection site at a 90-degree angle.
3. Grasp and raise the skin by 0.5 to 1 inch around the injection site.
4. Remove any air bubbles in the syringe.
5. Aspirate.
6. Insert the needle into the injection site at a 30-degree angle.

137. The physician issues the following order for a patient: 375 mg of ampicillin IV every 6 hours. The ampicillin is available at a concentration of 250 mg/mL. How many milliliters of ampicillin should the nurse administer?

1. 0.67 mL.
2. 1.0 mL.
3. 1.5 mL.
4. 3.0 mL.

138. Which statement by a 7-year-old client would indicate an understanding of when to take medication (via an inhaler)?

1. "When I remove the inhaler, I can exhale through my mouth."
2. "I need to inhale the medicine and then hold my breath to the count of 10."
3. "I need to depress the top of the inhaler as I begin to take a breath."
4. "After one puff, I can immediately give myself another puff."

139. Which emergency medication should the nurse administer to a child with ventricular tachycardia with a pulse and poor perfusion?

1. Epinephrine 0.01 mg/kg IV.
2. Amiodarone 5 mg/kg IV.
3. Atropine 0.02 mg/kg IV.
4. Dopamine 10 mcg/kg/min IV infusion.

140. Which instruction would be given to the parents of a child receiving oral Deltasone regarding when and how to take the medication?

1. On an empty stomach.
2. With breakfast.

3. Once a day with milk.
4. Before bedtime.

141. A 9-year-old client is receiving one unit of packed red blood cells. Which finding on assessment would indicate a possible hemolytic reaction? (Select all that apply.)

1. Temperature of 97.6°F.
2. Shaking.
3. Tightness in chest.
4. Bilateral crackles.
5. Red or black urine.
6. Flank pain.

142. A 3-year-old child weighs 33 pounds and is diagnosed with lower lobe pneumonia. The physician orders amoxicillin 175 mg by mouth every 8 hours. The oral suspension of amoxicillin is available at a concentration of 250 mg/5 mL. How many milliliters of amoxicillin should the nurse administer?

1. 3.5 mL.
2. 0.875 mL.
3. 7.0 mL.
4. 0.14 mL.

143. The physician orders Coumadin for a 15-year-old quadriplegic client who is confined to a wheelchair and has a past history of deep vein thrombosis. Which lab test should be done monthly?

1. Hemoglobin.
2. Prothrombin time.
3. Partial thromboplastin time.
4. Bleeding time.

144. A 6-month-old infant is scheduled for another diphtheria, tetanus, and pertussis (DPT) immunization. According to the mother, after the previous DPT immunization, the infant had a temperature of 102.8°F on the following day. Prior to administering this DPT vaccine, what would be the most appropriate nursing action?

1. Inform the physician.
2. Divide the dose in half, give half the dose now in one leg, and have the child come back tomorrow for the second dose in the other leg.
3. Administer the entire dose and instruct the mother to give the child acetaminophen (Tylenol) a total of three times every 4 to 6 hours.
4. Withhold the vaccine.

Identification

145. A 14-year-old client is admitted with diabetic ketoacidosis. The physician orders blood glucose testing every 4 hours and sliding-scale regular insulin.

Blood Glucose Level (mg/dL)	Regular Insulin Order
0–149	No insulin
150–199	4 units
200–249	6 units
250–300	8 units
> 300	Notify physician

At 2 P.M., the client's blood sugar is 262. On the syringe below, identify the appropriate amount of regular insulin that the client should receive.

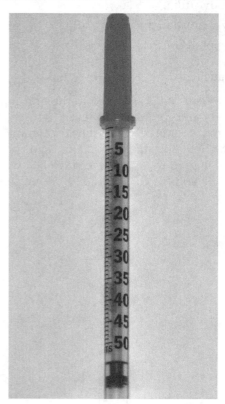

Multiple Choice

146. Which medication can be administered intravenously to reverse the effects of a benzodiazepine overdose?

1. Activated charcoal.
2. Flumazenil (Romazicon).
3. Nalozone (Narcan).
4. Pyridostigmine (Mestinon).

147. A 19-month-old child weighs 22 pounds and has an order for 200 mcg digoxin to be given intravenously. You have a vial of digoxin at a concentration of 0.1 mg/mL. How many milliliters of the solution will you need to deliver the ordered dose?

1. 0.002 mL.
2. 0.2 mL.
3. 0.22 mL.
4. 2.0 mL.

148. A 4-year-old client will be discharged and will receive total parenteral nutrition (TPN) at home. Which statement by the child's parent reflects a correct understanding of TPN administration?

1. "When the bag is empty, I can disconnect and wait for the home health nurse to arrive to begin the next bag."
2. "I will need to supplement my child's diet to provide the essential protein, glucose, vitamins, and minerals."
3. "Because the glucose concentration is high, it is important for me to do a finger prick three times a day to test blood sugar."
4. "The infusion rate can be adjusted to accommodate the home schedule and allow my child to rest uninterrupted."

149. A 22-month-old client is receiving Nystatin 200,000 units via oral swab every 6 hours. For which side effect should the nurse assess the client?

1. Oral thrush.
2. Thrombocytopenia.
3. Leukopenia.
4. Diarrhea.

Fill in the Blank

150. A 9-year-old weighs 55 pounds and is to receive cefuroxime sodium 750 mg IV every 6 hours. The recommended dose of cefuroxime sodium for children older than 1 month is 50–133 mg/kg every 24 hours. Is the ordered dose within the recommended limits? (Yes or No)

_____

Multiple Choice

151. A child is found to be in pulseless electrical activity, and immediate resuscitation is begun. Intravenous fluids and medications are ordered.

Which route should be used to administer the fluids and medications?

1. Subcutaneous.
2. Intramuscular.
3. Intraosseous.
4. Endotracheal.

152. A 9-year-old client is given his heparin injection on time, but it was administered intravenously instead of subcutaneously. The incident was discovered 2 hours after administration. Which plan would be most appropriate?

1. Assess for evidence of bleeding and notify the parents.
2. Document the event on an incident report, and notify the physician.
3. Hold the next scheduled heparin dose.
4. Order a PTT and INR levels, and notify the physician.

Identification

153. A 5-year-old child weighs 40 pounds and has a seizure disorder. The physician orders phenobarbital 60 mg by mouth three times a day as treatment. The elixir is available in the form of phenobarbital 15 mg/5 mL. On the medication cup below, locate the volume that would be administered to this client.

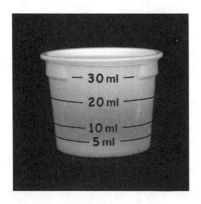

Multiple Choice

154. Which instruction would be included in a teaching plan for a caregiver of a client diagnosed with *Sarcoptes scabiei* infection who is to apply permethrin 5% cream (Elimite)?

1. The cream must remain on the client for 8–14 hours.
2. A total of two applications is needed.

3. The cream is applied only to areas with the rash.
4. The cream will also be effective for itching.

155. What lab test would be most important to monitor on a 6-year-old client who is receiving amphotericin B?

1. Blood glucose levels.
2. Serum calcium levels.
3. Serum creatinine levels.
4. Cardiac enzyme levels.

156. For which major side effect(s) should a nurse monitor the client when administering a loading dose of phenytoin sodium (Dilantin) to a 4-year-old child?

1. Hypertension.
2. Bradycardia.
3. Hypertension and bradycardia.
4. Hypotension and tachycardia.

Identification

157. A 16-year-old is admitted to the unit post-operatively and complains of severe nausea. The physician has ordered ondansetron (Zofran) 3 mg IV push. The medication is available at a concentration of 75 mg/50 mL. On the syringe below, identify the volume that would be administered to this client.

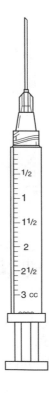

Multiple Choice

158. How would the nurse position the ear of a 2-year-old client while initiating eardrops?

1. Use an otoscope.
2. Pull the ear down and back.
3. Pull the ear up and back.
4. Touch chin to chest.

159. Which nursing action is most appropriate when inserting a rectal suppository in a 9-month-old infant?

1. There is no need to lubricate the suppository; just insert it into the rectal vault.
2. Using one finger, insert the suppository at least 4 inches so that it is beyond the internal sphincter.
3. Hold the buttocks together for at least 5 minutes to promote absorption and onset of action.
4. Instruct the child to lay still and squeeze the buttocks together for at least 5 minutes, and then encourage play.

REDUCTION OF RISK POTENTIAL

Multiple Choice

160. Which symptom is indicative of an increase in ineffective oxygenation in a 6-month-old infant with coarctation of the aorta?

1. Inspiratory wheeze bilaterally and pulse oximeter reading of 94%.
2. Restlessness and substernal retractions.
3. Heart rate of 130 and respiratory rate of 32.
4. Weight loss and pale, warm extremities.

161. A 5-year-old client receives blood transfusions every 4 weeks as treatment for β-thalassemia (Cooley's anemia). Which observation would the nurse identify as the desired response for this treatment?

1. Ability to play soccer.
2. Hemoglobin level of 6.0 g/dL.
3. Decreased appetite.
4. Frequent napping.

162. Which method is the best way for the nurse to evaluate the effectiveness of a 2-month-old infant's gavage feedings?

1. Consult with the nutritionist to determine the feedings' effectiveness.
2. Objective findings include an increased respiratory rate.

3. Weigh the client daily and note a 2-ounce weight gain.
4. The parents state that the infant appears more content and satisfied.

Identification

163. A nurse is assessing the apical impulse of a 4-year-old client. Identify the area where the nurse should place the stethoscope to locate the apical impulse of this client.

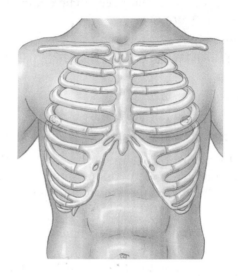

Multiple Choice

164. A 4-year-old child presents with possible rheumatic fever. Which findings will the nurse observe in this patient?

1. Macular rash that is pruritic.
2. Decreased antistreptolysin O titer.
3. Elevated C-reactive protein levels.
4. Decreased erythrocyte sedimentation rates.

165. Which assessment data would indicate that a 9-year-old client with chronic glomerulonephritis is in chronic renal failure?

1. Serum creatinine level of 1.0 mg/dL.
2. Urinary output of 20 mL/h.
3. Serum blood urea nitrogen level of 18 mg/dL.
4. Serum potassium level of 4.3 mEq/L.

166. A 12-year-old girl is diagnosed with systemic lupus erythematosus (SLE). Which statement made by the client would indicate a need for further teaching regarding minimizing exacerbations and complications associated with SLE?

1. "I should not skip taking my prednisone pills."
2. "I should wear a medic alert bracelet."

3. "I need to maximize my time outdoors and maintain a suntan."

4. "Taking hydroxchloroquine (Plaquenil) will help with my arthritis."

167. A 5-year-old client underwent a cardiac catheterization through the left femoral site. Which postprocedural nursing assessment(s) would justify calling the physician? (Select all that apply.)

1. Blood pressure of 72/50.

2. Intact dressing that needs to be reinforced due to bloody drainage.

3. Pulse of 92.

4. Left pedal pulse weaker than right pedal pulse.

5. Respirations of 26.

6. Equal, bilateral radial pulses.

7. Bilateral pink, warm toes.

168. A 14-month-old client with an Arnold-Chiari malformation has a ventriculoperitoneal shunt inserted. Which nursing assessment would indicate a malfunction in this shunt?

1. The infant cries but quiets when rocked or held.

2. The infant has a bulging anterior fontanel with opisthotonos.

3. The infant has increased abdominal girth.

4. The infant's pupils are equal with a brisk response to light.

169. A 6-year-old client receives midazolam and fentanyl in titrating amounts for conscious sedation during a chest tube insertion. The nurse reviews the following information:

Heart rate: 88

Respirations: 14

Pulse oximeter: 93%

Based on this assessment, which nursing action is appropriate?

1. Withhold further administration of midazolam only.

2. Withhold further administration of both medications.

3. Administer more midazolam and fentanyl.

4. Change to propofol because it is shorter acting.

170. A 7-year-old client is diagnosed with complete heart block, and a permanent demand pacemaker set at a rate of 80 is implanted. Which nursing

assessment would indicate a malfunction in the pacemaker?

1. Radial pulse rate of 150 and regular.

2. Blood pressure of 95/62.

3. Apical pulse rate of 74 and regular.

4. Outline of the pacemaker generator is noticeable under the skin.

171. Which finding(s) would the nurse anticipate in a 14-year-old client with Addison's disease? (Select all that apply.)

1. Blood glucose of 160 mg/dL.

2. Hyperpigmentation.

3. Blood pressure of 88/40.

4. Cold, clammy skin.

5. Petechial hemorrhages.

6. Insomnia.

172. A newborn has tested positive for phenylketonuria. What information would the nurse include in the teaching plan for the parents prior to the infant's discharge?

1. It is necessary to feed the child a formula containing increased protein.

2. The child may need to be fed a formula containing tyrosine.

3. Breastfeeding is an absolute contraindication.

4. It is important to maintain phenylalanine levels at more than 6 mg/dL.

173. A 14-year-old child presents with hyperparathyroidism. Which findings will the nurse observe with this client?

1. Positive Chvostek sign.

2. Serum calcium of 10.2 mg/dL.

3. Easily fatigued.

4. Serum sodium of 150 mEq/L.

174. A 2-month-old infant is 2 days postoperative tracheoesophageal fistula repair. A complete blood count reveals a hemoglobin of 8.6 g/dL and an erythrocyte count of 2.5 million/mm³. Which symptoms would the nurse most likely find on assessment?

1. Tachycardia and flushing.

2. Slight pallor and tires easily while crying.

3. Projectile vomiting after oral bottle feeding.

4. Sluggish capillary refill and hypotension.

Identification

175. A nurse is eliciting reflexes in a 6-week-old child during a physical examination. Identify the area the nurse would touch to elicit a rooting reflex.

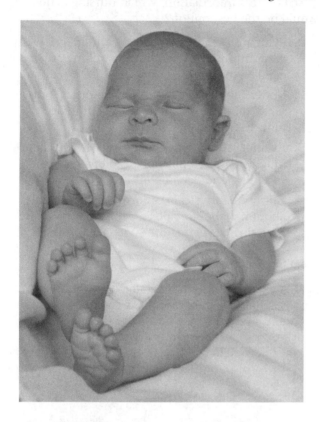

Multiple Choice

176. A 4-month-old client is in congestive heart failure and is receiving furosemide (Lasix) twice a day. Which assessment is the best technique to detect the effectiveness of this medication?

1. Assess for bulging fontanels.
2. Count and weigh the number of diapers.
3. Measure intake and output.
4. Weigh the infant daily.

177. A 7-year-old client is scheduled for a cardiac catheterization. Which priority nursing assessment finding should be reported to the physician?

1. The child insists on taking a stuffed teddy bear to the procedure.
2. The child has diminished palpable pedal pulses bilaterally.
3. The child has an allergic reaction of hives to shellfish.

4. The child has cool lower extremities with brisk capillary refill bilaterally.

178. Which nursing goal would be appropriate for a 6-year-old client with sepsis who has developed acute respiratory distress syndrome?

1. Prevention of hypoxia associated with the increased permeability of the alveolar-capillary membrane.
2. Preparation of the child and parents for anticipated surgery to remove damaged lung tissue.
3. Decreased inflammatory response of the sepsis cascade.
4. Increased intravascular volume so as to maintain cardiac output and sustain blood pressure.

179. Which actions should the nurse take when feeding an infant through an orogastric tube? (Select all that apply.)

1. Use petroleum jelly to lubricate the feeding tube.
2. Aspirate the stomach contents.
3. Auscultate with a stethoscope to determine tube placement.
4. Confirm each tube placement with an x-ray.
5. Deliver feedings through a syringe barrel attached to the feeding tube.
6. Prior to inserting the feeding tube, measure the tube from the tip of the child's nose to the earlobe to the umbilicus.

180. Which observation would alert the nurse to the initial development and onset of toxic shock syndrome in a 15-year-old female?

1. Fever of 101°F.
2. Desquamation of the palms and soles.
3. Presence of macular erythroderma.
4. Hypertension with syncope and dizziness.

181. What would be the highest priority when providing care to a 7-year-old client admitted to the hospital with sickle cell crisis?

1. Administer prophylactic antibiotics.
2. Initiate intravenous fluids to maximize hydration.
3. Insist the client rest instead of reading a book.
4. Insert a urinary catheter to assist in measuring accurate output.

SECTION I
SECTION II
SECTION III
SECTION IV
SECTION V
SECTION VI
SECTION VII
SECTION VIII
SECTION IX
SECTION X

182. A 4-year-old has a tracheostomy and is in the intensive care unit on a volume-cycled positive ventilator. The high-volume alarm sounds and the child is observed to be quite agitated. Which finding should the nurse expect?

1. The child is breathing over the ventilator settings.
2. The ventilator tubing is disconnected from the tracheostomy tube.
3. The child is biting the endotracheal tube.
4. There is a leak in the endotracheal tube cuff.

Identification

183. A 3-week-old infant is being evaluated for a patent ductus arteriosus (PDA). Identify the area where a PDA occurs.

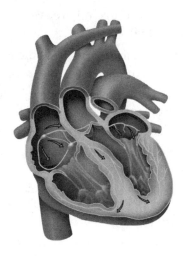

Multiple Choice

184. A 9-year-old client is admitted to the hospital after sustaining a basilar skull fracture. Which nursing assessment would support the complication of the skull fracture?

1. Pupils equal and respond briskly to light.
2. Clear drainage from the nose.
3. Ecchymosis on the face but most prominent under the eyes.
4. Temperature of 97.5°F.

185. The nurse is caring for an 11-year-old client with a thoracic spinal cord injury. Vital signs and laboratory results on this child are as follows:

Blood pressure: 104/62

Heart rate: 67

Respiratory rate: 12

Arterial pH: 7.2

Arterial pCO_2: 58 mm Hg

Arterial pO_2: 88 mm Hg

Arterial HCO_3: 30 mEq/L

Based on this information, which nursing action would be the best option?

1. Evaluate the airway patency, administer pain medication, and encourage coughing and deep breathing.
2. Notify the physician, request an order for a sedative, and reevaluate the client in 30 minutes.
3. Evaluate the airway patency, place the client in high Fowler's position, and encourage coughing and deep breathing.
4. Notify the physician, inform the physician about metabolic acidosis, and anticipate initiating oxygen at 60% via face mask.

Identification

186. A 2-month-old infant is diagnosed with aortic stenosis. Identify the area where the nurse should place the stethoscope to ausculate the midsystolic murmur associated with this condition.

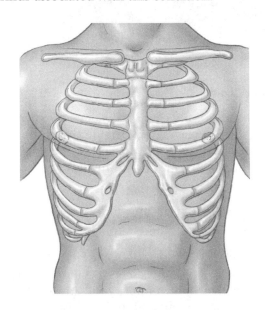

Multiple Choice

187. A 5-year-old boy with acute lymphoid leukemia (ALL) is admitted to the hospital. Vital signs and laboratory results on admission are as follows:

Blood pressure: 90/60

Heart rate: 116

Respiratory rate: 28

Pulse oximeter: 94%

Temperature: 98.8°F

RBC: 4.2 million/mm³

Platelets: 120,000/μL

WBC: 8,000/μL

Based on this nursing assessment, what is the most appropriate nursing diagnosis?

1. Impaired gas exchange related to decreased RBCs.
2. Potential for injury related to decreased platelets.
3. Activity intolerance related to altered respiratory function.
4. Potential for infection related to altered immune system.

188. A 14-month-old child is admitted with suspected pneumonia. The chest x-ray reveals a right lower lob consolidation. During auscultation of the right lower lobe, which finding related to the lungs would the nurse expect on assessment?

1. Inspiratory wheeze.
2. Bronchovesicular sounds.
3. Diminished breath sounds.
4. Tympanic hyperresonance.

189. A 4-month-old child has been hospitalized with Hirschsprung disease. The infant is lethargic, has a temperature of 101.4°F, and has experienced diarrhea and vomiting for the past 2 days. Which nursing action is most appropriate in evaluating this infant for fluid volume deficit?

1. Obtain the infant's weight daily, and assess for gain or loss.
2. Determine the infant's osmolality from urinalysis and blood work.
3. Assess the quality of skin turgor and amount of tenting.
4. Maintain strict recording of the infant's intake and output.

190. The nurse is preparing to do a postoperative assessment on a 5-year-old child who has undergone a tonsillectomy. During the assessment, the nurse should be alert for bleeding. Which signs and symptoms would indicate active bleeding? (Select all that apply.)

1. Frequent swallowing.
2. Drowsiness.
3. Heart rate of 90 beats/min.
4. Frequent clearing of throat.
5. Mouth breathing.
6. Dark red vomitus.

191. A 9-year-old child sustained a right hemothorax in a motor vehicle crash. Which assessment would determine the effective functioning of the chest drainage system?

1. Clots and bloody drainage in the chest tube.
2. Bubbling in the suction chamber.
3. Intermittent bubbling in the water seal chamber.
4. Blood leaking around the chest tube insertion site.

192. You are caring for a 7-year-old client who sustained severe burns and is intubated and on the ventilator at 40% FiO₂. You notice that the child is anxious and attempting to cough, and the respiratory rate is 40. What is your first action?

1. Increase the amount of oxygen.
2. Administer pain medication.
3. Call the physician and prepare for bronchoscopy.
4. Auscultate lung sounds and suction if needed.

PHYSIOLOGICAL ADAPTATION

Multiple Choice

193. A 9-year-old client is experiencing sepsis. The physician has ordered the child's medication to be regulated to maintain a mean arterial pressure (MAP) between 65 and 75 mm Hg. Which of the child's blood pressure readings meet this prescribed goal?

1. 80/45.
2. 85/50.
3. 85/60.
4. 90/50.

194. A child weighing 27 kg is admitted to the burn unit with third-degree burns to the chest, face, and extremities. During the acute phase (i.e., first 48 hours) of a major burn injury, which assessment findings should the nurse immediately report?

1. Temperature of 100°F.
2. Edema of the hands and feet.
3. Urinary output of 150 mL in 8 hours.
4. Decreased sensation in the extremities.

195. Which action would be the first priority in a 6-year-old child with anaphylaxis?

1. Prevent future antigen exposure.
2. Administer oxygen via face mask.
3. Obtain vascular access.
4. Administer an antibiotic.

196. Organize the following steps for synchronized cardioversion in chronological order (with 1 being the first step in this procedure).

1. Consider sedation.
2. Observe for markers on the R wave.
3. Press the synch button.
4. Attach the monitor leads.
5. Make sure everyone is clear.
6. Apply the conductor pads.

197. A 3-year-old child is admitted to the hospital with a moderate concussion after falling down a flight of stairs. Which physician's order should the nurse question?

1. Keep the head of the bed elevated by 15–30 degrees.
2. NPO and initiate IV fluids at 20 mL/h.
3. Vital signs and neuro checks every shift.
4. Acetaminophen 250 mg PO, every 4–6 hours PRN pain.

198. While the nurse is administering IV chemotherapy to a 6-year-old client with leukemia, the child suddenly begins to itch and wheeze. What should the nurse do next?

1. Stop the infusion immediately.
2. Slow the rate of the infusion.
3. Observe the child continuously for the next 15 minutes.
4. Explain to the child that this is normal.

199. A 4-year-old client is admitted with acute respiratory distress and is diagnosed with asthma. On assessment, you find the child sitting upright and sweating profusely; the client has wheezing that is audible without a stethoscope, and diminished breath sounds upon auscultation. What is your first action?

1. Check the chart to determine the last nebulizer treatment.
2. Notify the physician and encourage the child to lie down.

3. Stay with the child, call for help, and administer oxygen.
4. Administer epinephrine and oxygen while waiting for the physician.

200. A 9-month-old child is admitted with a fever and cough, and *Mycobacterium tuberculosis* infection is the suspected diagnosis. Select all of the infection control precautions that the nurse should implement when caring for this client.

1. Allow the door of the room to remain open.
2. Have the client wear a mask when leaving the room.
3. Wear sterile gloves when entering the room.
4. Place the client in a semi-private room.
5. Wear a mask when working within 3 feet of the client.
6. Place the client in a negative-pressure room.

201. Which assessment finding indicates effective chest compressions during CPR?

1. Palpable carotid pulse.
2. Dilated pupils bilaterally.
3. Sluggish capillary refill.
4. Pink mucous membranes.

202. A 6-month-old client is admitted for suspected Hirschsprung disease. Which assessment data would you expect the nurse to obtain?

1. Rectal bleeding, persistent diarrhea, and weight loss.
2. Diarrhea, abdominal distention, and history of constipation.
3. Irritability, bloody diarrhea, and severe dehydration.
4. History of colic, explosive bloody diarrhea, and vomiting.

203. During the suctioning of a 5-year-old client with an endotracheal tube, the heart rate decreases from 108 to 60 beats/min. What would be the priority nursing action?

1. Finish suctioning the child.
2. Stop suctioning and reconnect the child to the ventilator.
3. Administer epinephrine IV.
4. Stop suctioning and assess the breath sounds.

204. A 7-year-old child is diagnosed with insulin-dependent diabetes mellitus. The child and parents are being taught what should occur if the child presents with signs and symptoms of hypoglycemia. Which statement made by the parents would indicate an understanding of the teaching?

1. "It is important for the child to eat 4–6 Lifesavers candies or drink orange juice."
2. "It is important to increase activity prior to insulin administration."
3. "It is important to decrease the amount of long-acting insulin."
4. "It is important for the child to rest in bed until the symptoms subside."

Identification

205. A 7-month-old infant is brought to the Emergency Department in cardiac arrest. Cardiopulmonary resuscitation (CPR) is being performed. Identify the area where the pulse should be checked.

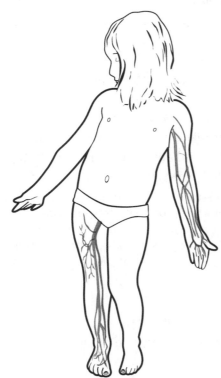

Multiple Choice

206. The physician admits a 4-year-old client to the hospital for severe dehydration with diarrhea, vomiting, and fever. Which method is most appropriate for rehydrating the child?

1. Give Pedialyte orally.
2. Give soft drinks and juices that have been diluted.

3. Initiate continuous intravenous fluids.
4. Give small amounts of gelatin and clear liquids.

207. A child is admitted in sickle cell crisis. Which action would be the highest priority for this client?

1. Administer morphine intravenously.
2. Administer prophylactic antibiotics.
3. Transfuse with 1 unit of packed red blood cells.
4. Initiate intravenous fluids.

208. The nurse is caring for an 8-year-old client who has undergone a cardiac catheterization. The child complains that the bandage is wet. The nurse finds the bandage and bed soaked with blood. Based on this information, which nursing intervention would be most appropriate?

1. Call the physician and change the bed linens.
2. Monitor vital signs and document findings.
3. Call the physician and place the child in Trendelenburg position.
4. Apply direct pressure to the wound site and notify the physician.

209. Which assessment findings indicate an early problem with shock in a 4-year-old child with severe second- and third-degree burns of the chest?

1. Widening pulse pressure and bradycardia.
2. Lethargy and cool, clammy skin.
3. Tachycardia and Kussmaul respirations.
4. Pain and progressive wound healing.

210. The nurse is monitoring a 5-year-old client's ECG strip and notes supraventricular tachycardia at a rate of 200–210. Which medication should the nurse administer?

1. Adenosine (Adenocard) IV.
2. Atropine sulfate (Atropine) IV.
3. Epinephrine IV.
4. Lidocaine hydrochloride (Xylocaine) IV.

211. A 3-year-old child is brought to the Emergency Department in respiratory distress. The physician informs you that the client will need to be intubated. In preparing to assist the physician, which equipment is appropriate for this procedure? (Select all that apply.)

1. Cuffed endotracheal tube.
2. Ambu bag.
3. Oral suction.

SECTION I

SECTION II

SECTION III

SECTION IV

SECTION V

SECTION VI

SECTION VII

SECTION VIII

SECTION IX

SECTION X

4. Face mask.

5. Sterile gloves.

6. Laryngoscope.

212. A 22-month-old child is hospitalized for heart failure. During the night, the child awakens crying and calling for the mother. The nurse assesses the child and notes dyspnea, jugular vein distention, crackles, and pink, frothy sputum. After the nurse begins oxygen by 40% face mask, which action should be taken next?

1. Place the child in a crib with a blanket and notify the physician.

2. Dim the lights and allow the mother to rock the child to sleep.

3. Stay with the child and call for assistance to notify the physician.

4. Continue to monitor the client frequently and increase IV fluid rate.

213. A 10-year-old child begins to choke and cough on a piece of candy. Which priority nursing action should the nurse implement?

1. Provide abdominal thrusts.

2. Give 5 back slaps, followed by 5 abdominal thrusts.

3. Look in the mouth and perform a blind finger sweep.

4. Allow a child to expel the candy by himself or herself.

214. A 4-year-old child enters the emergency room with an acute asthma attack. Admission vital signs are as follows:

Pulse: 120

Blood pressure: 95/62

Respiratory rate: 50, with substernal retractions and inspiratory and expiratory wheezes

Temperature: 99.5°F

Pulse oximeter: 92%

In which position should the nurse place the child?

1. High Fowler's.

2. Supine.

3. Trendelenburg.

4. Modified Sims'.

215. The nurse is caring for a child with acute renal failure who is in the intensive care unit. Which assessment finding would indicate a sign of hyperkalemia?

1. Dyspnea.

2. Seizure.

3. Oliguria.

4. ECG changes.

Fill in the Blank

216. A nurse is the first person on the scene of a motor vehicle crash and approaches a child who is lying on the ground. What is the first action the nurse should take in basic life support?

_____

Multiple Choice

217. A 3-year-old client is admitted for suspected meningitis. In delivering nursing care to this child, what would the priority action be?

1. Administer antibiotic therapy when the diagnosis is confirmed.

2. Administer analgesics as needed.

3. Immediately initiate isolation precautions.

4. Initiate isolation precautions when the diagnosis is confirmed.

218. An 18-month-old client is admitted to the hospital with a fever of 104°F, respirations of 56/min, suprasternal retractions, and a pulse oximeter reading of 85%; the infant is also drooling. Acute epiglottitis is suspected. Which equipment would be important to have at the bedside?

1. Code cart.

2. Tracheostomy tray.

3. Intravenous infusion pump.

4. Defibrillator.

219. You are caring for a 7-year-old client with a brain tumor. Which observation would alert you to the possible development of syndrome of inappropriate antidiuretic hormone secretion (SIADH)?

1. Peripheral edema.

2. Urinary output of 30 mL/h.

3. Serum sodium of 130 mEq/L.

4. Weight loss.

220. A 3-year-old client is admitted with a nephroblastoma (Wilm's tumor). Which nursing action would be most important to include when planning this client's care?

  1. Post a sign that reads "Do Not Palpate Abdomen."
  2. Prepare the patient for surgery within the next 24 hours.
  3. Prepare the parents for the initiation of chemotherapy after surgery.
  4. Initiate intravenous fluids as ordered.

221. The physician has determined that a 5-year-old client who is in respiratory distress needs intubation. In preparing to assist the physician with rapid-sequence intubation, organize the following steps in chronological order (with 1 being the first step in this procedure).

  1. Preoxygenate with 100% oxygen.
  2. Monitor the child's ECG and pulse oximeter readings.
  3. Apply crichoid pressure if needed.
  4. Administer sedation.
  5. Obtain a baseline assessment.
  6. Auscultate the breath sounds bilaterally.

222. During the initial assessment of a child with a major burn injury of the chest and face, what is the nurse's first action?

  1. Assess the airway patency.
  2. Assess the presence of pulses.
  3. Determine the percentage of burn area.
  4. Initiate intravenous fluid replacement.

ANSWERS AND RATIONALES

MANAGEMENT OF CARE

1. **Correct Answer: 3**

   Rationale: At the 2-month visit, scheduled immunizations include DTP (diphtheria, tetanus, and pertussis), IPV (inactivated polio), Hib (*Haemophilus influenzae* type B), and PCV (pneumococcal).

2. **Correct Answers: 1 and 6**

   Rationale: Medications are delivered through a gastrostomy tube with a syringe and are flushed with the tube clamped after administration. Medications are delivered at room temperature and usually mixed with water if too viscous. Tablets are crushed to a fine powder. Enteric-coated medications are never crushed.

3. **Correct Answer: 2**

   Rationale: A client in sickle cell crisis is the priority because oxygenation is the problem to be addressed. Oxygen needs to be initiated, and an IV needs to be started so that fluids can be infused for hydration. The client with acute appendicitis will need to be prepared for surgery. The other two clients have chronic conditions.

4. **Correct Answer: 3**

   Rationale: Any suspected abuse must be reported to the local authorities. Healthcare providers have various mechanisms available by which they can make such reports. Some use social workers; others directly inform the child abuse hotline. Documentation of assessment findings is crucial, as it assists in putting the case together.

5. **Correct Answer: Physical therapy**

   Rationale: Physical therapists will assist in recommending exercises and will be an integral part in teaching the client how to use assistive devices.

6. **Correct Answer: 1**

   Rationale: While starting an IV, administering appropriate antibiotics is important. The child also needs to be isolated from other children to prevent possible spread of the infection. In addition, the child will need a lumbar puncture to obtain a CSF culture so as to make a definitive diagnosis and determine the most appropriate antibiotic to be administered.

7. **Correct Answer: 3**

   Rationale: Bathing is an activity that CNAs can perform as long as the client is not compromised or needs a licensed professional.

8. **Correct Answer: 3**

   Rationale: The informed consent process is an active, shared decision-making process between the surgeon and the client and his or her family. The surgeon must provide adequate disclosure of the proposed procedure. Then, there must be clear understanding and comprehension of the procedure to be done. Finally, the consent must be voluntary and not forced.

9. **Correct Answer: 1**

   Rationale: Information sharing between parents and the healthcare team should be unbiased, supportive, and constant. Family-centered care focuses on the components of respect, collaboration, and support.

10. **Correct Answers: 2 and 4**

    Rationale: IV fluids are ordered to infuse continuously, so the continuous IV fluids would not be disconnected. The IV piggyback fluids would be connected to the primary IV fluid set at the port closest to the primary fluid bag and would need to be hung higher than the primary fluid bag.

11. **Correct Answer: 4**

    Rationale: NPH insulin is an intermediate-acting insulin. It is important that the client eat at normal times because the onset of action for this insulin is 1–3 hours and the peak action occurs 8 hours following its administration.

12. **Correct Answer: 3**

    Rationale: The client in skin traction requires routine care and ongoing assessment. The other clients need initial assessment, initial teaching, and specialized IV and medication training.

13. **Correct Answer: 1**

    Rationale: An immunosuppressed patient has a decreased number of white blood cells and is at increased risk for infection.

14. Correct Answers: **1, 2, 3, and 6**

    Rationale: Hands should be washed prior to beginning a dressing change. Next, gloves should be donned and worn as the old dressing is removed and discarded. A dressing kit is typically used that contains new gloves and all essential supplies. A Groshong catheter is a type of central venous line that is external to the body. After inspecting the site, the skin should be cleaned by using a circular motion with an antiseptic swab; a dressing is then reapplied.

15. Correct Answer: **3**

    Rationale: Given the situation, the best way to handle the situation is for the RN not to embarrass the LPN in front of the client but to use the opportunity as a teaching moment to ensure that the procedure is done correctly.

16. Correct Answer: **1**

    Rationale: A true contraindication for MMR immunization is known altered immunodeficiency. Current antimicrobial therapy is not a contraindication to receiving the vaccine.

17. Correct Answer: **2**

    Rationale: A person's autonomy and ability to make decisions that affect his or her care need to be considered and honored if the decision is the most beneficial and least harmful.

18. Correct Answer: **2**

    Rationale: Both clients can be cared for by the same nurse, in the same room. There is no need to move either one, as both clients are within the same age range and neither requires isolation. A nurse providing care to any client would be expected to adhere to standard precautions.

19. Correct Answers: **1, 2, 3, and 5**

    Rationale: Management of a client returning from surgery with a chest tube includes being prepared to apply wall suction to the ordered amount and being prepared for a possible disconnection or abrupt discontinuation of the chest tube.

20. Correct Answer: **3**

    Rationale: The planning phase of the nursing process includes developing the goals and specifying the outcomes that assist in creating the nursing care plan or plan of care for the client.

21. Correct Answer: **2**

    Rationale: When involved with the direct care of a burn client, staff must wear gloves, caps, gowns, and masks to prevent an infection. Burn patients are susceptible to infections. Nevertheless, antibiotics are not administered until specific cultures and organisms are identified.

22. Correct Answer: **3**

    Rationale: The five "rights" for medication administration include right patient and right dose.

23. Correct Answers: **2, 3, 4, 6, and 7**

    Rationale: Room temperature and PO intake are not critical to communicate in report. The client is not taking anything orally, because nutritional support is being given through enteric feedings.

24. Correct Answer: **3**

    Rationale: Upon arrival back to the unit, vital signs would need to be performed. Assessment of the child should include also observing the dressing and assessing for the presence of pain.

25. Correct Answer: **3**

    Rationale: Written consent must be obtained prior to any release of information. Client privacy must be assured.

26. Correct Answer: **4**

    Rationale: Everyone involved in this type of client care should be informed of this information as it directly affects the care of these clients.

27. Correct Answers: **2 and 4**

    Rationale: Have the child's father stay to assist, hold, and comfort the child.

28. Correct Answer: **3**

    Rationale: Peritoneal dialysis involves placement of a peritoneal catheter through which dialysate is infused into the peritoneal cavity; the indwelling catheter allows for exchange of fluid and electrolytes. The client's weight should be measured before and after dialysis, and a description of the fluid drained should be documented.

29. Correct Answer: **2**

    Rationale: The case manager would coordinate the healthcare services that the client and family need.

SECTION I

SECTION II

SECTION III

SECTION IV

SECTION V

SECTION VI

SECTION VII

SECTION VIII

SECTION IX

SECTION X

30. Correct Answer: **1**

    Rationale: Because pulmonary infections are common with cystic fibrosis, the desired outcome of performing accurate and adequate CPT would be a reduction in hospitalizations for pneumonia.

31. Correct Answers: **1, 3, and 5**

    Rationale: Colostomy care consists of washing the hands, removing the pouch and skin barrier, observing the site and skin for redness or irritation, and reapplying the barrier and pouch. Powder and antimicrobial ointment are not used, and sterile gloves are not indicated.

32. Correct Answer: **3**

    Rationale: A history of allergy to bananas is a risk factor suggesting that the client could be allergic to latex. Latex is a substance that is commonly found in surgical gloves.

33. Correct Answer: **2**

    Rationale: The most important aspect of aseptic technique is good hand washing.

34. Correct Answers: **1, 2, 4, and 5**

    Rationale: Most blood products require a microaggregate filter during their administration. Clotting factors are an exception, as the components in these factors would be filtered out by such a screening device.

35. Correct Answer: **3**

    Rationale: Varicella-zoster is highly contagious and is transmitted by direct contact and airborne. The child needs to be isolated, and strict isolation procedures need to be maintained.

36. Correct Answer: **2**

    Rationale: Air embolism is a complication that can occur during a blood transfusion. It is manifested by sudden difficulty in breathing, apprehension, and a sharp pain in the chest.

37. Correct Answer: **3**

    Rationale: Smoke inhalation most likely includes a thermal injury to the tracheobronchial tree. Swelling will occur, so the client's respiratory status needs to be monitored closely. Sometimes endotracheal intubation is necessary to maintain a patent airway.

38. Correct Answer: **1**

    Rationale: The other 3 clients require an initial assessment and complex medication administration and assessment.

39. Correct Answer: **1**

    Rationale: Slight swelling could indicate fluid seeping into the tissues and possibly infiltration.

40. Correct Answer: **2**

    Rationale: To perform eye irrigation, wash hands prior to beginning, and then position the client with the head tilted toward the affected eye so the irritant will be expelled from the eye. Irrigation should continue until the irritant has been washed from the eye.

41. Correct Answer: **3**

    Rationale: Insertion of a urinary catheter is a sterile procedure. To reduce the likelihood of introducing bacteria into the bladder, a new catheter would need to be obtained. Assistance would also be needed to make the procedure as atraumatic as possible.

42. Correct Answer: **4**

    Rationale: When a fire is suspected or confirmed, the nurse's first action should be to remove clients who are in immediate danger and then to activate the fire alarm. One should never yell, "Fire!" An attempt at extinguishing a fire can be made if the proper extinguisher is used—but only after everyone has been removed.

43. Correct Answer: **2**

    Rationale: The last recommended scheduled immunizations would have occurred at the 6-month visit and would have included DPT, Hib, and PCV immunizations. The total number of DPT immunizations would be 3; the number of IPV immunizations would be 2. MMR is not scheduled to be given until the child's next visit.

44. Correct Answer: **1**

    Rationale: The correct technique for administering eardrops to clients who are 3 years old or younger is to pull the earlobe down and back.

SAFETY AND INFECTION CONTROL

45. Correct Answer: 4

Rationale: The 6-month-old infant is the most mobile of the group of infants listed and might inadvertently come across agents that could pose a poisoning risk.

46. Correct Answer: 3

Rationale: A spiral fracture is not the type of injury that would have occurred had a bookcase fallen on the infant. Spiral fracture indicates a twisting of an extremity, which is more indicative of maltreatment.

47. Correct Answer: 4

Rationale: For this procedure, the child needs to be in a side-lying position, with the back closest to the edge of the bed so that the physician can access the site with ease. For everyone's safety, the nurse can position one arm behind the child's neck and the other behind the knees to stabilize the child from sudden movement.

48. Correct Answers: 1, 3, 4, 5, and 6

Rationale: Patient safety is the primary goal. To prevent medication errors, five "rights" related to medication administration are identified: right patient, right medication, right time, right dose, and right route.

49. Correct Answer: 2

Rationale: Medicines—both over-the-counter and prescription—need to be placed in a location that is not accessible to the child. They should also have child-resistant lids to make them more difficult to open.

50. Correct Answer: 3

Rationale: Methamphetamine is a central nervous system stimulant. Symptoms of its overdose include increased blood pressure and heart rate. The heart muscle is irritable, so cardiac arrhythmias can also occur.

51. Correct Answer: 3

Rationale: The car seat needs to be appropriate for an infant, securely anchored with a harness that fits snugly, and placed in the back passenger seat in a rear-facing position.

52. Correct Answers: 2 and 4

Rationale: If a seizure occurs, it is important to stay with the child and remain calm while observing the seizure. Allow the seizure to occur without interference, but protect the child by removing any hazards or hard objects. Do not place anything in the child's mouth, but keep suction available in case the child vomits or excessive saliva is present. Because the patient has a known history of seizures, the side rails of the bed should be padded as a precaution.

53. Correct Answer: 4

Rationale: All toys strung across the top of the crib, such as a mobile, should be removed, because children of this age are able to push up on their hands and knees and could fall.

54. Correct Answer: 1

Rationale: Eggs are not one of the first solid foods introduced. In addition, the consistency of the food could potentially induce choking.

55. Correct Answer: 3

Rationale: Because the child is older than 5 years of age, skateboards can be used with safety gear (helmet plus protective equipment—knee and elbow pads and wrist guards).

56. Correct Answers: 1, 2, 3, 4, and 6

Rationale: During early childhood, a child is very active and needs to be attended to while in a shopping cart. Household doors, cupboards, and cabinets should be locked. Medications need to be locked up, and preventive measures such as child-resistant caps need to placed on bottles. In-line skating should not be done until a child is at least 5 years old.

57. Correct Answer: 2

Rationale: The medical record is a legal document, and standards for charting must be followed when errors in documentation are made. An error should not be covered up, but can be corrected by drawing a single line through the entry and writing "error" and your initials above or beside the entry.

58. Correct Answer: 3

Rationale: Tinea capitis is a fungal infection that can be transmitted on a person-to-person basis through use of personal items, such as a hat or comb/brush. It may also be transmitted from household pets, especially cats.

59. Correct Answer: 1

Rationale: A toothbrush with soft bristles will minimize trauma and bleeding to the gums.

60. Correct Answer: **3**

    Rationale: With head lice, everything washable should be washed in hot water and dried in a hot dryer. Non-washable items should be either dry cleaned or placed in a plastic bag for 14 days to ensure that all eggs have hatched.

61. Correct Answers: **2, 4, and 5**

    Rationale: Buck's traction is a form of skeletal traction.

62. Correct Answer: **2**

    Rationale: A sterile dressing change requires scrubbing for the procedure and maintaining a sterile field.

63. Correct Answer: **3**

    Rationale: Airborne precautions include standard precautions equipment plus the use of a mask.

64. Correct Answer: **1**

    Rationale: Crust and debris from the infected lesions can be carefully removed after they have been softened with a 1:20 Burrow solution compress.

65. Correct Answer: **2**

    Rationale: This order needs to be checked for its accuracy.

66. Correct Answer: **3**

    Rationale: As part of the five "rights" to medication administration, the nurse needs to verify that the medication is being administered to the right patient.

HEALTH PROMOTION AND MAINTENANCE

67. Correct Answer: **2**

    Rationale: Foods should be introduced at an interval of 4 to 7 days to identify food allergies. For a 6-month-old child, the order for introducing foods is cereal first, followed by vegetables, fruits, and meat. Chopped table food or commercially prepared junior foods should not be introduced until the child is 9 to 12 months of age.

68. Correct Answer: **3**

    Rationale: Scoliosis is suspected when an Adam's test is performed with the child bending over and arms hanging and a noticeable asymmetry of the ribs is noted.

69. Correct Answer: **4**

    Rationale: Only a few teeth at a time should be brushed using 6–8 strokes before moving to the next few teeth. A dentist should be seen by the time the child is 18 months of age. The use of a fluoridated mouthwash is not recommended until the child is at least 6 years old.

70. Correct Answer: **4**

    Rationale: Classic symptoms of type 1 diabetes mellitus include polyphagia, polyuria, and polydipsia.

71. Correct Answer: **1**

    Rationale: A 3-year-old child should have conversation that is 75% intelligible; 50% intelligible is typical of a 2-year-old.

72. Correct Answers: **1, 2, 3, 5, and 6**

    Rationale: The number of wet diapers should decrease; dryness is an indicator of voluntary urethral sphincter control.

73. Correct Answer: **3**

    Rationale: It is best to be informed and be able to effectively communicate and make decisions when in a pressured situation.

74. Correct Answer: **4**

    Rationale: At this age, the child is developing a sense of autonomy and this behavior is to be expected.

75. Correct Answer: **2**

    Rationale: Imaginary friends are created in times of loneliness. Imaginary friends usually disappear once the child enters school.

76. Correct Answer: **2**

    Rationale: Duchenne muscular dystrophy is an X chromosome-linked recessive trait.

77. Correct Answer: **1**

    Rationale: It is important to acknowledge the perception and make a referral if needed. This teenager's height and weight are appropriate.

78. Correct Answers: **2, 4, and 6**

    Rationale: Normal physical assessment and developmental aspects for an infant aged 6 months include presence of the anterior fontanel, which will close between 12 and 18 months of life. Weight from birth should double by 6 months and triple by 1 year of age. The infant should be able to sit without support and begin to grab and manipulate toys and objects.

79. Correct Answer: 2

Rationale: The immunization schedule between the ages of 4 and 6 years old includes a DPT, IPV, and second MMR vaccination.

80. Correct Answer: 4

Rationale: Teething pain is caused by inflammation; application of cold is soothing.

81. Correct Answer: 2

Rationale: A heart rate up to 220 beats/min is indicative of fever. Normal resting heart rate for a newborn is 100–180.

82. Correct Answer: 1

Rationale: One should stand up straight when measuring with a peak expiratory flow meter.

83. Correct Answer: 1

Rationale: Hip movement toward the side of the spine touched is called a trunk incurvation or Galant reflex; it disappears by 4 weeks of age.

84. Correct Answers: 1, 3, 4, and 5

Rationale: A toddler enjoys coloring and finger painting, stringing beads, and watching television. Riding in a wagon is not an appropriate activity for a child in traction. Squeaky toys and animals are appropriate for infants.

85. Correct Answer: 4

Rationale: This behavior is normal for a toddler. A transitional object contributes to this child's security.

86. Correct Answers: 1 and 6

Rationale: The rooting reflex is assessed by stroking the cheek alongside the mouth. The infant should respond by turning the head toward that side and beginning to suck.

PSYCHOSOCIAL INTEGRITY

87. Correct Answer: 3

Rationale: Open communication and effective listening skills are the approach that must be used when caring for a client who may have experienced sexual abuse.

88. Correct Answer: 2

Rationale: A comprehensive history will need to be obtained, and aggressive behaviors and their frequency need to be described. Such information will be used to set limits and outcomes for the behavior modification program.

89. Correct Answer: 2

Rationale: No matter the level of cognitive impairment, a child can learn certain things. He or she must be assessed for readiness to learn and possible achievement of goals.

90. Correct Answer: 3

Rationale: Open communication is the best intervention to use and is facilitated by this response.

91. Correct Answers: 1, 3, 5, and 6

Rationale: Attention-deficit/hyperactivity disorder is characterized by difficulty with attention span, lack of attentiveness to work, easily distracted, talks excessively and thrives on activity and is often restless.

92. Correct Answer: 1

Rationale: Encouraging open communication among the child and family about what to expect as the child dies will provide the most support to the child and family.

93. Correct Answer: 2

Rationale: This meal selection is the only one that does not contain pork products. Muslims prohibit consumption of all pork products.

94. Correct Answer: 3

Rationale: An attempt at suicide indicates an immediate need for safety precautions and protection against harming oneself.

95. Correct Answer: 3

Rationale: Ritalin blocks the reuptake mechanism of dopaminergic neurons. Thus, in children with attention-deficit/hyperactivity disorder, it should decrease their symptoms. In this case, the ability to complete household chores is an accomplishment.

96. Correct Answer: 3

Rationale: An accomplishment with anorexia nervosa is the client beginning to eat and gain weight.

97. Correct Answers: 1, 3, and 6

Rationale: Oppositional defiant behaviors need behavior modification. For a 4-year-old child, that would consist of colorful charts to see accomplishments and setting limits with consequences.

SECTION I

SECTION II

SECTION III

SECTION IV

SECTION V

SECTION VI

SECTION VII

SECTION VIII

SECTION IX

SECTION X

98. Correct Answer: **1**

Rationale: During the protest phase of separation anxiety, a toddler would cry, scream, cling to the parent, and reject contact with strangers.

99. Correct Answer: **3**

Rationale: Therapeutic play is how nursing interventions take place when dealing with a child with depression. Play is considered a child's work. The nurse will observe the child in play where he or she expresses thoughts, feelings, fears, and frustrations.

100. Correct Answer: **2**

Rationale: Cocaine is consumed intravenously and through inhalation. The most common physical signs of inhalation are swelling and ulcerations of the nasal passages. The drug abuser may also demonstrate behavioral changes and irritability.

101. Correct Answer: **3**

Rationale: Developing a trusting relationship consists of sharing one's innermost feelings.

102. Correct Answer: **Enuresis**

Rationale: Enuresis is a common disorder among boys where there is an involuntary passage of urine.

103. Correct Answer: **4**

Rationale: This comment indicates that the parents want to start bonding with their baby.

104. Correct Answer: **1**

Rationale: A newborn going through neonatal abstinence syndrome needs decreased stimuli. Wrapping the infant snugly and rocking the child decreases the likelihood of the newborn performing self-stimulation.

105. Correct Answers: **2, 4, and 6**

Rationale: These attributes are positive responses moving the child toward good nutrition and growth.

106. Correct Answer: **2**

Rationale: A family needs to say good-bye to their child and should be allowed to rock and hold the child as long as they wish.

BASIC CARE AND COMFORT

107. Correct Answer: **2**

Rationale: Constipation is first managed by increasing the amount of fiber and fluid, plus promoting good toileting habits by responding to urges. An enema could be given for persistent constipation on an occasional basis.

108. Correct Answer: **3**

Rationale: A client with Graves' disease has hyperthyroidism and needs a quiet, unstimulating environment with frequent rest periods.

109. Correct Answer: **3**

Rationale: Pain is challenging to assess in children who cannot talk, and the nurse must rely on astute assessment skills. Common physiologic responses to pain include increased pulse, blood pressure, and respirations; restlessness; and crying.

110. Correct Answer: **2**

Rationale: Any infant with oxygenation problems during feeding should be fed small volumes every 2–3 hours; this plan allows for adequate rest between feedings. Feeding every 4 hours increases the volume of feeding, and the infant will tire easily.

111. Correct Answer: **4**

Rationale: The left side-lying position is optimal for maximum gas exchange, as it increases blood flow to the left lung.

112. Correct Answer: **4**

Rationale: Acute epiglottitis is typically characterized by three manifestations: irritability, drooling, and absence of spontaneous cough. Other clinical manifestations may include stridor when supine, high fever, tachycardia, and tachypnea.

113. Correct Answers: **3 and 5**

Rationale: Decerebrate posturing is extension of the upper extremities in response to noxious stimuli and is a sign of further neurological deterioration. Clear fluid that drains from the nose or ears with a basilar skull fracture could be cerebrospinal fluid, and the nurse should make the physician aware of this symptom.

114. Correct Answer: 1

Rationale: Increased ICP can cause the anterior fontanel to bulge. The posterior fontanel should have closed by the second month after birth.

115. Correct Answer: 3

Rationale: An infant younger than age 6 months receives nutrition through formula (breast or bottle feeding). Similac contains an increased amount of calories per ounce and provides the essential nutrients required by the infant.

116. Correct Answer: 1

Rationale: An adolescent should void 700–1,400 mL/day. Oliguria could potentiate other problems such as urinary retention, urinary tract infection, or the formation of renal calculi.

117. Correct Answer: 1

Rationale: Aortic stenosis is manifested as decreased cardiac output, faint pulses, hypotension, and tachycardia.

118. Correct Answer: 3

Rationale: A pheochromocytoma is an adrenal tumor that secretes catecholamines, which in turn increase pulse and blood pressure. Severe hypertension is a concern in these clients.

119. Correct Answer: 3→1→5→2→6→4

Rationale: The child is placed in a supine position with the head in a sniffing position. Next, the tube is measured for approximate insertion length. The tube is lubricated. It is passed first through the nose and then straight back. If child can swallow, he or she should be asked to assist with the insertion. Once the tube is in place, confirm its correct placement and secure the tube.

120. Correct Answer: 4

Rationale: Severe depletion of serum calcium leads to tetany and spasms of muscles including those in the larynx, which would be life-threatening.

121. Correct Answer: 2

Rationale: A total neurovascular assessment needs to be completed and compared bilaterally and to previous assessments to determine whether a change has occurred.

122. Correct Answer: 3

Rationale: The procedure is similar to a cardiac catheterization, except that the catheter is inserted into the femoral or antecubital site. Post-procedure care involves checking pulses, vital signs, and the dressing. The extremity also needs to be kept straight for at least 4 hours to allow adequate time for a clot to form over the puncture wound of the vessel.

123. Correct Answer: **High Fowler's**

Rationale: In the high Fowler's position, the client is positioned at 90 degrees, which promotes maximum lung and chest wall expansion.

124. Correct Answer: 1

Rationale: Preventing rupture and infection of the meningocele sac is the highest priority. It is best accomplished by positioning the infant prone and applying sterile, moist, nonadherent dressings over the sac.

125. Correct Answer: 4

Rationale: Because the client's white blood cell count is low, it is important to take steps to prevent infection and to monitor for early signs of a possible infection.

126. Correct Answers: **1, 2, and 6**

Rationale: In a three-point gait, only one foot (in this case, the left) is used for weight bearing; the other foot serves as a balance. The hands and arms should support the body weight on the crutches, not the axillary area.

PHARMACOLOGICAL AND PARENTERAL THERAPIES

127. Correct Answer: 3

Rationale: The medication is appropriate. The child is not experiencing any adverse effects from the medication and is ready for the debridement procedure.

128. Correct Answer: 4

Rationale: After identifying the patient and verifying the donor and recipient blood group and type, the first 50 mL of blood should be administered slowly while the child is monitored for complications. Blood should be used within 30 minutes of its arrival and should be infused within 4 hours. Its transfusion should be regulated to prevent fluid overload.

SECTION I

SECTION II

SECTION III

SECTION IV

SECTION V

SECTION VI

SECTION VII

SECTION VIII

SECTION IX

SECTION X

129. Correct Answer: **2**

Rationale: Total 250 mL to infuse over 6 hours. 250 mL/6 h = 41.5 mL/h = 42 mL/h.

130. Correct Answer: **1**

Rationale: Exercise and activity can lower blood glucose levels. Either additional food is needed or the amount of insulin should be decreased.

131. Correct Answer: **12 mL/h**

Rationale:
$$66 \text{ lb}/2.2 \text{ kg} = 30 \text{ kg}; 12{,}500 \text{ U}/250 \text{ mL}$$
$$= 50 \text{ U/mL}$$
$$20 \text{ U/kg/h} = 50 \text{ U/mL}$$
$$20 \text{ U}/30 \text{ kg/h} = 50 \text{ U/mL}$$
$$600 \text{ U/h} = 50 \text{ U/mL} = 12 \text{ mL/h}$$

132. Correct Answer: **4**

Rationale: The development of a rash is a possible sign of an allergic reaction to the medication. The medication should be discontinued and the child needs to be evaluated.

133. Correct Answer: **2**

Rationale: Sulfasalazine decreases the absorption of folic acid, so daily supplements must be given to meet the body's daily requirement for folic acid.

134. Correct Answer: **3**

Rationale: The client's heart rate must be checked prior to administration of digoxin. The medication would be withheld if the heart rate for a 1-year-old child was less than 90–110 beats/min.

135. Correct Answer: **3**

Rationale: Applying a topical anesthetic can minimize the pain of the injection by numbing the skin at the injection site. A 1-inch needle length is the appropriate needle size for infants. The injection site is the vastus lateralis or ventrogluteal muscle in children younger than 18 months old.

136. Correct Answers: **2, 3, 4, and 5**

Rationale: The MMR vaccine is administered subcutaneously. The method for giving a subcutaneous injection is to grasp and raise the skin up, and then give the injectate in the subcutaneous tissue. Aspiration should occur to confirm that the injection is not going into the bloodstream.

137. Correct Answer: **3**

Rationale:
$$250 \text{ mg}/1 \text{ mL} = 375 \text{ mg}/x$$
$$250x/250 = 375/250$$
$$x = 1.5 \text{ mL}$$

138. Correct Answer: **2**

Rationale: Holding the breath for 5–10 seconds after inhaling the aerosol allows the medicine to reach the lungs.

139. Correct Answer: **2**

Rationale: Amiodarone is administered after synchronized cardioversion.

140. Correct Answer: **2**

Rationale: Glucocorticoids are best taken in the morning with food to prevent insomnia and gastrointestinal upset.

141. Correct Answers: **2, 3, 5, and 6**

Rationale: A hemolytic reaction is the most severe reaction and is due to incompatible blood types. Clinical manifestations of a hemolytic reaction include chills, shaking, fever, headache, red or black urine, flank pain, nausea and vomiting, tightness in chest, and pain at the needle site.

142. Correct Answer: **1**

Rationale:
$$250 \text{ mg}/5 \text{ mL} = 175 \text{ mg}/x$$
$$250x/250 = 875/250$$
$$x = 3.5$$

143. Correct Answer: **2**

Rationale: A prothrombin time (PT) and international normalized ratio (INR) are monitored to determine the effectiveness of Coumadin therapy.

144. Correct Answer: **3**

Rationale: Prophylactic use of acetaminophen (Tylenol) is recommended to help offset the adverse effect of fever.

145. Correct Answer: **8 units**

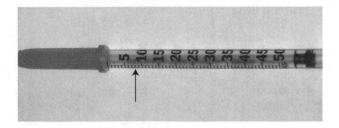

146. Correct Answer: <u>2</u>

Rationale: Frequently used benzodiazepines include intravenous midazolam (Versed); the antidote is flumazenil (Romazicon).

147. Correct Answer: <u>4</u>

Rationale:

$$1{,}000 \text{ mcg}/1 \text{ mg} = 200 \text{ mcg}/x$$
$$1{,}000x/1{,}000 = 200/1{,}000$$
$$x = 0.2 \text{ mg}$$
$$\text{Medication vial} = 0.1 \text{ mg}/1 \text{ mL} = 0.2 \text{ mg}/x$$
$$0.1x/0.1 = 0.2/0.1$$
$$x = 2.0 \text{ mL}$$

148. Correct Answer: <u>3</u>

Rationale: Hyperglycemia and hypoglycemia are side effects that require monitoring. TPN should be infused at a constant rate.

149. Correct Answer: <u>4</u>

Rationale: Nystatin is given for candidal infections such as oral thrush. A common side effect is diarrhea.

150. Correct Answer: <u>Yes</u>

Rationale: 55 lb = 25 kg

Recommended 24-hour dose range = [(lower dose range) 50 × 25] to [(higher dose) 133 × 25]

= 1,250 mg to 3,325 mg

Medication order: 750 mg × 4 times a day = 3,000 mg/day

Dose is within acceptable limits.

151. Correct Answer: <u>3</u>

Rationale: In resuscitation, intravenous or intraosseous routes are preferred for rapid delivery and absorption.

152. Correct Answer: <u>2</u>

Rationale: Any medication error must be reported and the physician notified.

153. Correct Answer: <u>20 mL</u>

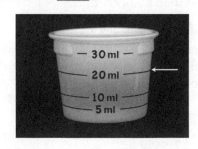

154. Correct Answer: <u>1</u>

Rationale: Scabies is caused by a mite that is killed by the application of Elimite. The cream application, once applied, should remain on the skin 8–14 hours before being washed off. One application is sufficient. The itch and rash that accompany scabies will not be relieved by the cream.

155. Correct Answer: <u>3</u>

Rationale: Amphotericin B affects the renal function, so BUN and creatinine need to be monitored closely.

156. Correct Answer: <u>2</u>

Rationale: Major side effects encountered when administering Dilantin include bradycardia and hypotension.

157. Correct Answer: <u>2 mL</u>

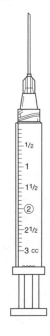

Rationale:

$$75 \text{ mg}/50 \text{ mL} = 3 \text{ mg}/x$$
$$75x/75 = 150/75$$
$$x = 2 \text{ mL}$$

158. Correct Answer: <u>2</u>

Rationale: For a child younger than age 3 years, the earlobe should be pulled down and back to straighten the ear canal and allow the medication to enter.

159. Correct Answer: **3**

Rationale: A 9-month-old infant is too young to follow directions. The caregiver would need to hold the buttocks together after inserting the suppository 1–2 inches to assure the effectiveness of the suppository.

REDUCTION OF RISK POTENTIAL

160. Correct Answer: **2**

Rationale: One of the earliest signs of an oxygenation problem is restlessness. In infants, substernal retractions also indicate an increased effort to maintain oxygenation.

161. Correct Answer: **1**

Rationale: The goal for hemoglobin levels with frequent transfusions is more than 9.5 g/dL. With effective treatment, the child will have improved physical abilities—in this case, the ability to play soccer.

162. Correct Answer: **3**

Rationale: The best method for evaluating the effectiveness and adequacy of gavage feeding is to weigh the client and document any weight gain.

163. Correct Answer:

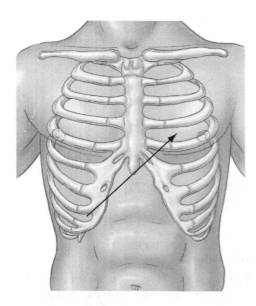

Rationale: In a child younger than 7 years, the apical impulse is located just left and lateral to the left midclavicular line and fourth intercostal space.

164. Correct Answer: **3**

Rationale: Rheumatic fever presents with a macular rash that is nonpruritic. Laboratory values include elevated ASO titers, C-reactive protein levels, and erythrocyte sedimentation rates.

165. Correct Answer: **1**

Rationale: Chronic renal failure presents with decreased urinary output and increased serum BUN, creatinine, and potassium levels. In this case, the serum creatinine level is elevated and everything else is within normal limits.

166. Correct Answer: **3**

Rationale: A client with SLE should avoid extended exposure to the sun, as it might lead to an exacerbation of SLE.

167. Correct Answers: **1, 2, and 4**

Rationale: Assessment findings warranting a call to the physician include signs and symptoms of bleeding and possible perfusion problems. In this case, the decreased blood pressure for a child of this age, the increased amount of blood drainage, and asymmetrical pulses are reasons to call the physician.

168. Correct Answer: **2**

Rationale: Signs of increased intracranial pressure would be manifested—in this case, a bulging fontanel and the presence of opisthotonos.

169. Correct Answer: **2**

Rationale: Based on the assessment findings, this client is beginning to show manifestations of respiratory depression. Both medications should be withheld.

170. Correct Answer: **3**

Rationale: The pacemaker is set in the demand mode at a rate of 80, which means that the pacemaker would fire anytime the heart rate was less than 80 beats/min.

171. Correct Answers: **2, 3, and 4**

Rationale: Addison's disease is caused by adrenocortical insufficiency and manifests with (among other things) hypotension; tachycardia; cold, clammy skin; increased sleepiness; and hypoglycemia.

172. Correct Answer: 2

Rationale: PKU is an inborn metabolism error caused by a deficiency in tyrosine; tyrosine metabolizes the essential amino acid phenylalanine. Breastfeeding can occur as long as the mother monitors both her own and the baby's phenylalanine levels. Most commonly, the formula that needs to be used will not contain any phenylalanine but will contain tyrosine.

173. Correct Answer: 3

Rationale: Clients with hyperparathyroidism will be easily fatigued because they have a deficient production of parathyroid hormone (PTH), decreased serum calcium, and increased serum phosphorus.

174. Correct Answer: 2

Rationale: While both the hemoglobin and erythrocyte levels are slightly below normal, they are not severe enough to cause a hemodynamic response consisting of hypotension and tachycardia. Instead, the client might exhibit slight pallor. Because of the decrease in oxygen-carrying capacity, the client will also tire easily.

175. Correct Answer:

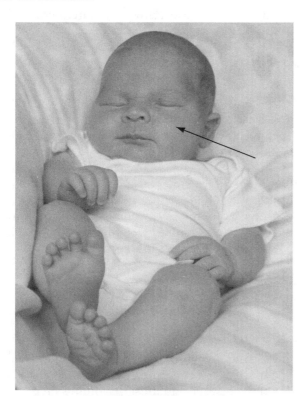

Rationale: The rooting reflex is elicited by stroking the cheek of the infant. The infant should turn the head toward the side and begin to suck.

176. Correct Answer: 4

Rationale: Weighing is the most accurate assessment technique to determine the effectiveness of fluid loss from furosemide.

177. Correct Answer: 3

Rationale: An allergy to seafood is linked to iodine, which is a component of the radiographic dye. Given that this client has a known allergic reaction to seafood, its use during cardiac catheterization could precipitate an anaphylactic reaction while the client is undergoing the procedure.

178: Correct Answer: 1

Rationale: The primary (and priority) concern for a client in acute respiratory distress syndrome (ARDS) is maintaining oxygenation. ARDS affects the alveolar-capillary membrane and surfactant production, making the lungs stiff and difficult to ventilate.

179. Correct Answers: 2, 3, 5, and 6

Rationale: Water or a water-soluble lubricant is used to insert the tube. An x-ray would determine the placement, but is unnecessary (and costly) in this case.

180. Correct Answer: 3

Rationale: Toxic shock syndrome is caused by the toxin *Staphylococcus aureus* and presents with a high fever (greater than 102°F), a diffuse sunburn-like rash, hypotension with orthostatic syncope, and dizziness. Desquamation of the palms and soles occurs 1–2 weeks after the initial onset of toxic shock syndrome.

181. Correct Answer: 2

Rationale: Maintaining hydration reduces the viscosity of the sickled blood cells.

182. Correct Answer: 3

Rationale: A high-pressure alarm would mean resistance within the system.

SECTION I
SECTION II
SECTION III
SECTION IV
SECTION V
SECTION VI
SECTION VII
SECTION VIII
SECTION IX
SECTION X

183. Correct Answer:

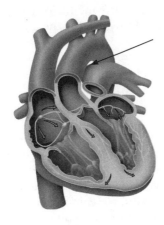

Rationale: A PDA is the failure of the opening between the aorta and pulmonary artery to close.

184. Correct Answer: **2**

Rationale: Clear drainage from the nose is most likely cerebrospinal fluid and would be a complication of a skull fracture.

185. Correct Answer: **3**

Rationale: The airway must be evaluated. The lab results reveal the client is in respiratory acidosis. The client should be stimulated to breathe deeply so pCO_2 does not continue to increase.

186. Correct Answer:

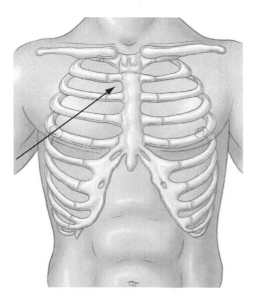

Rationale: The murmur is heard during systole and is most readily heard over the aortic valve area, which is the second intercostal space at the right sternal border.

187. Correct Answer: **2**

Rationale: Based on the lab results, the platelet count is low.

188. Correct Answer: **3**

Rationale: Consolidation will result in diminished lung sounds over the lobe.

189. Correct Answer: **1**

Rationale: Weighing the client is the most accurate method of determining overall fluid gain or loss.

190. Correct Answers: **1 and 4**

Rationale: Active bleeding would be indicated by frequent swallowing and clearing of the throat. Vomitus would be bright red in color in case of active bleeding. Dark red vomitus most likely includes blood swallowed in surgery and is indicative of old blood.

191. Correct Answer: **4**

Rationale: If the system is working properly, blood would not leak around the insertion site.

192. Correct Answer: **4**

Rationale: The nurse must assess the client further to determine the problem before notifying the physician or performing other interventions.

PHYSIOLOGICAL ADAPTATION

193. Correct Answer: **3**

Rationale: The MAP on this blood pressure is 68 mm Hg, which is within the parameter. MAP = [SBP + 2(DBP)]/3.

194. Correct Answer: **3**

Rationale: Fluid volume replacement and urinary output are extremely important in a burn client. Children weighing less than 30 kg should produce 1–2 mL/kg/h of urine.

195. Correct Answer: **2**

Rationale: The first action is to establish an airway and administer oxygen.

196. Correct Answer: **1→4→3→2→6→5**

Rationale: Synchronized cardioversion is used for unstable tachycardia. It discharges a shock on the R wave and must be administered in the "synch" mode. One first begins by considering sedation if there is time.

197. Correct Answer: **3**

Rationale: Vital signs and neuro checks should be performed at more frequent intervals because the child has a moderate concussion and is at risk of developing increased intracranial pressure.

198. Correct Answer: **1**

Rationale: The wheezing and itching could indicate anaphylaxis. The infusion must be stopped immediately.

199. Correct Answer: **3**

Rationale: The child is in acute distress. The nurse should stay with the child, call for help, and begin oxygen until help arrives.

200. Correct Answers: **2 and 6**

Rationale: A client with suspected tuberculosis will be placed on airborne precautions, which require the client to be placed in a private, negative-pressure room with the door closed at all times. Anyone entering the room must wear a mask and clean, nonsterile gloves, and perform good hand washing before and after caring for the client. If the client needs to leave the room, he or she must wear a mask.

201. Correct Answer: **1**

Rationale: The best evidence of chest compression effectiveness during CPR is a palpable carotid pulse during CPR.

202. Correct Answer: **2**

Rationale: During infancy, clinical manifestations of Hirschsprung disease include failure to thrive, constipation, abdominal distention, and episodes of diarrhea and vomiting.

203. Correct Answer: **2**

Rationale: Acute bradycardia during suctioning is indicative of hypoxia. In this case, suctioning should be stopped and the child reconnected to the ventilator to receive supplemental oxygen.

204. Correct Answer: **1**

Rationale: If the child exhibits signs and symptoms of hypoglycemia, then this problem must be corrected immediately. In this case, Lifesavers or orange juice can quickly increase the blood glucose levels and reverse the signs and symptoms of hypoglycemia.

205. Correct Answer:

Rationale: On an infant younger than 1 year of age, the brachial pulse is the pulse that is assessed during CPR.

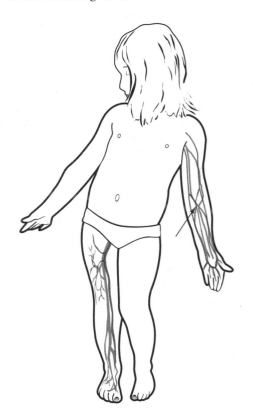

206. Correct Answer: **3**

Rationale: The child is severely dehydrated and has been vomiting, so this client most likely will not be able to keep down the fluids or solids taken orally. The most appropriate method to ensure proper rehydration is intravenous fluids.

207. Correct Answer: **1**

Rationale: The crisis manifests as a painful episode. One of the goals of medical management of sickle cell crisis is to relieve the pain through opioid administration.

208. Correct Answer: **4**

Rationale: The child is actively bleeding from the insertion site; the nurse should apply direct pressure. The physician also needs to be notified of the active bleeding.

SECTION I

SECTION II

SECTION III

SECTION IV

SECTION V

SECTION VI

SECTION VII

SECTION VIII

SECTION IX

SECTION X

209. Correct Answer: **2**

Rationale: A change in mental status and shunting of blood inward could be indicative of shock. Burn clients are susceptible to sepsis, which would be manifested initially as tachycardia; a change in mental status; cool, clammy skin; tachypnea; and WBC count abnormalities.

210. Correct Answer: **1**

Rationale: Adenosine is administered for supraventricular tachycardia with rates of 180 beats/min or more in children.

211. Correct Answers: **2, 3, 4, and 6**

Rationale: When preparing to intubate a child younger than 8 years of age, the equipment needed includes an uncuffed endotracheal tube, ambu bag and face mask to oxygenate the client, and a laryngoscope. Sterile gloves are not necessary, but clean nonsterile gloves and other personal protective equipment should be used during the procedure.

212. Correct Answer: **3**

Rationale: The child is in distress, and both parent and child should be reassured. The nurse should call for assistance, and the physician needs to be notified of the change in the client's condition.

213. Correct Answer: **1**

Rationale: When a conscious child is choking, abdominal thrusts should be performed until the object is expelled or the child loses consciousness.

214. Correct Answer: **1**

Rationale: The child is in distress, and oxygenation must be maximized. The child should be placed in an upright sitting position at a 90-degree angle (high Fowler's position).

215. Correct Answer: **4**

Rationale: Hyperkalemia causes ECG changes such as tall, peaked T waves.

216. Correct Answer: **Establish unresponsiveness**

Rationale: Once unresponsiveness has been verified, the nurse would activate EMS and focus on the ABCs of cardiopulmonary resuscitation.

217. Correct Answer: **3**

Rationale: Meningitis is extremely contagious. Clients with suspected meningitis must be isolated.

218. Correct Answer: **2**

Rationale: The child is in need of a patent, secured airway, which would be accomplished by intubation or tracheostomy.

219. Correct Answer: **3**

Rationale: SIADH is characterized by hypersecretion of ADH, which causes fluid to be retained and dilutes the serum sodium. Urinary output decreases owing to the reabsorption of fluid. Edema is not manifested in children, however, because the circulatory system accommodates the expanded circulatory volume.

220. Correct Answer: **1**

Rationale: Wilm's tumor is a malignant renal and intra-abdominal tumor. Manipulation of the mass may cause dissemination of cancer cells.

221. Correct Answer: **5→2→1→4→3→6**

Rationale: Rapid-sequence intubation begins by obtaining the baseline status of the client and performing continuous monitoring throughout the procedure. The client is preoxygenated, and then medication is administered to assist in the relaxation. Crichoid pressure may be necessary to assist in visualizing the landmarks for intubation. Once the endotracheal tube is in place, the presence of bilateral breath sounds should be auscultated.

222. Correct Answer: **1**

Rationale: Airway patency is in jeopardy with a major burn of the chest and face secondary to edema and suspected inhalation injury.

Care of Adults

MANAGEMENT OF CARE

Multiple Choice

1. Implementing which client's plan of care first would indicate that the nurse has an appropriate understanding of how to prioritize the workload?

1. A 58-year-old client admitted with acute pancreatitis.
2. A 68-year-old client admitted with acute pulmonary edema.
3. A 72-year-old client with resolving transient ischemic attack.
4. A 64-year-old client with dilated cardiomyopathy.

2. What must the nurse know about a certified nursing assistant (CNA) prior to delegating responsibilities to him or her?

1. The person's age.
2. The person's competency level.
3. The length of time employed on the unit.
4. The person's ethnic background.

3. A nurse is demonstrating colostomy care to a client with a new colostomy. Which actions would the nurse teach the client to perform? (Select all that apply.)

1. Use antimicrobial ointment on the skin.
2. Apply talcum powder.
3. Wash the hands.
4. Observe for any irritation.
5. Cut the skin barrier to size.
6. Wear sterile gloves.

4. In caring for a 74-year-old client in the terminal stages of lung cancer who refuses any further treatment, the nurse should provide ethical care that

1. Requires treatment be continued.
2. Ensures a cure and benefits the family.
3. Promotes equity and prevents litigation.
4. Allows the client to determine his or her care.

5. During a preoperative assessment of a client undergoing a laminectomy, the nurse identifies a risk for latex allergy when the client reports an allergy to the following substance?

1. Tomatoes.
2. Apples.
3. Milk.
4. Bananas.

6. Which duty would be most appropriate to assign to the certified nursing assistant?

1. Assist in bathing a client with Guillain-Barré syndrome who is on the ventilator.
2. Assist in bathing a client with pneumonia who is acutely short of breath.
3. Assist in ambulating a client with a hemothorax and chest tube to water seal.
4. Assist in feeding a client with a stroke and swallowing difficulties.

7. During the planning phase of the nursing process for a client admitted for a craniotomy, what should the nurse do?

1. Establish outcomes.
2. Collect information about past medical problems.
3. Determine that the goal has been met.
4. Identify the problem and nursing diagnosis.

8. When assessing the presence of a deep vein thrombosis, which clinical manifestations should the nurse expect to be present? (Select all that apply.)

1. Throbbing in the extremity.
2. Absence of a peripheral pulse.
3. Swelling of the affected extremity.
4. Extremity is cool to the touch.
5. Increased extremity circumference.
6. Positive Homan's sign.

9. A client is admitted to the hospital for repair of an abdominal aortic aneurysm. This client's insurance coverage comes from an HMO. After the initial treatment and surgery, who would coordinate the client's ongoing and specific needs for care?

1. The charge nurse.
2. The case manager.
3. The vascular surgeon.
4. Home healthcare nurses.

10. A client has undergone a total laryngectomy with radical neck dissection. While caring for the client postoperatively, the nurse observes the client to be restless with a respiratory rate of 26 breaths/min and audible gurgling. What should the nurse do?

1. Suction the client's tracheostomy.
2. Suction the client's mouth.
3. Apply oxygen by mask at 4 L/minute.
4. Notify the physician immediately.

11. When the nurse manager receives information that is pertinent to a current performance improvement project on reducing the number of methicillin-resistant *Staphylococcus aureus* infections, the nurse manager may

1. Share the information at a monthly unit staff meeting.

2. Share the information with the multidisciplinary team that provides care on the unit.
3. Share the information only with the unit's performance improvement committee.
4. Display the information on the bulletin board in the unit's locker room and bathroom.

12. The nurse presents an informed consent form for insertion of a ventricular peritoneal shunt to a client. The client tells the nurse that he is confused about what the neurosurgeon said about the procedure. Which nursing action is appropriate?

1. Have the client sign the form so surgery is not delayed.
2. Explain the procedure to the client and have him or her sign the form.
3. Have the client sign the form and tell the client that you will call the surgeon.
4. Notify the surgeon that the client has questions and that the form is not signed.

13. Which interventions would be most appropriate when performing central line site care? (Select all that apply.)

1. No dressing change is needed—this device is implanted.
2. Wash the hands.
3. Don gloves, remove the dressing, and discard the dressing.
4. Use a circular motion, going from the insertion site outward, with each antiseptic swab.
5. Inspect the skin and insertion site, and document the findings.
6. Don gloves, remove the dressing, and discard the dressing and the gloves.

14. A father who is a member of a prominent family in the community is admitted to the hospital following a motor vehicle crash. A reporter for the local television station telephones the nursing unit and asks for an update on the client's status. Prior to providing information to the reporter, what should the nurse do?

1. Obtain a signed client authorization.
2. Answer each question.
3. File a complaint with the television station.
4. Confirm the reporter's identity.

15. Which nursing action has the highest priority for a client who is admitted with full-thickness burns covering 60% of the body and smoke inhalation?

1. Administer antibiotics.
2. Maintain strict fluid restriction.
3. Monitor respiratory status.
4. Encourage fluid and food intake.

16. A nurse is preparing to administer oral Dilantin (phenytoin) to a client who is experiencing seizures. Before administering the medication, which action is the most important for the nurse to perform?

1. Document that the medication was administered.
2. Count the available medication on hand and sign for the medication.
3. Initiate an IV with normal saline infusing.
4. Check the medication dose and the client's identification.

17. Which of these client's would be the most appropriate assignment for a licensed practical nurse (LPN)?

1. A 67-year-old client admitted to the unit with recurring angina.
2. A 48-year-old client with emphysema and pneumonia who is receiving oxygen.
3. A 55-year-old client with breast cancer who is receiving chemotherapy.
4. A 69-year-old client admitted to the unit with a cerebrovascular accident.

18. A client is on a ventilator, has a tracheostomy tube, and has a gastrostomy tube for enteric feedings. Which information is critical to communicate to the next nurse caring for this client? (Select all that apply.)

1. PO intake.
2. Vital signs.
3. Room temperature.
4. New orders.
5. Ventilator settings.
6. Arterial blood gas results.
7. Tracheal secretion characteristics.

19. During a preoperative assessment of a client who is undergoing an aneurysm clipping, the nurse identifies a risk for increased bleeding when the client reports taking

1. A daily multivitamin.
2. Garlic.
3. Echinacea.
4. Vitamin K.

20. A client is admitted with full-thickness burns of the back and posterior thighs. Multiple dressing changes to the burns will be performed as part of the patient's care, and the expected client outcome while hospitalized is absence of a wound infection. Which intervention is most appropriate in meeting this outcome?

1. Gloves, gowns, masks, and caps must be worn during the care of this client and sterile gloves must be worn for the dressing changes.
2. The use of good hand washing technique is the only intervention that is needed.
3. Intubation and aggressive ventilatory management are needed to reverse the effects of an inhalation burn injury.
4. Prophylactic antibiotics must be administered to prevent an infection and colonization of wounds.

21. During the insertion of a urinary catheter, the tip of the catheter brushes against the arm of the nurse. Which nursing action is most appropriate?

1. Wipe the catheter with Betadine and continue the catheter insertion.
2. Soak catheter in sterile saline solution for 15 minutes and then reattempt insertion.
3. Continue with the catheter insertion.
4. Obtain a new catheter and reattempt insertion.

22. Which nursing action is a priority for a client who is admitted to the hospital with suspected tuberculosis?

1. Place the client on airborne precautions.
2. Administer the prescribed antibiotic.
3. Initiate intravenous fluids.
4. Place the client on droplet precautions.

Identification

23. The most important aspect of aseptic technique is _____.

Multiple Choice

24. A client is discharged and needs to perform dressing changes at home. Which statement made by the client indicates a correct understanding of aseptic technique?

1. "I should wash my hands and use an over-the-counter antimicrobial ointment to help the healing process."
2. "I should wash my hands prior to removing the old dressing and again before redressing the wound."
3. "I need to take a pain pill 30 minutes before changing the dressing."
4. "I should wear sterile gloves when I apply the new dressing."

25. The nurse on the unit observes smoke billowing from a room. Which action should first be taken by the nurse?

1. Close the client's door.
2. Evacuate all clients in the room.
3. Yell "fire."
4. Grab the fire extinguisher.

26. An RN assigns the care of a client to an LPN. This client has a wound requiring a sterile dressing change every 6 hours. As the nurse walks into the room, the LPN is observed not using clean gloves to perform the dressing change. How should the RN handle the situation?

1. Use the situation to teach the LPN how to perform the procedure correctly and, upon exiting the client's room, counsel the LPN.
2. Inform the LPN that the nurse is doing the procedure incorrectly and that a report will be filed after the RN finishes the dressing change.
3. Document the LPN's actions in a report to be placed in the nurse's personnel folder.
4. Inform the LPN that they need to talk after the dressing change is completed.

27. A client is returning from surgery after a thoracotomy procedure for a left lower lobectomy. A chest tube is in place. To care for this client postoperatively, which equipment should be at the bedside? (Select all that apply.)

1. Sterile petroleum-covered gauze.
2. Endotracheal tube.
3. Sterile gloves.
4. Thoracotomy tray.
5. Sterile glass bottles.
6. Wall suction.
7. Sterile gauze.

28. In performing a chart audit, the nurse evaluates the nursing documentation. Which data should be present in the chart for a client in left-sided heart failure and acute renal failure who is receiving continuous venovenous hemofiltration?

1. Client weight, blood pressure, dialysate, and amount of fluid removed.
2. Client weight, lab values, and urinary output.
3. Dialysate, dwell time, and description of fluid drained.
4. Peritoneal site appearance and amount of fluid removed.

29. The charge nurse is making assignments for the next shift. Client A, who is currently in a semi-private room, has a suspected subarachnoid hemorrhage. Client B has a possible cerebrovascular accident and delirium.

1. Assign one nurse to client A and another nurse to client B.
2. Assign the same nurse to care for both clients in the same room.
3. Place client A in a private room, and assign different nurses to care for client A and client B.
4. Place client B in a room at the end of the hall, and assign the same nurse to care for both client A and client B.

30. Before administering a subcutaneous injection of NPH insulin to a client with type 1 diabetes mellitus at 4 P.M., what should the nurse do?

1. Check the client's glycosated hemoglobin value.
2. Instruct the client to eat dinner and a bedtime snack.
3. Test the urine for ketones.
4. Document the client's vital signs.

31. Select the blood products that would require use of a microaggregate filter when infusing multiple types of blood products in a client with disseminated intravascular coagulopathy.

1. Packed red blood cells.
2. Clotting factors (VIII, IX).
3. Whole blood.
4. Platelets.
5. Fresh frozen plasma.

32. A client complains about burning around an IV site in the arm. Which symptom would cause a nurse to become concerned about possible IV infiltration?

1. Softness at the IV site and the surrounding tissue.
2. Slight swelling.
3. Cool skin.
4. No redness around the IV site.

33. A 72-year-old client was admitted yesterday and placed in a room with another client who has cancer and is receiving chemotherapy. Now, the 72-year-old client presents with a rash that itches and is oozing. Shingles (varicella-zoster infection) is suspected. Which measure should the nurse take to prevent the spread of the virus?

1. Place this client in a private room and adhere to strict isolation precautions.
2. No isolation precautions are necessary, but place the client in a private room.
3. Observe good hand washing technique and move the client with cancer.
4. The client with suspected shingles can be left in the semi-private room with the other client.

34. The client's physician informs him that he must receive chemotherapy or the client will die within 6 weeks. The client expresses to the nurse that he does not want the treatment. As the client's advocate, the nurse should recognize that the client

1. Has the right to refuse the treatment to the extent permitted by law.
2. Must recognize the physician's expertise and agree to the treatment.
3. Has the right to ask for an early death.
4. Has an obligation to himself and his family to accept the life-saving treatment.

35. Which assignment would be most appropriate for a certified nursing assistant (CNA)?

1. Performing a venipuncture for laboratory blood tests.
2. Bathing a client who is in Russell's traction.
3. Administering acetaminophen to a client with a temperature of 99.8°F.
4. Changing a triple-lumen central line dressing.

36. Which interventions would be most appropriate when giving home care instructions on how to administer medications through a gastrostomy tube? (Select all that apply.)

1. Clamp the tube after flushing it.
2. Cut a tablet in half and push it through the tube.
3. Mix the medication with the enteral formula in a medication cup.
4. Warm the medication in a microwave oven.
5. It is appropriate to crush an enteric-coated aspirin.
6. Pour the medication into a syringe.

37. The charge nurse is making shift assignments. Which client assignment to an LPN indicates that the charge nurse understands appropriate delegation?

1. A client needing to receive conscious sedation.
2. A client just admitted with multiple rib fractures.
3. A client receiving a bone marrow transplant.
4. A client with dehydration and inflammatory bowel disease.

38. The nurse is providing care to a client who has undergone a mastectomy and has just been received from the recovery room. Which sequence of care is correct for caring for this client?

1. Assess the urinary output, change the client's gown, and obtain a warm blanket.
2. Check the vital signs, administer pain medications, and assess the dressing.
3. Administer pain medications, check the vital signs, and assess the dressing.
4. Check the vital signs, assess the dressing, and assess for the presence of pain.

39. Home health nurses are visiting the family of a client with chronic obstructive pulmonary disease (COPD) and a tracheostomy to assist in reinforcing the teaching of chest physiotherapy (CPT). What would the desired evaluation and outcome management for this family include?

1. Completion of a satisfaction survey on the home health nurses.
2. A reduction in hospitalizations for pneumonia.
3. The ability to use an inhaler to deliver a bronchodilator.
4. Physical activity and dietary intake.

SECTION I
SECTION II
SECTION III
SECTION IV
SECTION V
SECTION VI
SECTION VII
SECTION VIII
SECTION IX
SECTION X

40. A nurse is assigned to care for several clients. Which client should be the first to receive care at the start of the nurse's shift?

   1. A client with gastroenteritis and dehydration.
   2. A client with cirrhosis.
   3. A client with graft-versus-host disease.
   4. A client with tertiary syphilis.

41. An intravenous infusion has been initiated to deliver continuous IV fluids and antibiotic therapy. To administer the first IV in piggyback fashion, select the steps that would be needed to infuse the antibiotic.

   1. Connect the antibiotic IV tubing to the port located closest to the continuous fluid IV bag.
   2. Hang the IV antibiotic bag higher than the continuous IV fluid bag.
   3. Connect the antibiotic IV tubing to the port located closest to the client.
   4. Hang the IV antibiotic bag lower than the continuous IV fluid bag.
   5. Detach the primary IV fluid bag and insert the antibiotic fluid bag.

42. Which nursing observation would indicate a major complication in a client who is receiving a packed red blood cell transfusion?

   1. Difficulty breathing.
   2. Brisk capillary refill.
   3. Temperature of 98.5°F.
   4. Sleeping soundly.

43. During the acute phase of Guillain-Barré syndrome, the major nursing goals are to monitor and detect disease progression and to maintain

   1. Good hand washing techniques to avoid a septic rebound reaction.
   2. Passive range of motion to enhance joint mobility and prevent contractures.
   3. Fluid and nutritional intake by mouth.
   4. Respiratory and cardiovascular function.

44. The charge nurse is determining in which room to place a client who is being admitted with hyperthyroidism. Which room assignment would be the best for this client?

   1. A semi-private room near the elevators.
   2. A private room near the end of the hall.
   3. A private room near the nurses' station.
   4. A multibed room with one shared bathroom.

SAFETY AND INFECTION CONTROL

Multiple Choice

45. To promote safety, the nurse would implement which safety measure to decrease the risk of a client developing septic shock?

   1. Perform a thorough hand washing.
   2. Restrict visitors.
   3. Administer antibiotics.
   4. Implement strict isolation procedures.

46. A client received a tracheostomy 3 days ago. To maintain client safety, which equipment should be readily available when providing tracheostomy care?

   1. Distilled water.
   2. Cotton gauze.
   3. Obturator.
   4. Suction catheter.

47. A client is admitted after being thrown from a motorcycle, and the use of cocaine is suspected as a factor in the accident. Which assessment findings would indicate this client has a possible overdose of cocaine?

   1. Hypertension, bradycardia, and hallucinations.
   2. Hypertension, tachycardia, and cardiac arrhythmias.
   3. Hypotension, tachycardia, and dilated pupils.
   4. Hypotension, bradycardia, and cardiac arrhythmias.

48. A client is admitted with epilepsy. To promote safety, which equipment should be in use or available at the bedside? (Select all that apply.)

   1. Suction.
   2. Padded side rails.
   3. Pulse oximeter.
   4. Tongue depressor.
   5. Restraints.
   6. Code cart.

49. Which statement concerning the transmission of herpes simplex virus, type 2, would be most important for the nurse to teach?

   1. It is a fungal infection that is spread by skin-to-skin contact.
   2. It is a viral infection that requires prompt treatment with acyclovir.

3. It is a bacterial infection has been linked to the development of cervical cancer.

4. It is a viral infection that requires treatment with azithromycin (Zithromax).

50. Which nursing approach would be most appropriate for following airborne precautions?

1. Place the client in a semi-private room, and wear a gown when in the room.

2. Place the client in a private room, and wear gloves and a gown when in the room.

3. Place the client in a private room, and wear gloves, a mask, and a gown when in the room.

4. Place the client in a private room, and wear gloves and a mask when entering the room.

51. A client returns to the unit from a cerebral angiography with a left femoral dressing that is dry and intact. What positioning considerations should the nurse apply?

1. Restrict the head movement.

2. Keep the client supine for 12 hours.

3. Keep the left leg straight.

4. Position the client on the right side.

52. In planning care for a client with diabetic peripheral neuropathy, what would the nurse teach the client to do?

1. Massage a thick layer of cream or lotion on the feet and between the toes twice a day.

2. Soak the feet in hot water for 30 minutes twice a day and pat them dry with an absorbent towel.

3. Wear open-toed, rubber- or plastic-soled shoes.

4. Inspect the feet twice a day and wear soft, absorbent socks.

53. A client is admitted and is confused, disoriented, and combative. Which measures should the nurse take initially to reduce the potential for the client harming himself or herself? (Select all that apply.)

1. Keep the bed in a low position.

2. Administer a sedative and an antipsychotic.

3. Place the client in a vest restraint.

4. Encourage the family to stay with the client.

5. Activate the bed alarm.

6. Place all four side rails in the up position.

54. The nurse is caring for a client who is comatose and is on intermittent gastrostomy feedings. Which action indicates that the nurse has an understanding of safe medication administration in this situation?

1. Contact the physician to clarify possible adverse reactions prior to administering any medications.

2. Prior to administering the medication at the bedside, confirm the client's identity by checking the arm band.

3. Confirm the order by checking it against the medication package and chart after the medication has been administered.

4. Add the medication to the feeding formula to ensure that the total dose is administered.

55. A client is admitted with suspected meningitis. In delivering nursing care to this client, what would be the priority action?

1. Initiate isolation precautions once the diagnosis is confirmed.

2. Immediately initiate isolation precautions.

3. Administer analgesics as needed.

4. Once the diagnosis is confirmed, administer antibiotic therapy.

56. To promote safety in the environment of a client with Von Willebrand's disease, which actions would the nurse take?

1. Administer ibuprofen if the client has a temperature of 101.5°F or experiences pain.

2. Advise the client to wear gloves while doing household chores.

3. Provide oral care and recommend daily flossing.

4. Administer vitamins C and K on a daily basis.

57. While the nurse is caring for a client on a ventilator, the low-pressure ventilator alarm sounds. What should the nurse's first action be?

1. Suction the secretions from the endotracheal tube.

2. Check the client and ventilator connections.

3. Administer intravenous sedation and analgesia.

4. Reassure the client and instruct him or her not to bite on the tube.

58. What "rights" pertain to administering medications to an adult client. (Select all that apply.)

1. Right physician.
2. Right dose.
3. Right route.
4. Right time.
5. Right medication.
6. Right client.

59. During the assessment of a client who has been diagnosed with a brain tumor in the left frontal lobe, the nurse would expect to find

1. Ataxic gait and complaints of dizziness.
2. Vision disturbances and complaints of a headache.
3. Changes in personality and impaired judgment.
4. Inability to communicate needs appropriately.

60. A nurse is caring for a client with mild dehydration. The physician's order reads as follows: "1,000 mL normal saline with 50 mEq KCl to infuse in 30 minutes." What is the nurse's first action?

1. Initiate a second IV line.
2. Assess breath sounds.
3. Call and verify the order with the pharmacist.
4. Call and verify the order with the physician.

61. A client is scheduled for a sterile dressing change. Which action is necessary to prevent sepsis?

1. If the new dressing is ready to be applied and a piece falls on the outer aspect of the sterile field, it may be left there until the dressing change is completed.
2. After the hands are washed, sterile gloves are applied and the dressing change is begun by first removing the existing dressing.
3. If sterile solution splashes onto the sterile field while pouring the solution into the dressing tray, the nurse must start the procedure over.
4. After removing the existing dressing, it is appropriate to place it on the outermost portion of the sterile field and then discard it when the dressing change is finished.

Identification

62. When caring for all clients, which type of precautions should the nurse observe?

___ STANDARD precautions

Multiple Choice

63. A client is in a halo brace. Before administering pin site care, what should the nurse check?

1. The tightness of the brace.
2. The client's mental status.
3. The appearance of the pin sites.
4. The availability of a halo vest wrench.

64. The nurse is preparing a client to undergo a computed tomography of the head with contrast medium. What follow-up care should the nurse be prepared to provide?

1. Immobilization of the head for 4 hours.
2. Pressure to the injection extremity.
3. Fluid replacement.
4. Administering sedation.

65. To protect a client who has undergone a bone marrow transplant from potential sources of infection, what should the nurse do?

1. Allow the client to have flowers in the room.
2. Restrict a friend from visiting who is coughing.
3. Isolate the client using contact precautions.
4. Administer prophylactic antibiotics.

66. Multiple documentation entries have been made in the progress notes of a client's chart by multiple healthcare providers. Now an error is made when documenting a new entry in the progress notes. Which method would be the best way to correct the documentation error?

1. Draw a single line through the entry, and write "error" and your initials above the entry.
2. Discard the page where the error occurred, and begin documentation on a new page after hand-copying the previous entries.
3. Use a black marker to cover up the entry, and continue to chart.
4. Use correction fluid to cover the entry, and write over the correction fluid once it dries.

HEALTH PROMOTION AND MAINTENANCE

Multiple Choice

67. A client presents with a complaint of chest pain after physical exertion. The nurse explains to the client that in most cases angina pectoris is due to

1. Hypertension.
2. Atherosclerosis.
3. Smoking.
4. Dysrhythmias.

68. Which behavior by a postoperative client would be most indicative of positive relief from analgesia administration?

1. The client is difficult to arouse from a sound sleep.
2. The client verbalizes a decrease in level of pain.
3. The client refuses more medication.
4. The client is loud and aggressive with visitors.

Identification

69. A client is admitted with suspected hepatitis. Which type of hepatitis is spread by consuming contaminated food?

_A_____

Multiple Choice

70. While taking the history for a young male client, which information would indicate that the client has a high risk for developing testicular cancer?

1. Undescended right testicle.
2. Recent genital herpes exposure.
3. Occurrence of a hydrocele at birth.
4. Measles as a child.

71. A client is admitted to rule out a myocardial infarction. The nurse teaches the client about lifestyle modification. Which risk factors are considered to be modifiable?

1. Gender and 20 pounds overweight.
2. Mother has hyperlipidemia and hypertension.
3. Hypertension and family history of angina.
4. Hyperlipidemia and hypertension.

72. A client receives a tuberculin skin test; 24 hours later, the site reveals an induration of 12 mm. How would the result of the skin test be interpreted?

1. Not significant.
2. Might be significant.
3. Significant.
4. The client is definitely infectious.

73. To help prevent polypharmacy interactions in a client who is taking multiple prescriptions, what instruction would the nurse give to the client?

1. Inform a family member of the names and uses of all medications.
2. Abstain from taking any over-the-counter medications in addition to the medication you are already taking.
3. Use a dispensing system as a reminder to take medications on a schedule.
4. Bring all medications, including supplements and herbal remedies, to your doctor's appointments.

74. While taking the history for a client, which information would indicate that the client is at high risk for developing breast cancer? (Select all that apply.)

1. Mother-in-law has breast cancer.
2. Early age of onset for menses.
3. Nulliparity.
4. Late age of menopause.
5. Obesity.
6. Consumption of a low-fat diet.

75. Which client is at the greatest risk of developing a deep vein thrombophlebitis?

1. A 25-year-old, overweight woman who is hospitalized for an acute asthma attack.
2. A 35-year-old woman who exercises regularly, smokes, and takes aspirin frequently for headaches.
3. A 62-year-old man who has a cerebrovascular accident with left-sided paralysis.
4. A 75-year-old man who has hypertension and is ambulating four times daily after surgery.

76. After a cesium implant treatment, a client is discharged home. The nurse is teaching the client how to use a vaginal dilator to prevent vaginal stenosis. What instruction would the nurse deliver?

1. Avoid the use of the vaginal dilator if intercourse is resumed once a month.
2. Gently insert the vaginal dilator as deep as possible for 15 minutes, three times a week.
3. Gently insert the vaginal dilator three times a day for 6 months.
4. Avoid intercourse and insert the vaginal dilator to a depth of 1 inch for 15 minutes, three times a week.

77. Upon the client's admission to the unit, the nurse discovers that the client is unable to read. In developing a discharge teaching plan for the client the nurse should

1. Determine the client's degree of motivation to learn.
2. Determine the client's ability to understand information.
3. Determine the client's instructional preferences for learning.
4. Recognize that the family must be included.

78. Why should the nurse who is caring for a client with chronic obstructive pulmonary disease encourage the client to quit smoking?

1. Smoking decreases the amount of mucus production.
2. Smoking allows hemoglobin to become highly oxygenated.
3. Smoking shrinks the alveoli in the lungs.
4. Smoking damages the ciliary cleaning mechanism.

Identification

79. What kind of diet should a client who is attempting to modify his or her risk factors for hypertension consume?

Low Na intake

Multiple Choice

80. When teaching a young adult client, when should the nurse stress that breast self-examination is best performed?

1. Anytime during the month.
2. Five to seven days after menses.
3. On the first day of every month.
4. On the first day of menstruation.

81. A postoperative client informs the nurse that it hurts too much to use the incentive spirometer and cough, so the client refuses to perform the activity. What is the best intervention for the nurse to implement?

1. Respect the client's wishes.
2. Notify the physician.
3. Explain the importance of the activity.
4. Withhold pain medication.

82. A client is receiving instruction from the nurse on ways to minimize the effects of fibrocystic breast disease. Which statement by the client requires clarification by the nurse?

1. "I'll continue to do my monthly breast self-exam."

2. "Because limiting my caffeine might help, I will decrease my coffee intake."
3. "I'll start limiting my intake of vitamin E and discontinue my hormones."
4. "It's a good thing that I do not smoke."

83. What equipment would be necessary for the nurse to complete an evaluation of cranial nerve III during a physical assessment?

1. A safety pin.
2. A tongue depressor.
3. A pen light.
4. A cotton swab.

84. An adult client is inquiring about vaccinations against communicable diseases. Which vaccines are available to prevent or minimize the effects of contracting communicable diseases? (Select all that apply.)

1. Hepatitis A vaccine.
2. Influenza vaccine.
3. Hepatitis B vaccine.
4. Pneumococcal vaccine.
5. Hepatitis C vaccine.
6. *Helicobacter pylori* vaccine.

85. While taking the history for a client, which information would indicate that the client is at high risk for developing cervical cancer?

1. Began sexual activity at an early age.
2. Early age of onset for menarche.
3. Nulliparity.
4. BRCA-1 and BRCA-2 mutations.

86. A client is diagnosed with degenerative joint disease and osteoarthritis of the hip. Which conditions might potentially exacerbate the symptoms of degenerative joint disease?

1. Smoking.
2. Hypertension.
3. Overweight.
4. Steady exercise.

PSYCHOSOCIAL INTEGRITY

Multiple Choice

87. The nurse interviewing a newly admitted client asks the client to explain how he happened to come to the hospital today. What is the purpose of obtaining this information from the client?

1. To identify the client's level of stress related to the admission process.

2. To report correct information to the client's physician.

3. To determine the client's perception of the illness.

4. To accurately document the admission findings.

88. A client presents with a 20-year history of alcohol and nicotine dependence; she is also separated from her husband and has difficulties managing everyday activities. What is an appropriate nursing diagnosis for this client?

1. Ineffective denial.

2. Risk for loneliness.

3. Ineffective individual coping.

4. Powerlessness.

89. The probable occurrence of withdrawal symptoms in a client with a history of chronic alcoholism is most accurately assessed by identifying which of the following factors? (Select all that apply.)

1. Blood alcohol level.

2. Drinking history.

3. Type of alcoholic beverage last consumed.

4. Time that last alcoholic beverage was consumed.

5. Quantity of alcohol last consumed.

6. Experiences following previous episodes of withdrawal.

90. A client is admitted to an inpatient psychiatric unit after attempting suicide. What is the initial nursing priority?

1. Ensure the client's safety.

2. Establish a therapeutic group session.

3. Increase the client's self-esteem and promote his or her identity.

4. Establish a therapy schedule.

91. Four days following surgery for a brain tumor, the client's dressing is removed. The nurse finds the client crying. The client informs the nurse that she looks and feels awful. The nurse recognizes this behavior is related to

1. Mental and emotional residual effects from surgery.

2. Altered self-esteem due to the change in appearance.

3. Effects of surgical trauma and swelling in the brain tissue.

4. An improvement in the client's condition with increased awareness of self.

92. A client is admitted for pneumonia and has a history of drug abuse. The nurse observes tremulousness, anorexia, hypertension, and confusion in the client. What do these symptoms indicate?

1. Wernecke's encephalopathy.

2. Delirium tremens.

3. Alcoholic hallucinations.

4. Korsakoff's syndrome.

93. During a group session, the members of the group are discussing the types of stressors that affect their lives. Which individual is experiencing a psychological stressor in his or her life?

1. A 32-year-old person who was exposed to extreme cold while skiing.

2. A 52-year-old person who has just learned that her job is being eliminated.

3. A 68-year-old person who has a history of hypertension now controlled.

4. A 47-year-old person who has a family history of lung and bone cancer.

Identification

94. A client is admitted and treated for a myocardial infarction. Now the client tells the nurse that he is feeling better and would like to go home. The nurse reinforces the diagnosis to the client, but he is adamant that he wants to go home. Which defense mechanism is the client exhibiting?

Multiple Choice

95. A client is admitted to the inpatient psychiatric unit with a diagnosis of an adjustment disorder. What is the primary goal of nursing care?

1. Include the family members in the treatment plan.

2. Reduce the client's level of anxiety to prevent escalation.

3. Identify the stressful event and current problems.

4. Include pertinent information and data in the chart.

96. A client with ulcerative colitis tells the nurse, "I can't take this anymore! I'm in constant pain, and I need to stay close to the toilet all the time. I don't know how to deal with this problem." Based on the client's comments, what is the most appropriate nursing diagnosis?

    1. Impaired physical mobility.

    2. Altered thought processes.

    3. Social isolation.

    4. Ineffective individual coping.

97. Which action should be included in the plan of care for a 14-year-old client who is admitted following a sexual abuse incident?

    1. Medicate the client with Ativan (lorazepam).

    2. Limit communication with parents and reinforce the secrets.

    3. Encourage communication and listen attentively.

    4. Encourage the client to immediately engage in normal routines and social activities.

98. A client has just received news that surgery will be performed tomorrow for an ostomy placement. The client responds, "I'd rather die than become disfigured!" How should the nurse respond?

    1. "It's okay—a lot of clients have ostomies."

    2. "You sound very upset about the possibility of an ostomy."

    3. "If I had to have an ostomy, I would be very upset, too."

    4. "Remember, this measure is only temporary, not permanent."

99. Which clinical findings might confirm the suspicion of elder abuse? (Select all that apply.)

    1. Malnourishment.

    2. Client is disoriented.

    3. Disheveled appearance.

    4. Excessive bruising.

    5. Withdrawn.

    6. Recent fractured arm.

100. A lung cancer client is in the terminal stages of lung cancer. Which nursing action would provide the most support to the client and family during this time?

    1. Promote client rest by limiting visitation.

    2. Begin decreasing the current treatment regimen.

    3. Promote open communication about what to expect.

    4. Prevent information overload by communicating once a week.

101. The nurse is caring for a client who is newly admitted with a traumatic spinal cord injury. The client is tearful, complains constantly, and uses the nurse call button frequently. What is the most likely source of the client's attention-seeking behaviors?

    1. Sensory overload.

    2. Vulnerability.

    3. Social isolation.

    4. Anger.

102. The spouse of a client who has had a brain tumor removed voices concern that the client is in restraints and is confused and combative. The client's spouse asks the nurse why the client is behaving this way. Which statement would be the nurse's most appropriate explanation?

    1. "I don't know why your spouse is behaving this way, but I am sure the client is fine."

    2. "The client hit me once and might hit me again; that is why the client is tied down."

    3. "If this is too upsetting for you, then maybe you should just go home for a few days."

    4. "Sometimes after brain surgery, clients go through confusion and demonstrate difficult behavior."

103. A trusting relationship is crucial in providing client care. Which behavior indicates that a client with schizophrenia is developing a trusting relationship?

    1. The client openly describes his feelings to the nurse during a therapeutic session.

    2. The client openly describes his vivid hallucinations during group therapy.

    3. The client mimics the same behavior and follows the nurse around the unit.

    4. During group therapy, the client openly states that he feels normal and is ready to go home.

Identification

104. A client who was admitted to the hospital for alcoholism is being discharged. To which outpatient group should the nurse refer the client?

_____

Multiple Choice

105. Which approach should be included in the plan of care for a client who was admitted to the hospital following a rape attack?

1. Limit communication with the family.
2. Encourage the client to immediately engage in normal routines and social activities.
3. Medicate the client with Ativan (lorazepam) 5 mg IV.
4. Encourage communication and listen attentively.

106. When evaluating a client's drug use, the nurse assesses the presence of tolerance as indicated by the client's

1. Ability to adapt to adverse side effects.
2. Need to consume drugs and alcohol on a regular basis.
3. Need for increased amounts of the drug to produce the desired effect.
4. Physiological and psychological dependence on the substance.

BASIC CARE AND COMFORT

Multiple Choice

107. In planning care for a client with increased intracranial pressure, which steps would the nurse take?

1. Keep the head of the bed flat, and not use a pillow for head support.
2. Elevate the head of the bed by 30 to 45 degrees, and keep the client's head in a neutral position.
3. Elevate the head of the bed by 90 degrees, and support the client's knees with a pillow.
4. Position the client on the right side, and use a pillow to support the client's neck.

108. A client who is receiving chemotherapy develops mild stomatitis. The nurse should encourage the client to

1. Swish and spit with full-strength hydrogen peroxide.
2. Swish and spit a mixture of Xylocaine, Benadryl, and Maalox.
3. Drink hot tea with honey before and after each meal.
4. Brush the teeth after each meal, and use dental floss twice a day.

109. The nurse is caring for a client who was recently hospitalized for a peptic ulcer. Which assessment findings would suggest possible perforation of the ulcer?

1. Bradycardia.
2. Anorexia.
3. Right shoulder pain.
4. Soft abdomen.

110. A client needs instruction on how to use a cane prior to being discharged. Which instructions would be included? (Select all that apply.)

1. The cane is held on the client's weaker side.
2. The weaker leg is advanced first.
3. The cane's height should be at the client's waist.
4. The stronger leg is advanced first.
5. The cane is held on the client's stronger side.
6. The cane is advanced 15 to 20 inches for every stride.

111. Which measures should nursing care of a client with hypothyroidism include?

1. Providing a cool environment.
2. Encouraging the use of a heating pad.
3. Providing a low-calorie, high-protein diet.
4. Planning frequent rest periods.

112. The nurse determines that teaching regarding the prevention of urinary tract infections for a client with cystitis has been effective when the client states:

1. "I will limit my fluid intake to 1 liter per day to prevent symptoms of frequency and urgency."
2. "I will increase my fluid intake and empty my bladder every 2 to 3 hours throughout the day."
3. "I will use an antiseptic vaginal deodorant spray twice a day to reduce the bacterial growth."
4. "I will wash my perineal area with soap and water after each bowel movement and before and after sexual intercourse."

113. Which nursing diagnosis would be appropriate for a client who is experiencing a vitamin K deficiency related to cirrhosis?

1. Activity intolerance.
2. High risk for injury.
3. Altered thought processes.
4. Ineffective breathing pattern.

114. When teaching a client with myasthenia gravis about the management of the disease, what advice should the nurse give to the client?

1. Arrange a routine to accommodate frequent visits to the doctor's office.
2. Perform structured, active exercises at least twice a week to prevent muscle atrophy.
3. Perform necessary physically demanding activities in the morning.
4. Protect extremities from injury due to decreased sensory perception.

Identification

115. A client is admitted with acute respiratory distress. An audible wheeze is heard on auscultation, and the client exhibits substernal retractions and use of accessory muscles. In which position should the nurse place the client to maximize oxygenation?

_____

Multiple Choice

116. After receiving a total left hip replacement, the client returns to the unit with an abductor pillow in place. The client informs the nurse that he would be more comfortable without the pillow. What is the nurse's best response?

1. "The pillow is intended to prevent the contact of both knees and reduce the risk that pressure ulcers will form."
2. "The pillow is intended to prevent the inadvertent movement of the left leg too far away from the body."
3. "The pillow is intended to prevent the inadvertent movement of the left leg beyond the body's midline."
4. "The pillow is intended to prevent early ambulation if you should wake up confused."

117. A client returns to the unit from the recovery room following a laryngoscopy. Which position would be most effective in helping the client breathe?

1. Low Fowler's position.
2. Side-lying position.
3. Trendelenberg position.
4. Sim's position.

118. Which menu selection would be most appropriate for a client with cholelithiasis?

1. Two eggs, two slices of toast with margarine, and a glass of whole milk.
2. Grilled cheese sandwich, steamed vegetables with butter, and a cup of coffee.
3. Roasted chicken breast, baked potato with margarine and chives, and skim milk.
4. Baked fish, steamed broccoli with salt and pepper, and a glass of iced tea.

119. Which assessment finding most strongly suggests urinary catheter occlusion?

1. Increased urinary output.
2. Increased urge to void.
3. Complaint of urethral pressure.
4. Bladder distention.

120. A client is admitted with a closed head injury. At the time of admission, the client is unconscious and exhibits decorticate posturing to noxious stimulation. One hour later, the nurse assesses the client. Which findings should the nurse report to the physician? (Select all that apply.)

1. Bilateral flexion of the upper extremities to noxious stimuli.
2. Small, reactive pupils bilaterally.
3. Slight drainage from facial lacerations.
4. Lethargic state of the client.
5. Bilateral extension of the upper extremities to noxious stimuli.
6. Clear fluid draining from the nostrils.
7. Diminished visual acuity.

121. A client has chronic osteomyelitis of the femur and is being discharged from the hospital with self-administration of IV antibiotics. On a home visit, the nurse identifies ineffective management of the therapeutic regimen when the client reports

1. Using a heating pad over the affected area for comfort.
2. Using crutches to avoid weight-bearing on the affected leg.
3. Frustration with the length of time the treatment is taking.
4. Afebrile readings for daily morning and evening temperatures.

122. Lactulose (Cephulac) is prescribed for a client with advanced cirrhosis. The client complains that the medication causes diarrhea and refuses to take the next dose. Which response by the nurse provides the best explanation to the client regarding the importance of this medication?

1. "You are receiving the medication to decrease abdominal bloating."
2. "You are receiving the medication to prevent constipation."
3. "The medication will prevent you from developing a gastrointestinal ulcer."
4. "The medication will improve your mental function and help you think more clearly."

123. A client is diagnosed with a peptic ulcer. In providing discharge instructions regarding dietary modifications, what would the nurse's teaching include?

1. Encourage consumption of a well-balanced diet consisting of three large meals per day. ✗
2. Encourage intake of caffeinated beverages. ✗
3. Encourage consumption of a bland diet consisting of six small meals per day.
4. Encourage consumption of foods high in fiber and roughage.

124. A nasogastric tube is ordered to be placed in a client. Organize the following steps in chronological order as they relate to this procedure:

1. Lubricate the tube.
2. Measure the tube for approximate placement length.
3. Place the client in a high Fowler's position.
4. Advance the tube downward and backward.
5. Insert the tube along the base of the nose.
6. Check the position of the tube, and secure the tube.

125. A client returns to the unit after undergoing a right modified radical mastectomy with dissection of the axillary lymph nodes. Which measure is an appropriate intervention for the nurse to include in the client's postoperative care?

1. Instruct the client to watch the clock and use the PCA pump every 10 minutes.
2. Insist that the client examine the surgical incision when the surgical dressings are removed.
3. Post a sign at the bedside to avoid pressure measurements or venipunctures in the right arm.
4. Encourage the client to obtain a permanent breast prosthesis upon discharge from the hospital.

126. A client is experiencing a severe migraine headache. When providing care to this client, which intervention should the nurse implement?

1. Position the head of the bed flat.
2. Encourage the client to watch television.
3. Dim the lights.
4. Identify the headache trigger.

PHARMACOLOGICAL AND PARENTERAL THERAPIES

Multiple Choice

127. The physician orders 1 g of oxacillin sodium IV every 6 hours. The pharmacy sends a vial of oxacillin sodium powder for reconstitution with the following directions: For IM injection, IV direct (bolus) injection, or IV infusion, add 10 mL sterile water for injection. Shake well. Provides a concentration of 125 mg/mL. How many milliliters of medication will the nurse administer to the client?

1. 1.25 mL.
2. 4.0 mL.
3. 8.0 mL.
4. 10.0 mL.

128. The physician orders Coumadin for a client who has undergone a hip replacement and has a past history of deep vein thrombosis. Which lab test should be done monthly?

1. Bleeding time.
2. Hemoglobin.
3. International normalized ratio.
4. Partial thromboplastin time.

129. A client is admitted with frequent premature ventricular contractions. The physician orders a lidocaine infusion to be initiated at 30 mL/h. The IV solution contains 1 g of lidocaine in 500 mL D_5W. How much lidocaine per hour will the client receive?

1. 15 mg.
2. 30 mg.
3. 45 mg.
4. 60 mg.

130. A client is receiving a unit of packed red blood cells. Which assessment would indicate a possible hemolytic reaction? (Select all that apply.)

1. Shaking.
2. Bilateral crackles.
3. Flank pain.

4. Temperature of 102.5°F.

5. Tightness in chest.

6. Red or black urine.

131. A client is being discharged on total parenteral nutrition (TPN). Which statement by the client's caregiver reflects an understanding of TPN administration?

1. "I will need to supplement the diet to provide essential nutrients and protein."

2. "The infusion rate can be adjusted to accommodate the client's home schedule."

3. "When the bag is finished, I can disconnect it and wait for the home health nurse to arrive."

4. "Because the glucose concentration is high, it is important to test the client's blood sugar three times a day."

132. A client is receiving a dopamine infusion of 13 mcg/kg/min to assist in maintaining a mean arterial pressure of 70–80 mm Hg. How does this medication affect the patient's afterload?

1. Increases afterload.

2. Decreases afterload.

3. No effect on afterload.

4. Counteracts all other medications.

133. One gram of aminophylline is added to 500 mL normal saline. The physician orders aminophylline to be infused over 10 hours. How much aminophylline per hour will the client receive?

1. 50 mg.

2. 60 mg.

3. 75 mg.

4. 100 mg.

134. Which parameter should the nurse check before administering digoxin to a client?

1. Blood pressure.

2. Heart rate.

3. Potassium level.

4. Weight.

Identification

135. A client is to receive Solu-Medrol 75 mg IM. The drug on hand is available as 125 mg Solu-Medrol in a 2-mL vial. How much should the nurse administer?

Multiple Choice

136. Which medication can be administered intravenously to reverse the effects of a midazolam (Versed) overdose?

1. Activated charcoal.

2. Epinephrine.

3. Flumazenil (Romazicon).

4. Naloxone (Narcan).

137. A client is admitted to the unit with profound and symptomatic bradycardia with a blood pressure of 82/36 mm Hg and a heart rate of 40 beats/min. What effect would the nurse expect an epinephrine infusion at 2 mcg/min to have on the client's cardiac output?

1. Cardiac output will increase.

2. Cardiac output will decrease.

3. There will be no effect on cardiac output.

4. The client will progress to cardiac arrest.

138. A client has an order for IV fluid of D_5 0.45 normal saline, 500 mL, to infuse from 12 midnight to 6 A.M. At what rate would the nurse set the infusion pump?

1. 21 mL/h.

2. 42 mL/h.

3. 83 mL/h.

4. 120 mL/h.

139. Two hours after a client receives a scheduled heparin injection, it is discovered that the medication was administered intravenously instead of subcutaneously. Which plan would be most appropriate?

1. Hold the next scheduled heparin dose.

2. Assess for evidence of bleeding.

3. Order a PTT and INR level, and notify the physician.

4. Notify the physician, and document the event on an incident report.

140. Which emergency medication should the nurse initially administer to a client in pulseless electrical activity?

1. Epinephrine 1.0 mg IV push.

2. Amiodarone 300 mg IV push.

3. Atropine 1.0 mg IV push.

4. Lidocaine 4 mg/min IV infusion.

Identification

141. A client is to receive ondansetron (Zofran) 4 mg IV push. The medication is currently available in the form of 32 mg/50 mL. Calculate what volume would be administered to this client.

_____

Multiple Choice

142. After taking two doses of ampicillin, the client develops a chest rash. What is the nurse's most appropriate action?

1. Instruct the client to take diphenhydramine prior to taking the next dose.
2. Instruct the client to decrease the dose by half for the next dose.
3. Inform the physician, and instruct the client to stop the medication.
4. Instruct the client to adhere to the schedule for taking the ampicillin.

143. The nurse is caring for a client who is scheduled to receive insulin. The order reads as follows: "30 units of regular insulin with 70 units of NPH insulin." When administering the insulin to the client, the nurse should

1. Draw the regular (unmodified) insulin into the syringe first.
2. Inform the client that mixing the insulins will facilitate insulin production in the body.
3. Use the same injection site as used for the previous dose.
4. Use a 23- to 25-gauge syringe with a 1-inch needle for maximum absorption.

144. Which measurements would be most important to monitor in an adult client who is receiving amphotericin B for a systemic fungal infection?

1. Blood glucose levels.
2. Cardiac enzyme levels.
3. Serum calcium levels.
4. Serum creatinine levels.

Identification

145. A client who weighs 80 kg is admitted to the hospital. The client is hypotensive after numerous IV fluid boluses, and a dopamine infusion is ordered. Currently, the infusion is proceeding at 5 mcg/kg/min. The IV bag contains 400 mg dopamine in 250 mL normal saline. Calculate how many milliliters of dopamine per hour are being delivered.

_____

Multiple Choice

146. How would the nurse position the earlobe of an adult while administering eardrops?

1. Pull the ear down and back.
2. Pull the ear up and back.
3. Touch the chin to the chest.
4. Use an otoscope.

147. A client is to receive 1,000 mL of IV fluid over 10 hours. The IV tubing set calibration is 15 gtt/mL. How many drops per minute would the nurse give?

1. 25 gtt/min.
2. 100 gtt/min.
3. 115 gtt/min.
4. 125 gtt/min.

148. Which instruction would be given to a client who is receiving oral methylprednisolone regarding when and how to take the medication?

1. The medication once a day with breakfast.
2. The medication once a day before bedtime.
3. Consume 10–12 glasses of water per day.
4. The medication once a day on an empty stomach.

149. Which observation indicates that the nurse should withhold a scheduled dose of diltiazem (Cardizem)?

1. Heart rate 98 beats/min.
2. Heart rate 120 beats/min.
3. Blood pressure 90/60 mm Hg.
4. Blood pressure 160/98 mm Hg.

Identification

150. A client is admitted with hyperosmolar hyperglycemic nonketotic syndrome There is an order for blood glucose testing every 4 hours and administration of sliding-scale regular insulin as follows:

Blood Glucose Level (mg/dL)	Regular Insulin Order
0–149	No insulin
150–199	4 units
200–249	6 units
250–300	8 units
>300	Notify physician

SECTION I

SECTION II

SECTION III

SECTION IV

SECTION V

SECTION VI

SECTION VII

SECTION VIII

SECTION IX

SECTION X

The client's blood sugar reading is 246. You have available a tuberculin (1 mL) syringe. What amount of insulin should be drawn for administration?

_____

Multiple Choice

151. Which statement made by a client with newly diagnosed type 2 diabetes indicates an understanding of daily diabetes management?

1. "I need to take my insulin faithfully."
2. "I need to eat a snack prior to exercising."
3. "I can eat anything I want."
4. "I need to prick my finger four times a day."

152. Which major side effect(s) of phenytoin sodium (Dilantin) should a nurse monitor for when administering a loading dose of this medication intravenously?

1. Bradycardia.
2. Hypertension.
3. Hypertension and bradycardia.
4. Hypotension and tachycardia.

153. A client is admitted in sickle cell crisis and is receiving IV morphine by PCA pump. The nurse makes the following observations:

> Pulse: 73
>
> Respirations: 6
>
> Blood pressure: 112/72 mm Hg
>
> Client is sleeping quietly

Which nursing action is most appropriate?

1. Administer 100% oxygen.
2. Keep the code cart at the bedside.
3. Allow the client to sleep quietly.
4. Administer naloxone (Narcan).

Identification

154. An order reads as follows: "Heparin 25,000 U in 250 mL of D_5W intravenously. Infuse at 20 U/kg/hr." The client weighs 186 pounds. What is the flow rate in milliliters per hour?

_____

Multiple Choice

155. What are the nurse's first actions for a client who is experiencing unrelieved chest pain?

1. Administer morphine 5 mg IV and monitor the ECG tracing.
2. Administer morphine 5 mg IV and elevate the head of the bed.
3. Provide oxygen and encourage the client to hyperventilate.
4. Provide oxygen and offer a nitroglycerin tablet.

156. A client is being discharged from the hospital, and the physician has ordered minoxidil 0.04 g once a day for hypertension. The bottle has 100 tablets in it; each tablet contains 10 mg of minoxidil. How many tablets would the client be instructed to take?

1. 25 tablets.
2. 10 tablets.
3. 4 tablets.
4. 2.5 tablets.

157. A client is ordered to take ibuprofen (Motrin) for left hip pain. What instructions should be included in the client's teaching plan?

1. Drink large amounts of fluid daily.
2. Notify the physician if you develop bleeding gums.
3. Take the medication on an empty stomach.
4. Decrease the dosage by half if nausea occurs.

158. A client with myasthenia gravis is instructed to take the anticholinesterase medications on time and to eat meals 45–60 minutes later. The client asks the nurse why the timing of the medications is so important. What is the nurse's best response?

1. "The timing allows the medication to have its greatest effect so it is easier for you to chew, swallow, and not choke."
2. "The timing prevents your blood sugar level from dropping too low and causing you to be at risk for falling."
3. "The medication is very irritating to your stomach and you could develop ulcers if you take it too early before meals."
4. "The medication can cause nausea and vomiting. By waiting a while to eat after you have taken the medication, you are less likely to vomit."

Identification

159. K-Lor elixir 15 mEq is ordered to be given once daily. The elixir is currently available as K-Lor 20 mEq in 15 mL. Calculate the amount of K-Lor that would be administered to this client.

_____

REDUCTION OF RISK POTENTIAL

Multiple Choice

160. A client has been receiving intravenous heparin therapy for the treatment of a deep vein thrombophlebitis. In addition, the physician orders warfarin sodium (Coumadin) without discontinuing the heparin infusion. The client questions the nurse about the simultaneous use of both medications. What is the nurse's best response?

1. "I will check with the doctor about this issue. You are certainly at greater risk for bleeding with both of these medications."
2. "Because you are at risk of experiencing a pulmonary embolism, it is important for you to have additional anticoagulation."
3. "It takes several days for the Coumadin to have an effect, so we need to keep you on heparin for a few more days."
4. "Because you are allowed more activity now, the heparin is metabolized more quickly and needs to be supplemented with Coumadin."

161. Which assessment data would indicate that a client is manifesting chronic renal failure?

1. Urinary output of 876 mL over 24 hours.
2. Serum potassium level of 4.2 mEq/L.
3. Serum creatinine level of 1.1 mg/dL.
4. Serum blood urea nitrogen level of 25 mg/dL.

162. A client presents with hypoparathyroidism. Which assessments will the nurse make with this client?

1. Serum calcium level of 6.8 mg/dL.
2. Positive Chvostek's sign.
3. Serum phosphorus level of 5.2 mg/dL.
4. Nephrolithiasis.

163. A client underwent a cerebral angiogram through the right femoral site. Which post-procedural nursing assessment(s) would justify calling the physician? (Select all that apply.)

1. Intact dressing that needs reinforcement due to bloody drainage.
2. Right pedal pulse weaker than left pedal pulse.
3. Equal, bilateral radial pulses.
4. Bilateral pink, warm toes.
5. Blood pressure 88/52 mm Hg.
6. Pulse 122.
7. Respirations 22.

164. Which nursing goal would be appropriate for a client with sepsis who has developed acute respiratory distress syndrome?

1. To decrease the inflammatory response of the sepsis cascade.
2. To prevent hypoxia associated with increased alveolar-capillary membrane permeability.
3. To increase the intravascular volume so as to maintain cardiac output and sustain blood pressure.
4. To prepare the client and family members for anticipated surgery to remove the damaged lung tissue.

165. A client is receiving plasmapheresis treatments for myasthenia gravis. Which observation would the nurse identify as the desired response for this treatment?

1. Need for frequent rest periods.
2. Ability to consume an entire meal.
3. Increased ptosis.
4. Decreased functional residual capacity.

166. A client is admitted with suspected pneumonia. The chest x-ray reveals right middle and lower lung consolidation. During auscultation of the right middle and lower lobes, which finding related to the pulmonary system would the nurse anticipate?

1. Diminished breath sounds.
2. Inspiratory and expiratory wheezing.
3. Bronchovesicular sounds.
4. Tympanic hyperresonance.

Identification

167. A nurse is assessing the apical impulse of an adult client. In which anatomical area would the nurse auscultate this impulse?

_____

Multiple Choice

168. A client with left-sided heart failure is receiving furosemide (Lasix) twice a day. Which assessment is the best technique to detect the effectiveness of this medication?

1. Measure the client's intake and output.
2. Weigh the client daily.
3. Assess the client for the presence of crackles.
4. Assess the client for the presence of dependent edema.

SECTION I
SECTION II
SECTION III
SECTION IV
SECTION V
SECTION VI
SECTION VII
SECTION VIII
SECTION IX
SECTION X

169. Which observation would alert the nurse to the initial development of compensatory shock?

   1. Hypotension.
   2. Bradycardia.
   3. Increased urinary output.
   4. Mental status change.

170. A client is receiving midazolam and propofol in titrating amounts for conscious sedation during a bedside procedure. The nurse reviews the following information:

   Heart rate: 76 beats/min

   Respirations: 12

   Pulse oximeter: 91%

Based on this assessment, which nursing action is appropriate?

   1. Administer more midazolam and propofol.
   2. Withhold further administration of midazolam only.
   3. Withhold further administration of both medications.
   4. Change to fentanyl because it is shorter acting.

171. A client is admitted to the hospital after falling from a ladder and sustaining a basilar skull fracture. Which nursing assessment would support the complication of the skull fracture?

   1. Clear rhinorrhea.
   2. Raccoon eyes.
   3. Temperature of 99.2°F.
   4. Pupils round and equal, and respond briskly to light.

172. The nurse is preparing to do a shift assessment on a client who was admitted with an upper gastrointestinal bleed. Which signs and symptoms would indicate active bleeding? (Select all that apply.)

   1. Heart rate 128 beats/min.
   2. Hemoglobin 18 g/dL.
   3. Respirations 32 and shallow.
   4. Stool black and tarry.
   5. Hematocrit 32%.
   6. Blood pressure 80/52 mm Hg.

173. Which method is the best way for the nurse to evaluate the effectiveness of a client's enteral gastric gavage feedings?

   1. Objective findings include a decrease in the amount of gastric residual.
   2. Weigh the client daily and note a 1-pound weight gain in 10 days.
   3. Consult with the dietician to determine the feeding formula effectiveness.
   4. Objective findings include normal laboratory values for albumin and electrolytes.

174. Which symptom is indicative of an increase in ineffective oxygenation in a client with aortic valve regurgitation?

   1. Diastolic murmur and crackles.
   2. Inspiratory wheeze bilaterally.
   3. Restlessness and use of accessory muscles.
   4. Fatigue and exertional dyspnea.

175. A client has a right-side pneumothorax, and a chest tube has been inserted. Which finding would indicate that the chest drainage system is functioning effectively?

   1. Bubbling in the suction chamber.
   2. Blood leaking around the chest tube insertion site.
   3. Constant bubbling in the water seal chamber.
   4. Absence of breath sounds on the right side.

176. The nurse is caring for a client with a cervical spinal cord injury. Vital signs and laboratory results for this client are as follows:

   Blood pressure: 128/72 mm Hg

   Heart rate: 94 beats/min

   Respiratory rate: 28

   Arterial pH: 7.3

   Arterial pCO_2: 60 mm Hg

   Arterial pO_2: 75 mm Hg

   Arterial HCO_3: 35 mEq/L

Based on this information, which nursing action would be the best option?

   1. Notify the physician, inform the physician about the client's metabolic acidosis, and anticipate initiating a sodium bicarbonate continuous infusion.
   2. Notify the physician, request an order for midazolam, and reevaluate the client in 30 minutes.
   3. Evaluate airway patency, administer pain medication, and encourage coughing and deep breathing.

4. Evaluate airway patency, place the client in the high Fowler's position, and encourage coughing and deep breathing.

177. Which findings would the nurse expect in a client with Graves' disease? (Select all that apply.)

1. Exophthalmos.
2. Hypotension.
3. Tachycardia.
4. Bounding pulses.
5. Decreased appetite.
6. Nervousness.

178. A client with sick sinus syndrome has a permanent pacemaker implanted. This ventricular demand pacemaker is set at a rate of 70. Which nursing assessment would indicate a malfunction in the pacemaker?

1. Blood pressure of 130/84 mm Hg.
2. Apical pulse of 90 and irregular.
3. Outline of pacemaker generator under skin under left clavicle.
4. Apical pulse of 64 and regular.

179. A client presents with possible systemic lupus erythematosus (SLE). Which findings would the nurse expect with this client?

1. Leukoplakia.
2. Facial butterfly rash.
3. Generalized dermatitis.
4. Chloasma.

180. A client is scheduled for a cardiac catheterization. Which is a priority nursing assessment finding to report to the physician in this case?

1. Diminished palpable pedal pulses bilaterally.
2. Cool lower extremities with bilateral brisk capillary refill.
3. An allergic reaction of hives to shellfish.
4. A serum creatinine level of 0.8 mg/dL.

181. What is the highest priority in providing care to a client who is admitted to the hospital with sickle cell crisis?

1. Initiate intravenous fluids to maximize hydration.
2. Insert a urinary catheter to measure accurate output.

3. Administer prophylactic antibiotics.
4. Insist that the client rest instead of visiting with family.

182. When assessing a client with an S_3 heart sound, identify the assessment techniques that would be used. (Select all that apply.)

1. Sound auscultated at the apex.
2. Client placed in a supine position.
3. Bell of the stethoscope used.
4. Sound auscultated at the second intercostal space, left sternal border.
5. Diaphragm of the stethoscope used.
6. Heard best on inspiration.

183. After a cholecycstectomy, a client's serial vital signs for the past 4 hours are as follows:

Blood pressure (mm Hg): 112/82, 110/82, 112/80, 114/82

Heart rate (beats/min): 76, 78, 78, 80

Respiratory rate: 22, 24, 24, 26

Pulse oximeter: 92%, 89%, 91%, 88%

The client is sleepy but awakens easily and is oriented. Based on this nursing assessment, what is the nurse's most appropriate action?

1. Assess the client's pain level and administer pain medication.
2. Check the client's temperature and apply warm blankets.
3. Encourage the client to take deep breaths and cough.
4. Position the client in a recumbent lateral position.

184. Laboratory tests are obtained on a client who has been prescribed high-dose aspirin and corticosteroids for treatment of rheumatoid arthritis symptoms. The nurse recognizes that a complication of the drug therapy may be indicated by

1. Positive guiac (hemoccult) of stool.
2. Elevated serum liver enzymes.
3. Increased blood urea nitrogen.
4. An increased erythrocyte sedimentation rate (ESR).

185. Which nursing diagnosis would be a priority for a client who is admitted to the unit with left-sided heart failure?

SECTION I
SECTION II
SECTION III
SECTION IV
SECTION V
SECTION VI
SECTION VII
SECTION VIII
SECTION IX
SECTION X

1. High risk for infection related to stasis of secretions in the alveoli.

2. Impaired skin integrity related to dependent edema and pressure.

3. Activity intolerance related to oxygen supply-and-demand imbalance.

4. Constipation related to immobility and decreased fluid intake and output.

186. A client with metastatic breast cancer is being followed in the clinic after completing chemotherapy. Laboratory results reveal a white blood cell count of 6,000/μL and a platelet count of 75,000/μL. Based on these findings, the nurse knows that discharge teaching has been effective if the client

1. Has no bleeding episodes.

2. Has remained free of infection.

3. Has no evidence of skin breakdown.

4. Has decreased fatigue.

187. What actions should the nurse take when performing intermittent nasogastric (NG) feedings in a client? (Select all that apply.)

1. Aspirate the stomach contents.

2. Deliver feedings through a syringe barrel attached to the NG tube.

3. Keep the head of the bed elevated at 15 degrees.

4. Clamp the NG tube once the feeding is complete.

5. Deliver the feeding by pushing on the syringe plunger.

6. Irrigate the NG tube prior to initiating feeding.

188. A client is prescribed warfarin sodium (Coumadin) to be taken daily. Which instructions should the patient be given?

1. Monitor the blood pressure weekly.

2. Observe for signs and symptoms of infection.

3. Discontinue the medication if bruising occurs.

4. Avoid using products that contain aspirin.

189. On the second day after a subtotal thyroidectomy, the client informs the nurse that she is experiencing numbness and tingling around her mouth. What is the nurse's best first action?

1. Offer mouth care.

2. Loosen the neck dressing.

3. Notify the physician.

4. Order a thyroid-stimulating hormone level.

190. A client is suspected of being in progressive renal failure. When reviewing the client's chart, which measurement(s) would be the best indicator of the client's renal function?

1. Serum creatinine and blood urea nitrogen levels.

2. 24-hour urine output measurement.

3. Complete blood count results.

4. Urinalysis and client's weight.

191. A client is admitted with primary hyperparathyroidism. Laboratory values are as follows:

Serum calcium: 14 mg/dL

Serum phosphorus: 1.7 mg/dL

Serum creatinine: 1.7 mg/dL

Urine calcium: High

Based on these findings, what should the nurse do?

1. Institute seizure precautions and have oxygen available.

2. Encourage the client to drink at least 2 L of fluid daily.

3. Order a diet that includes foods and beverages rich in calcium.

4. Assess the client for a positive Trousseau's sign.

192. Which finding(s) would the nurse anticipate in a client with syndrome of inappropriate antidiuretic hormone secretion (SIADH)? (Select all that apply.)

1. 24-hour weight loss of 5 kg.

2. Serum sodium level of 130 mEq/L.

3. Urine specific gravity of 1.008.

4. Serum sodium level of 149 mEq/L.

5. 24-hour weight gain of 3 kg.

6. Urine specific gravity of 1.003.

PHYSIOLOGICAL ADAPTATION

Multiple Choice

193. A client with deep vein thrombophlebitis suddenly develops dyspnea, tachypnea, and chest pain. What is the nurse's initial, most appropriate action?

1. Auscultate for abnormal heart sounds.

2. Assess the client's blood pressure and heart rate.

3. Apply 100% oxygen via a face mask.

4. Obtain a 12-lead ECG.

194. The nurse is monitoring a client's ECG monitor and notes supraventricular tachycardia at a rate of 170. Which medication should the nurse administer?

1. Atropine sulfate (Atropine) IV.
2. Adenosine (Adenocard) IV.
3. Epinephrine IV.
4. Lidocaine hydrochloride (Xylocaine) IV.

195. While administering IV chemotherapy to an adult client with lung cancer, the client begins to itch and wheeze. What should the nurse do next?

1. Slow the rate of the infusion.
2. Explain to the client that this reaction is normal.
3. Discontinue the infusion immediately.
4. Observe the client continuously for the next 15 minutes.

196. The physician informs the nurse that a client needs to be intubated. In preparing for the physician to perform the intubation, which equipment is appropriate for this procedure? (Select all that apply.)

1. Ambu bag.
2. Face mask.
3. Laryngoscope.
4. Uncuffed endotracheal tube.
5. Oral suction.
6. Sterile gloves.

197. On admission, the vital signs of a client with a closed head injury were temperature 98.6°F, blood pressure 128/68 mm Hg, heart rate 110 beats/min, and respirations 26. One hour after admission, the nurse observes that the client may be experiencing Cushing's triad. Which vital signs are indicative of Cushing's triad?

1. Blood pressure 130/72, mm Hg, heart rate 90 beats/min, respirations 24.
2. Blood pressure 150/70, mm Hg, heart rate 80 beats/min, respirations 14.
3. Blood pressure 110/70, mm Hg, heart rate 120 beats/min, respirations 30.
4. Blood pressure 152/88, mm Hg, heart rate 122 beats/min, respirations 16.

198. The initial treatment for ventricular fibrillation, besides performing CPR, would include

1. Administering lidocaine hydrochloride (Xylocaine) IV.
2. Drawing an arterial blood gas sample.
3. Defibrillation at 360 joules (monophasic defibrillator).
4. Preparing for intubation.

199. The nurse is caring for a client who sustained severe burns and has an inhalational thermal injury. The client is intubated and on the ventilator at 60% FiO_2. The nurse notices that the client is restless, thrashing, and attempting to cough; the respiratory rate is 34. What should the nurse's first action be?

1. Notify the physician and prepare for immediate surgery.
2. Administer pain medication.
3. Increase the FiO_2 setting to 100%.
4. Auscultate lung sounds and suction if needed.

200. Which arterial blood gas results would alert the nurse to the initial development and onset of acute respiratory distress syndrome?

1. pH 7.38, PaO_2 72, PCO_2 44, HCO_3 22.
2. pH 7.50, PaO_2 60, PCO_2 28, HCO_3 21.
3. pH 7.28, PaO_2 64, PCO_2 32, HCO_3 17.
4. pH 7.42, PaO_2 75, PCO_2 40, HCO_3 25.

201. Organize the following steps for synchronized cardioversion in chronological order (with 1 being the first step in this procedure):

1. Observe for markers on the R wave.
2. Attach the monitor leads.
3. Apply the conductor pads.
4. Consider sedation.
5. Press the synch button.
6. Make sure everyone is clear.

202. A client is recovering from surgery for repair of an abdominal aortic aneurysm. Nitroprusside sodium (Nipride) is currently infusing at a rate of 1.8 mcg/kg/min. The current hemodynamic readings are as follows:

Heart rate: 80 beats/min

Arterial line: 229/110 mm Hg

Pulmonary artery pressure: 18/8 mm Hg

Pulse oximeter: 93%

Based on the hemodynamic data, which nursing action is most appropriate when caring for this client?

1. Increase the rate of nitroprusside sodium infusion to 2.3 mcg/kg/min.
2. Decrease the rate of nitroprusside sodium infusion to 1.5 mcg/kg/min.
3. Administer 1,000 mL of normal saline IV fluid bolus.
4. Due nothing and continue to monitor client closely.

203. Which assessment finding indicates effective chest compressions during CPR?

1. Dilated and fixed pupils bilaterally.
2. Palpable femoral pulse during compressions.
3. Warm skin and pink mucous membranes.
4. Sluggish capillary refill.

204. A client is admitted with a complaint of chest pain. When assessing the client, the nurse expects which client description of pain to be most indicative of an acute coronary syndrome?

1. "The pain is in my chest, but it goes away when I sit down and rest."
2. "The pain is in my upper back and radiates down my left leg."
3. "The pain is in the middle of my chest, and I feel like I am being crushed."
4. "The pain started after eating; it is now right below my ribcage and is burning."

205. The nurse assesses a client to have blood pressure 70/42 mm Hg, respiratory rate 28, and heart rate 130 beats/min; frequent premature ventricular contractions are observed on the cardiac monitor. Based on these data, what is the highest-priority nursing diagnosis for this client?

1. Ineffective breathing pattern.
2. Decreased cardiac output.
3. Ineffective thermoregulation.
4. Impaired urinary elimination.

206. The physician has determined that a client in respiratory distress requires intubation. Organize the following steps in preparing to assist the physician with rapid-sequence intubation in chronological order (with 1 being the first step in this procedure):

1. Monitor the client's ECG and pulse oximeter readings.
2. Administer sedation.
3. Auscultate breath sounds bilaterally.
4. Preoxygenate with 100% oxygen.
5. Apply cricoid pressure if needed.
6. Obtain a baseline assessment.

207. The nurse is caring for a client postoperatively following removal of a pituitary tumor. Which observation would alert the nurse to the possible development of diabetes insipidus (DI)?

1. Peripheral edema.
2. Urinary output greater than 200 mL/h.

3. Serum sodium of 150 mEq/L.
4. Weight gain.

208. Which action would be the first priority when caring for a client in anaphylaxis?

1. Obtaining vascular access.
2. Preventing future antigen exposure.
3. Administering oxygen via face mask.
4. Administering an antibiotic.

209. A client with a severe closed head injury has a systemic blood pressure of 100/60 mm Hg and an ICP reading of 24 mm Hg. What does the cerebral perfusion pressure of this client indicate?

1. Increased blood flow to the brain.
2. Normal intracranial pressure.
3. Impaired blood flow to the brain.
4. Adequate autoregulation of cerebral blood flow.

210. Twelve hours after a total thyroidectomy, the client develops stridor on exhalation. What is the nurse's best first action?

1. Reassure the client that the voice change is temporary.
2. Document the finding as the only action.
3. Hyperextend the client's neck.
4. Call for emergency assistance.

Identification

211. A nurse notices ventricular tachycardia on the cardiac monitor at the nurses' station and goes to the client's room. What is the first action the nurse should take in assisting this client?

_____

Multiple Choice

212. A client is brought to the emergency room after a motor vehicle accident that resulted in the client sustaining a head injury. Which assessments should the nurse perform immediately?

1. Assessment of pupils.
2. Assessment of motor function.
3. Assessment of respiratory status.
4. Assessment of short-term memory.

213. A nurse is caring for a client with a spinal cord injury. Which observations would indicate this client is exhibiting neurogenic shock?

1. Heart rate of 115 beats/min.
2. Heart rate of 52 beats/min.
3. Cool, moist skin.
4. Temperature of 102.5°F.

214. In planning care for a client with cirrhosis who was admitted with bleeding esophageal varices, to which goal should the nurse assign the highest priority?

1. Control the bleeding.
2. Maintain airway patency.
3. Maintain fluid volume.
4. Relieve the client's anxiety.

215. A client is being prepared for surgical repair of an abdominal aortic aneurysm. The nurse suspects complete aortic dissection when

1. The client complains of severe leg and arm pain.
2. The client becomes hypotensive and unresponsive.
3. A bruit and thrill are palpable at the aneurysm site.
4. The client becomes hypertensive and tachycardic.

216. A client is admitted with a fever and cough, and infection with *Mycobacterium tuberculosis* is suspected. Which infection control precautions should the nurse implement when caring for this client? (Select all that apply.)

1. Have the client wear a mask when leaving the room.
2. Place the client in a semi-private room.
3. Place the client in a negative-pressure room.
4. Allow the door of the client's room to remain open.
5. Wear sterile gloves when entering the client's room.
6. Wear a mask when working within 3 feet of the client.

217. A client is experiencing sepsis. The physician has ordered a medication infusion to be regulated to maintain a mean arterial pressure (MAP) between 65 and 75 mm Hg. Which of the client's blood pressure readings meet this prescribed goal?

1. 95/52 mm Hg.
2. 98/40 mm Hg.
3. 122/88 mm Hg.
4. 90/50 mm Hg.

218. Which clinical manifestation would lead the nurse to suspect that the client might be in disseminated intravascular coagulopathy (DIC)?

1. Diminished bowel sounds.
2. Oozing of serous drainage from venipuncture sites.
3. Positive Homan's sign.
4. Platelet count 175,000/µL.

219. A client who has been diagnosed with insulin-dependent diabetes mellitus is being taught what to do when signs and symptoms of hypoglycemia occur. Which statement made by the client would indicate an understanding of the teaching?

1. "It is important to increase my activity prior to insulin administration."
2. "It is important to rest in bed until the symptoms subside."
3. "It is important to eat 4–6 Lifesavers candies or drink a glass of orange juice."
4. "It is important to decrease the amount of long-acting insulin."

220. The intraparenchymal ICP monitor on a client with a closed head injury shows a sustained pressure of 20 mm Hg. What should the nurse's first action be?

1. Notify the physician immediately, and prepare the client for ventriculostomy placement.
2. Immediately lower the ventriculostomy drainage bag, and drain the CSF until the ICP is 12 mm Hg.
3. Document the reading, and reassess the client in 30 minutes.
4. Eliminate all stimuli, and elevate the head of the bed while maintaining head alignment.

Identification

221. An adult client is brought into the Emergency Department in cardiac arrest. Cardiopulmonary resuscitation (CPR) is being performed. Name the area where the pulse should be checked.

_____

Multiple Choice

222. A client is admitted to the burn unit with third-degree burns to the chest, face, and upper extremities. During the acute phase (i.e., first 48 hours) of a major burn injury, which assessment findings should the nurse report immediately?

1. Edema of the hands.
2. Urinary output of 200 mL over 8 hours.
3. Temperature of 100°F.
4. Decreased sensation in the extremities.

MANAGEMENT OF CARE

1. Correct Answer: **2**

Rationale: A client with acute pulmonary edema is the priority because oxygenation is the problem to be addressed.

2. Correct Answer: **2**

Rationale: The level of competency determines which activities and responsibilities a person can perform.

3. Correct Answers: **3, 4, and 5**

Rationale: Colostomy care consists of washing the hands, removing the pouch and skin barrier, observing the site and skin for redness or irritation, and reapplying the barrier and pouch. Powder and antimicrobial ointments are not used, and the use of sterile gloves is not indicated.

4. Correct Answer: **4**

Rationale: A client's autonomy and ability to make decisions that affect his or her care must be considered and honored if it is the most beneficial and least harmful course of action.

5. Correct Answer: **4**

Rationale: A history of an allergy to bananas is a risk factor suggesting that the client could be allergic to latex. Latex is a substance that is commonly found in surgical gloves.

6. Correct Answer: **3**

Rationale: The lowest-priority client in this instance is the one with a hemothorax and a chest tube, which does not require that the client be connected to suction. All of the other clients have conditions that require the assessment and attention of the registered nurse.

7. Correct Answer: **1**

Rationale: The planning phase of the nursing process includes developing goals and outcomes that assist in creating the nursing care plan or plan of care for the client.

8. Correct Answers: **1, 3, 5, and 6**

Rationale: The presence of a deep vein thrombosis is usually manifested by swelling, an increase in circumference, throbbing, and a positive Homan's sign. A pulse will be present because this is a venous problem. The extremity is usually very warm to the touch; it would be cool if the client was experiencing an arterial problem.

9. Correct Answer: **2**

Rationale: The case manager would coordinate the healthcare services needed by the client.

10. Correct Answer: **1**

Rationale: The primary goal is to maintain a patent airway. Given the presence of audible gurgling, this client needs to be suctioned first through the tracheostomy that is present for this type of surgical procedure.

11. Correct Answer: **2**

Rationale: Everyone involved in this type of client care should be informed of this information, as it directly affects all client care.

12. Correct Answer: **4**

Rationale: Obtaining informed consent is an active, shared decision-making process between the surgeon and the client. The surgeon must provide adequate disclosure of the benefits and risks of the proposed procedure. In addition, the client must have a clear understanding and comprehension of the procedure to be done. Lastly, the consent must be voluntary and not forced.

13. Correct Answers: **2, 4, 5, and 6**

Rationale: The hands should be washed prior to beginning a dressing change. Next, gloves should be donned and worn as the old dressing is removed and discarded. A dressing kit is typically used for this purpose; it contains new gloves and all essential supplies. After inspecting the site, the skin is cleaned by using a circular motion with an antiseptic swab, and then a new dressing is applied.

14. Correct Answer: **4**

Rationale: Written consent must be obtained prior to any release of information. Client privacy must be assured.

15. Correct Answer: **3**

Rationale: Smoke inhalation most likely includes a thermal injury to the tracheobronchial tree. Swelling will occur quickly, so the client's respiratory status needs to be monitored closely. Sometimes, endotracheal intubation is necessary to maintain a patent airway.

16. Correct Answer: **4**

Rationale: The five "rights" for medication administration include the right client and the right dose.

17. Correct Answer: **2**

Rationale: A current client who requires routine care and ongoing assessment is most appropriate for an LPN assignment. The other clients listed here need initial assessment, and their care requires specialized IV and medication training.

18. Correct Answers: **2, 4, 5, 6, and 7**

Rationale: Room temperature and PO intake are not critical information to communicate in the report. This client is not taking anything orally because the nutritional support occurs through enteric feedings.

19. Correct Answer: **2**

Rationale: Garlic is a supplement that can interfere with clotting. Its use should be discontinued 2–3 weeks before surgery.

20. Correct Answer: **1**

Rationale: When providing direct care to a burn client, staff must wear gloves, caps, gowns, and masks to prevent an infection. Although burn clients are susceptible to infections, administration of antibiotics is not ordered until specific cultures and organisms are identified.

21. Correct Answer: **4**

Rationale: Insertion of a urinary catheter is a sterile procedure. To reduce the likelihood of introducing bacteria into the bladder, a new catheter would need to be obtained in this scenario.

22. Correct Answer: **1**

Rationale: This client needs to be placed on airborne precautions to prevent spread of the infection.

23. Correct Answer: **Good hand washing**

Rationale: Hand washing is the most effective way to prevent the spread of infectious organisms.

24. Correct Answer: **2**

Rationale: The most important aspect of aseptic technique is good hand washing.

25. Correct Answer: **2**

Rationale: When a fire is suspected or confirmed, the nurse's first action should be to remove clients who are in immediate danger and then activate the fire alarm.

26. Correct Answer: **1**

Rationale: The best way for the RN to handle this situation is to not embarrass the LPN in front of the client, but to use the opportunity as a teaching moment to ensure that the procedure is done correctly.

27. Correct Answers: **1, 3, 6, and 7**

Rationale: Management of a client who returns from surgery with a chest tube includes being prepared to apply wall suction to the ordered amount and being prepared for a possible disconnection or abrupt discontinuation of the chest tube.

28. Correct Answer: **1**

Rationale: Continuous venovenous hemofiltration involves continuous hemofiltration through the venous system. The client's weight should be measured before and after dialysis, and then daily if the client remains on continuous venovenous hemofiltration. In addition, the client's blood pressure should be monitored, as only hemodynamically unstable clients require this type of dialysis. Finally, the type of dialysate used and the amount of fluid removed should be documented.

29. Correct Answer: **3**

Rationale: Both clients can be cared for by the same nurse. Client A should be moved to a quiet room—preferably a private room, if one is available. Bleeding into the subarachnoid space causes headaches, so this client needs a quiet, dark room in which to rest.

30. Correct Answer: **2**

Rationale: NPH insulin is an intermediate-acting insulin. It is important that the client eat at normal times, because the onset for this type of insulin is 1–3 hours and the peak action occurs 8 hours following its administration.

31. Correct Answers: 1, 3, 4, and 5

Rationale: Most blood products require a micro-aggregate filter when they are administered to clients. The exception is clotting factors, for which such filtering would remove the needed components in these factors.

32. Correct Answer: 2

Rationale: Slight swelling could indicate fluid seeping into the tissues and possible infiltration.

33. Correct Answer: 1

Rationale: Varicella-zoster is highly contagious and is transmitted by direct contact and airborne. The client needs to be isolated, and strict isolation procedures need to be maintained.

34. Correct Answer: 1

Rationale: Clients have the right to be autonomous and make their own choices.

35. Correct Answer: 2

Rationale: Bathing is an activity that CNAs can perform as long as the client is not compromised or does not need a licensed professional.

36. Correct Answers: 1 and 6

Rationale: Medications are delivered through a gastrostomy tube with a syringe and are flushed with the tube clamped after administration. Medications are delivered at room temperature and are often mixed with water if they are highly viscous. Tablets are crushed to a fine powder. Enteric-coated medications are never crushed, however.

37. Correct Answer: 4

Rationale: The other three clients require an initial assessment or complex medication administration and assessment.

38. Correct Answer: 4

Rationale: Upon the client's arrival on the unit from the recovery room, the client's vital signs should be taken and an assessment performed, to include observing the dressing and assessing for the presence of pain.

39. Correct Answer: 2

Rationale: Because pulmonary infections are common with this disease process and in the presence of a tracheostomy, the desired outcome of performing accurate and adequate CPT would be a reduction in pneumonia-related hospitalizations.

40. Correct Answer: 3

Rationale: An immunosuppressed client has a decreased number of white blood cells and is at an increased risk for infection.

41. Correct Answers: 2 and 3

Rationale: IV fluids are ordered to infuse continuously so the continuous IV fluids would not be disconnected. Instead, the IV piggyback fluids would be connected to the primary IV fluid set at the port closest to the primary fluid bag; the bag containing these fluids would need to be hung higher than the primary fluid bag.

42. Correct Answer: 1

Rationale: Air embolism is a complication that can occur during a transfusion. It is manifested as sudden difficulty in breathing, apprehension, and a sharp pain in the chest.

43. Correct Answer: 4

Rationale: During the acute phase of Guillain-Barré syndrome, the major nursing goal is to detect respiratory and cardiac dysfunction and to assist in treating the client as the disease progresses.

44. Correct Answer: 2

Rationale: Hyperthyroidism is characterized by excessive release of thyroid hormone, which makes the client nervous, hyperexcitable, irritable, and apprehensive. Therefore, the nurse would want to assign this client to a private room that is located far away from the activity of the nurses' station and traffic flow on the unit.

SAFETY AND INFECTION CONTROL

45. Correct Answer: 1

Rationale: The best way to prevent any infection is to perform thorough hand washing.

46. Correct Answer: 3

Rationale: An obturator should be available to insert into the stoma if the tracheostomy tube becomes dislodged.

47. Correct Answer: 2

Rationale: Cocaine is a central nervous system stimulant. Symptoms of a cocaine overdose include increased blood pressure and heart rate. The heart muscle is irritable, so arrhythmias may also occur.

48. Correct Answers: **1 and 2**

    Rationale: If a seizure occurs, it is important to remain with the client and to stay calm while observing the seizure. Allow the seizure to proceed without interference, but protect the client by removing any hazards or hard objects in the vicinity. Do not place anything in the client's mouth, but keep suction available in case the client vomits or excessive saliva is present. Because this client has a known history of seizures, the side rails of the bed should be padded as a precaution.

49. Correct Answer: **2**

    Rationale: Herpes simplex virus, type 2 (also known as genital herpes), is highly contagious when lesions are present and must be treated promptly. Acyclovir is an antiviral agent used to treat this condition.

50. Correct Answer: **3**

    Rationale: Airborne precautions include standard precaution equipment plus the use of a mask.

51. Correct Answer: **3**

    Rationale: The arterial access through the femoral artery is prone to bleeding. The client should be positioned in such a way as to prevent increased pressure on the site and allow for adequate clotting.

52. Correct Answer: **4**

    Rationale: Preventive foot care includes properly bathing, drying, and lubricating the feet. Hot water should not be used because the client has neuropathy and cannot feel the extent of the temperature of the water. Shoes should fit well and be closed-toe.

53. Correct Answers: **1, 4, and 5**

    Rationale: With a confused client, the nurse would initially institute measures that are not considered restraints. Restraints are used as a last resort when other measures do not work.

54. Correct Answer: **2**

    Rationale: As part of the five "rights" to medication administration, the nurse needs to verify

that the medication is being administered to the right client.

55. Correct Answer: **2**

    Rationale: Meningitis is extremely contagious. Any client with suspected meningitis must be isolated.

56. Correct Answer: **2**

    Rationale: In clients with Von Willebrand's disease (also known as hemophilia), trauma and bleeding occurrences need to be minimized.

57. Correct Answer: **2**

    Rationale: A low-pressure ventilator alarm most likely signals a disconnection from the ventilator.

58. Correct Answers: **2, 3, 4, 5, and 6**

    Rationale: Client safety is the primary goal. To prevent medication errors, five "rights" to medication administration are observed: right client, right medication, right time, right dose, and right route.

59. Correct Answer: **3**

    Rationale: Damage to the frontal lobe may result in inappropriate behavior, inattentiveness, impaired judgment, inappropriate social behavior, and flat affect.

60. Correct Answer: **4**

    Rationale: This order needs to be checked for its accuracy.

61. Correct Answer: **1**

    Rationale: A sterile dressing change requires scrubbing for the procedure and maintaining a sterile field at all times until the dressing change is complete.

62. Correct Answer: **Standard precautions**

    Rationale: Standard precautions are used in the care of all clients, regardless of their diagnoses.

63. Correct Answer: **3**

    Rationale: Each pin site should be examined carefully to detect any signs of infection, such as redness or drainage.

64. Correct Answer: **3**

    Rationale: If contrast medium is used, the resultant diuresis may require fluid replacement.

SECTION I
SECTION II
SECTION III
SECTION IV
SECTION V
SECTION VI
SECTION VII
SECTION VIII
SECTION IX
SECTION X

65. Correct Answer: **2**

Rationale: A bone marrow transplant recipient has a compromised immune system due to immunosuppression and needs to be protected from other individuals who might be contagious.

66. Correct Answer: **1**

Rationale: The medical record is a legal document, so standards for charting must be followed when errors in documentation occur. To correct a documentation error, the nurse would draw a single line through the entry and then write "error" and his or her initials above or beside the entry.

HEALTH PROMOTION AND MAINTENANCE

67. Correct Answer: **2**

Rationale: Atherosclerosis is the pathophysiological cause that contributes to angina.

68. Correct Answer: **2**

Rationale: Positive relief from analgesia administration would mean that the pain medication is working.

69. Correct Answer: **Hepatitis A**

Rationale: Hepatitis A is typically spread through consumption of contaminated food.

70. Correct Answer: **1**

Rationale: The greatest risk factor for developing testicular cancer is the presence of an undescended testicle.

71. Correct Answer: **4**

Rationale: Modifiable risk factors can be changed in a positive way, such as by controlling lipid levels and blood pressure.

72. Correct Answer: **3**

Rationale: A tuberculin skin test is considered positive when the induration is greater than 5 mm.

73. Correct Answer: **4**

Rationale: To prevent polypharmacy interactions, it is essential that the physician be aware of all medications and supplements that the client is taking.

74. Correct Answers: **2, 3, 4, and 5**

Rationale: Risk factors for breast cancer include age, previous history of breast cancer, prolifera-tive breast disease, early onset of menses, late age for menopause, first-degree relative with breast cancer, genetic link with the BRCA-1 and BRCA-2 mutations, obesity, and consumption of a high-fat diet.

75. Correct Answer: **3**

Rationale: The client with left-sided paralysis is older than age 40 and is immobile and not able to move around, which puts him at greater risk for developing DVT.

76. Correct Answer: **2**

Rationale: Vaginal stenosis is best prevented by providing frequent tissue expansion.

77. Correct Answer: **3**

Rationale: Because the client cannot read, another instructional strategy must be used. To be most effective, this strategy should be one that the client prefers.

78. Correct Answer: **4**

Rationale: Smoking damages the ciliary action in the respiratory tract, which is a protective mechanism.

79. Correct Answer: **Low sodium or low salt**

Rationale: High sodium levels lead to increased water retention and thus increased intra-vascular volume, which in turn contributes to increased blood pressure.

80. Correct Answer: **2**

Rationale: A breast self-exam is best performed 5–7 days after menses—a time when less fluid is retained in the breast tissue.

81. Correct Answer: **3**

Rationale: Explaining the importance and reason for the activity will assist the client in understanding the importance of the activity.

82. Correct Answer: **3**

Rationale: Fibrocystic breast disease can be minimized by dietary changes such as increasing consumption of vitamin E and taking hormone therapy. Limiting coffee consumption may also help because it leads to a lower intake of methylxanthine (caffeine is not the important factor here).

83. Correct Answer: **3**

Rationale: Cranial nerve III deals with occulomotor function. The pupil size, shape, and reaction are tested in this case.

84. Correct Answers: <u>**1, 2, 3, and 4**</u>

    Rationale: Currently available adult vaccines include those for hepatitis A and B, influenza, and pneumonia. No vaccine is available for hepatitis C or *H. pylori.*

85. Correct Answer: <u>**1**</u>

    Rationale: The most important risk factors for developing cervical cancer are early sexual activity, multiple sexual partners, smoking, and infection with HPV.

86. Correct Answer: <u>**3**</u>

    Rationale: Obesity can contribute to degenerative joint disease and is considered a modifiable risk factor.

PSYCHOSOCIAL INTEGRITY

87. Correct Answer: <u>**3**</u>

    Rationale: Asking a client to state in his or her own words the reason for seeking care provides the overall perception the client has regarding being admitted.

88. Correct Answer: <u>**3**</u>

    Rationale: This client is exhibiting signs that she is unable to cope and function through chemical dependencies and managing everyday life.

89. Correct Answers: <u>**2, 4, and 5**</u>

    Rationale: To best determine the probable occurrence of alcohol withdrawal symptoms, an assessment of the individual's drinking history and the time and quantity of the last alcohol consumption are important pieces of information to be collected.

90. Correct Answer: <u>**1**</u>

    Rationale: An attempt at suicide points to an immediate need for protection and safety from harming self.

91. Correct Answer: <u>**2**</u>

    Rationale: The client is having difficulty with the change in her appearance, as evidenced by her crying and verbalizations.

92. Correct Answer: <u>**2**</u>

Rationale: Delirium tremens is manifested by tremulousness, anorexia, hypertension, and confusion.

93. Correct Answer: <u>**2**</u>

    Rationale: A psychological stressor is something that is personally emotional.

94. Correct Answer: <u>**Denial**</u>

    Rationale: Denial is used as a protective reaction to increased anxiety.

95. Correct Answer: <u>**3**</u>

    Rationale: Adjustment disorders result from a failure of existing coping skills. The primary goal of treatment is to assist the client in identifying the stressful event and current problems.

96. Correct Answer: <u>**4**</u>

    Rationale: Understanding and emotional support are essential because the client is expressing ineffective coping—the client feels isolated, helpless, and out of control.

97. Correct Answer: <u>**3**</u>

    Rationale: Open communication and effective listening skills must be used when caring for a client who may have been the victim of sexual abuse.

98. Correct Answer: <u>**2**</u>

    Rationale: This response validates what has been expressed by the client and encourages further exploration of the client's feelings and perceptions.

99. Correct Answers: <u>**1, 3, 4, and 5**</u>

    Rationale: Possible signs of elder abuse may include poor nutrition, poor hygiene and unkempt appearance, and unexplained medical signs and symptoms such as excessive bruising. Disorientation might be due to age and needs further testing. Recent fractures might be secondary to a fall and osteoporosis.

100. Correct Answer: <u>**3**</u>

    Rationale: Encouraging open communication about what to expect as the client dies provides the greatest support to the client and family.

101. Correct Answer: <u>**2**</u>

    Rationale: The client is coming to terms with the physical impairment from the spinal cord injury and the loss of independence.

SECTION I

SECTION II

SECTION III

SECTION IV

SECTION V

SECTION VI

SECTION VII

SECTION VIII

SECTION IX

SECTION X

102. Correct Answer: **4**

Rationale: This statement addresses the spouse's concerns accurately.

103. Correct Answer: **1**

Rationale: Developing a trusting relationship includes sharing one's innermost feelings.

104. Correct Answer: **Alcoholics Anonymous**

Rationale: The preferred outpatient support group for recovering alcoholics is Alcoholics Anonymous.

105. Correct Answer: **4**

Rationale: Open communication and effective listening skills must be used when caring for a possible rape victim.

106. Correct Answer: **3**

Rationale: Tolerance means that a larger dose is now needed to achieve the same effects once experienced with the original dose.

BASIC CARE AND COMFORT

107. Correct Answer: **2**

Rationale: The head of the bed should be elevated at least 30 degrees and the client should be in a neutral position to promote venous outflow. There should be no flexion or extension of the neck or hips.

108. Correct Answer: **2**

Rationale: A client with mild stomatitis is in discomfort and needs items that will soothe (and not irritate) the mouth and gum tissue.

109. Correct Answer: **3**

Rationale: A perforated ulcer will manifest suddenly and dramatically. A client will report severe, upper abdominal pain and possibly shoulder pain if gastric contents spill out and irritate the phrenic nerve.

110. Correct Answers: **2 and 5**

Rationale: The cane is held on the client's stronger side and is advanced 4–12 inches for every stride. The weaker leg moves first until it is parallel to the cane.

111. Correct Answer: **3**

Rationale: A client with hypothyroidism has a slow metabolism. The client is typically inactive and has most likely experienced a weight gain.

112. Correct Answer: **2**

Rationale: Cystitis is an inflammation of the bladder. Urinary tract infections are best prevented by decreasing the likelihood of urinary stasis.

113. Correct Answer: **2**

Rationale: The client is at risk for bleeding related to the vitamin K deficiency and the altered liver functions.

114. Correct Answer: **3**

Rationale: The client should be taught to participate in activities early in the day or during the energy peaks that follow medication administration.

115. Correct Answer: **High Fowler's position**

Rationale: In the high Fowler's position, the client sits at a 90-degree angle, which promotes maximum lung and chest wall expansion.

116. Correct Answer: **3**

Rationale: Adduction beyond the midline could dislodge the newly implanted prosthesis.

117. Correct Answer: **1**

Rationale: The head of the bed should be elevated to assist with breathing and to maintain the airway.

118. Correct Answer: **3**

Rationale: Clients with cholelithiasis should avoid consumption of foods high in cholesterol, such as whole milk, butter, fried foods, and gas-forming vegetables.

119. Correct Answer: **4**

Rationale: A urinary catheter occlusion would cause a decrease in the amount of urine in the collection bag. The most indicative assessment finding would be the distended bladder.

120. Correct Answers: **5 and 6**

Rationale: Decerebrate posturing—the extension of the upper extremities in response to noxious stimuli—represents further neurological deterioration. Clear drainage from the nose or ears in conjunction with a basilar skull fracture could be cerebrospinal fluid and necessitates notification of the physician.

121. Correct Answer: **1**

Rationale: The infection might be spread with the application of heat to the affected area.

122. Correct Answer: **4**

Rationale: Lactulose causes diarrhea, which is how excess ammonia is excreted; thus this medication should help improve the client's mental functioning.

123. Correct Answer: **3**

Rationale: Small, frequent, bland meals are less irritating.

124. Correct Answer: $3 \rightarrow 2 \rightarrow 1 \rightarrow 5 \rightarrow 4 \rightarrow 6$

Rationale: First, the client is placed in the high Fowler's position. Next, the tube is measured for approximate insertion length. The tube is lubricated and passed through the nose first, and then downward and straight back. If the client can swallow, he or she should be asked to assist in this procedure. Once the tube is in place, confirm its placement and secure the tube.

125. Correct Answer: **3**

Rationale: Postoperative care of a client following a modified radical mastectomy includes not taking the blood pressure or performing venipunctures on the operative side.

126. Correct Answer: **3**

Rationale: A client suffering from a migraine should seek a quiet environment with the lights dimmed.

PHARMACOLOGICAL AND PARENTERAL THERAPIES

127. Correct Answer: **3**

Rationale:

$$125 \text{ mg}/1 \text{ mL} = 1,000 \text{ mg}/x$$
$$x = 8.0 \text{ mL}$$

128. Correct Answer: **3**

Rationale: The prothrombin time (PT) and international normalized ratio (INR) are monitored to ascertain the effectiveness of Coumadin therapy.

129. Correct Answer: **4**

Rationale:

$$1,000 \text{ mg}/500 \text{ mL} = x \text{ mg}/30 \text{ mL}$$
$$x = 60 \text{ mg}$$

130. Correct Answers: **1, 3, 4, 5, and 6**

Rationale: A hemolytic reaction is the most severe reaction and occurs in the event of an incompatible blood transfusion. Clinical manifestations of a hemolytic reaction include chills, shaking, fever, headache, red or black urine, flank pain, nausea and vomiting, tightness in the chest, and pain at the needle site.

131. Correct Answer: **4**

Rationale: Hyperglycemia and hypoglycemia are common side effects that should be monitored with TPN administration. TPN should be delivered at a constant rate and should not be discontinued for long periods of time.

132. Correct Answer: **1**

Rationale: Afterload will be increased because dopamine infused at this dose causes vasoconstriction, making it a little more difficult for the heart to pump, and leads to increased blood pressure and mean arterial pressure.

133. Correct Answer: **4**

Rationale:

$$500 \text{ mL}/10 \text{ h} = 50 \text{ mL/h}$$
$$1,000 \text{ mg}/500 \text{ mL} = x \text{ mg}/50 \text{ mL}$$
$$x = 100 \text{ mg}/50 \text{ mL}$$

134. Correct Answer: **2**

Rationale: The client's heart rate must be checked prior to the administration of digoxin. The medication would be withheld if the heart rate of an adult client is less than 60 beats/min.

135. Correct Answer: **1.2 mL**

Rationale:

$$125 \text{ mg}/2 \text{ mL} = 75 \text{ mg}/x$$
$$125x/125 = 150/125$$
$$x = 1.2 \text{ mL}$$

136. Correct Answer: **3**

Rationale: The antidote for a benzodiazepine overdose is flumazenil (Romazicon).

137. Correct Answer: **1**

Rationale: Cardiac output is severely compromised in this client owing to the profound and symptomatic bradycardia. Cardiac output = stroke volume × heart rate. Epinephrine will increase the heart rate and cause vasoconstriction, which in turn will increase afterload and thus assist in increasing cardiac output.

138. Correct Answer: **3**

Rationale: 500 mL/6 h = 83.3 mL/h ≈ 83 mL/h

SECTION I

SECTION II

SECTION III

SECTION IV

SECTION V

SECTION VI

SECTION VII

SECTION VIII

SECTION IX

SECTION X

139. Correct Answer: 4

Rationale: The route of administration was incorrect and could lead to an adverse effect—namely, bleeding. The physician should be notified and the incident documented.

140. Correct Answer: 1

Rationale: Epinephrine is the initial medication administered in a code situation where the client is in pulseless electrical activity.

141. Correct Answer: 6.25 mL

Rationale:

$$32 \text{ mg}/50 \text{ mL} = 4 \text{ mg}/x$$
$$x = 6.25 \text{ mL}$$

142. Correct Answer: 3

Rationale: The development of a rash is a possible sign of an allergic reaction to the medication. The medication should be discontinued.

143. Correct Answer: 1

Rationale: Regular (short-acting) insulin should be drawn up first in case contamination of the vials occurs.

144. Correct Answer: 4

Rationale: Amphotericin B affects renal function and is nephrotoxic. BUN and serum creatinine levels must be monitored closely in this client.

145. Correct Answer: 15 mL/h

Rationale:

$$\text{Concentration} = 400 \text{ mg} \div 250 \text{ mL} \times 1,000$$
$$= 1.6 \times 1,000$$
$$= 1,600 \text{ mcg/mL}$$

$$\text{Rate in mL/h} = \frac{\text{mcg/kg/min to be given} \times 60 \times \text{kg}}{\text{Drip concentration in mcg/mL}}$$

$$= \frac{5 \times 60 \times 80}{1,600}$$

$$= \frac{24,000}{1,600}$$

$$= 15 \text{ mL/h}$$

146. Correct Answer: 2

Rationale: For an adult, the earlobe should be pulled up and back to straighten the ear canal and allow the medication to enter.

147. Correct Answer: 1

Rationale:

$$\text{gtt/min} = \frac{\text{total} \times \text{drop factor}}{\text{time (min)}} = \frac{1,000 \text{ mL} \times 15}{10 \times 60}$$

$$= \frac{15,000}{600} = 25 \text{ gtt/min}$$

148. Correct Answer: 1

Rationale: Glucocorticoids are best taken in the morning with food to prevent insomnia and gastrointestinal upset.

149. Correct Answer: 3

Rationale: Diltiazem is a calcium-channel blocker that is prescribed for hypertension and fast-rate atrial fibrillation. Adverse effects associated with this agent include hypotension and bradycardia.

150. Correct Answer: 0.08 mL

Rationale: Insulin comes in a vial with a concentration of 100 U/mL. In this case, the amount needed is calculated to be 0.08 mL.

151. Correct Answer: 2

Rationale: Exercise and activity can lower blood glucose levels, so additional food is needed in case of exertion. A client with type 2 diabetes usually takes an oral agent and is considered non-insulin-dependent.

152. Correct Answer: 1

Rationale: Bradycardia and hypotension are the major systemic side effects encountered when administering Dilantin intravenously.

153. Correct Answer: 4

Rationale: The client has had too much morphine and needs to be given an antagonist to reverse its effects. The narcotic antagonist to be administered is naloxone.

154. Correct Answer: 17 mL/h

Rationale:

$$\frac{187 \text{ lb}}{2.2 \text{ kg}} = 85 \text{ kg} \qquad \frac{25,000 \text{ U}}{250 \text{ mL}} = 100 \text{ U/mL}$$

$$20 \text{ U/kg/h} = 100 \text{ U/mL}$$
$$20 \text{ U/85 kg/h} = 100 \text{ U/mL}$$

$$\frac{1,700 \text{ U/h}}{100} = \frac{100 \text{ U/mL}}{100}$$

$$= 17 \text{ mL/h}$$

155. Correct Answer: 4

Rationale: Unrelieved chest pain is best treated with oxygen, nitroglycerin, morphine, and aspirin.

156. Correct Answer: 3

Rationale:

$$\frac{1\,g}{1,000\,mg} = \frac{0.04\,g}{x\,mg} \quad x = 40\,mg$$

$$\frac{10\,mg}{1\,tab} = \frac{40\,mg}{x\,tab} \quad x = 4\,tablets$$

157. Correct Answer: 2

Rationale: A potential side effect of ibuprofen is bleeding.

158. Correct Answer: 1

Rationale: The skeletal muscle weakness extends to the ability to chew and swallow, so clients with myasthenia gravis are at risk for aspiration during meals. The majority of the meal should be eaten at a time when the medication is having its peak effect, thereby enhancing the client's chewing and swallowing abilities.

159. Correct Answer: 11.25 mL

Rationale:

$$15\,mEq/x = 20\,mEq/15\,mL$$
$$x = 11.25\,mL$$

REDUCTION AND RISK POTENTIAL

160. Correct Answer: 3

Rationale: The client will remain on both medications until the appropriate international normalized ratio (INR) is reached. At that point, the heparin infusion will be discontinued.

161. Correct Answer: 4

Rationale: Chronic renal failure presents with decreased urinary output and increased serum BUN, creatinine, and potassium levels. In this case, the serum BUN level is elevated and everything else is within normal limits.

162. Correct Answer: 2

Rationale: Clients with hypoparathyroidism will manifest with increased serum phosphorus levels and decreased serum calcium levels. The decreased amount of calcium leads to muscle tetany, as evidenced by a positive Chvostek's sign.

163. Correct Answers: 1, 2, 5, and 6

Rationale: Assessment findings warranting a call to the physician include signs and symptoms of bleeding and possible perfusion problems. In this case, the client's decreased blood pressure, increased heart rate, increased amount of blood drainage, and asymmetrical pulses would necessitate notification of the physician.

164. Correct Answer: 2

Rationale: The primary and priority concern for a client with acute respiratory distress syndrome is maintaining oxygenation and preventing hypoxia.

165. Correct Answer: 2

Rationale: Plasmapheresis may help in improving the clinical manifestations of myasthenia gravis.

166. Correct Answer: 1

Rationale: Consolidation will result in diminished breath sounds over the lobes involved.

167. Correct Answer: Mitral area or fifth intercostal space at the left midclavicular line.

168. Correct Answer: 2

Rationale: Weighing the client is the most accurate assessment technique to determine effectiveness of (i.e., fluid loss from) furosemide.

169. Correct Answer: 4

Rationale: The first change in tissue perfusion will be manifested as a change in the client's level of consciousness. In compensatory shock, blood pressure will be normal and the client will be tachycardic with urinary output beginning to diminish.

170. Correct Answer: 3

Rationale: Based on the assessment findings, this client appears to be showing signs of respiratory depression. Both medications should be withheld.

171. Correct Answer: 1

Rationale: Clear drainage from the nose is most likely cerebrospinal fluid (CSF) and would be a complication in this case.

172. Correct Answers: 1, 3, 5, and 6

Rationale: Active bleeding would result in tachycardia, decreased blood pressure, increased respirations, and decreased hemoglobin and hematocrit levels.

173. Correct Answer: 2

Rationale: The best method for evaluating the effectiveness and adequacy of gavage feeding is to weigh the client and observe a weight gain.

174. Correct Answer: 3

Rationale: One of the earliest signs of an oxygenation problem is restlessness. The client's use of accessory muscles for breathing also means that the client is making an increased effort to maintain oxygenation.

175. Correct Answer: 1

Rationale: Bubbling in the suction chamber is normal and indicates that the drainage system is connected to suction.

176. Correct Answer: 4

Rationale: The airway must be evaluated. The lab results indicate that the client is in respiratory acidosis and needs to be stimulated to breathe deeply so pCO_2 does not continue to increase.

177. Correct Answers: 1, 3, 4, and 6

Rationale: Graves' disease results from hyperthyroidism and is characterized by nervousness, hyperactivity, exophthalamos, hypertension, tachycardia, bounding peripheral pulses, and weight loss, among other signs and symptoms.

178. Correct Answer: 4

Rationale: The pacemaker is set in the demand mode at a rate of 70, which means that the pacemaker will fire whenever the heart rate falls below 70 beats/min.

179. Correct Answer: 2

Rationale: A facial butterfly rash is very characteristic of SLE. Lab findings include leukocytosis or leucopenia.

180. Correct Answer: 3

Rationale: An allergy to shellfish indicates a sensitivity to iodine, which is a component of the radiographic dye used in cardiac catheterization. The client's allergic reaction to shellfish could precipitate an anaphylactic reaction while the client is undergoing this procedure.

181. Correct Answer: 1

Rationale: Maintaining hydration reduces the viscosity of the sickled blood.

182. Correct Answers: 1, 2, and 6

Rationale: An S_3 heart sound is most readily heard when the client is in the supine or left lateral position and the bell of the stethoscope is used. The sound increases on inspiration and is heard most clearly at the apex.

183. Correct Answer: 3

Rationale: Oxygenation is the problem in this case. The most appropriate action is to have the client take some deep breaths and cough.

184. Correct Answer: 1

Rationale: Both medications have a tendency to contribute to gastrointestinal bleeding.

185. Correct Answer: 3

Rationale: Activity intolerance is the priority diagnosis, as there is an imbalance between oxygen supply and demand in this client.

186. Correct Answer: 1

Rationale: The platelet lab value is abnormally low, indicating that the client is at risk for bleeding.

187. Correct Answers: 1, 2, and 4

Rationale: When delivering intermittent feedings by NG tube, one would first position the client with the head of the bed elevated at least 30 degrees. Then gastric contents would be aspirated, followed by using an open system flow of feeding from a syringe barrel (no plunger). The feeding would be complete when the tube is flushed with 30–60 mL of water and then clamped until the next feeding.

188. Correct Answer: 4

Rationale: Coumadin is a blood thinner (anticoagulant), and bruising is a common side effect that does not prompt discontinuation of the medication. Products containing aspirin should be avoided because they can aggravate the tendency to bleed.

189. Correct Answer: 3

Rationale: Numbness and tingling around the mouth or in the fingers and toes are manifestations of hypocalcemia, which may potentially progress to muscle tetany and seizure activity.

190. Correct Answer: 1

Rationale: Serum creatinine measures the effectiveness of renal function. BUN is an index of renal function.

191. Correct Answer: **2**

Rationale: Hyperparathyroidism results in acute hypercalcemia. To flush the extra calcium out of the system, fluid is required.

192. Correct Answers: **2, 3, and 5**

Rationale: Clients with SIADH exhibit a decreased serum sodium level, a urine specific gravity greater than 1.005, and a weight gain.

PHYSIOLOGICAL ADAPTATION

193. Correct Answer: **3**

Rationale: This client is exhibiting signs and symptoms of a pulmonary embolism. The nurse's first action would be to apply oxygen and notify the physician.

194. Correct Answer: **2**

Rationale: Adenosine is administered for supraventricular tachycardia.

195. Correct Answer: **3**

Rationale: The wheezing and itching could indicate anaphylaxis, so the infusion must be discontinued.

196. Correct Answers: **1, 2, 3, and 5**

Rationale: When preparing to intubate an adult client, the equipment needed includes a cuffed (not uncuffed) endotracheal tube, an ambu bag and face mask to oxygenate the client, and a laryngoscope. Sterile gloves are not necessary, but clean nonsterile gloves and other personal protective equipment should be used during the procedure.

197. Correct Answer: **2**

Rationale: Cushing's triad is a late sign of increased intracranial pressure. It consists of severe hypertension, widened pulse pressure, bradycardia, and slowed, irregular respirations.

198. Correct Answer: **3**

Rationale: The initial treatment for ventricular fibrillation is to defibrillate at 360 joules using a monophasic defibrillator.

199. Correct Answer: **4**

Rationale: The nurse must assess the client further to determine the problem before notifying the physician or performing other interventions.

200. Correct Answer: **2**

Rationale: The early-onset stage of acute respiratory distress syndrome will be characterized by respiratory alkalosis.

201. Correct Answer: **4 → 2 → 5 → 1 → 3 → 6**

Rationale: Synchronized cardioversion is used for unstable tachycardia. It discharges a shock on the R wave and must be delivered in the "synch" mode. One first begins by considering the administration of sedation if there is time.

202. Correct Answer: **1**

Rationale: Nitroprusside sodium is a potent, rapid-acting hypertensive agent that causes vasodilation. This client is hypertensive, and the blood pressure abnormality needs to be treated.

203. Correct Answer: **2**

Rationale: The best determinant of chest compression effectiveness during CPR is a palpable femoral pulse with each compression.

204. Correct Answer: **3**

Rationale: The chest pain typically associated with acute coronary syndrome is described as crushing and vise-like.

205. Correct Answer: **2**

Rationale: This client is manifesting signs and symptoms of hypovolemic shock. The decreased blood pressure is leading to decreased cardiac output, which is the highest treatment priority for the nurse.

206. Correct Answer: **6 → 1 → 4 → 2 → 5 → 3**

Rationale: Rapid-sequence intubation begins with determining the baseline for the client and includes continuous monitoring throughout the procedure. The client is preoxygenated, and then medication is administered to assist in the client's relaxation. Crichoid pressure may be applied to assist in visualizing the landmarks for intubation. Once the endotracheal tube is in place, the presence of bilateral breath sounds should be auscultated.

207. Correct Answer: **2**

Rationale: DI involves a deficiency in the production or secretion of ADH, resulting in increased urinary output, weight loss, hypernatremia, low specific gravity of the urine, low urine osmolality, and elevated serum osmolality.

SECTION I

SECTION II

SECTION III

SECTION IV

SECTION V

SECTION VI

SECTION VII

SECTION VIII

SECTION IX

SECTION X

208. Correct Answer: **3**

Rationale: The first action is to establish an airway and administer oxygen.

209. Correct Answer: **3**

Rationale: The CPP of this client is 49 mm Hg, which indicates a decreased blood flow to the brain. A CPP exceeding 70 mm Hg is needed to satisfy the body's metabolic needs.

210. Correct Answer: **4**

Rationale: Stridor on exhalation is a hallmark of respiratory distress, usually caused by obstruction resulting from tissue edema. A tracheostomy set is usually kept at the bedside in case of such emergencies, and the physician is summoned at the first indication of respiratory distress.

211. Correct Answer: **Establish unresponsiveness**

Rationale: Once unresponsiveness has been verified, the nurse would call for help and begin the ABCs of cardiopulmonary resuscitation. Clients in ventricular tachycardia may or may not have a pulse, and each case is treated differently.

212. Correct Answer: **3**

Rationale: The highest-priority assessment is the ABCs (airway, breathing, and circulation). Injuries to the brain stem can cause changes in the client's breathing pattern.

213. Correct Answer: **2**

Rationale: Neurogenic shock occurs due to a disruption in the sympathetic nervous system. It is manifested as bradycardia, which leads to decreased tissue perfusion.

214. Correct Answer: **2**

Rationale: The highest priority is the ABCs (airway, breathing, and circulation). Of first and foremost concern is the airway. Bleeding from esophageal varices is difficult to control.

215. Correct Answer: **2**

Rationale: When aortic dissection occurs, there is a rapid decrease in blood pressure and the client quickly loses consciousness.

216. Correct Answers: **1 and 3**

Rationale: A client with suspected tuberculosis will be placed on airborne precautions, which requires that the client be placed in a private, negative-pressure room with the door kept closed at all times. Anyone entering the room must wear a mask and clean nonsterile gloves, and must perform good hand washing prior to and after caring for the client. If the client needs to leave the room, he or she must wear a mask.

217. Correct Answer: **1**

Rationale: The MAP on this blood pressure is 66 mm Hg, which is within the parameter. MAP = [SBP + 2(DBP)]/3.

218. Correct Answer: **2**

Rationale: DIC is a bleeding disorder. One of its first clinical manifestations is serous oozing from venipuncture sites.

219. Correct Answer: **3**

Rationale: If the client is experiencing signs and symptoms of hypoglycemia, then this problem must be corrected through the quick intake of a substance with sugar.

220. Correct Answer: **4**

Rationale: The ICP reading has increased and is being maintained at this level, so measures need to be taken to decrease ICP. The easiest thing for the nurse to do is to eliminate any external stimuli and elevate the head of the bed to 30 degrees with proper head alignment.

221. Correct Answer: **On an adult, the femoral or carotid pulse is assessed during CPR.**

222. Correct Answer: **2**

Rationale: Fluid volume replacement and urinary output are extremely important in a burn client. The urinary output of an adult burn client should be in the range of 30–50 mL/h.

Care of Patients with Psychiatric and Mental Health Problems

MANAGEMENT OF CARE

Multiple Choice

1. Your patient has an admitting diagnosis of alcohol withdrawal syndrome. You receive a phone call at the nurses' station from a person who says he is the patient's minister and wants to know if the patient "fell off the wagon again" and when visitation hours are. What is your best response?

1. "Yes, the patient drank too much, but he should be fine in a few days. Visiting hours are 9 A.M. to 6 P.M."
2. "We do not give out any information. Visitation hours in the hospital are from 9 A.M. to 6 P.M. daily."
3. "Please pray for the patient; he is in bad shape. You can visit him anytime between 9 A.M. and 6 P.M. daily."
4. "Please contact the hospital's chief executive officer, who can give you the information you are requesting."

2. Your patient has been hospitalized for acute alcohol withdrawal. It is the fifth day, and he is having visual hallucinations followed by a seizure. What is the most likely source of the patient's problem?

1. Autonomic dysreflexia (AD).
2. A brain tumor.
3. Sleep deprivation.
4. Delirium tremens (DTs).

3. Which of the following assessments is used to confirm alcohol intake?

1. Pupil dilation.
2. Serum sample.
3. Hair shaft analysis.
4. Sputum sample.

4. Which of the following questions is most appropriate to ask in screening for a potential problem of high alcohol intake?

1. "Have you felt you should cut down on your alcohol consumption?"
2. "Do you enjoy getting smashed?"
3. "Have you ever thought about killing someone?"
4. "In the last week, have you had a glass of wine?"

Identification

5. Which of the following are behavioral symptoms of a child with autism? (Circle the three correct answers.)

Short attention span

Inability of body to roll over

Spins a toy constantly

Temper tantrums

Repeated voiding in clothes

Psychosis

Multiple Choice

6. Your patient in the Emergency Department has a diagnosis of acute alcohol withdrawal syndrome (AWS). He is acting euphoric, yet shy. The APN has prescribed the following care: CAGE questionnaire, serum for toxicology, IV of D_5 ½ NS and 1 amp multivitamin (MVI) at 75 mL/h, neuro check q 1 h. What is your first priority?

1. Administer the CAGE questionnaire.
2. Start the IV.
3. Do the neuro check.
4. Obtain a serum blood sample.

7. Your patient sees you at a preplanned postoperative visit 4 weeks after being hospitalized for acute alcohol withdrawal. Upon questioning, she states that her husband is abusive, so she drinks to "drown out his yelling." The patient also complains of depression and severe pain in the epigastric region that radiates to her back and has been constant since yesterday. She has vomited twice in the past 12 hours. What is your first priority?

1. Refer her immediately for treatment of depression.
2. Call social services and report spousal abuse.
3. Assess her for pancreatitis.
4. Administer a test or scale that assesses alcohol withdrawal.

Identification

8. Which of the following symptoms are associated with acute alcohol withdrawal syndrome? (Circle all that apply.)

Tremor

Big toe pain

Tachycardia

Confusion

Seizures

Hypotension

Multiple Choice

9. Prolonged alcohol ingestion can cause disorders of the liver such as

1. Pancreatitis.
2. Hypomagnesemia.
3. Cirrhosis.
4. Colitis.

True/False

10. Adolescent suicide has increased over the past and is among the top five causes of death in U.S. adolescents.

11. Alcohol tolerance develops as a result of the central nervous system's adaptive mechanisms.

Multiple Choice

12. Your patient experienced alcohol withdrawal syndrome and now admits he "needs help." Which of the following is the most appropriate resource to which you should direct the patient?

1. Reach to Recovery.
2. Alcoholics Anonymous.
3. Depression support group.
4. Suicide support group.

Identification

13. Which of the following include comorbidities associated with eating disorders? (Circle the two correct answers.)

Anxiety

Chronic obstructive pulmonary disorder (COPD)

Headache

Diabetes mellitus

Depression

Bilateral leg edema

Multiple Choice

14. Which of the following is a common symptom of a major depressive episode?

1. Loss of hearing.
2. Increased energy.
3. Hopelessness.
4. Recurrent thoughts of well-being.

15. Which of the following statements would indicate a depressed mood?

1. "I can't wait to go to the ballgame today; it should be fun."
2. "I feel sad today, just like yesterday."
3. "I feel like going to the gym for a workout today, then maybe to a movie."
4. "Since it's raining outside, how about a game of chess?"

16. Which of the following medical conditions has similar signs and symptoms as those seen in a major depressive episode?

1. Pancreatitis.
2. Cholecystitis.
3. Tuberculosis.
4. Hypothyroidism.

17. Once a patient is diagnosed with a major depressive episode, the primary nursing intervention should be associated with

1. Safety.
2. Pharmacology.
3. Administration of gastric lavage.
4. Hemodialysis.

Identification

18. Fill in the blank with one of the words listed below to make the statement true.

_____ is (are) often (a) lethal companion(s) to suicidal acts as it (they) lower(s) inhibition and quicken(s) impulsivity.

> *Words*
> Guns
> Lack of social support
> Sexual dysfunctions
> Compulsive disorders
> Drugs
> Eating disorders

Multiple Choice

19. A 35-year-old male patient has been brought to your hospital unit after making a suicide attempt at his workplace. Which of the following interventions can you legally implement?

1. Call the patient's girlfriend and inform her of his admission and visiting hours.
2. Physically search the patient for weapons and harmful materials.
3. Call the patient's boss at work and report him as in need of extended medical leave.
4. Place the patient in four-point restraints and begin an IV for sedation.

20. Your patient has just received his sixth electroconvulsant therapy outpatient treatment. He tells you that he plans to drive himself home because his wife is working at her part-time job today. What is your best response?

1. "Be careful and drive slowly."
2. "You need to wait 30 minutes and then you will be safe to drive."
3. "Let me take your vital signs; if they are stable, then you can drive."
4. "You cannot drive. I can call you a cab, or would you prefer to call your wife or someone for a ride home?"

Identification

21. Fill in the blank with one of the words listed below to make the following statement true:

Your patient has a confirmed and new diagnosis of HIV. He tells you, "I don't care what the doctors say, there is no way I can have HIV, and I don't need treatment for something I don't have." The most appropriate nursing diagnosis for this patient is _____.

> *Words*
> Ineffective coping
> Denial
> Anxiety
> Social isolation

Multiple Choice

22. Which of the following patients is at risk for depression?

1. A patient with history of diabetes mellitus.
2. A patient with a depressive genetic predisposition.
3. A patient who recently bought a puppy.
4. A patient who had only 6 hours of sleep last night due to watching a TV movie.

23. A patient has been admitted to your unit with a drug overdose, and you need to assess for acidosis and hypoxemia. Which test should you perform?

1. Complete blood count (CBC).
2. Serum electrolytes.
3. Partial thromboplastin time (PTT).
4. Arterial blood gases (ABG).

24. Which of the following is an example of a bite/sting that can cause a poison exposure?

1. Butterfly.
2. Grass seed.
3. Jellyfish.
4. Fly.

25. When a patient shares with a psychiatrist that he plans to harm a specific person and includes the person's name, the health professional must notify the intended identified victim. What is this rule called?

1. Seclusion and restraints rule.
2. Voluntary commitment rule.
3. Right to treatment rule.
4. Duty to warn rule.

26. When documenting the behavior of a patient with a mental health diagnosis, which chart entry includes the patient's action and responses?

1. The patient is less expressive today in group therapy.
2. The patient appears to drift in and out of reality.
3. The patient is wearing shorts and a sleeveless top even though it's January and wintertime. When asked about her clothing choices, she states, "The devil told me what to wear. To make things different, I need an exorcism."
4. The patient is wearing pants and a long-sleeved shirt, is appropriately dressed for group therapy, and refrains from sleeping as she did in last group sessions.

27. During a group session, one patient states that he will be released soon because he is superior to his therapist, who is a female. This is an example of which bias or prejudice?

1. Racism.
2. Sexism.
3. Ageism.
4. Neonatalism.

28. A 48-year-old Hispanic woman is seen by a psychiatric clinical nurse specialist after receiving a call by her son. According to the son, since his father's death 7 months ago, his mother has lost 30 pounds and can't sleep. During her initial visit, the patient states, "My husband talks to me in his visits, but his words make no sense to me. I don't understand what he wants me to do." What is an appropriate nursing diagnosis?

1. Ineffective denial.
2. Bipolar mood disorder.
3. Hyper-religiosity.
4. Grieving.

29. Your neighbor's husband comes to talk to you. He says his wife has not left the house in 2 weeks, has a flat mood, and has lost interest in her usual activities. You recognize these as the primary symptoms of

1. Depression.
2. Schizophrenia.
3. Suicidal ideation.
4. Bipolar manic episodes.

Identification

30. Which of the following are appropriate coping forms for patients with HIV? (Circle all that apply.)

Alcohol

Meditation

Hypoglycemic diet

Marijuana

Guided imagery

Coffee-ground enemas

Multiple Choice

31. Your patient is ready for discharge after a 30-day hospitalization for manic depression. About 30 minutes before his discharge, his roommate comes to you and says, "He is talking crazy." When you ask your patient how he is feeling, he states, "I feel like Superman. I can do anything. I can fly home today and then become a U.S. Senator." Which type of mania-related symptoms is this patient exhibiting?

1. Social.
2. Cognitive.
3. Behavioral.
4. Perceptual.

32. You need to assess whether a patient who has a mood disorder is ready for discharge. Which statement would indicate readiness for discharge?

1. "Right now, I can't bathe myself or dress myself, but I feel good about that."
2. "Going home will be fun, but if it isn't fun, I can always make my mother help me or tell her to do so. She better help me."
3. "I will take my medicines as I should and know to call the number you gave me if I have bad thoughts."
4. "Taking care of myself is important, but it's okay if I don't want to do anything."

33. A 22-year-old female was admitted to the mental health unit with major depression and suicidal ideation. She has a history of cutting her wrists intermittently throughout the last 2 years. On days 1 and 2, the patient stays in her room and eats only 20% of her meals. On day 3, she eats 80% of her meals and is talking to others in group. The nurse should consider that the patient is

1. Showing improvement.
2. Highly suicidal.
3. Exhibiting mood swings.
4. In need of electroshock therapy.

34. A 21-year-old patient has a diagnosis of schizophrenia and is stuporous, yet exhibits sudden, excessive motor activity with repetitive sit-ups. What is this behavior called?

1. Delusional.
2. Hallucinogenic.
3. Paranoid.
4. Catatonic.

35. A 16-year-old girl is admitted for her first psychotic break. Her parents feel very guilty. What is your best nursing response?

1. "No one really knows the cause of schizophrenia. It is not your fault and is not due to anything you did in the past. It is important to understand this, to support your daughter, and to find support for yourselves."
2. "Does anyone in your family have schizophrenia, as this disease is known to be genetic?"
3. "You may feel bad now, but there are so many other bad things out there, such as cancer and paralysis."
4. "Let me share with you some websites to help you deal with your guilt."

True/False

36. A physical indicator of possible abuse in a battered woman would be a fracture of the distal bones, such as the skull, face, or extremities.

Multiple Choice

37. Which of the following statements indicates that your patient, who has schizophrenia, is ready to manage a relapse?

1. "I will think of a plan of action before I get these racing thoughts again."

2. "I will not drink alcohol and will exercise daily. This will help me stay well."
3. "If I start feeling badly and don't sleep very much, then I will tell my friend Sandy and talk to her. She or I will call my therapist."
4. "When I feel stressed, I will sit near my bed and wait to feel better."

38. Your patient has a diagnosis of schizophrenia and believes that his thoughts are broadcast from his head. What is the most appropriate nursing diagnosis?

1. Risk for self-directed violence.
2. Disturbed sensory perception.
3. Impaired verbal communication.
4. Disturbed thought processes.

39. As a nurse, you wish to reinforce functional behavior in your schizophrenic patient. Which intervention will accomplish reinforcement?

1. Praise the patient for reality-based perceptions and cessation of acting-out behaviors.
2. Educate the patient about the symptoms of schizophrenia.
3. Facilitate learning about the importance of medication compliance using written materials for reinforcing medication use.
4. Focus on the feelings of delusion to reinforce reality and decrease false beliefs by talking to the patient.

40. Your patient is preoccupied with perfection and control, has difficulty relaxing, exhibits rule-conscious behavior, and cannot discard anything. What type of personality disorder does this behavior reflect?

1. Antisocial personality.
2. Obsessive-compulsive personality.
3. Manic behavior.
4. Anxiety disorder.

41. Which of the following questions is appropriate to assess for disturbances in a patient's relationships?

1. What are your main worries?
2. Have you ever used alcohol or illegal drugs?
3. How has your appetite been in the past month?
4. What do you talk about with friends?

42. Which type of therapy helps patients with personality disorders explore ways to enjoy themselves and increase their socialization skills?

1. Occupational therapy.
2. Recreational therapy.
3. Music therapy.
4. Medication therapy.

43. Which of the following symptoms of alcohol detoxification would you be most concerned about?

1. Vitamin and mineral depletion.
2. Diaphoresis.
3. Increased heart rate.
4. Hallucinations and delusions.

44. What is the priority nursing intervention to help orient a patient who has Alzheimer's disease?

1. Post a schedule in the dining room of daily activities.
2. Use an overhead loudspeaker to announce upcoming events.
3. Provide a daily routine and easy-to-read clocks.
4. Have the patient live alone in a private room.

SAFETY AND INFECTION CONTROL

Multiple Choice

45. You are caring for a patient and pour out his evening risperidone (Risperdal) 2 mg tablet. The pill falls on the countertop. What is your next intervention?

1. Pick the pill up from the counter and place it in a cup.
2. Wash the pill off with alcohol and place it in a cup.
3. Discard the pill and repour the medication.
4. Call the patient up to the pill line to receive his medication.

46. Your patient has just shown you some fresh, self-inflicted, superficial cuts—eight of them going up and down his right arm. What is your initial intervention based on infection control principles?

1. Send the patient back to his room as part of behavioral modification.
2. Suture the cuts using a large-bore needle and nondissolving sutures.

3. Cleanse the wounds with soap and water.
4. Administer tetanus toxoid injection intramuscularly.

47. A hypomanic patient tells you that she has been "picking up energy from my car engine and car CD player" while driving and has received five speeding tickets in the past 6 months. What would be one effective intervention to avoid fast driving?

1. Make a contract not to drive more than 55 miles per hour and drive with the CD player turned off.
2. Call the local police and alert them to the patient's car license plate number and the make and model of her car.
3. Ask the patient to "hand over the keys" to you, and tell her that now she must use a cab or other public transportation until your next session.
4. Share with the patient that she cannot drink and drive.

48. Patients who require close surveillance due to the potential for safety hazards give up the right of

1. Continued confusion.
2. Decision making.
3. Social contact.
4. Privacy.

Identification

49. When preparing to administer an oral medication to a patient who has a history of chronic depression, what should you do *first*? (Circle the correct answer.)

Validate the patient's home address.

Validate the patient's insurance status.

Make sure the intravenous site is patent.

Assess the Depakote (valproic acid) lab value.

Wash your hands.

Assess temperature.

Multiple Choice

50. A patient is extremely agitated and is throwing body fluids at anyone who comes near him. What is the best way to protect yourself as you and others physically restrain the patient?

1. Wash your clothes within 30 minutes of becoming soiled with body fluids.
2. Wear protective eyewear and a face shield.

3. Check that your tetanus and hepatitis B titers are within normal limits.

4. Wear a gown over your clothes and shoe covers.

51. A patient who is psychotic has a formed bowel movement on the floor of his room. How should you clean up this excrement?

1. Use a thick diaper or pad.

2. Wear gloves and use some paper towels or toilet paper.

3. Wear gloves, use toilet paper, and wash the area with a 1:10 bleach solution.

4. Wear a gown, shoe covers, mask, and chemotherapy-impervious gloves, and wash the area with an ammonia with bleach 1:1 solution.

52. Your patient is scheduled for a one-on-one therapy session. Upon his entry into your office, you note that the patient has a cough, is sweating, is coughing up a small amount of blood, and has a fever. What is your initial intervention regarding infection control?

1. Wash all of the patient's sheets and clothes.

2. Place a mask on the patient and yourself.

3. Take the patient's temperature.

4. Place resuscitation equipment in the patient's room.

53. You have just given your patient an intramuscular injection of fluphenazine (Prolixin) with a syringe that does not have a safety lock. What is your next step?

1. Recap the needle.

2. Snap the needle off and place it in the needle box.

3. Immediately place the syringe in a nearby impermeable container.

4. Clip the needle off with a syringe needle cutter (SNC).

True/False

54. In an inpatient acute psychiatric unit, it is important to shut and lock the unit door behind you.

Multiple Choice

55. You drive up to the house of your patient, who is known to have schizophrenia with manic episodes. This is your fifth visit. On this occasion, the patient is sitting on his front porch in a rocking chair with a shotgun in his arms. What should your next intervention be?

1. Beep your car horn to get your patient's attention.

2. Yell your patient's name out your car window and wave at him to say hello.

3. Keep driving in a path that is going away from the patient's house.

4. Stop the car in the patient's driveway and call your boss on your cell phone.

56. Your patient, who is in a community psychiatric program, shows up at your home peeping through your kitchen window. You also noticed the patient yesterday when you went to the grocery story and the hairdresser. You believe he is stalking you. What should you do?

1. Call the local police and report your suspicion of stalking.

2. Call the patient's spouse and discuss his behavior.

3. Invite the patient to have a cup of coffee with you at a local café to discuss his behavior.

4. Wait until the patient's next group meeting to discuss his stalking behavior.

57. Your patient's auditory, visual, and tactile hallucinations are controlled with bimonthly injections of haloperidol (Haldol) that the community health nurse administers during home visits. You are the new nurse on this case; the previous nurse has retired. The previous nurse has stated in her care plan that the patient will let the nurse in the house only if the nurse carries a public health-issued blue bag and wears black pants. You are scheduled to visit this patient tomorrow. What should you do?

1. Call the patient and tell her that you are a new nurse and will be wearing white pants.

2. Show up as scheduled carrying only a stethoscope, vial, alcohol wipe, and medication syringe.

3. Show up as scheduled with a police officer.

4. Telephone the patient, introduce yourself, and show up carrying a blue bag and wearing black pants.

58. An angry patient is in the community room. She picks up a chair and uses it to hit another patient on the head. When you come into the community room, what should your first response to the patient holding the chair be?

1. "Are you crazy? Hitting people can hurt them!"

2. "Hitting others is unacceptable. Please put the chair completely down on the floor."

3. "How would you like it if I hit you over the head with a chair?"

4. "You're in big trouble now. It's probably prison you are looking at!"

Identification

59. You have a psychiatric patient who is aggressive. What is an appropriate distance that would be therapeutic between you and the patient? (Circle the correct answer.)

2 to 3 inches

6 inches

8 feet

1 arm's length

12 inches

12 feet

Multiple Choice

60. A 22-year-old female is admitted to the unit following a suicide attempt. She has a 2-week history of depression as well as a history of abusing multiple substances and anorexia nervosa. What is your first nursing priority?

1. Socialization.

2. Contracting for eating behavior.

3. Safety.

4. Administering the Beck depression scale.

61. Gerald was admitted to the psychiatric acute care unit because he stood in the center of a main two-way street in his underwear and a T-shirt, shouting, "I am being held against my will. I have personal rights." Gerald was diagnosed with bipolar disorder, manic type. Which of the following interventions will add to everyone's safety in the acute care environment?

1. Have hectic surroundings.

2. Have consistent unit routines.

3. Minimize staff interventions.

4. Medicate the patient only if he has private health insurance.

62. Your patient has just been physically cleaned up after slicing his left arm 8 times. To show an appropriate evaluative response, which of the following would be your best statement?

1. "I could care less if you cut yourself. It doesn't hurt me."

2. "If you wouldn't cut yourself, you would have a much happier life."

3. "You are lucky someone found you in time. Now you can help us make you better."

4. "The behavior of cutting is not acceptable."

63. Which of the following is an acceptable reason for placing a person in restraints?

1. Continued, acute self-mutilation.

2. Coercion.

3. Discipline for throwing food at staff.

4. Punishment for verbal abuse.

64. A son petitioned the court to place his father in a state psychiatric hospital for care for the father's own safety. The father has refused care. The son is asking for

1. A right to refuse treatment.

2. Protection and duty to warn.

3. Involuntary commitment.

4. Privileged communication.

65. Your patient on the psychiatric unit is being asked to participate in a research study. Which of the following is normally included in informed consent and is associated with safety?

1. The name of the company that prints the questionnaires used in the study.

2. A statement that participation is mandatory.

3. The telephone number of the appropriate U.S. Congress member for the state where the study is being implemented.

4. Disclosure of risks and benefits.

Identification

66. Which body position in relation to your patient indicates that you are not aggressive? (Choose one of the pictures below.)

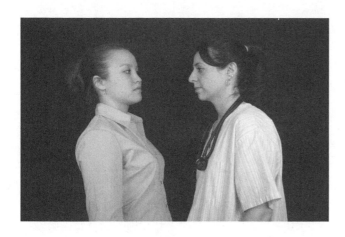

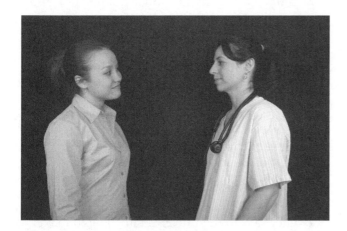

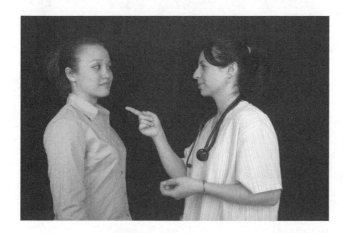

HEALTH PROMOTION AND MAINTENANCE

Multiple Choice

67. Which nursing diagnosis best reflects that your patient is ready to go back home and begin living within her societal environment once again?

1. Readiness for enhanced community coping.
2. Readiness for enhanced communication.
3. Risk for other-directed violence.
4. Risk for loneliness.

68. Which of the following assessments best reflects a nursing assessment of environmental maintenance?

1. Sleep-rest patterns.
2. Peripheral circulation.
3. Ability to cook.
4. Possession of a weapon.

69. To promote better health, one needs to identify stressors. Which of the following questions will help the nurse identify potential stressors?

1. Do you have a car?
2. How do you get along with people at work?
3. What do you want to feel like at the time of discharge?
4. What are your goals for yourself?

Identification

70. Which of the following experiences place a person at great risk for suicide? (Circle all that apply.)

Hallucinations

Depression

Delusions

Lasting friendships

Multiple Choice

71. To promote health in Native American patients who are living in the United States, the nurse needs to respect Native Americans'

1. Stigma placed on poor horsemanship.
2. Traditions.
3. Heritage of Taoism and Buddhism.
4. Matriarchal structure.

72. To best promote health in members of African American communities in the United States, you need to understand that African American families often have what type of structure?

SECTION I

SECTION II

SECTION III

SECTION IV

SECTION V

SECTION VI

SECTION VII

SECTION VIII

SECTION IX

SECTION X

1. Matriarchal.
2. Patriarchal.
3. Idiosyncratic.
4. Code of silence.

73. You are asked to speak to the local community church group on health promotion for good mental health. What is an appropriate topic?

1. How to speak in tongues.
2. How to be able to enter heaven.
3. Reducing stressors in your life.
4. Ultimate authority in torment and natural disasters.

74. Which statement by Mrs. Smotik, who has a history of depression, indicates that she continues to maintain good health after 30 days' discharge to her home?

1. "Oh, I don't care about much. It's all around me, too much to handle."
2. "I've been a little tired after work, but not all the time. It's been nice to cook what I want, too."
3. "I just don't have the energy to go to work, but I learn a lot when I watch television programs."
4. "No matter what I do, it's just not right. I don't know what I'll do if things don't turn around!"

75. Education about health promotion is often effective during periods of role transitions. Which of the following is a role transition?

1. Moving into a new house in the same neighborhood.
2. Going grocery shopping.
3. Buying a new car.
4. Retirement.

Identification

76. Choose the correct word from those provided to make the following sentence true: Patients with HIV can maintain positive coping and reduce stress by the use of _____.

> *Words*
> Alcohol
> A low-sugar diet
> Meditation

Multiple Choice

77. To promote better health in older adults related to heart disease, hypertension, and diabetes, what would the nurse recommend?

1. A diet high in carbohydrates.
2. Calcium, folic acid, and seaweed supplements twice daily.
3. Exercise.
4. Reach to Recovery meetings weekly.

78. Which statement by a 70-year-old male reflects healthy adaptation a year after his wife has died?

1. "My wife was wonderful. I'm nothing without her."
2. "I'm enjoying my new hobby of bowling and spending time with my kids."
3. "I worked my whole life, and none of my kids visit me. I wasted my life."
4. "Since my hip surgery, I can't do what I want to do. This is not living."

79. Lucy is a 34-year-old married woman with chronic low self-esteem. Which action by Lucy demonstrates assertive behavior and positive interpersonal relationships?

1. Lucy says to the nurse, "My husband's behavior gives me headaches, so I sleep a lot."
2. Lucy says to the nurse, "I am going to make other people's lives as miserable as mine is."
3. Lucy cries for 28 minutes of the 30-minute therapy session.
4. Lucy requests that her husband join her weekly sessions to deal with the husband's use of alcohol and extramarital affair.

True/False

80. In an effort to maintain health, patients diagnosed with HIV infection need to have their CD4 counts evaluated periodically.

Multiple Choice

81. Which statement by a patient with a history of major depression indicates that he is not maintaining good health in his current environment?

1. "I had a great trip to the Smokey Mountains. It was fun."
2. "Going back to work, well, it's not bad; it's okay."

3. "I just don't like going to the movies like I did before."

4. "I can't wait to go to my son's wedding next weekend. It will be nice to have the whole family together."

82. Which subject would you discuss with recent mothers to promote health and encourage them to maintain a safe environment for their babies?

1. Hypertension.

2. Postpartum mood disorder.

3. Seasonal affective disorder.

4. Hyperactivity depressive mood disorder.

83. To maintain health in your patient who has a mood disorder, you need to assist the patient in promoting structure. Which statement by the patient indicates she is promoting structure?

1. "Today I will go to group, speak about my feelings, and then go to art therapy and dinner."

2. "I might go to group or maybe watch television. I don't know. I'll figure it out later."

3. "Today, I will see what it brings. Maybe I will see. Maybe I won't see."

4. "I might as well do something today so the staff will get off my back."

84. Your patient has a problem with health maintenance associated with sleep disturbance. Which areas of nursing care do you need to assess?

1. Potential for falls and sexuality.

2. Harm to self and serum iron laboratory test.

3. Spiritual distress and deferred psoriasis.

4. Activities of daily living (ADLs) and diet.

True/False

85. Nursing care for patients with cognitive disorders should be done in collaboration with the patients' caregivers.

Multiple Choice

86. To maintain health and avoid relapse in a 20-year-old patient who is chronically mentally ill, the patient needs to avoid

1. Medication noncompliance.

2. Obtaining a job.

3. Outpatient progress.

4. State-funded institutions.

PSYCHOSOCIAL INTEGRITY

Identification

87. Mr. Williamson is being treated for depression with imipramine hydrochloride (Tofranil) 200 mg orally as a total daily dose, with half the dose taken in the morning and half the dose taken in the evening. The pharmacist dispenses Tofranil in 25-mg tablets. How many tablets do you give Mr. Williamson in the morning?

Multiple Choice

88. Smoking cigarettes increases the metabolism of some psychiatric medications. In such a case, if the patient smokes, how should the medication dose be adjusted?

1. Decrease the dose.

2. Increase the dose.

3. Administer the entire dose of medication in the morning.

4. Administer the entire dose of medication at bedtime.

89. Mr. Yeh is manic depressive and is being treated with lithium carbonate (Eskalith) for this condition. He is also anxious and has been prescribed diazepam (Valium) for this disorder. These two medications can interact and cause hypothermia as a side effect. To assess for this potential side effect, what would you ask the patient?

1. "Have you been feeling dizzy?"

2. "Do you have a skin rash anywhere on your body?"

3. "Have you been going to the bathroom a lot?"

4. "Have you been feeling cold?"

90. Mrs. Allison is being treated with olanzapine (Zyprexa) 7.5 mg daily orally for her schizophrenia. The pharmacy dispenses Zyprexa as 2.5-mg tablets. How many tablets do you give Mrs. Allison daily?

1. 2 tablets.

2. 3 tablets.

3. 4 tablets.

4. 6 tablets.

Fill in the Blank

91. Mrs. Peabody has been taking a tricyclic antidepressant for the last few days and experiences dizziness upon getting out of a chair or bed. Her physician assesses her blood pressure while she is standing and sitting, and finds that Mrs. Peabody's

SECTION I
SECTION II
SECTION III
SECTION IV
SECTION V
SECTION VI
SECTION VII
SECTION VIII
SECTION IX
SECTION X

blood pressure is much lower when she stands up. This medication side effect on blood pressure is called _____ hypotension.

Multiple Choice

92. Mr. Collins is receiving Aripiprazole 15 mg orally daily. The pharmacy dispenses Aripiprazole as 15-mg tablets. How many tablets do you give Mr. Collins daily?

1. 0.5 tablet.
2. 1 tablet.
3. 2 tablets.
4. 3 tablets.

93. Ms. Fluoski is prescribed fluoxetine hydrochloride (Prozac) 30 mg orally daily. The pharmacy dispenses 10-mg capsules of Prozac. How many capsules do you educate Ms. Fluoski to take daily?

1. 1 capsule.
2. 2 capsules.
3. 3 capsules.
4. 5 capsules.

Identification

94. Your patient has a tendency to experience gastric irritation from taking medications. What could you suggest the patient take with the medication so it will cause less gastric irritation?

Multiple Choice

95. Mr. Mohammed is being treated with buspirone hydrochloride (BuSpar) for anxiety. He is prescribed BuSpar 5 mg twice a day, once in the morning and once in the evening. The pharmacy dispenses 10-mg scored tablets. How many tablets of BuSpar do you administer to Mr. Mohammed in the morning?

1. 0.5 tablet.
2. 1 tablet.
3. 2 tablets.
4. 4 tablets.

96. Mr. Lordin is prescribed valproic acid (Depakene) 750 mg orally every morning for treatment of his bipolar disorder. The pharmacy dispenses valproic acid as 250-mg capsules. How many capsules do you give Mr. Lordin every morning?

1. 2 capsules.
2. 3 capsules.
3. 6 capsules.
4. 8 capsules.

97. Mrs. Washington is prescribed chlordiazepoxide (Librium) 200 mg orally now for treatment of alcohol withdrawal. The pharmacy dispenses Librium as 25-mg tablets. How many tablets of Librium do you give Mrs. Washington now?

1. 2 tablets.
2. 3 tablets.
3. 4 tablets.
4. 8 tablets.

98. Mrs. McCormick has acute psychosis and is being treated with chlorpromazine hydrochloride (Thorazine) 10 mg four times per day. What is her total daily dose of Thorazine?

1. 20 mg.
2. 30 mg.
3. 40 mg.
4. 60 mg.

Identification

99. Your patient complains of insomnia as a side effect of his medication. When would be a good time to administer the medication to try to prevent this side effect?

Multiple Choice

100. Mr. White has been taking risperidone (Risperdal) for treatment of his schizophrenia. He receives 2 mg of Risperdal in the morning and 3 mg in the evening. What is the total dose of Risperdal that Mr. White receives daily?

1. 1.5 mg.
2. 4 mg.
3. 7 mg.
4. 5 mg.

101. Mr. Merriweather has his psychosis treated with trifluoperazine (Stelazine) 2 mg tablets orally daily. The pharmacy dispenses trifluridine (Viroptic 1%). How many tablets do you administer daily?

1. None.
2. 1 tablet.
3. 0.5 tablet.
4. 2 tablets.

102. Charlie Eagle is a 38-year-old Native American who is being treated with haloperidol (Haldol) 1.5 mg orally, twice per day, for schizophrenia. His pharmacist dispenses Haldol tablets in 1-mg tablets. How many tablets should Mr. Eagle take in the morning?

    1. 0.5 tablet.

    2. 1.5 tablets.

    3. 3 tablets.

    4. 6 tablets.

103. Ms. Gszewski is prescribed amitriptyline hydrochloride (Elavil) 150 mg orally at bedtime daily to treat her depression. The pharmacist dispenses 75-mg tablets of Elavil. How many tablets should Ms. Gszewski take at bedtime?

    1. 2 tablets.

    2. 3 tablets.

    3. 4 tablets.

    4. 0.5 tablet.

104. Mr. Lazarus is being treated for anxiety with clorazepate dipotassium (Tranxene) 22.5 mg orally every morning. The pharmacy dispenses Tranxene as 7.5-mg tablets. How many tablets should Mr. Lazarus receive every morning?

    1. 2 tablets.

    2. 3 tablets.

    3. 5 tablets.

    4. 6 tablets.

105. Mr. Johnson is prescribed 200 mg daily of desipramine hydrochloride (Norpramin) for treatment of cocaine withdrawal. The pharmacy dispenses Norpramin as 100-mg tablets. How many tablets do you administer to Mr. Johnson daily?

    1. None.

    2. 0.5 tablet.

    3. 1 tablet.

    4. 2 tablets.

106. Mr. Alfred is clinically depressed, and his physician has recently prescribed nefazodone hydrochloride (Serzone) 300 mg daily, orally. The pharmacy dispenses 150-mg tablets. How many tablets of Serzone should Mr. Alfred take daily?

    1. 0.5 tablet.

    2. 2 tablets.

    3. 4 tablets.

    4. 10 tablets.

BASIC CARE AND COMFORT

Identification

107. Circle the two basic preliminary tests to be completed prior to electroconvulsive therapy (ECT).

    Electrocardiogram (EKG or ECG)

    Serum steroid

    Serum parathyroid hormone

    Complete blood count (CBC)

    Colonoscopy

    Urine for oxycodone analysis

Multiple Choice

108. Prior to electroconvulsive therapy (ECT) treatment, the patient receives an injection of a medication that reduces secretions and protects against vagal bradycardia. Which medication will you administer?

    1. Diphenhydramine (Benadryl).

    2. Atropine.

    3. Epinephrine (Adrenalin).

    4. Fluoxetine (Prozac).

Identification

109. You are in charge of setting up the electroconvulsive therapy (ECT) room with essential monitoring equipment. Circle the three pieces of equipment that are appropriate to set up.

    Electroencephalogram (EEG) monitor ✓

    Blood pressure monitor ✓

    Rigid sigmoidoscopy

    Cardiac monitor ✓

    Ventriculostomy monitor

    Hemoccult test pad

Multiple Choice

110. Which of the following items is used during electroconvulsive therapy (ECT) to prevent oral damage and maintain airway?

    1. Tracheostomy tube.

    2. Esophageal monitor.

    3. Nasal trumpet.

    4. Mouth guard.

SECTION I

SECTION II

SECTION III

SECTION IV

SECTION V

SECTION VI

SECTION VII

SECTION VIII

SECTION IX

SECTION X

111. Which of the following therapies would you recommend for your patient if the goal is to focus on the performance of tasks?

1. Occupational therapy.
2. Electroconvulsive therapy.
3. Family therapy.
4. Group therapy.

Identification

112. Circle the three complementary and alternative medical (CAM) therapies that are effective in preventing and managing disease processes.

Diet

Otic rectal irrigation

Peroxide and cinnamon IV bolus

Exercise

Stress-reduction therapies

Radiation normotherapy

Multiple Choice

113. Mrs. Wommelburg has a diagnosis of acute depression. She is 5 feet 4 inches tall, weighs 280 pounds, and smokes one-half pack of cigarettes per day. In preparing for her care, you note that health promotion and education are warranted in the following areas:

1. Tobacco abuse, substance abuse, and violence.
2. Responsible sexual behavior, mental health, and obesity.
3. Injury, tobacco abuse, and immunizations.
4. Obesity, tobacco abuse, and physical activity.

114. Mrs. Forintu is a devout Orthodox Catholic who has a diagnosis of acute depression. She has been admitted yearly for her depression over the last 5 years. Which mind–body intervention might be appropriate when you are caring for her?

1. Drama therapy.
2. Prayer.
3. Yoga.
4. Humor therapy.

115. Mrs. Sadan is from Egypt. Upon admission for acute anxiety, she tells you that she responds well to zone therapy to the feet, a manual massage healing method that is based on the premise that feet and hands are mirrors of the body. What name is given to this intervention?

1. Osteopathic massage.
2. Accupressure.

3. Foot reflexology.
4. Ayurveda.

116. Which of the following physical manifestations are common in patients undergoing grief?

1. Nausea, headache, and chest pain.
2. Fatigue, exhaustion, and insomnia.
3. Diarrhea, vomiting, and hypertension.
4. Thought disturbances, constipation, and dry mouth.

117. Grief increases a person's vulnerability to which physical illness?

1. Myocardial infarction.
2. Systemic lupus erythematosus (SLE).
3. Hip fractures.
4. Obsessive-compulsive disorder.

118. You need to assess Mrs. Wolberg for chronic grief. What physical disturbances would indicate the patient is in chronic grief?

1. Anxiety and sinus pain.
2. Amnesia and overeating.
3. Bilateral lower leg pain and visual cloudiness.
4. Cardiovascular and gastrointestinal problems.

119. Mr. Stevers is in the last stages of AIDS and has diarrhea. Which of the following nursing intervention(s) would be related to providing comfort?

1. Medicate with milk of magnesia and Haldol.
2. Give a back rub every 6 hours, and clip the patient's toenails.
3. Change diapers when necessary, and provide skin care.
4. Place an occlusive dressing over the patient's buttocks every 8 hours.

120. You are providing care for a patient diagnosed with HIV who has fatigue, difficulty concentrating, and forgetfulness. Your assessment indicates the patient has

1. Dementia.
2. Psychosis.
3. Anxiety.
4. Depression.

121. A person comes to the Emergency Department who is high on street drugs and is homeless. Which physical integrity should you assess to determine whether infection or inflammation is present in this patient?

1. Self-esteem integrity.
2. Skin integrity.
3. Elimination.
4. Hormonal/metabolic patterns.

122. Patients with psychosis often have trouble attending to activities of daily living (ADLs). Which area of care would include ADLs?

1. Automobile care.
2. Hygiene.
3. Isolation for infection.
4. Leukopenia serum laboratory venipuncture.

123. Mr. Allen has psychosis and has been treated with haloperidol (Haldol). You need to assess him for movement disorders as a side effect of Haldol. What is another name for these movement disorders?

1. Extrapyramidal reactions.
2. Autonomic dysreflexia.
3. Biologic rigidity reactions.
4. Delusional etiologies.

Identification

124. Circle all self-care activities that persons should be able to perform prior to discharge to home.

Hygiene

Bathing

Car oil change

Banking

Dressing

Grooming

True/False

125. Independent function in activities of daily living preserves dignity and self-esteem.

Multiple Choice

126. Mr. Hawkins is depressed and has a skin wound on his left arm that is 1 cm by 2 cm by $\frac{1}{4}$ cm. To promote healing, which type of diet should Mr. Hawkins consume?

1. High protein.
2. High vitamin K.
3. High calcium.
4. Low iron.

PHARMACOLOGICAL AND PARENTERAL THERAPIES

Multiple Choice

127. Which of the following side effects is related to the effects of anticholinergic medications?

1. Pain in great toes.
2. Vomiting.
3. Dry mouth.
4. Diarrhea.

128. Mrs. Mirion is prescribed 300 mg of Mellaril every morning. The pharmacy sends up thioridazine (Mellaril) in the form of 100-mg tablets. How many tablets do you give Mrs. Mirion?

1. 1 tablet.
2. 2 tablets.
3. 3 tablets.
4. 4 tablets.

129. Mr. Bennett is prescribed 10 mg of olanzapine (Zyprexa) every morning. The pharmacy sends up 5-mg tablets of Zyprexa. How many tablets do you give Mr. Bennett?

1. 1 tablet.
2. 2 tablets.
3. 3 tablets.
4. $\frac{1}{2}$ tablet.

True/False

130. Gastric lavage with ice water is a reliable way to rapidly reduce serum lithium blood levels.

Multiple Choice

131. Mr. Abdullah is prescribed 3 mg of risperidone (Risperdal) every evening. The pharmacy sends up 2-mg tablets of Risperdal. How many tablets of Risperdal do you give Mr. Abdullah in the evening?

1. 1 tablet.
2. $1\frac{1}{2}$ tablets.
3. 2 tablets.
4. $\frac{3}{4}$ tablet.

132. Ms. Shoman is prescribed 4 mg haloperidol lactate orally now. The pharmacy sends up the medication in the form of 2 mg/mL of haloperidol lactate liquid. How much haloperidol lactate do you give Ms. Shoman?

SECTION I

SECTION II

SECTION III

SECTION IV

SECTION V

SECTION VI

SECTION VII

SECTION VIII

SECTION IX

SECTION X

1. 0.5 mL.

2. 1 mL.

3. 2 mL.

4. 4 mL.

133. Ms. Tunner is prescribed a monthly injection of 25 mg haloperidol decanoate to treat her psychosis. The pharmacy sends up the medication in the form of haloperidol decanoate injectable 50 mg/mL. How much haloperidol decanoate do you draw up to give the patient?

1. 0.25 mL.

2. 0.5 mL.

3. 2 mL.

4. 20 mL.

Identification

134. What of the following potential side effects is (are) related to the gastrointestinal tract? (Circle all that apply.)

Nausea

Vomiting

Diarrhea

Dyspepsia

Osteoporosis

Otitis

Multiple Choice

135. Mrs. Luccille is prescribed the antipsychotic olanzapine (Zyprexa) 20 mg total daily, to be given in two equally divided doses every 12 hours. How much Zyprexa do you give with each dose every 12 hours?

1. 10 mg.

2. 20 mg.

3. 40 mg.

4. 0.5 mg.

136. Mr. Holloway has just received his first dose of the antipsychotic medication perphenazine (Trilafon). You know that the response time to the medication for cognitive and perceptive symptoms, such as hallucinations, delusions, and thought broadcasting, may take how long?

1. Up to 3 minutes.

2. Up to 30 minutes.

3. From 2 to 8 weeks.

4. From 28 to 52 weeks.

Identification

137. Which of the following are aggressive symptoms of psychosis? (Circle all that apply.)

Catatonia

Hostility

Thought disorder

Verbal abuse

Depression

Worry

Fill in the Blank

138. Mr. Jejun is prescribed carbamazapine (Tegretol) ER tablets for the treatment of bipolar mania. The "ER" stands for _____.

Multiple Choice

139. Sedation is a common side effect of antipsychotics. For this reason, which medications should patients avoid if they are taking antipsychotics?

1. Antidiarrheals.

2. Acetaminophen (Tylenol).

3. Antihypertensives.

4. Antihistamines.

140. Mr. Albertson is experiencing dystonia as a side effect of his antipsychotic medication perphenazine (Trilafon). The nurse practitioner prescribes 1 mg of benztropine (Cogentin) intramuscularly now to prevent a recurrence of dystonia. The pharmacy sends up benztropine in the form of 1 mg/mL for IM use. How much medication do you draw up for Mr. Albertson's injection?

1. 0.25 mL.

2. 0.5 mL.

3. 1 mL.

4. 2 mL.

141. Mrs. Tonnilski is prescribed 50 mg diphenhydramine (Benadryl) orally for extrapyramidal side effects due to the antipsychotic medication trifluoperazine (Stelazine) she is prescribed. The pharmacy sends up diphenhydramine in the form of 25-mg capsules. How many capsules of Benadryl do you give Mrs. Tonnilski?

1. None; you cannot give half of a capsule.

2. 1 capsule.

3. 2 capsules.

4. 4 capsules.

142. Mr. Harris is prescribed 75 mg of Symmetrel liquid now, to be given orally, as a dopamine agonist to treat extrapyramidal side effects from his antipsychotic medications. The pharmacy sends up amantadine (Symmetrel) in the form of 50 mg/5 mL liquid packs. How much amantadine do you pour to give Mr. Harris?

1. 3 mL.
2. 5 mL.
3. 7.5 mL.
4. 12 mL.

143. Your patient is receiving a medication once a day that is causing him sedation. The medication is required to be given. What intervention would help manage the side effect of sedation?

1. Give the medication with a 6-ounce glass of milk.
2. Give one-half pill with breakfast and one-half pill with lunch.
3. Allow the patient to take the medication anytime he wants as long as he takes 7 pills per week.
4. Give the medication at bedtime.

144. Your patient, Mr. Wallenberg, is experiencing postural hypotension as a side effect of his low-potency antipsychotic medication chlorpromazine (Thorazine). What would be an appropriate intervention to teach the patient associated with postural hypotension?

1. Assess the blood sugar every 2 hours.
2. Read in well-lighted areas.
3. Count the calories with each meal.
4. Rise from bed slowly.

145. While Mrs. Cruz is taking a phenothiazine medication, she goes to the beach and within 1 hour has a bad sunburn. What is this medication-induced reaction called?

1. Photosensitivity.
2. Gynecomastia.
3. Akathisia.
4. Dystonia.

146. Maintenance dosages of haloperidol by injection are equivalent to 10 times the daily oral dose. If your patient is receiving 0.5 mg orally daily of haloperidol, how much should he receive as a maintenance dose by injection?

1. 2.5 mg.
2. 5 mg.
3. 50 mg.
4. 20 mg.

147. Mrs. Hondu is taking clozapine and has a 1% to 3% chance of developing agranulocytosis. Which laboratory value should you monitor to assess for agranulocytosis?

1. Red blood cell count.
2. White blood cell count.
3. Platelet count.
4. Prothrombin time.

148. You reconstitute ziprasidone with 1.2 mL of sterile water for injection into the vial, which produces a resulting volume of 20 mg ziprasidone per 1 mL solution. The physician prescribes 10 mg ziprasidone intramuscularly now. How much of the medication do you draw up in the syringe?

1. 0.2 mL.
2. 0.3 mL.
3. 0.5 mL.
4. 2 mL.

Fill in the Blank

149. Gabapentin (Neurontin) is a mood stabilizer that requires good renal function; therefore, prior to administration of this medication, the nurse must assess the results of the _____ clearance urinary test.

Multiple Choice

150. Mr. Barry is taking a monoamine oxidase inhibitor (MAOI) as part of his treatment for depression. You should educate him to avoid which food?

1. Oatmeal cookies.
2. Diet soda.
3. Orange juice.
4. Aged cheese.

151. Mrs. Wallace, who has been diagnosed with schizophrenia, has a fever, is confused, and has rigid muscles. These effects may be symptoms of

1. Alcohol withdrawal.
2. Grand mal seizure.
3. Neuroleptic malignant syndrome.
4. Tardive dyskinesia.

SECTION I

SECTION II

SECTION III

SECTION IV

SECTION V

SECTION VI

SECTION VII

SECTION VIII

SECTION IX

SECTION X

True/False

152. Patients with bipolar disorder usually require lifelong medication therapy.

Multiple Choice

153. Mrs. Tungen, who has been diagnosed with bipolar disorder, is receiving lithium and outpatient therapy. She now complains of diarrhea, vomiting, thirst, and coarsening hand tremors. What should the nurse's first intervention be?

  1. Hold the lithium, and call for an order to obtain a lithium level.

  2. Administer an antidiarrheal medication.

  3. Obtain a stool sample for culture.

  4. Begin an intravenous drip of D_5 $\frac{1}{2}$ NS with 20 mg potassium chloride to infuse at 125 mL/h.

154. Mrs. Roberts has been receiving buspirone (BuSpar) for 4 weeks for generalized anxiety disorder. Which statement indicates that she is improving?

  1. "Let me rest. I'm too tired to go to group therapy."

  2. "I just can't seem to sit still."

  3. "I'm able to sleep a full 8 hours at night now."

  4. "I have no idea what I want to do today. I'm a little foggy anyway."

Identification

155. Mr. Ran is prescribed alprazolam 2 mg orally on day 1, with the dose to be increased by 5 mg/day beginning on day 2. What is Mr. Ran's dose of alprazolam on day 3?

Multiple Choice

156. Mr. Cook is receiving nefazodone to treat his depression. The half-life of this drug is short, so how should it be taken?

  1. Once per day only.

  2. Two or three times per day.

  3. Once per month.

  4. By intramuscular route only.

157. Mr. Goldstein is receiving trazadone for treatment of his depression. He complains that he has a painful and persistent penile erection that is not a result of sexual stimulation. What is the name given to this emergent condition?

  1. Angioedema.

  2. Petechiae.

  3. Priapism.

  4. Erythema.

158. Mrs. Turnon is prescribed 300 mg lithium orally three times per day. The pharmacy fills her medication draw for 24 hours at a time. Lithium is dispensed from the pharmacy in 150-mg capsules. How many capsules should be in Mrs. Turnon's medication draw for a 24-hour supply of lithium?

  1. 3 capsules.

  2. 5 capsules.

  3. 6 capsules.

  4. 9 capsules.

159. Mrs. Andrews is a diagnosed schizophrenic who has just received a new prescription for quetiapine (Seroquel) to be taken as 50 mg, by tablet form, three times per day for 3 days, then increase dose to 100 mg three times per day times 27 days. Her prescription is filled by the pharmacy as Seroquel 25 mg per tablet. On day 1, how many total tablets should Mrs. Andrews take that day?

  1. 3 tablets.

  2. 5 tablets.

  3. 6 tablets.

  4. 9 tablets.

REDUCTION OF RISK POTENTIAL

Multiple Choice

160. Mr. Zionetti's medication profile reveals that three of his four prescribed medications can cause constipation. His last bowel movement was yesterday. What is an appropriate nursing diagnosis based on these data?

  1. The patient is at risk for trauma.

  2. The patient has constipation related to age and prescribed narcotics.

  3. The patient is at risk for constipation related to medications.

  4. The patient has constipation related to his refusal to drink water.

161. Which of the following is a complete nursing diagnosis because it contains both a risk problem and a risk factor?

  1. Trauma related to risk for other directed violence.

2. Memory loss related to chronic confusion.

3. Risk for loneliness related to social isolation.

4. Impaired socialization related to anxiety.

162. Mrs. Codo is admitted from the Emergency Department to the psychiatric mental health unit post rape. She is very anxious and very talkative. What is an appropriate nursing diagnosis based on these data?

1. The patient is at risk for violence related to physical isolation.

2. The patient has anxiety related to repetitive nightmares and intrusive thoughts.

3. The patient is at risk for impaired parenting related to her risk for trauma.

4. The patient has post-trauma syndrome related to anxiety secondary to rape.

163. Mr. Lobonowitz is at risk for constipation related to his prescribed tricyclic antidepressant medications. Which nursing intervention will help reduce the risk of constipation?

1. Consume a high-carbohydrate diet.

2. Increase fluid intake.

3. Administer furosemide (Lasix) orally, 40 mg.

4. Consume a diet high in iron and vitamin B_{12}.

164. Mrs. Wallace is at risk for self-directed violence. Which verbalization indicates a positive outcome?

1. "I don't need a bath today—you need one, though."

2. "I still like to play with knives; it's exhilarating."

3. "At most I will just take a razor and cut myself."

4. "I realize that killing myself is not right. I don't want to hurt myself."

Identification

165. Circle the three outcome statements associated with a nursing diagnosis of risk for self-directed harm.

Grooms self in morning

Verbalizes absence of suicidal thoughts

Interacts socially

Complies with medication regimen

Mucous membranes intact

Urinary continence

Multiple Choice

166. Which of the following actions by the nurse will help predict that an outcome will be attained?

1. Identify a specific target date for the outcome.

2. Choose a patient who is not angry.

3. The nurse should be well groomed.

4. Evaluate the prescribed medication with the pharmacist.

Identification

167. Circle the three risk factors associated with the nursing diagnosis of risk for loneliness.

Physical isolation

Social isolation

Urinary continence

Cast on right arm

Diabetes mellitus

Long-term institutionalization

Multiple Choice

168. Mr. Oliphant has a diagnosis of anxiety. Which behavior would indicate a reduction in anxiety?

1. The patient paces the floor.

2. The patient fidgets with his hands and walks the halls with a scanning motion.

3. The patient talks continuously to whoever is nearest.

4. The patient is able to sit calmly for 10 minutes.

169. A 19-year-old patient has just been admitted to the detoxification unit after drinking a quart of vodka every day for the past 3 weeks. What is the most important nursing intervention on the day of admission to reduce the risk of harm to this patient?

1. Administer Librium as prescribed.

2. Explain the addictive process to the patient.

3. Give the patient a meeting schedule for Alcoholics Anonymous.

4. Encourage the patient to attend group therapy sessions.

170. A 15-year-old patient with anorexia nervosa has a diagnosis of imbalanced nutrition—that is, less nutrition than the body requires. Which behavior would indicate a decreased risk for this diagnosis?

SECTION I
SECTION II
SECTION III
SECTION IV
SECTION V
SECTION VI
SECTION VII
SECTION VIII
SECTION IX
SECTION X

1. Patient performs continuous excessive exercise.
2. Patient eats meals in the dining room.
3. Patient verbalizes importance of increased vitamin intake.
4. Patient experiences a weight loss of only $\frac{1}{2}$ pound over the last 2 weeks.

Short Answer

171. Post-traumatic stress disorder (PTSD) is associated with increased risk for substance abuse. Which area must be assessed in patients with PTSD?

172. Hyperreflexia is a symptom of anxiety. Which physical assessment test would be appropriate to assess for hyperreflexia?

Multiple Choice

173. Which of the following statements by the patient indicates that he is at increased risk for self-mutilation?

1. "Today is a gray day—not black, not white, just gray."
2. "I think I'll go to art therapy today and make something nice."
3. "My voices are telling me to hit people who have red hair."
4. "A razor, I need it. I know what to do with it. Cut, cut, cut."

174. Which of the following nursing actions will help reduce a patient's anxious feelings and impulses?

1. Avoid any eye contact with the patient.
2. Use brief, directive verbal instructions.
3. Explain to the patient that only medication will help anxiety, so he should sit still and wait.
4. Explain to the patient that exercise will counteract anxiety.

175. Your patient is 84 years old, has a 3-year history of dementia, and has just begun taking antipsychotic and antianxiety medications for a diagnosis of anxiety and related disorders. These data place the patient at high risk for

1. Hypertension.
2. Cardiac dysrhythmias.
3. Falls.
4. Somatized disorder.

176. Twenty-two-year-old Samantha Barker is being discharged from an inpatient psychiatric mental health unit, where she received a diagnosis of schizophrenia and was started on antipsychotic medications. She is planning to live with her sister and hopes to return to college. To reduce this patient's risk of readmission, what should the nursing discharge teaching include?

1. Information about vocation training opportunities.
2. Information about family relationships.
3. Information about medication side effects.
4. Information about support groups for the chronically mentally ill.

177. A 40-year-old male psychiatric inpatient with dual diagnoses of depression and alcohol abuse told his nurse that when he is released he plans to kill his ex-wife with whom he was involved in a child custody battle. The nurse shares this information with the treatment team. What is the team's legal duty in this scenario?

1. Keep the patient hospitalized indefinitely.
2. Warn the patient's ex-wife of the threat.
3. Maintain strict patient confidentiality.
4. Transfer the patient to a state hospital.

178. Mrs. Robinson is a 38-year-old woman being treated on an outpatient basis for depression. Three months ago, her husband revealed that he was having an affair with her best friend and planned to file for divorce. Three weeks ago, Mrs. Robinson's 14-year-old son (her only child) committed suicide on an inpatient psychiatric mental health unit. In today's therapy session, Mrs. Robinson reveals to her nurse therapist that she is seriously contemplating suicide herself. What action should the therapist take?

1. None, because people who speak of committing suicide seldom do it.
2. Request permission to speak with the husband to suggest marriage counseling.
3. Arrange for voluntary hospitalization, if the patient is willing.
4. Arrange for immediate hospitalization.

179. A 35-year-old patient with a diagnosis of bipolar disorder is receiving Librium and preparing for discharge from the inpatient mental health unit. Which of the following is a critical part of the nursing discharge instruction?

1. Providing information on support groups for people with mood disorders.

2. Providing information about the importance of medication compliance, including regular blood draws to determine lithium levels.

3. Providing referral information for marital therapy.

4. Providing information about other types of mood disorders.

True/False

180. People with the diagnosis of schizophrenia rarely attempt suicide.

Multiple Choice

181. Which of the following treatments would *not* ordinarily be used to reduce the risk of further self-harm in a patient with a personality disorder?

1. Journaling about intense feelings.

2. Electroshock therapy.

3. Cognitive therapy.

4. Antianxiety or antipsychotic medication.

182. Ms. Sullivan is a 28-year-old psychiatric nurse who is working in an outpatient clinic. Her new patient is an attractive 33-year-old man who has recently moved to this city and has sought treatment because he is lonely and feeling "low." Which of the following interventions is *not* appropriate to include in the treatment plan?

1. Assess the depth of the patient's depression.

2. Determine whether the patient has experienced similar problems in the past.

3. Assess the presence of suicidal ideation or plans.

4. Invite the patient to join the nurse for "happy hour" after the session ends, as she is also new in town.

183. A personality disorder

1. Is a long-standing pervasive pattern of maladaptive behavior that is so severe that it is always an Axis I diagnosis.

2. Is caused solely by biological factors.

3. Often includes the risk of violence toward self and others.

4. Is a "hopeless" diagnosis, as patients with this diagnosis never show any improvement.

184. It is important for women in substance abuse programs who are pregnant or who may become pregnant to be educated about the risks of drinking alcohol during pregnancy. What is the most serious of these risks?

1. Having a child with fetal alcohol syndrome.

2. Developing gestational diabetes.

3. Gaining too much weight from drinking beer.

4. Setting a poor example for her children.

185. A psychiatric consultation was requested for a 78-year-old man who was 2 days postoperative for a fractured hip when he suddenly became confused, restless, and agitated and insisted that he was in the Atlanta airport. To determine the appropriate treatment, an accurate diagnosis is needed. Which of the following is most likely the diagnosis?

1. Sudden-onset Alzheimer's disease.

2. Major depression.

3. Creutzfeldt-Jakob disease.

4. Delirium.

186. During the third stage of Alzheimer's disease, it is important to monitor eating behavior because of the increased risk of

1. Weight loss.

2. Weight gain.

3. Aspiration.

4. Spitting at others.

True/False

187. Suicide is one of the leading causes of death in adolescents.

Multiple Choice

188. Children younger than age 14 years are at risk for several adult psychiatric diagnoses. What is the most common of these diagnoses?

1. Anxiety disorder.

2. Depression.

3. Schizophrenia.

4. Bipolar disorder.

SECTION I
SECTION II
SECTION III
SECTION IV
SECTION V
SECTION VI
SECTION VII
SECTION VIII
SECTION IX
SECTION X

Fill in the Blank

189. Complete this sentence by choosing the one correct response to make the statement true: The highest mortality rate found in any psychiatric diagnosis is found in _____.

> *Words*
>
> Schizophrenia
>
> Anorexia nervosa
>
> Obsessive-compulsive disorder

Multiple Choice

190. Psychiatric medications have side effects associated with varying degrees of risk. Which of the following side effects always represents a medical emergency?

1. Tardive dyskinesia.
2. Neuroleptic malignant syndrome.
3. Pseudoparkinsonism.
4. Postural hypotension.

191. Which of the following is a major risk factor for child sexual abuse?

1. Low income.
2. Drug-related crime in the neighborhood.
3. Having two or more older siblings.
4. A parent who was sexually abused as a child.

Identification

192. Which three of the following symptoms suggest that a severely and persistently mentally ill person may be at risk of violence toward self or others?

> Tardive dyskinesia
>
> Paranoid delusions
>
> Homelessness
>
> Failure to take medications
>
> Command hallucinations
>
> History of violence
>
> Apathy
>
> Diuresis

PHYSIOLOGICAL ADAPTATION

Multiple Choice

193. A 78-year-old patient with diagnosed bipolar disorder has been doing well the last few months, but he does complain about no longer being able to read the newspaper or his favorite book series.

Which nursing intervention might help this patient?

1. Obtain a hearing aid.
2. Obtain large-print books and newspapers.
3. Place extra salt on his food.
4. Patch one eye during reading time.

194. Mr. Ranny, a 70-year-old patient who has been diagnosed with anxiety, is scheduled to visit you in the clinic. His wife calls and states, "He just walked in front of a car that beeped its horn, but he's okay." When Mr. Ranny shows up 20 minutes later, what should you assess him for?

1. Obsessive-compulsive disorder.
2. Midlife transition.
3. Hearing problems.
4. Denial through fantasy.

195. Mrs. Shoemaker is taking antipsychotic medications and is a heavy cigarette smoker (3 packs per day). You know that cigarette smoking tends to activate hepatic enzymes that cause medications to be metabolized more quickly. Therefore, how should the antipsychotic medications be prescribed to Mrs. Shoemaker?

1. At a higher dose.
2. At a lower dose.
3. Every 2 hours, with around-the-clock frequency.
4. At 4-hour intervals, to be taken with an antacid.

196. Ms. Jarrell is placed on the antipsychotic thioridazine (Mellaril) and complains of feeling tired after her first week of medication therapy. Which education should the nurse provide to Ms. Jarrell?

1. Hallucinations will occur in 1 week, but are acceptable.
2. Her blood levels must be evaluated on a biweekly basis to assess for anemia.
3. Common ECG changes of bradycardia are normal, and she should sit down for 10 minutes during periods of tiredness.
4. Drowsiness is a common treatment side effect of antipsychotics during the first 2 weeks of therapy.

197. Mrs. Walton is started on antipsychotic medications in divided doses, to be taken 4 times per day. Once the medication effectiveness level is reached, her regimen is reduced to a once-daily dose. This reduced frequency of administration increases the likelihood of

1. Extrapyramidal side effects.
2. Compliance with the medication regimen.
3. Catatonia.
4. Delusions.

198. Mr. Hernandez has been taking antipsychotic medications for 3 weeks and comes to see you in clinic for his weekly session. You realize he is adapting to his home environment when he states:

1. "For the last several days, I've taken a shower and dressed myself."
2. "I just stare into space mostly. I talk to the dog sometimes."
3. "I saw a television commercial on having vegetables with your dinner."
4. "I want to get up and go and do something, but it never happens."

199. Your patient is taking the antipsychotic medications clozapine and divalproex sodium (Depakote), both of which cause weight gain. What should this patient be carefully monitored for?

1. Decreased serum calcium.
2. Urine nitrates.
3. Decreased blood pressure.
4. Increased blood glucose.

200. Mrs. Irinowitz is taking a low-potency antipsychotic, chlorpromazine, and is experiencing the anticholinergic side effect of constipation. Which nursing intervention will best help alleviate this side effect?

1. Use of sugarless gum or ice chips.
2. Docusate sodium (Colace), orally, once daily.
3. Oxybutynin (Ditropan), 1 mg intravenously now.
4. Oxycodone 5/325 (Percocet), one tablet orally daily.

201. Mr. Cruz is experiencing the side effect of dry mouth from taking the low-potency antipsychotic chlorpromazine. Which nursing intervention is most appropriate to deal with this side effect?

1. Use of nasal decongestants.
2. Exercise.
3. Use of ice chips and sugarless candies.
4. Administer docusate sodium (Colace), orally, once daily.

202. Your patient is prescribed thioridazine (Mellaril) and ziprasidone (Geodon) to treat his mental health disorders. He complains of heart palpitations. What should your first nursing intervention be?

1. Obtain an electrocardiogram (ECG, EKG) as prescribed.
2. Have the patient lie down, and assess his respirations.
3. Place the patient in the Trendelenberg position, and assess his blood pressure.
4. Administer dopamine hydrochloride, intravenously, 1 mg/kg, as prescribed.

203. Mr. Koo is prescribed chlorpromazine (Thorazine) as an antipsychotic medication. When he comes to the pill line in the hospital, he reports that he has taken 2 days' worth of the medication as prescribed and is now experiencing dizziness. What should your first nursing intervention be?

1. Obtain pulmonary function tests, stat.
2. Obtain a complete blood count and serum ammonia level as prescribed.
3. Assess blood pressure with the patient in both the lying and standing positions.
4. Assess the optic chiasm using an ophthalmoscope.

Fill in the Blank

204. Choose the correct word to make the statement true: _____ is a condition that results in hyperprolactinemia due to dopamine blockade resulting from the administration of antipsychotic medications.

> *Words*
> Gynecomastia
> Poikilothermia
> Photosensitivity

205. Choose the correct word to make the statement true: Neuroleptic malignant syndrome (NMS) includes the laboratory finding of increased white blood cell count known as _____.

> *Words*
> Pancytopenia
> Leukocytosis
> Myoglobinuria

Multiple Choice

206. As a result of neuroleptic malignant syndrome (NMS), your patient has hyperthermia. Which of the following nursing interventions would be most appropriate to treat hyperthermia?

1. Infuse dantrolene (Dantrium) for muscle relaxation.
2. Administer acetaminophen (Tylenol).
3. Administer a dopaminergic drug such as bromocriptine (Parlodel).
4. Cover the patient with three or more blankets.

207. Mr. Robinson is taking clozapine for treatment of schizophrenia. He has hypersalivation as a side effect of this medication. Which type of medication could be given to alleviate this side effect?

1. Anticholinergic.
2. Antihypertensive.
3. Dopamine antagonist.
4. Serotonin inhibitor.

208. Your patient has akathisia as a result of treatment with perphenazine (Trilafon) and is placed on propranolol (Inderal) 40 mg orally twice daily to help control this side effect. Which vital sign should you monitor based on the patient's treatment?

1. Temperature.
2. Pain.
3. Heart rate.
4. Blood pressure.

True/False

209. Oxybutynin (Ditropan) is a medication used to treat urinary retention, a side effect that is sometimes seen in patients who are treated with antipsychotics.

Identification

210. Which two of the following anticholinergic side effects are possible with the use of low-potency conventional antipsychotics?

Dry mouth
Ototoxicity
Seizures
Constipation
Diarrhea
Hypotension

Multiple Choice

211. Mr. Smart is scheduled to be converted from oral haloperidol daily to decanoate injections. This conversion includes administering 10 times the daily oral dose of haloperidol as a maintenance dose. If Mr. Smart's current haloperidol dose is 5 mg daily, what should his maintenance dose be?

1. 2 mg.
2. 25 mg.
3. 50 mg.
4. 0.5 mg.

212. Mr. Rabins is placed on quetiapine, an antipsychotic whose side effects include elevated cholesterol. Which laboratory test should you monitor related to this side effect?

1. Serum digoxin.
2. Complete blood count (CBC).
3. Liver function tests.
4. Lipid profile.

Identification

213. Of the following gastrointestinal side effects, which two are commonly seen with antipsychotic medications?

Hypotension
Sweating
Skin rash
Inverted QT wave
Dyspepsia
Nausea

Fill in the Blank

214. Fill in the blank with six letters to make an eight-letter word that makes the statement true: One side effect of selective serotonin reuptake inhibitors (SSRIs) is an inability to sleep, which is called "in_ _ _ _ _ _."

Multiple Choice

215. One of the side effects of antidepressants can be disturbance of near vision. What is another name for this side effect?

1. Pilocarpinemia.
2. Presbyopia.
3. Petechiae.
4. Priapism.

216. A rare side effect of taking trazadone is a prolonged, painful, nonsexual erection. What is this medical emergency called?

1. Priapism.
2. Cardiac blockade.
3. Presbyopia.
4. Petechiae.

217. Monoamine oxidase inhibitors (MAOIs) can cause numbness, prickling, or tingling feelings, which are called

1. Orthostatic hypotension.
2. Paresthesias.
3. Edema.
4. Melancholia.

218. Mr. Rogers has been taking lithium therapy and has the persistent side effect of edema. Which medication would be the most appropriate to give to manage this side effect?

1. Docusate sodium (Colace).
2. Digoxin (Lanoxin).
3. Furosemide (Lasix).
4. Albuterol (Proventil) inhaler.

219. Patients who take valproic acid (Depakote) are at risk for hepatotoxicity. Which laboratory values should you monitor associated with this risk?

1. Pulmonary function tests.
2. Liver function tests.
3. Thyroid function tests.
4. Pancreatic enzymes.

220. Mrs. Swim is taking carbamazepine (Tegretol) and complains of nausea as a side effect. Which of the following interventions might help her manage this side effect?

1. Drink 32 ounces of milk of magnesia before each meal.
2. Administer St. John's wort (an herbal medication) daily as prescribed.
3. Take the medication with 4 ounces of hot tea.
4. Take the medication immediately before or after meals.

221. Hyponatremia is a major concern in persons taking oxycarbazepine therapy. Which laboratory serum value should you monitor for this side effect?

1. Sodium.
2. Potassium.
3. Magnesium.
4. Thyroxine.

222. Ms. Daniels is taking gabapentin (Neurontin) as a mood stabilizer and complains of fatigue, headache, diplopia, impaired concentration, and tremor. These are common side effects related to which system?

1. Autonomic nervous system (ANS).
2. Central nervous system (CNS).
3. Hypothalmic-vagal neuronal system (HVNS).
4. Krebs-glycemic system (KGS).

SECTION I

SECTION II

SECTION III

SECTION IV

SECTION V

SECTION VI

SECTION VII

SECTION VIII

SECTION IX

SECTION X

MANAGEMENT OF CARE

1. Correct Answer: **2**

   Rationale: Patient confidentiality is required, and there is no way to verify the identity of the person calling.

2. Correct Answer: **4**

   Rationale: Delirium tremens occurs as acute alcohol withdrawal progresses. It includes symptoms such as clouding of sensorium, hallucinations, seizures, and autonomic hyperactivity.

3. Correct Answer: **2**

   Rationale: Urine and serum samples are toxicology specimens used to assess and monitor alcohol withdrawal.

4. Correct Answer: **1**

   Rationale: Screening requires questions associated with cutting down, feelings of guilt about drinking, and having a first drink in the morning.

5. Correct Answer: **Behavior manifestations of autism include hyperactivity, short attention span, impulsivity, aggressiveness, self-injurious behavior, temper tantrums, and recurrent actions.**

6. Correct Answer: **4**

   Rationale: Obtain a toxicology sample, as the patient is too euphoric to answer the CAGE questionnaire. The IV and neuro checks can wait.

7. Correct Answer: **3**

   Rationale: Approximately 65% of cases of pancreatitis are related to alcohol. This patient is exhibiting the classic symptoms of this disease.

8. Correct Answer: **Tremor, tachycardia, confusion, seizures are signs of acute alcohol withdrawal syndrome along with insomnia, vivid dreams, headache, sweating, restlessness, and nausea and vomiting.**

9. Correct Answer: **3**

   Rationale: Cirrhosis is a liver disorder that can result from prolonged ingestion of alcohol.

10. Correct Answer: **True**

    Rationale: Adolescent suicides have quadrupled since 1950 and are the third leading cause of death in U.S. adolescents.

11. Correct Answer: **True**

    Rationale: The central nervous system adapts, so more alcohol is needed to obtain the initial effects of alcohol ingestion, especially euphoria.

12. Correct Answer: **2**

    Rationale: Alcoholics Anonymous is the most appropriate resource for alcoholism, although depression may or may not be involved in this case.

13. Correct Answer: **Depression and anxiety**

    Rationale: Comorbidities include depression, anxiety, obsessive-compulsive disorder, panic, dissociative disorder, and substance abuse.

14. Correct Answer: **3**

    Rationale: Hopelessness, loss of pleasure, and a profound sense of sadness are symptoms of a major depressive episode.

15. Correct Answer: **2**

    Rationale: A subjective report of feeling sad or empty is a sign of depression.

16. Correct Answer: **4**

    Rationale: Signs and symptoms of hypothyroidism include changes in weight, sleep disturbances, decreased energy, and difficulty in thinking—just like in depression.

17. Correct Answer: **1**

    Rationale: Safety is the primary focus for an intervention, as 25% to 30% of depressed patients are at risk for suicide.

18. Correct Answer: **Use of drugs often accompanies suicide because they contribute to poor, impulsive decisions due to lowering inhibitions and quickening impulsivity.**

19. Correct Answer: **2**

    Rationale: A suicide attempt is a serious and self-destructive behavior that demands searching for weapons and harmful materials to increase safety.

20. Correct Answer: **4**

    Rationale: Patients cannot drive after ECT, as its effects can include disorientation, muscle pain, central nervous system depression, and cardiac dysrhythmias.

21. Correct Answer: **Denial**

    Rationale: The patient's statement includes a lack of recognition of the disease with accompanying denial of treatment.

22. Correct Answer: **2**

    Rationale: Risk factors include genetic predisposition, a recent loss or trauma, and a feeling of sadness or hopelessness.

23. Correct Answer: **4**

    Rationale: ABGs assess for acidosis [pH, bicarbonate, and hypoxemia (pO_2)].

24. Correct Answer: **3**

    Rationale: A jellyfish sting can cause a poison exposure.

25. Correct Answer: **4**

    Rationale: Duty to warn is a protective privilege and ends where public peril begins, so an intended, identifiable victim needs to be notified.

26. Correct Answer: **3**

    Rationale: Action and responses include what one does and says.

27. Correct Answer: **2**

    Rationale: Sexism is the belief that members of one sex are superior to members of the other sex.

28. Correct Answer: **4**

    Rationale: Grieving may be characterized by weight loss, sleep disturbances, and messages from beyond.

29. Correct Answer: **1**

    Rationale: Depressed mood and anhedonia (loss of interest or pleasure in activities) are the primary symptoms of major depression.

30. Correct Answer: **Stress reduction techniques such as meditation and guided imagery help patients cope.**

31. Correct Answer: **2**

    Rationale: Cognitive symptoms include inflated self-esteem and grandiosity.

32. Correct Answer: **3**

    Rationale: Verbalization of a plan for help and demonstration of care are realistic discharge criteria.

33. Correct Answer: **1**

    Rationale: The patient improvement is based on increased socialization and increased appetite.

34. Correct Answer: **4**

    Rationale: Catatonic schizophrenia occurs suddenly and includes motor immobility or excessive motor activity.

35. Correct Answer: **1**

    Rationale: Schizophrenia has a multifocal origin and its cause may include a genetic component. Support is needed for both patients and caregivers.

36. Correct Answer: **True**

    Rationale: Musculoskeletal fractures and sprains, especially of distal versus proximal bones, are indications of battering. Also assess for dislocated shoulders and old fractures.

37. Correct Answer: **3**

    Rationale: Managing a relapse includes a plan of action, involvement of a friend or family member, and, after identification of signs, notification of a therapist.

38. Correct Answer: **4**

    Rationale: Thought broadcasting and thought withdrawal are disturbed thought processes.

39. Correct Answer: **1**

    Rationale: Reinforcement by praise increases functional behavior.

40. Correct Answer: **2**

    Rationale: Obsessive-compulsive disorder is a personality disorder that includes perfection, control, procrastination, excessive devotion to work, difficulty relaxing, rule-conscious behavior, and inability to discard anything.

41. Correct Answer: **4**

    Rationale: Asking what the patient talks about with family or friends and what types of activities he or she engages in can help assess relationships.

SECTION I

SECTION II

SECTION III

SECTION IV

SECTION V

SECTION VI

SECTION VII

SECTION VIII

SECTION IX

SECTION X

42. Correct Answer: **2**

Rationale: Recreational therapy helps patients explore ways to enjoy themselves without using alcohol or drugs and strengthens social skills.

43. Correct Answer: **4**

Rationale: Hallucinations and delusions can result in problems with safety and possibly lead to suicide.

44. Correct Answer: **3**

Rationale: Daily routines and large clocks help patients' functional status.

SAFETY AND INFECTION CONTROL

45. Correct Answer: **3**

Rationale: The pill is contaminated once dropped, so for infection control purposes you discard it and repour the medication.

46. Correct Answer: **3**

Rationale: Cleansing the wound with soap and water is the initial intervention.

47. Correct Answer: **1**

Rationale: Contracts can see a patient through period of hypomanic agitation.

48. Correct Answer: **4**

Rationale: Privacy and autonomy are often given up for the sake of safety.

49. Correct Answer: **First, wash your hands when preparing medications.**

50. Correct Answer: **2**

Rationale: Protective gear helps prevent infections that may gain entry through openings in the skin, the eyes, or the mouth.

51. Correct Answer: **3**

Rationale: Clean all body fluids with an appropriate disinfectant such as 1:10 bleach solution, using universal precautions.

52. Correct Answer: **2**

Rationale: The patient might have tuberculosis, so wear a mask, especially given that the patient is coughing.

53. Correct Answer: **3**

Rationale: Place the syringe in a nearby container specific for needles. Do not recap, bend, clip, or manipulate the needle in any way.

54. Correct Answer: **True**

Rationale: This behavior enhances safety.

55. Correct Answer: **3**

Rationale: Safety includes not placing yourself in vulnerable situations.

56. Correct Answer: **1**

Rationale: Stalking behavior needs to be dealt with by the police for your safety.

57. Correct Answer: **4**

Rationale: The patient needs her medication, and following the care plan is the optimal course of action.

58. Correct Answer: **2**

Rationale: Use words to indicate your lack of acceptance of the patient's behavior in a nonthreatening voice or tone.

59. Correct Answer: **1 arm's length.**

Rationale: One arm's length is enough length for safety in case the patient becomes physical such as hitting.

60. Correct Answer: **3**

Rationale: Safety is the major principle underlying psychiatric nursing.

61. Correct Answer: **2**

Rationale: Quiet environments with consistent routines will help calm patients and add to safety.

62. Correct Answer: **4**

Rationale: Focus on the behavior, not the person. Be neutral, but not indifferent.

63. Correct Answer: **1**

Rationale: Safety is an acceptable reason to restrain a patient. Coercion, discipline, punishment, and nursing convenience are unacceptable reasons for employing restraints.

64. Correct Answer: **3**

Rationale: Involuntary commitment results from petitioning the court, which then determines that the evidence indicates treatment is necessary.

65. Correct Answer: **4**

Rationale: Risks and benefits, including compensation and medical treatments, are stated in an informed consent.

66. Correct Answer:

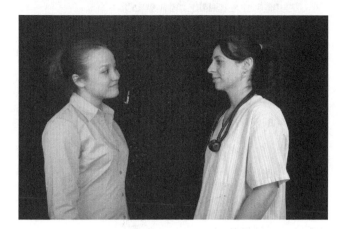

Rationale: Standing at a side angle indicates attentiveness whereas standing real close is assertive and indicative of not respectful of space and pointing your finger is angry and/or aggressive.

HEALTH PROMOTION AND MAINTENANCE

67. Correct Answer: **1**

Rationale: "Readiness for enhanced" is the prefix for a higher level of functioning, with "community" indicating society.

68. Correct Answer: **4**

Rationale: Environmental maintenance includes assessing for risk of injury, violence, and possession of weapons.

69. Correct Answer: **2**

Rationale: Usual stressors include work and relationships.

70. Correct Answer: **Hallucinations, depression, and delusions.**

Rationale: Lasting friendships are support mechanisms and do not increase risk for suicide.

71. Correct Answer: **2**

Rationale: Respect for tradition and community organizations are values that characterize Native American culture.

72. Correct Answer: **1**

Rationale: Many African American families have strong matriarchal structure and feature large extended family networks.

73. Correct Answer: **3**

Rationale: Reducing stress helps promote good mental health and is universal to local groups.

74. Correct Answer: **2**

Rationale: Coping and positivism are ways of maintaining good health post-discharge.

75. Correct Answer: **4**

Rationale: Widowhood, retirement, and grandparenting are role transitions.

76. Correct Answer: **Meditation and guided imagery are stress reducers and may enhance coping. Use of alcohol and a low sugar diet can lead to metabolic alterations and harm.**

77. Correct Answer: **3**

Rationale: Exercise helps prevent and combat heart disease, hypertension, and diabetes.

78. Correct Answer: **2**

Rationale: Involvement in hobbies, social life, and family reflects health adaptations.

79. Correct Answer: **4**

Rationale: Initiation of requests and specific identification of problems are positive and assertive behaviors.

80. Correct Answer: **True**

Rationale: CD4 counts help healthcare personnel care for patients with HIV infection, as they are an indication of immune status.

81. Correct Answer: **3**

Rationale: Anhedonia—the loss of interest and pleasure in activities—is a sign of depression.

82. Correct Answer: **2**

Rationale: Postpartum depression or mood disorder occurs in 10% to 15% of women after they give birth.

83. Correct Answer: **1**

Rationale: Establishing goals and expectations promotes structure and helps minimize anxiety.

84. Correct Answer: **4**

Rationale: Health maintenance measures related to sleep disturbances includes assessment of ADLs, diet, medications, and laboratory tests (i.e., chem 19, CBC, UA, toxicology, and TSH).

85. Correct Answer: **True**

Rationale: To maintain health, the caregiver is key to implementing effective strategies and evaluating the patient's responses.

86. Correct Answer: **1**

Rationale: Medication noncompliance and alcohol/drug abuse are leading causes of relapse in chronically mentally ill patients.

PSYCHOSOCIAL INTEGRITY

87. Correct Answer: **4 tablets**

Rationale: $25 \times 4 = 100$

88. Correct Answer: **2**

Rationale: Increasing the dose will help maintain blood levels based on increased metabolism.

89. Correct Answer: **4**

Rationale: Hypothermia is feeling cold from low body temperature.

90. Correct Answer: **2**

Rationale: Ratio is $2.5:1 = 7.5:x$; $x = 7.5/2.5 = 3$.

91. Correct Answer: **Orthostatic**

92. Correct Answer: **2**

Rationale: Ratio is $15:1 = 15:x$; $x = 15/15 = 1$.

93. Correct Answer: **3**

Rationale: Ratio is $10:1 = 30:x$; $x = 30/10 = 3$.

94. Correct Answer: **Food**

Rationale: Gastric irritation is a result of stomach acid secretion and utilization, so if you have food in your stomach the acid will eat the food and not your stomach lining or a small amount of medication.

95. Correct Answer: **1**

Rationale: Ratio is $10:1 = 5:x$; $x = 5/10 = 0.5$.

96. Correct Answer: **2**

Rationale: Ratio is $250:1 = 750:x$; $x = 750/250 = 3$.

97. Correct Answer: **4**

Rationale: Ratio is $25:1 = 200:x$; $x = 200/25 = 8$.

98. Correct Answer: **3**

Rationale: $10 \times 4 = 40$

99. Correct Answer: **Administer the medication during the waking hours, usually the morning.**

Rationale: If medication causes disruption in sleep, then give the medication upon rising in the morning so you have the entire day being awake when the medication is most effective.

100. Correct Answer: **4**

Rationale: $2 + 3 = 5$

101. Correct Answer: **1**

Rationale: You administer none, because the pharmacy has dispensed the wrong medication in the wrong form.

102. Correct Answer: **2**

Rationale: Ratio is $1:1 = 1.5:x$; $x = 1.5/1 = 1.5$.

103. Correct Answer: **1**

Rationale: Ratio is $75:1 = 150:x$; $x = 150/75 = 2$.

104. Correct Answer: **2**

Rationale: Ratio is $7.5:1 = 22.5:x$; $x = 22.5/7.5 = 3$.

105. Correct Answer: **4**

Rationale: Ratio is $100:1 = 200:x$; $x = 200/100 = 2$.

106. Correct Answer: **2**

Rationale: Ratio is $150:1 = 300:x$; $x = 300/150 = 2$.

BASIC CARE AND COMFORT

107. Correct Answers: **EKG and CBC**

Rationale: Tests prior to electroconvulsive therapy include a complete blood count and evaluation of the heart by an EKG. There is no need to determine serum steroids, parathyroid hormone, or urine for drug analysis such as with oxycodone as these will have no effect on therapy. There is also no need to assess the colon via a diagnostic colonoscopy as this has no effect on treatment.

108. Correct Answer: **2**

Rationale: Atropine has a vagolytic effect as well as blocks muscarinic responses and has selective depression of central nervous system. Benadryl is an H-1 receptor antagonist and antihistamine with anticholinergic activity and does not protect against vagal bradycardia. Adrenalin is a catecholamine that constricts bronchioles and inhibits histamine release, and Prozac is a antidepressant.

109. Correct Answers: <u>**EEG, blood pressure monitor, cardiac monitor.**</u>

Rationale: A sigmoidoscopy is used to assess the intestine up to the sigmoid colon, a ventriculostomy is placed in the ventricles of the brain for monitoring pressures, and hemoccult is for assessing blood in the stool, which makes these tests not appropriate for ECT therapy.

110. Correct Answer: <u>**4**</u>

Rationale: A mouth guard prevents damage to the oral cavity and helps in delivering oxygen.

111. Correct Answer: <u>**1.**</u>

Rationale: Occupational therapy focuses on tasks particular to work and jobs. ECT is therapy for mental illness, family therapy deals with family issues not the performance of tasks and group therapy does not focus on specific tasks associated with job/work but on dynamics within groups.

112. Correct Answers: <u>**Diet, exercise, stress-reduction therapies.**</u>

Rationale: Diet, exercise, and stress-reduction therapies are all scientifically proven ways that are effective in preventing and managing diseases such as heart disease and diabetes. Otic rectal irrigation is flushing of the eyes and rectum which is not a known therapy. Radiation normotherapy is also not a known therapy. Peroxide and cinnamon IV bolus is made up and theoretically can be very dangerous.

113. Correct Answer: <u>**4**</u>

Rationale: The patient's height and weight indicate that she is obese, smoking is tobacco abuse, and obesity requires physical activity.

114. Correct Answer: <u>**2**</u>

Rationale: Prayer can be a therapeutic tool and is associated with the Catholic faith.

115. Correct Answer: <u>**3**</u>

Rationale: Foot reflexology is a known method of massage to the feet. Osteopathic massage is a made up combination of words and is not a known method, acupressure is the use of pressure points and Ayurveda is a healing method common in India that includes herbs, nutrition, panchakarma cleansing, acupressure massage, Yoga, Sanskrit, and Jyotish.

116. Correct Answer: <u>**2**</u>

Rationale: Fatigue, exhaustion, and insomnia are common manifestations, along with shortness of breath, chest tightness, dry mouth, and gastrointestinal disturbances.

117. Correct Answer: <u>**1**</u>

Rationale: Grief increases vulnerability to myocardial infarction, hypertension, depression, drug abuse, malnutrition, and rheumatoid arthritis.

118. Correct Answer: <u>**4**</u>

Rationale: Cardiovascular and gastrointestinal problems are common in chronic grief. Acute grief is often characterized by weakness, anorexia, tight chest, dry mouth, and gastrointestinal disturbances.

119. Correct Answer: <u>**3**</u>

Rationale: Skin care and diaper changes are essential for comfort.

120. Correct Answer: <u>**1**</u>

Rationale: AIDS-associated dementia includes fatigue, forgetfulness, and problems with concentration.

121. Correct Answer: <u>**2**</u>

Rationale: A skin integrity assessment will identify abrasions, bruises, lacerations, and possible infection.

122. Correct Answer: <u>**2**</u>

Rationale: Bathing, hygiene, dressing, and food preparation are examples of ADLs.

123. Correct Answer: <u>**1**</u>

Rationale: Extrapyramidal reactions include movement disorders such as dystonia, tardive dyskinesia, and pseudoparkinsonism.

124. Correct Answers: <u>**Hygiene, dressing, grooming and bathing are activities of daily living.**</u>

125. Correct Answer: <u>**True**</u>

Rationale: Self-esteem is possibly associated with independence.

126. Correct Answer: <u>**1**</u>

Rationale: Healing is promoted by high protein, iron, and vitamin C intake.

SECTION I
SECTION II
SECTION III
SECTION IV
SECTION V
SECTION VI
SECTION VII
SECTION VIII
SECTION IX
SECTION X

PHARMACOLOGICAL AND PARENTERAL THERAPIES

127. Correct Answer: **3**

Rationale: Common side effects of anticholinergics include dry mouth, blurred vision, urinary retention, and constipation.

128. Correct Answer: **3**

Rationale: 300/100 = 3 tablets.

129. Correct Answer: **2**

Rationale: 10/5 = 2 tablets.

130. Correct Answer: **False**

Rationale: Hemodialysis is the only reliable method to decrease serum lithium levels.

131. Correct Answer: **2**

Rationale: 3/2 = 1.5 tablets.

132. Correct Answer: **3**

Rationale: 4/2 = 2 mL.

133. Correct Answer: **2**

Rationale: 25/50 = 0.5 mL.

134. Correct Answers: **Nausea, vomiting, diarrhea, dyspepsia.**

Rationale: Osteoporosis is a disease of the bone, and otitis refers to the ears.

135. Correct Answer: **1**

Rationale: 20/2 = 10 mg.

136. Correct Answer: **3**

Rationale: Cognitive and perceptive symptoms have a response of 2–8 weeks.

137. Correct Answer: **Hostility and verbal abuse. Assault, sexual acting out, and poor impulse control are other aggressive symptoms of psychosis.**

138. Correct Answer: **Extended release**

139. Correct Answer: **4**

Rationale: Alcohol, antihistamines, and sleeping aids should be avoided in persons who are taking antipsychotic medications.

140. Correct Answer: **3**

Rationale: 1/1 = 1 mL.

141. Correct Answer: **3**

Rationale: 50/25 = 2 capsules.

142. Correct Answer: **3**

Rationale: $50/5 = 75/x$; $375 = 50x$; $x = 7.5$ mL.

143. Correct Answer: **4**

Rationale: Giving the medication at bedtime or decreasing the dose will help in his sedation.

144. Correct Answer: **4**

Rationale: Sudden changes in position lead to dizziness associated with postural hypotension.

145. Correct Answer: **1**

Rationale: Photosensitivity is a general term used to describe phototoxic or photoallergenic reactions.

146. Correct Answer: **2**

Rationale: $10 \times 0.5 = 5$ mg.

147. Correct Answer: **2**

Rationale: The WBC count will indicate agranulocytosis.

148. Correct Answer: **3**

Rationale: $20/1 = 10/x$; $20x = 10$; $x = 0.5$ mL.

149. Correct Answer: **Creatinine**

150. Correct Answer: **4**

Rationale: Aged or fermented foods such as cheese are high in tyramine and may cause hypertensive crisis.

151. Correct Answer: **3**

Rationale: Neuroleptic malignant syndrome includes confusion, fever, and muscle rigidity.

152. Correct Answer: **True**

Rationale: The need for lifelong medication often leads to a high noncompliance rate of taking medications as prescribed.

153. Correct Answer: **1**

Rationale: Unsteady gait, slurred speech, nausea, vomiting, diarrhea, thirst, and coarsening of hand tremors indicate lithium toxicity.

154. Correct Answer: **3**

Rationale: Ability to sleep and going to therapy are indicators of anxiety disorder being controlled.

155. Correct Answer: **12 mg**

Rationale: 2 mg + 5 mg + 5 mg = 12 mg.

156. Correct Answer: <u>2</u>

Rationale: Drugs with a short half-life need to be taken several times a day to maintain an effective level in the patient's blood.

157. Correct Answer: <u>3</u>

Rationale: Priapism is painful and persistent erection that requires immediate medical attention.

158. Correct Answer: <u>3</u>

Rationale: $300 \times 3 = 900$; $900/150 = 6$.

159. Correct Answer: <u>3</u>

Rationale: $25 \text{ mg} \times 2 = 50 \text{ mg}$; $2 \times 3 = 6$ tablets.

REDUCTION OF RISK POTENTIAL

160. Correct Answer: <u>3</u>

Rationale: It is not certain what his age is.

161. Correct Answer: <u>3</u>

Rationale: Risk for loneliness is a nursing diagnosis/problem, and social isolation is a risk factor for it.

162. Correct Answer: <u>4</u>

Rationale: Post-traumatic stress syndrome is a nursing diagnosis with an etiologic factor of anxiety secondary to rape.

163. Correct Answer: <u>2</u>

Rationale: Increased fluids will help liquefy stool.

164. Correct Answer: <u>4</u>

Rationale: Verbalization of the absence of suicidal intent indicates a positive outcome.

165. Correct Answers: <u>**Outcome statements include those that patient will do and are not nursing interventions. Outcomes here include "interacts socially," "verbalizes absence of suicidal thoughts," and "complies with medication regimen."**</u>

166. Correct Answer: <u>1</u>

Rationale: A specific target date will help predict that an outcome is attained.

167. Correct Answers: <u>**Risk factors include physical and social isolation and long-term institutionalization.**</u>

168. Correct Answer: <u>4</u>

Rationale: Reduced anxiety can be seen in the activity of sitting calmly.

169. Correct Answer: <u>1</u>

Rationale: By administering Librium, you will prevent delirium tremens and possibly harm during the process.

170. Correct Answer: <u>2</u>

Rationale: Eating meals and eating in a socialized environment will increase body requirements.

171. Correct Answer: <u>**Drug abuse or substance abuse or use.**</u>

172. Correct Answer: <u>**Assess reflexes using a reflex hammer.**</u>

173. Correct Answer: <u>4</u>

Rationale: Verbal threats and a plan for use indicate increased risk.

174. Correct Answer: <u>2</u>

Rationale: Use of brief, directive verbal instructions will help patient gain control of his or her overwhelming feelings and impulses.

175. Correct Answer: <u>3</u>

Rationale: Age, dementia, and antipsychotic/anti-anxiety medications can lead to hypotension and a high risk for falls.

176. Correct Answer: <u>3</u>

Rationale: Awareness of medication-related side effects reduces the risk of noncompliance, which itself could cause a recurrence of symptoms.

177. Correct Answer: <u>2</u>

Rationale: Under the "Tarasoff ruling," the hospital has the "duty to warn" the ex-wife of the threat.

178. Correct Answer: <u>4</u>

Rationale: The suicide of her son puts this patient at high risk of suicide. This risk is exacerbated by the betrayal of her husband and best friend.

179. Correct Answer: <u>2</u>

Rationale: A person on lithium can move from the effective to the toxic range very quickly.

180. Correct Answer: <u>**False**</u>

Rationale: Studies show that approximately 50% of people with schizophrenia will attempt suicide at some point.

SECTION I

SECTION II

SECTION III

SECTION IV

SECTION V

SECTION VI

SECTION VII

SECTION VIII

SECTION IX

SECTION X

181. Correct Answer: **2**

Rationale: Electroshock treatment is used for the treatment of some types of depression.

182. Correct Answer: **4**

Rationale: Socialization with patients goes against all professional codes of ethics.

183. Correct Answer: **3**

Rationale: The lack of impulse control that characterizes some personality disorders leads to the risk of violence toward self and others.

184. Correct Answer: **1**

Rationale: Children who are exposed to alcohol in utero run a high risk of developing fetal alcohol syndrome. This syndrome is characterized by growth retardation, facial deformity, and neurological deficits including mental retardation.

185. Correct Answer: **4**

Rationale: The reported prevalence of delirium in elderly hospitalized patients ranges from 4% to 53%. Failure to recognize delirium can lead to treatment delays and increased morbidity and mortality.

186. Correct Answer: **3**

Rationale: Aspiration is a high-risk behavior because it can quickly lead to aspiration pneumonia and death.

187. Correct Answer: **True**

Rationale: As of 2004, suicide was the third leading cause of death in U.S. adolescents.

188. Correct Answer: **1**

Rationale: Anxiety disorders in childhood include social phobias, simple phobias, anxiety, overanxious disorder, and obsessive-compulsive disorder.

189. Correct Answer: **Anorexia nervosa**

Rationale: Lifetime mortality rates are reported to be in the range of 15% to 20%.

190. Correct Answer: **2**

Rationale: Neuroleptic malignant syndrome is a potentially fatal reaction that occurs in approximately 1% of people who take antipsychotic medications. The case fatality rate is approximately 10%.

191. Correct Answer: **4**

Rationale: Parents who were sexually abused as children are at high risk of abusing their own children.

192. Correct Answers: **History of violence, paranoid delusions, and command hallucinations.**

Rationale: These factors, particularly when combined with failure to take medications, are all predictors of violence in severely and persistently mentally ill persons.

PHYSIOLOGICAL ADAPTATION

193. Correct Answer: **2**

Rationale: Large-print books will help in case of visual problems.

194. Correct Answer: **3**

Rationale: Hearing problems are common in the elderly.

195. Correct Answer: **1**

Rationale: Higher doses will counteract the smoking effect.

196. Correct Answer: **4**

Rationale: Drowsiness is most common during the first days of treatment and disappears in 1–2 weeks.

197. Correct Answer: **2**

Rationale: The need to take medication only once or twice daily increases compliance.

198. Correct Answer: **1**

Rationale: Adaptation includes self-care and return to ADLs.

199. Correct Answer: **4**

Rationale: This patient is at increased risk for adult-onset diabetes, so monitor glucose.

200. Correct Answer: **2**

Rationale: Colace is a stool softener.

201. Correct Answer: **3**

Rationale: Use of ice chips, artificial saliva, and sugarless gums and candies may help decrease dry mouth.

202. Correct Answer: <u>1</u>

Rationale: Arrhythmias and palpitations are known to occur when patients take combination drug regimens, such as the Mellaril/Geodon combination.

203. Correct Answer: <u>3</u>

Rationale: Postural hypotension can be a result of dizziness owing to the use of low-potency antipsychotics such as chlorpromazine or thioridazine.

204. Correct Answer: <u>**Gynecomastia (enlarged breasts)**</u>

205. Correct Answer: <u>**Leukocytosis**</u>

206. Correct Answer: <u>2</u>

Rationale: Acetaminophen is an antipyretic and will help decrease fever.

207. Correct Answer: <u>1</u>

Rationale: Anticholinergics decrease saliva production.

208. Correct Answer: <u>4</u>

Rationale: Blood pressure should be monitored for Inderal treatment.

209. Correct Answer: <u>**True**</u>

Rationale: Ditropan is often given to patients undergoing antipsychotic medication treatment because antipsychotics can cause urinary retention which can lead to infection of the urinary tract and kidneys as well as sepsis.

210. Correct Answers: <u>**Dry mouth, constipation.**</u>

Rationale: Anticholinergic side effects include dry mouth and constipation and loss of taste. Ototoxicity is hearing problems, seizures and diarrhea or stool and hypotension or low blood pressure are also not anticholinergic effects.

211. Correct Answer: <u>3</u>

Rationale: $10 \times 5 = 50$ mg

212. Correct Answer: <u>4</u>

Rationale: A lipid profile includes cholesterol.

213. Correct Answers: <u>**Dyspepsia and nausea.**</u>

214. Correct Answer: <u>**Somnia (insomnia)**</u>

215. Correct Answer: <u>2</u>

Rationale: Presbyopia is a disturbance of near vision.

216. Correct Answer: <u>1</u>

Rationale: Priapism is a medical emergency for a sexual dysfunction.

217. Correct Answer: <u>2</u>

Rationale: MAOI-induced paresthesias are a result of vitamin B_6 (pyridoxine) deficiency.

218. Correct Answer: <u>3</u>

Rationale: Furosemide is a diuretic.

219. Correct Answer: <u>2</u>

Rationale: Liver function tests are used to monitor for liver dysfunction (i.e., hepatotoxicity).

220. Correct Answer: <u>4</u>

Rationale: Taking medication with meals, dividing the doses, or changing to a sustained-release formulation are appropriate interventions to decrease nausea.

221. Correct Answer: <u>1</u>

Rationale: Monitor serum sodium to assess for decreased serum sodium (i.e., hyponatremia).

222. Correct Answer: <u>2</u>

Rationale: CNS side effects include fatigue, headache, diplopia, impaired concentration or memory, nystagmus, abnormal speech, and tremors.

SECTION I

SECTION II

SECTION III

SECTION IV

SECTION V

SECTION VI

SECTION VII

SECTION VIII

SECTION IX

SECTION X

Trends and Current Issues in Nursing

MANAGEMENT OF CARE

Selection

1. Select all the statements about the Health Insurance Portability and Accountability Act (HIPAA) that are true.

1. Information about a patient can be disclosed to family members at any time.

2. HIPAA established regulations that address the use and disclosure of individually identifiable health information in verbal, electronic, or written form.

3. A patient's address would be an example of personally identifiable information.

4. Health information can no longer be transmitted to insurance companies for payment purposes.

5. HIPAA is a law passed by individual states that regulates health information.

6. HIPAA is a federal law.

Matching

A patient has experienced a stroke affecting the left side of the brain. Clinical manifestations of the stroke include right-side hemiplegia and expressive aphasia. Identify the actions that the members of the interdisciplinary healthcare team might take in the care of the patient.

2. Dietician

3. Home health aide

4. Social worker

5. Speech therapist

6. Physician

7. Physical therapist

1. Assistance with personal care and hygiene.

2. Evaluation of nutritional status.

3. Assessment of swallowing ability.

4. Follow-up and monitoring of medical condition.

5. Light housekeeping and meal preparation.

6. Referral to community resources such as a local stroke support group.

7. Gait training.

8. Treatment of medical complications associated with the stroke.

9. Securing financial resources for disability.

10. Assessment of caloric requirements.

11. Improvement of expressive abilities.

12. Improvement of musculoskeletal strength.

Match the type of nursing care delivery system with the scenario.

8. The nurse is assigned to administer all patient medications for the shift.

9. The registered nurse rounds and assesses all patients who are assigned to his or her care. The RN then assigns and delegates care to the licensed practical nurse and the certified nursing assistant care based on the assessment.

1. Primary nursing.
2. Team nursing.
3. Functional nursing.

Multiple Choice

10. The nurse is caring for a surgical patient who has been placed on a multidisciplinary treatment plan or critical pathway. One outcome identified by the plan is that the patient will ambulate on the first postoperative day. The patient was unable to ambulate on postoperative day 1. Which term is used to describe the deviation from the critical pathway?

1. Incident.
2. Root cause.
3. Variance.
4. Sentinel event.

11. When is the most appropriate time to begin discharge planning for a patient who is admitted to an acute care facility?

1. 48 hours before discharge.
2. Once the discharge order is written.
3. Upon the patient's admission to the facility.
4. Once the insurance company approves discharge coverage.

12. The nurse is completing the preoperative teaching for a patient who is to undergo a gastrectomy. Which teaching intervention would have the highest priority to ensure the prevention of postoperative complications?

1. Allowing the patient to tour the post-anesthesia care unit.
2. Applying a sequential compression device so the patient will know how the device will feel.
3. Discussing the visitation policy for the clinical unit.
4. Teaching the patient to splint the incision and to cough and deep breathe.

13. The nurse has received report and rounded on all assigned patients. It is now 8:00 A.M. Which patient should the nurse plan to care for first?

1. A patient who is ambulatory and going for an x-ray at 10:00 A.M.
2. A patient who is to be discharged at 11:00 A.M.
3. A postoperative patient who has just received pain medication.
4. A patient who is short of breath.

14. A new nurse asks the preceptor if personal professional liability insurance should be purchased. What is the preceptor's best response?

1. "Personal liability coverage is not needed, as the organization has insurance that will cover any malpractice litigation."
2. "Each nurse should purchase individual professional liability coverage."
3. "Coverage is not needed because liability insurance is very costly and the chance of a malpractice suit is low."
4. "Individual coverage for malpractice is not a good idea, as the hospital can then sue the nurse to recoup costs."

15. The nurse finds an unopened vial of morphine sulfate lying on the cabinet in a patient's room. What is the most appropriate action for the nurse to take first?

1. Secure the vial and return the medication to stock for future use.
2. Remove the vial from the patient's bedside and notify the nurse supervisor that an unsecured vial of a controlled substance was found.
3. Check with the other nurses to see if their patients have morphine orders and administer the medication to another patient to avoid waste.
4. Contact the organization's security department and have it investigate the crime scene.

16. On nursing rounds, a patient is found lying on the floor. Which statement would be most appropriate for the nurse to document in the patient's medical record?

1. "It is most likely that the patient attempted to climb over the side rails and fell."
2. "Upon entering the room, the patient was found lying on the floor."

3. "The patient had been restless all evening and was trying to get out of bed."

4. "The presence of a bed alarm could have prevented the fall."

17. After signing an informed consent form, the patient states, "I have changed my mind and do not want to have the procedure done." Which action would be most appropriate for the nurse to take first?

1. Remind the patient that a signed informed consent form is a legally binding document.

2. Notify the surgeon that the patient wishes to withdraw informed consent for the procedure.

3. Contact the operating room and tell the personnel there the patient's surgery has been cancelled.

4. Proceed with preparation of the patient for the surgical procedure.

18. Which action by a nurse could jeopardize the confidentiality of computerized medical records available at a nurses' station?

1. Log out and sign off all computer screens before leaving a terminal.

2. Share passwords for computer access with colleagues who have forgotten their own passwords.

3. Periodically change computer access passwords.

4. Prevent an unidentified healthcare worker from viewing computer records.

19. While at the grocery store, a nurse comes upon a shopper who has fallen. The nurse assists the woman and notices that she has slurred speech, facial drooping, and significant weakness on the right side as compared to the left. The shopper tells the nurse she is 70 years of age, has no allergies, and takes medication for high blood pressure. The woman asks, "What is wrong with me? I was fine just a few minutes ago." What is the priority action the nurse should take?

1. Obtain the number of the patient's primary care physician and offer to contact the physician's office.

2. Find a location where the patient can sit down and rest for a few minutes and offer to stay with the woman until a family member arrives.

3. Call 911 and notify the dispatcher that you have a person exhibiting clinical manifestations of a stroke.

4. Drive the patient to the nearest emergency treatment center for evaluation of her blood pressure.

20. The nurse is caring for a patient who has a traumatic brain injury. To promote continuity of care and a positive patient outcome, which finding would be most important for the nurse to report to the oncoming shift nurse?

1. Neurological assessment.

2. Patient complaints.

3. History of the injury.

4. Findings of a CT scan.

21. When transcribing medical orders, the nurse is unable to read a written order. What is the best action by the nurse?

1. Clarify the type of medication with the family.

2. Interpret the order based on the patient's history.

3. Ask the pharmacist for clarification.

4. Contact the prescriber to clarify the order.

22. Which nursing diagnosis has the highest priority for a patient with an open abdominal wound during the acute phase of care?

1. Altered body image.

2. Risk for infection.

3. Delayed surgical recovery.

4. Knowledge deficit about wound care.

23. Which patient would be most appropriate to assign to a private room?

1. A patient who is admitted with fever of unknown origin.

2. A patient who is expected to die within the next 24 hours.

3. A patient who has been diagnosed as HIV positive.

4. A patient with a stage II sacral pressure ulcer.

24. Which part of a research study would tell the nurse about the predicted relationship of the variables being tested?

1. Abstract.

2. Research question.

3. Hypothesis.

4. Review of the literature.

25. Who has the authority to revoke a professional nurse's license?

 1. A court of law.
 2. The chief nursing officer of a hospital.
 3. The state board of nursing.
 4. The state arm of the American Nurses Association.

26. The nurse arrives for her shift at 7:00 A.M. and receives her assignment. Which patient should the nurse assess first?

 1. A diabetic patient whose blood sugar at 6:50 A.M. was 40 and who just received 50% dextrose for a hypoglycemic episode.
 2. A patient who was admitted with chest pain; whose troponin I results were 0.6 ng/mL and 0.8 ng/mL at 24 and 48 hours after admission, respectively; and who is now complaining of indigestion.
 3. A patient who was treated for a temperature of 102°F at 4:00 A.M. and who has pneumonia and an SpO_2 of 94% on 2 L nasal cannula.
 4. A patient with peptic ulcer disease who has pulled out the peripheral IV catheter and is scheduled to receive a dose of famotidine (Pepcid) at 8:00 A.M.

27. An ethical conflict about a patient's care has developed, and the nurse is unable to resolve the conflict. Which hospital resource would be most appropriate for the nurse to consult about the ethical dilemma?

 1. Hospital ethics committee.
 2. Quality improvement committee.
 3. Chaplain.
 4. Nursing supervisor.

28. The nurse is unable to find coverage to leave the floor for a personal appointment outside the hospital. The nurse decides to leave her scheduled shift an hour early without permission and notification of the charge nurse. The patients assigned to the nurse are in stable condition. What type of legal tort could apply to the situation?

 1. Patient abandonment.
 2. Intentional infliction of emotional distress.
 3. Battery.
 4. Slander.

29. Two nurses are arguing over which one will go to lunch first. The charge nurse tells the pair of nurses that she is tired of hearing them argue and that she will cover patient care so both nurses can go to lunch together. Which type of conflict management style did the charge nurse use?

 1. Avoiding or withdrawing.
 2. Competing or forcing.
 3. Compromising or negotiating.
 4. Accommodating or smoothing.

30. The cardiac catheterization lab has established a procedure for achieving hemostasis of the cardiac catheter insertion site. Which type of standard does this exemplify?

 1. Structure.
 2. Process.
 3. Outcome.
 4. Performance.

31. A nurse works a full-time equivalent (1.0 FTE). How many hours per year are equal to 1.0 FTE?

 1. 2,080 hours.
 2. 2,000 hours.
 3. 1,872 hours.
 4. 1,040 hours.

32. A patient with sleep apnea is being prepared for discharge from the hospital on bilevel positive airway pressure (BiPAP) at night. Which healthcare team member would be helpful in educating the patient on the use of the home continuous positive airway pressure equipment?

 1. Occupational therapist.
 2. Physical therapist.
 3. Respiratory therapist.
 4. Case manager.

33. A nurse researcher is conducting a study. A notice is posted asking for volunteers to participate in the study. What type of a sample would be obtained with this technique?

 1. Random.
 2. Convenience.
 3. Quota.
 4. Network.

34. A patient requests that a nurse who was working on a previous shift not be allowed to provide the patient's care again. What is the most appropriate action by the nurse?

1. Document the issue on an incident report.
2. Address the patient's concern with the charge nurse.
3. Explain to the patient that the nurse was just having a bad day.
4. Notify the human resources department.

35. A new type of infusion pump is introduced to the nursing unit. In which type of educational setting would the nurse most likely learn about the operation and use of this equipment?

1. In-service education.
2. Continuing education.
3. Online education.
4. Undergraduate education.

36. The nurse determines that a patient's pain score is 8 on a scale of 0 to 10 (where 10 is the highest level of pain). The nurse administers pain medication to the patient. Based on this scenario, which parts of the nursing process did the nurse use?

1. Assessment and intervention.
2. Planning and evaluation.
3. Evaluation and analysis.
4. Intervention and evaluation.

37. Which statement gives an example of intrapersonal conflict?

1. Nurses on the day shift contend that nurses on the night shift should be responsible for daily weights, but nurses on the night shift argue that nurses on the day shift should do it, so they don't have to wake the patients so early.
2. Some members of the unit staff want 8-hour shifts, but others want 12-hour shifts.
3. Nurse Jones is torn between going to a professional meeting or attending the last night of a play.
4. Nurse Lee is professionally threatened by Nurse Doe, the new clinical nurse specialist, and refutes everything Nurse Doe says.

38. Which nursing action would contribute to the cost of care for a patient?

1. Delaying discharge from an inpatient care unit for 1 hour until the patient's transportation becomes available.
2. Encouraging a postoperative patient to turn, cough, and deep breathe every 2 hours.

3. Opening a dressing change kit to obtain a single sterile gauze.
4. Encouraging an elderly patient to obtain an annual flu vaccine.

39. A patient is newly diagnosed with type 1 diabetes. What would the nurse expect the most common disease management plan to include?

1. Oral hypoglycemic agents, dietary counseling, and an exercise plan.
2. Insulin replacement, nutrition management, and self-monitoring of blood glucose.
3. Insulin replacement, oral hypoglycemic agents, and a 1,200-calorie diet.
4. Pancreatic transplant, implantation of an insulin pump, and monitoring of glycated hemoglobin (HbA_{1c}).

40. Which patient would benefit most from a nurse advocate?

1. A patient who has previously undergone a procedure that is about to be performed for a second time.
2. A patient who has been educated on treatment options and chooses alternative treatments.
3. A cancer patient who makes an informed decision not to participate in chemotherapy treatment.
4. A geriatric patient with no family members who is uncertain about a decision of whether to have a gastrostomy tube inserted.

41. The nurse is looking for evidence on a practice-based question. Which tool would the nurse use to obtain the highest level of evidence?

1. Randomized controlled trial research study.
2. Descriptive research study.
3. Quasi-experimental study.
4. Case study.

42. The nurse has made a decision to resign from a staff nurse position because of dissatisfaction with the present working conditions. Which action should the nurse take first?

1. Write a letter of resignation.
2. Review the organizational policies for resignation.
3. Notify the charge nurse that the nurse has accepted another position and is leaving.
4. Constructively share concerns about the working environment in an exit interview.

43. A charge nurse hears a physician say to the staff nurse in a loud voice, "You are incompetent. You were expected to have everything ready for the procedure when I arrived on the unit." Which action should the charge nurse take?

1. Change the staff nurse's assignment.
2. Discuss appropriate alternative responses to the situation with the staff nurse.
3. Report the staff nurse to the nursing supervisor.
4. Discuss the inappropriate behavior with the physician.

44. A 42-year-old patient who is scheduled to have an elective surgical procedure tells the nurse that she wants to be designated as a "do not resuscitate" (DNR) case. Which response would be appropriate for the nurse to give?

1. "You're having a simple procedure. You need to discuss this issue with your anesthesiologist."
2. "There can be complications with any type of surgery but the surgery you are having is minor."
3. "I'll ask your family and the hospital lawyer to speak with you about this decision."
4. "Explain to me what you think DNR means."

SAFETY AND INFECTION CONTROL

Matching

Match the toxic or overdosed substance with the antidote that would be used to treat it.

45. Morphine overdose

46. Insulin-induced hypoglycemia

47. Acetaminophen overdose

48. Benzodiazepine overdose

1. Acetylcysteine (Mucomyst)
2. Naloxone (Narcan)
3. Glucagon
4. Flumazenil (Romazicon)

Multiple Choice

49. Which hand hygiene practice would be inappropriate for a nurse to use?

1. Use an alcohol-based hand rub when the hands are visibly soiled with body fluids.
2. Decontaminate the hands before inserting invasive devices.
3. Wash the hands with soap and water for a minimum of 15 seconds, using a vigorous rub.

4. Apply an alcohol-based hand rub after removing nonsterile gloves.

50. A four-tier triage system is used to test an organization's disaster preparedness. A 22-year-old patient with hemorrhagic shock from a punctured femoral artery presents to the triage nurse. What is the most appropriate triage classification?

1. Emergent.
2. Expectant.
3. Delayed.
4. Urgent.

51. The nurse has administered an intramuscular injection to a patient with hepatitis C. What is the safest action by the nurse to prevent transmission of the disease?

1. Recap the needle and dispose of it in a puncture-resistant container.
2. Place the cap on a table and then slide the needle into the cap.
3. Ask the patient to recap the needle before disposing of it in a sharps container.
4. Place the uncapped needle in a puncture-resistant container.

52. What is the method of choice for the removal of ingested poisons from the gastrointestinal tract?

1. Irrigation and gastric lavage.
2. Ingestion of syrup of ipecac.
3. Administration of osmotic diarrheal agents.
4. Administration of activated charcoal.

53. A patient is started on a continuous enteral feeding, using an open system. The feeding bag and formula are hung at 8 A.M. on Monday. To minimize bacterial growth, when should the feeding bag be changed?

1. 4 P.M. on Monday.
2. 8 A.M. on Tuesday.
3. 8 P.M. on Tuesday.
4. 8 A.M. on Wednesday.

54. Which statement depicts an inappropriate technique for the assessment of a blood pressure in an upper extremity using a sphygmomanometer?

1. Wrap the blood pressure cuff as smoothly and snugly as possible around the arm.
2. Place the patient in a standing position with the arm above the level of the heart.
3. Check the instrument gauge to make sure that the reading starts at zero.

4. Center the cuff bladder over the brachial artery, above the inner aspect of the elbow.

55. Which situation in a healthcare organization might exacerbate the potential for workplace violence?

1. Comfortable waiting areas that prevent overcrowding.
2. Well-lit facility corridors and access areas.
3. A response time standard of 2 to 5 minutes by hospital security staff.
4. Unrestricted movement of the public in and out of the facility.

56. A patient is diagnosed with genital herpes caused by infection with herpes simplex virus type 2. Which statement about sexual activity and disease transmission is incorrect?

1. Once his or her symptoms have resolved, the patient is no longer able to transmit the disease.
2. Transmission of the disease can occur both when symptoms are present and when they are absent.
3. The use of condoms will reduce the risk of viral transmission.
4. Valacyclovir (Valtrex) reduces, but does not eliminate, the risk of viral transmission.

57. One room is available that will accommodate a patient who needs airborne precautions. Which patient should be assigned to the room?

1. A patient with Guillain Barré syndrome who is on a ventilator.
2. A patient with community pneumonia who is having copious respiratory secretions.
3. A patient with a tracheostomy who has bronchitis.
4. A patient with an undetermined cause of pneumonia who has AIDS.

58. Which intervention would be most appropriate to use for an adult patient who is at risk for the development of ventilator-associated pneumonia?

1. Elevate the head of the bed by 30 to 45 degrees.
2. Change the ventilator circuits daily.
3. Turn the patient from side to side every 4 hours.
4. Administer prophylactic antibiotics.

59. To prevent medication errors, what is the safest way to write an order for a medication to be administered every day?

1. q.d.
2. daily
3. q. day
4. every d.

60. When transcribing medical orders, the nurse is unable to read a written order. What is the best action by the nurse?

1. Clarify the type of medication with the family.
2. Interpret the order based on the patient's history.
3. Ask the pharmacist for clarification.
4. Contact the prescriber to clarify the written order.

61. Which use of antibiotics would help to delay the emergence of antibiotic resistance?

1. Antibiotics are prescribed only when a viral infection is present.
2. Broad-spectrum antibiotics are used whenever possible.
3. Antibiotic dosages below the minimum inhibitory concentration are prescribed.
4. A specific pathogen is targeted with an antibiotic that is active against that organism.

62. Which individual is at highest risk for exposure to human immunodeficiency virus (HIV)?

1. A counselor who works with the families of HIV-infected patients.
2. A personal trainer who works with HIV-infected patients.
3. A phlebotomist who collects blood in a mobile donor unit.
4. A lab technician who collects saliva for ELISA testing for insurance companies.

63. The monophasic defibrillators in the cardiac catheterization lab have recently been replaced with biphasic defibrillators. Which statement about the operation of a biphasic defibrillator is true?

1. The nurse should expect to use more joules of energy when defibrillating a patient with a biphasic defibrillator.
2. The success rate for defibrillation with biphasic defibrillators is lower than that with monophasic defibrillators.

3. The recommended range for the termination of ventricular fibrillation with a biphasic defibrillator is 300 to 360 joules of energy.

4. The most effective initial shock for ventricular fibrillation using a biphasic defibrillator has not been determined.

64. Which equipment should the nurse have immediately available for a patient who is about to receive a neuromuscular blocking agent?

1. Bag valve mask device and oxygen.

2. Defibrillator and pacemaker.

3. Chest tube insertion equipment and drainage unit.

4. Central venous catheterization equipment and IV fluids.

65. Which action would be contraindicated for a patient on seizure precautions for tonic-clonic seizures?

1. Encourage the patient to perform his or her own personal hygiene.

2. Allow the patient to be ambulatory.

3. Assess the patient's oral temperature with a glass thermometer.

4. Give the patient only plastic eating utensils.

66. During the administration of an oral medication, an alert elderly patient states, "The pill I always take is green. I don't take an orange pill." What is the best response by the nurse?

1. "Sometimes the same pill comes in a different color."

2. "Let me explain the purpose of the medication."

3. "I will check your medication orders again."

4. "This is the medication that your doctor wants you to take."

HEALTH PROMOTION AND MAINTENANCE

Multiple Choice

67. Which statement about health literacy is incorrect?

1. If a patient is literate, he or she is also health literate.

2. A lack of health literacy can create barriers to achieving desired health outcomes.

3. Difficulty in understanding and using health information is a common problem in the United States.

4. One intervention for the problem of health literacy is to increase healthcare providers' awareness of this problem.

68. The nurse is providing discharge teaching to a patient who has been diagnosed with a latex allergy. What should the nurse instruct the patient to avoid?

1. Applying elastic bandages.

2. Ingesting leafy green vegetables.

3. Using cotton-tipped applicators.

4. Putting on Nitrile gloves.

Identification

69. Identify, in the proper sequence, the components of the abdominal physical examination.

_____ Inspection

_____ Auscultation

_____ Percussion

_____ Palpation

Multiple Choice

70. An increased number of cases of infection with West Nile virus have been noted in recent months. Which actions should be taken to prevent the transmission of the disease?

1. Encourage the use of mosquito repellant.

2. Exterminate the pigeon population in the area.

3. Increase pools of standing water around the home.

4. Check pets for ticks before bringing them into the home.

71. Which test would the nurse anticipate using to assess for a potential problem with cranial nerve II?

1. Use a Snellen chart to assess vision.

2. Touch a wisp of cotton to the cornea to assess for a corneal reflex.

3. Use substances with distinguishable scents to detect a problem with smell.

4. Ask the patient to drink from a glass of water to assess swallowing.

72. A nurse has multiple requests for an education program on prostate cancer screening. Which group should receive the presentation first, based on their level of risk?

1. Caucasian middle-class men.
2. African American men with a low socioeconomic status.
3. Asian men with a high socioeconomic status.
4. Hispanic men who are unemployed.

73. According to *Healthy People 2010,* which indicator will be used to measure the health of the people in the United States from the beginning of the twenty-first century until 2010? (Select all that apply.)

1. Physical activity.
2. Overweight and obesity.
3. Tobacco use.
4. Access to health care.
5. Responsible sexual behavior.
6. Environmental quality.

74. A patient is experiencing sleep disturbances and has established a goal of decreased caffeine consumption. Which beverage selection would be the best choice to help the patient meet this goal?

1. Lemon-lime soda.
2. Brewed iced tea.
3. Diet cola.
4. Chocolate milk.

75. A patient is allergic to dust mites. Which action would be appropriate for the nurse to include in patient/family education geared toward reducing the patient's exposure to the allergen?

1. Encase pillows and mattresses with covers.
2. Replace wooden or tiled floors with carpet.
3. Increase the room humidity to greater than 60%.
4. Wash bedding in cool water (70 to 80°F) on a weekly basis.

76. The nurse is teaching a patient with end-stage renal disease about diet. The patient expresses concern and frustration about compliance with the diet. Which action should the nurse take first?

1. Tell the patient that dietary compliance is essential.
2. Continue with the patient's dietary education.
3. Identify the cause of the patient's concern and frustration.
4. Direct the education to the patient's family members.

77. A nurse is providing discharge instructions for a patient who has undergone outpatient cataract surgery with insertion of an intraocular lens. Which instruction would the nurse want to provide the patient to promote self-care after discharge? (Select all that apply.)

1. Avoid pulling, pushing, or lifting objects that weigh more than 10 to 15 pounds.
2. Wear a protective shield on the affected eye as instructed by the physician.
3. Irrigate the eye with saline every 4 hours for 48 hours.
4. When sleeping on the first postoperative night, lie on the side the affected eye is on.
5. Avoid tub baths or showers for 5 days after the surgery.
6. Contact the physician for pain unrelieved by the prescribed analgesics.

78. The nurse is obtaining a health history on a patient. Which reported information would indicate a risk factor for hepatitis C?

1. Eating raw shellfish.
2. Intravenous drug abuse.
3. Employment in a child care center.
4. Recent travel to a developing country.

79. Which statement about upper body obesity is true?

1. It is also described as female obesity.
2. Patients with upper body obesity are at a higher risk of developing health problems.
3. Upper body obesity is associated with a lower incidence of complications than is lower body obesity.
4. This type of obesity is described as a "pear shape."

80. Which patient is at greatest risk for the development of an obesity-related disease?

1. A female with a body mass index of 24 and a waist circumference of 30 inches.
2. A male with a body mass index of 29 and a waist circumference of 38 inches.
3. A female with a body mass index of 32 and a waist circumference of 40 inches.
4. A male with a body mass index of 33 and a waist circumference of 42 inches.

81. During a routine gynecological exam, a Papanicolaou (Pap) test is completed and abnormal cells are identified. What type of community-based preventive care is a Pap test?

1. Primary.
2. Secondary.
3. Tertiary.
4. Quaternary.

82. Which person is a candidate for the meningococcal conjugate vaccine (Menactra)?

1. A 7-year-old child who attends day care before and after school.
2. An 18-year-old youth who lives in a college dormitory.
3. A 78-year-old person who lives in an assisted living home.
4. A 65-year-old person who volunteers at an elementary school.

Identification

83. The nurse is completing a physical exam and is assessing the liver. Identify the area of the abdomen where the nurse would palpate for the liver.

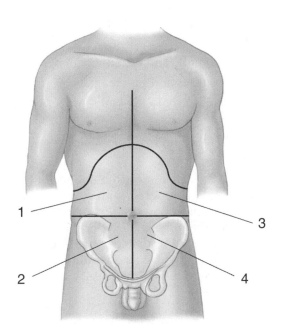

Multiple Choice

84. The nurse is developing a patient teaching brochure on testicular cancer. Which information would be most appropriate to include in the brochure?

1. The testicular exam is performed weekly at any time of the day.
2. It is unnecessary to palpate the epididymis when performing the exam.
3. A normal testicle should be smooth and uniform in consistency.
4. The exam should be completed biannually, using the heel of one hand.

85. Which statement best describes a health promotion activity that a nurse would implement?

1. Teach a patient with an extremity fracture to use crutches.
2. Volunteer time serving meals at a neighborhood soup kitchen.
3. Present a class to fifth-graders on the risks of tobacco use.
4. Refer a patient with a 20-year history of smoking to smoking cessation resources.

86. The nurse has conducted a health promotion class on sun protection. Which response by participants in the class demonstrates that the nurse provided effective teaching about the use of sunscreen?

1. Sunscreen does not need to be applied on a cloudy day.
2. Application of a sunscreen should occur 30 minutes to 2 hours before sun exposure.
3. A sunscreen with a minimum sun protection factor (SPF) of 10 should be chosen.
4. There is no need to reapply sunscreen after swimming or profuse sweating when a water-resistant product is used.

PSYCHOSOCIAL INTEGRITY

Matching

Match the eating disorder with the correct description of the disease.

87. An excessive concern over gaining weight and a refusal to maintain a minimally normal body weight.

1. Anorexia nervosa.
2. Bulimia nervosa.

88. Binge eating followed by self-induced vomiting, excessive exercise, or fasting, plus extreme concern over body shape and size.

Identification

Identify which of each pair of patients is more likely to adapt to the identified stressor.

89. A respiratory infection:

1. Patient A, who is 75 years old and has multisystem trauma.
2. Patient B, who is 20 years old and has multisystem trauma.

90. A diagnosis of liver cancer:

1. Patient A, who has a supportive family.
2. Patient B, who is homeless.

Multiple Choice

91. The nurse is caring for a patient who is confused in association with a neurological disorder. Which approach by the nurse would be most helpful for the patient?

1. Provide detailed explanations of medical procedures.
2. Increase environmental stimuli by turning on the television.
3. Keep familiar items at the bedside such as pictures.
4. Medicate the patient with an antipsychotic as needed.

92. A failed resuscitation attempt occurred for a patient whom a new nurse had frequently cared for. This was the first time a nurse had been involved in a resuscitation. The nurse confides to a colleague that she cannot stop thinking about the resuscitation and was unable to sleep last night. Which statement would be most therapeutic for the colleague to make?

1. "Why don't we take some time to talk about what happened?"
2. "Maybe you had better schedule an appointment with a psychiatrist."

3. "It's hard at first but you will get used to these things."
4. "Don't worry. We all go through these feelings; they will pass."

93. An intervention is scheduled for a nurse who is abusing alcohol. Which coping mechanism are the people involved in the intervention most likely to observe the nurse using?

1. Projection.
2. Rationalization.
3. Repression.
4. Denial.

94. A mental health nurse has been counseling a victim of spousal, physical violence for 1 week since the patient's discharge from an acute care facility. Which short-term outcome is the most appropriate goal for this patient?

1. Resolution of fears related to the incident.
2. Participation in the treatment plan.
3. Confrontation and incorporation of the abuser into the treatment plan.
4. Effective implementation of new coping skills.

95. The nurse is caring for a patient with presbycusis. Which intervention would be most appropriate for the nurse to use when caring for this patient?

1. Speak loudly and into the patient's good ear.
2. Use pictures and sign language.
3. Speak directly to the patient in a normal, clear voice.
4. Face the patient directly and speak very slowly.

96. A patient with chronic mental health problems has been making progress with treatment. During the most recent visit to the clinic, however, the patient tells the nurse he lost his job and feels useless because he is unable to provide for the family. Which nursing diagnosis would be most appropriate for this patient?

1. Anxiety.
2. Situational low self-esteem.
3. Social isolation.
4. Caregiver role strain.

97. Which statement by a patient would indicate that the patient is adapting well to changes in functional status after experiencing a spinal cord injury?

1. "My wife tries to get me to go to the grocery store, but I don't like to go out much."

2. "I have been using the modified feeding utensils at every meal. I still have spills, but I'm getting better."

3. "I tire easily when I use my wheelchair just around the house. I know I would get tired if I tried to leave the house."

4. "I have all the equipment to take a shower, but I prefer a bed bath, because it is easier."

98. At which developmental stage would the nurse expect to identify the clinical manifestations of autism?

1. Neonate.
2. Toddler.
3. Middle age.
4. Geriatric.

99. The psychiatric mental health nurse has referred a patient with an alcohol addiction to a 12-step Alcoholics Anonymous program. What is the first step of the 12-step program?

1. Admission that a drinking problem exists.
2. Detoxification from the addictive substance.
3. Identification of stimuli that promote drinking.
4. Inclusion of the family in counseling sessions.

100. A patient is diagnosed with attention-deficit hyperactivity disorder. What are the most common clinical manifestations of this disorder?

1. Avoidance, generalized emotional numbing, and withdrawal.
2. Periods of abnormally elevated moods, hyperactivity, and insomnia.
3. Difficulty concentrating, excessive anxiety, and inattention.
4. Inattention, hyperactivity, and impulsivity.

101. Which statement by a nurse in response to a patient would be an example of a reflective question or comment?

1. "You've been upset about your blood pressure."
2. "What time do you take your medication?"
3. "How do you feel when you take the medication?"
4. "Tell me what occurred first—did your symptoms occur before or after you took the medication?"

102. The nurse is providing smoking cessation information to a patient. Which statement by the patient would indicate a need for further education?

1. "Now that I have made the decision to quit smoking, I plan to go to the bar where I always used to smoke to see if I am strong enough to quit."
2. "I will distract myself by working on my woodworking hobby."
3. "I will call someone I know who has quit if I develop the urge to have a cigarette."
4. "I will keep a log of slips and near-slips to see what I can learn about my smoking habit and things that trigger the habit."

103. Which situation provides an example of a chronic, intermittent stressor?

1. A 68-year-old patient who is diagnosed with viral pneumonia.
2. A 22-year-old patient with type 1 diabetes.
3. A 59-year-old patient who is diagnosed with Stage II Alzheimer's disease.
4. A 40-year-old patient with genital herpes.

104. In which situation is the patient most likely to experience anticipatory grieving?

1. A patient finds out that her symptoms were from an ectopic pregnancy.
2. The patient experiences traumatic amputation of an extremity in an industrial accident.
3. A patient is brought into the Emergency Room and declared brain dead.
4. After diagnostic testing, a patient is diagnosed with metastatic liver cancer.

105. A patient was rescued from an apartment building a week after Hurricane Katrina. The patient's elderly mother died during the disaster. One year after the event, the patient presents to the outpatient mental health clinic with nightmares about being in the hurricane, feelings of survivor guilt, and increased difficulty concentrating. Which problem are the patient's symptoms clearly an example of?

1. Generalized anxiety disorder.
2. Post-traumatic stress syndrome.
3. Acute stress disorder.
4. Dissociative identity syndrome.

SECTION I
SECTION II
SECTION III
SECTION IV
SECTION V
SECTION VI
SECTION VII
SECTION VIII
SECTION IX
SECTION X

106. A 25-year-old woman is a victim of domestic violence. Which problem related to self-concept is she most likely to be at risk for?

1. Personal identity disturbance.
2. Body image disturbance.
3. Altered role performance.
4. Self-esteem disturbance.

BASIC CARE AND COMFORT

Matching

Match the herbal supplement on the left with its purported use on the right.

107. Saw palmetto (*Serenoa repens*).

108. Ginkgo (*Ginkgo biloba*).

109. St. John's wort (*Hypericum perforatum*).

110. Black cohosh (*Cimicifuga racemosa*).

1. Used to relieve depression.
2. Used to relieve symptoms associated with benign prostatic hypertrophy.
3. Used to improve memory, sharpen concentration, and promote clear thinking.
4. Used to relieve symptoms of menopause.

Multiple Choice

111. A nursing diagnosis of the potential for altered skin integrity is identified for a patient with ulcerative colitis who is experiencing frequent diarrheal stools. Which patient action would help prevent perianal breakdown?

1. A sitz bath is used for 20 minutes after each stool.
2. A soap suds enema is given to clear the colon of fecal matter.
3. The perianal area is cleansed using an antimicrobial scrub, rinsed, and dried.
4. The perianal area is cleansed with mild soap and water and dried.

112. The nurse is caring for a hospitalized patient who has a urine output of 250 cc in a 24-hour period. Which term would the nurse use when analyzing and documenting the patient's urine output?

1. Enuresis.
2. Anuria.
3. Azotemia.
4. Oliguria.

113. Which item is inappropriate for a patient whose dietary prescription is for clear liquids?

1. Ice cream.
2. Popsicle.
3. Gelatin.
4. Broth.

114. A patient is receiving enteral feedings via a gastrostomy tube. What is the priority nursing diagnosis for this patient?

1. Risk for constipation.
2. Impaired gas exchange.
3. Body image disturbance.
4. Risk for aspiration.

115. A patient has dysphagia. Which nursing action is most appropriate for this patient?

1. Monitor intake and output, and encourage fluid intake.
2. Elevate the head of the bed, and observe for signs of aspiration.
3. Ensure an emesis basin is available, and plan to administer an antiemetic if needed.
4. Prepare for the insertion of subclavian venous catheter for parenteral nutrition.

116. A patient with chronic renal failure who is on hemodialysis is placed on a low-protein diet. The patient asks, "Why do I have to be concerned with protein?" What is the best response by the nurse about the purpose of this diet?

1. Waste products, like urea, build up as a result of protein breakdown, and the kidneys are not able to rid the body of the wastes.
2. Because the kidneys have failed, a smaller amount of protein is needed to produce essential amino acids.
3. In the presence of renal disease, a normal amount of protein intake will cause hyperkalemia when the protein is broken down by the body.
4. A low-protein diet will cause hypoalbuminemia, which can increase colloid osmotic pressure and prevent fluid overload.

117. A patient has daily weights ordered. Which action should be avoided to ensure an accurate weight?

1. The same scale should be used.

2. The scale should be balanced at zero.

3. The patient's weight should be taken at different times each day.

4. The patient should wear the same clothing during each measurement.

118. The healthcare provider orders that the patient's temperature be taken every 4 hours. When the nurse attempts to obtain the patient's oral temperature, the patient informs the nurse that he has just had some ice chips. What is the most appropriate nursing action?

1. Wait 15 minutes and return to take the oral temperature.

2. Provide a sip of warm water, wait 5 minutes, and take the temperature.

3. Document that a temperature was unable to be obtained.

4. Proceed to take the oral temperature.

119. A patient is confused and has pulled out a peripheral IV catheter. Which alternative therapy might the nurse consider prior to using restraints?

1. Obtain an order for sedation.

2. Place mittens on the patient's hands.

3. Involve family members in reorienting the patient.

4. Apply additional tape to IV sites.

120. What is the best method for the assessment of fluid volume increases?

1. Daily weight.

2. Serum sodium.

3. Tissue turgor.

4. Intake and output.

121. What is the most appropriate site at which to assess a patient for central cyanosis?

1. Oral mucosa.

2. Nail beds.

3. Earlobes.

4. Eyelids.

122. What is the most appropriate site for a nurse to assess for jaundice on a dark-skinned patient?

1. Palms of the hands.

2. Around the mouth.

3. Sclera.

4. Trunk.

123. Which patient is most likely to receive total parenteral nutrition?

1. A patient with acute gastritis.

2. A patient with a complete bowel obstruction.

3. A patient who has been vomiting for the past hour.

4. A patient who has undergone a cholecystectomy.

124. The nurse is monitoring a postoperative patient who weighs 60 kilograms. What hourly urine output rate should the nurse report?

1. 20 mL/h

2. 60 mL/h

3. 100 mL/h

4. 140 mL/h

125. The nurse is discussing the side effects of an alkylating chemotherapy medication, cyclophosphamide (Cytoxan). The patient asks about hair loss associated with the medication. Which statement is accurate and should be included in the discussion?

1. "Most individuals do not lose their hair after taking the medication."

2. "Hair loss is common, including your eyebrows and eyelashes."

3. "Most patients get fitted for a wig, because the hair loss will be permanent."

4. "Individuals lose their hair, but it usually grows back nice and thick."

126. The nurse is preparing to insert an indwelling urinary catheter in a female patient who is being prepared for an operative procedure. Which statement about catheter insertion is true?

1. Clean technique should always be used for the insertion procedure.

2. The catheter balloon should be inflated with 20 cc of sterile water.

3. Advance the catheter 2 to 3 inches into the urinary meatus.

4. Lubrication of the catheter tip prior to its insertion can result in urinary tract infections.

PHARMACOLOGICAL AND PARENTERAL THERAPIES

Matching

A client with advanced cirrhosis of the liver has developed the complications of ascites, esophageal varices, and hepatic encephalopathy. Medications prescribed for the condition include: famotidine, lactulose, propranolol and spironolactone. Match the intervention on the left with the rationale for use on the right.

127. Albumin.

128. Lactulose (Cephulac).

129. Propanolol (Inderal).

130. Spironolactone (Aldactone).

1. Decreases portal venous pressure and reduces the risk of variceal bleeding.

2. Increases plasma colloid osmotic pressure and promotes the maintenance of intravascular volume.

3. Decreases the formation of ammonia by enhancing intestinal excretion of ammonia.

4. Blocks the action of aldosterone and increases the excretion of sodium to reduce edema.

Multiple Choice

131. Which statements about the use of drotrecogin alpha activated (Xigris) for the treatment of severe sepsis is correct?

1. The effectiveness of the drug has been established for pediatric, adult, and geriatric populations.

2. The drug acts by inhibiting protein synthesis in gram-negative microorganisms.

3. Bleeding is the most common adverse effect of the drug.

4. A daily dose of the medication is administered intravenously for a period of 10 days.

132. The school nurse is teaching a class that warns against the use of anabolic steroids to enhance athletic performance for high school athletes. Which statement by the nurse should be a focus of the presentation?

1. There is no athletic enhancement benefit for females from anabolic steroids.

2. Use of these prescription drugs for athletic enhancement is illegal.

3. Luteinizing hormone (LH) is the primary endogenous androgen found in anabolic steroids.

4. Anabolic steroids bring a decreased risk for the development of atherosclerosis caused by the lowering of LDL cholesterol and the elevation of HDL cholesterol.

133. A patient is seen in the clinic with an acute asthma exacerbation. Which medication should cause a reduction in the symptoms?

1. Cromolyn (Intal) via metered-dose inhaler.

2. Oral montelukast (Singular).

3. Budesonide (Pulmicort) via dry-powder inhaler.

4. Albuterol (Proventil) via jet nebulizer.

Identification

134. For which cardiac rhythm would it be appropriate for the nurse to administer vasopressin?

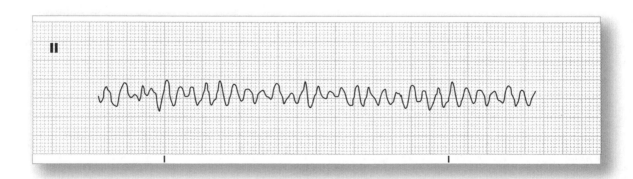

1.

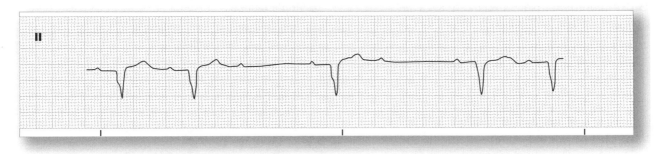

2.

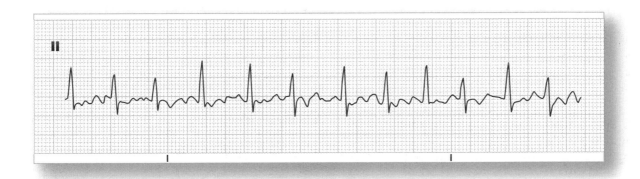

3.

Multiple Choice

135. Which drug used in the treatment of obesity acts by decreasing the absorption of dietary fat in the gastrointestinal tract?

1. Bupropion (Wellbutrin).
2. Sibutramine (Meridia).
3. Orlistat (Xenical).
4. Rimonabant (Acomplia).

136. The nurse is reading the drug insert for Humolog insulin. The insert states that the drug is produced by recombinant DNA technology. Which description applies to this technology?

1. Technology that inserts a chromosome into unicellular bacteria to produce endogenous substances.
2. Inoculation of genetic vehicles to stimulate stem cells to produce hormones and enzymes.
3. Genetic engineering that involves recombining genes into hybrid molecules that are then duplicated.

4. Reproduction of genetic maps to identify a hormone site in the body and stimulate substance production.

137. Which statement about the use of botulinum toxin Type A (Botox or Botox Cosmetic) is incorrect?

1. The botulinum toxin is a potent poison produced by the bacterium *Clostridium botulinum.*
2. Botox Cosmetic permanently eliminates glabellar lines.
3. Botulinum toxin type A is a neurotoxin that blocks the release of acetylcholine and blocks transmission at the neuromuscular junctions and cholinergic synapses.
4. Botox is approved for use in the ocular conditions strabismus (lazy eye) and blepharospasm (involuntary, intermittent forced closure of the eyelid).

SECTION
I

SECTION
II

SECTION
III

SECTION
IV

SECTION
V

SECTION
VI

SECTION
VII

SECTION
VIII

SECTION
IX

SECTION
X

138. Which patients is most likely to develop an iatrogenic effect of drug therapy?

1. A patient in the third trimester of pregnancy.
2. An elderly patient with a genetic defect of liver metabolism.
3. A patient taking an antipsychotic who develops pseudoParkinson's symptoms.
4. An adult patient who is being treated for cancer with chemotherapy.

139. Identify the anticancer drug that acts to suppress the formation of new blood vessels and deprive solid tumors of the blood supply needed for growth.

1. Trastuzumab (Herceptin).
2. Bevacizumab (Avastin).
3. Interferon alfa-2A (Roferon-A).
4. Tamoxifen (Nolvadex).

140. Which scheduled drug level indicates that the drug has accepted medical application and the least potential for abuse under the Controlled Substances Act?

1. Schedule 2.
2. Schedule 3.
3. Schedule 4.
4. Schedule 5.

Identification

141. A capillary blood glucose value of 205 mg/dL is obtained. The prescribed sliding scale insulin protocol reads:

> Blood glucose 120–150: Administer 2 units of regular insulin subcutaneously.
>
> Blood glucose 151–200: Administer 3 units of regular insulin subcutaneously.
>
> Blood glucose 201–250: Administer 4 units of regular insulin subcutaneously.
>
> Blood glucose 251–300: Administer 5 units of regular insulin subcutaneously.

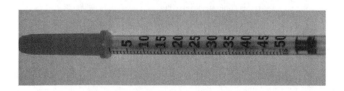

Indicate on the syringe the correct dosage of insulin you would administer.

Multiple Choice

142. Which statement about the administration of the smallpox vaccination is true?

1. The vaccination is given in the upper thigh.
2. The vaccine is introduced through multiple skin punctures.
3. Intramuscular injection is the route of administration.
4. A 22-gauge 5/8 needle should be used for administration of the vaccine.

143. Morphine sulfate 6 mg IV push is administered to a patient with postoperative pain. The patient is assessed 15 minutes after the morphine is administered. Which assessment finding represents an adverse effect of morphine administration?

1. Sleeping, but arouses when name is called.
2. Respiratory rate of 7 breaths/min.
3. Numerical scale pain report indicating that the pain level decreases from 6 to 4.
4. Pulse oximeter reading of SaO_2 equal to 96%.

144. The nurse is preparing to infuse nesiritide (Natrecor). What is the expected action of this medication?

1. Increase myocardial contractility.
2. Decrease preload.
3. Increase intravascular volume.
4. Promote vasodilation.

145. The nurse is caring for a patient with a history of chronic alcoholism. Based on the patient's history, which pharmacokinetic process will most likely be affected?

1. Excretion.
2. Absorption.
3. Metabolism.
4. Distribution.

146. A patient experiences anaphylactic shock in response to the administration of penicillin. Which medication would the nurse anticipate administering first?

1. Dobutamine.
2. Corticosteroids.
3. Furosemide.
4. Epinephrine.

147. A patient who underwent a kidney transplant is prescribed the medication Cyclosporine (Sandimmune). Identify how the immunosuppressant therapy works to prevent organ rejection.

1. Suppresses B- and T-cell proliferation by inhibiting DNA synthesis.
2. Inhibits antigen replication by suppressing RNA synthesis.
3. Selective inhibitor of B- and T-cell proliferation.
4. Inhibits production of interleukin-2.

Identification

148. Levothyroxine 0.1 milligram (mg) is ordered daily. The pharmacy sends 50 microgram (mcg) tablets. How many tablets will the nurse administer? _____

Multiple Choice

149. A patient with primary hypothyroidism is prescribed levothyroxine (Synthroid). Which statement should be included in the patient education?

1. "You will need to take this medication until your symptoms are gone. Then your dose will be tapered off and discontinued."
2. "Symptoms such as tremors, nervousness, and insomnia may indicate your dose is too high."
3. "You should begin to see your symptoms improve immediately after starting your medication."
4. "The reason for taking the drug is because the thyroid gland produces too much thyroxine."

150. Which use of estrogen hormone replacement therapy is no longer recommended?

1. Protection against cardiovascular disease.
2. Treatment of severe vasomotor symptoms of menopause.
3. Prevention of urogenital atrophy.
4. In combination with progestin for contraception.

151. The nurse is planning an in-service educational program on sildenafil (Viagra). Which statement should the nurse include in the in-service program?

1. The drug should be taken with grapefruit juice to promote its absorption.
2. Patients taking nitrates should not take sildenafil (Viagra).

3. Severe hypertension can be an adverse effect of the drug.
4. The medication has also been approved for use in women.

152. Vancomycin (Vancocin), linezolid (Zyvox), and dalfopristin/quinupristin (Synercid) are all antibiotics indicated for the treatment of infections caused by what organism?

1. *Pseudomonas aeruginosa.*
2. *Klebsiella.*
3. *Candida.*
4. Methicillin-resistant *Staphylococcus aureus.*

153. Identify the statement that correctly describes the action of a drug agonist.

1. The activation of the receptor site is blocked by the drug.
2. A partial drug effect is achieved due to a reduced action on the receptor site.
3. The drug competes with the body's chemicals at the receptor site and intensifies the response.
4. The drug binds with and activates the receptor site.

154. Oral hypoglycemic medications are recommended for patients who have which type of diabetes mellitus?

1. New-onset type 2 diabetes complicated by obesity and lack of activity.
2. New-onset type 1 diabetes in the honeymoon phase.
3. Gestational diabetes complicated by obesity.
4. Type 2 diabetes not controlled by dietary and activity modifications.

155. What is the purpose for administering donepezil (Aricept) to a patient with Alzheimer's disease?

1. To enhance transmission of cholinergic neurons in the central nervous system.
2. To decrease the transmission of gamma-aminobutyric acid (GABA) in the central nervous system.
3. To intensify the effects of dopamine at the neural junction.
4. To inhibit the influx of sodium into the neurons.

156. The nurse is reviewing a medication list for a patient with intrinsic (intra-renal) failure. Which medication should the nurse question because of the associated nephrotoxic adverse effects?

1. Vancomycin (Vancocin).
2. Amphotericin (Amphotec).
3. Erythropoietin (Epogen).
4. Furosemide (Lasix).

157. In which situation would the prophylactic use of antibiotics be inappropriate?

1. Fever of unknown origin in a patient with an intact immune system.
2. Neutropenia following cancer chemotherapy.
3. Following surgical debridement of an animal bite.
4. Emergency cesarean section.

158. What are the most common adverse effects from the use of inhaled glucocorticoids?

1. Elevation of blood sugar and potassium levels.
2. Hypertension and congestive heart failure.
3. Adrenocortical dysfunction and hyperglycemia.
4. Oropharyngeal candidiasis and dysphonia.

159. The nurse is caring for a single patient who was infected with aerosolized *Bacillus anthracis* (anthrax). What is the expected initial pharmacologic treatment for an infection with inhaled anthrax?

1. Intravenous ciprofloxacin (Cipro) or doxycycline (Vibramycin).
2. Oral fluconazole (Diflucan) or traconazole (Sporanox).
3. Intravenous tobramycin (Nebcin) or gentamycin (Garamycin).
4. Oral vancomycin (Vancocin) or dirithromycin (Dynabec).

REDUCTION OF RISK POTENTIAL

Multiple Choice

160. Which lab tests would most likely be used to aid in the diagnosis of metabolic syndrome X?

1. Liver function studies and bilirubin.
2. Fasting glucose and lipid profile.
3. Complete blood count (CBC) and blood urea nitrogen (BUN).
4. Basic metabolic profile and troponin I.

161. Which patient is at greatest risk for the development of teratogenic effects of drug therapy?

1. A patient in the first trimester of pregnancy.
2. An elderly patient with decreased renal function.
3. A neonate whose liver function is immature.
4. An adult patient who is being treated for cancer.

162. Which patient would be the most likely to receive continuous renal replacement therapy (CRRT)?

1. A 20-year-old, hemodynamically unstable, trauma patient in acute renal failure.
2. A 68-year-old patient with renal insufficiency and congestive heart failure.
3. A 45-year-old patient with post-renal failure.
4. A 39-year-old, hypertensive, diabetic patient with end-stage renal disease.

Identification

163. Which type of abnormal finding associated with the motor tracts of the spinal cord is depicted in the following illustration?

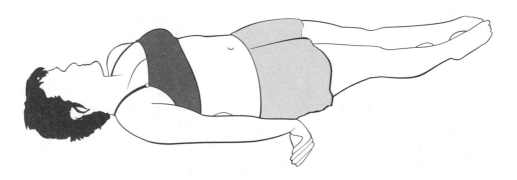

Multiple Choice

164. Which action will promote the best outcome for a patient who is experiencing pulseless electrical activity?

1. Initiation of CPR and rapid cardioversion.
2. Rapid defibrillation and administration of epinephrine.
3. Treatment of a potassium level of 7.0 mEq/dL with insulin and calcium.
4. Administration of sodium bicarbonate for a patient with a pH of 7.55.

165. A patient who is diagnosed with respiratory failure is intubated and being mechanically ventilated. The patient pulls out the endotracheal tube. What is the priority action for the nurse to take?

1. Administer oxygen via a 100% non-rebreather mask.
2. Ensure that the patient's airway is open.
3. Prepare for reintubation.
4. Provide nasotracheal suctioning.

166. A patient has a cerebral perfusion pressure (CPP) of 39. Based on the nurse's knowledge of cerebral perfusion pressures, which statement is true?

1. The increased pressure within the cerebral spinal fluid circulation could result in herniation.
2. According to the Monroe–Kellie hypothesis, the brain will accommodate for the elevated cerebral perfusion pressure.
3. Autoregulation of blood flow through the brain is maintained at a CPP of 39.
4. The pressure is too low, and the patient is experiencing impairment of cerebral perfusion.

167. Identify the person who would be at greatest risk for the development of an ischemic, embolic stroke?

1. A 44-year-old patient with uncontrolled hypertension.
2. A 68-year-old patient with chronic atrial fibrillation.
3. A 75-year-old patient with thrombocytopenia.
4. A 36-year-old patient with an arteriovenous malformation.

168. The nurse is caring for a patient with a serum potassium of 6.2 mEq/L. Which statement is true regarding appropriate treatment options for the patient?

1. An intravenous infusion of KCl is appropriate as long as the infusion rate doesn't exceed 10 mEq/h.
2. Intravenous calcium chloride is appropriate for the patient because it moves potassium out of the cells and into the extracellular fluid.
3. Dextrose and insulin are appropriate for the patient because they help the kidneys eliminate potassium from the body.
4. Sodium polystyrene sulfonate (Kayexalate) is appropriate for the patient because it is an exchange resin that can remove potassium from the body.

Identification

Based on the following Punnett square, which indicates that both parents are carriers of the autosomal recessive cystic fibrosis gene, answer the following questions.

Dad

		C	c
Mom	C	CC	Cc
	c	Cc	cc

C = dominant

c = recessive

169. What is the probability (percent chance) that a child will get the disease?

170. What is the probability (percent chance) that a child will be a carrier of the disease?

171. What is the probability (percent chance) that a child will not have the disease or be a carrier?

Multiple Choice

172. A patient who is diagnosed with anorexia nervosa experiences amenorrhea, decreased breast size, and a loss of pubic hair. What is the cause of these clinical manifestations?

1. Lack of dietary protein.

2. Decreasing estrogen levels.

3. Lack of calcium and phosphorus in the diet.

4. Increasing levels of progestin.

173. Which assessment parameters should the nurse consider as the most reliable indicator of the existence and intensity of acute pain?

1. Vital signs.

2. Self-report of pain.

3. Severity of the condition.

4. Nonverbal behavior.

174. Which person is at the highest risk for development of erectile dysfunction?

1. A 35-year-old CEO of a company with a huge debt.

2. A 40-year-old smoker who drinks socially.

3. A 60-year-old man with a 15-year history of uncontrolled diabetes.

4. A 55-year-old man with diet-controlled hypertension.

175. Upon physical examination of a patient who has been on prolonged bed rest, the nurse identifies that the patient has wasting of the muscles from disuse. Which term would be appropriate for the nurse to use to document the finding?

1. Atrophy.

2. Apraxia.

3. Hemiparesis.

4. Dyskinesia.

176. Upon inspection of the skin, the nurse identifies an area of injury that is reddened, but the skin is not torn. Which finding would the nurse document in the patient's record?

1. Hematoma.

2. Laceration.

3. Contusion.

4. Petechiae.

177. Which electrolyte and acid–base imbalances are associated with acute renal failure?

1. Hypokalemia, hyponatremia, and respiratory acidosis.

2. Hypermagnesemia, hypernatremia, and metabolic alkalosis.

3. Hyperkalemia, hypocalcemia, and metabolic acidosis.

4. Hyperphosphatemia, hypocalcemia, and respiratory alkalosis.

178. An adult patient has been diagnosed with type 2 diabetes and needs to begin daily medications and blood glucose monitoring. The patient's response was, "This is not possible. How can I have diabetes when I'm not sick?" What is the most appropriate response by the nurse?

1. "Type 2 diabetes has a latent period when blood glucose levels are very high but the body has not experienced enough deterioration to make you very ill."

2. "You are in denial, which is preventing you from experiencing many of the symptoms."

3. "Type 2 diabetes is often asymptomatic, and the best way to understand the body's actual response to managing glucose is to monitor your blood sugar at home for a period of time."

4. "Patients with newly diagnosed diabetes are very ill with nausea, vomiting, weight loss, and confusion, along with thirst and frequent urination. You should feel encouraged that you have few symptoms."

Calculation

179. Calculate the cerebral perfusion pressure for a patient with an intracranial pressure of 40 mm Hg and a blood pressure of 100/60 mm Hg.

180. Is the finding in Question 179 normal or abnormal?

Multiple Choice

181. A patient is receiving total parenteral nutrition (TPN). The nurse reviews the following lab values:

Glucose = 72 mg/dL

Chloride = 98 mEq/L

Sodium = 138 mEq/L

Potassium = 3.0 mEq/L

Based on the nurse's review of the lab values, which nursing action is appropriate?

1. Discontinue the TPN administration.

2. Notify the physician and discuss the need for potassium replacement.

3. Administer 50% dextrose immediately.

4. Assess the patient's vital signs and perform a physical assessment.

182. The nurse would observe a patient diagnosed with anorexia nervosa for which complication?

1. Heavy menstrual cycles.
2. Osteoporosis.
3. Enhanced sexual characteristics.
4. Heat intolerance.

183. A 57-year-old homeless man is being evaluated in a mobile clinic. He has recently immigrated to the United States from Southeast Asia. He presents with fatigue, anorexia, fever, night sweats, and cough. What is the most probable cause of his symptoms?

1. Tuberculosis.
2. Emphysema.
3. Pneumonia.
4. Pulmonary embolus.

184. The nurse is caring for a patient following a thyroidectomy. During the postoperative period, the nurse notes that the patient's serum calcium is low. For which signs and symptoms would it be most appropriate for the nurse to monitor the patient?

1. Muscle weakness and constipation.
2. Facial spasms and hyperreflexia.
3. Abdominal pain and nausea.
4. Anorexia, nausea, and vomiting.

185. The nurse is caring for a patient who has just been admitted to the hospital with severe dehydration over the past 72 hours. Which type of renal failure is this patient at risk for developing?

1. Pre-renal failure.
2. Intra-renal failure.
3. Post-renal failure.
4. Extrinsic renal failure.

186. The nurse is caring for a patient with end-stage renal disease. The patient has experienced weight gain, peripheral edema, hypertension, and jugular neck vein distention. Which finding best explains this patient's symptoms?

1. Hypovolemia.
2. Hypervolemia.
3. Hyperkalemia.
4. Hyponatremia.

Identification

187. The nurse is assessing a patient who experienced blunt head trauma; to do so, the nurse uses the Glasgow Coma Scale. The patient responds by opening his eyes when a noxious stimulus is applied and attempts to remove the offending stimulus. The patient is unable to identify the date or year and calls the nurse "Mom." What is the patient's score on the Glasgow Coma Scale?

_____

Test	Score
Eye Opening	
Spontaneous	4
To call	3
To pain	2
None	1
Motor Response	
Obeys commands	6
Localizes pain	5
Normal flexion (withdrawal)	4
Abnormal flexion (decortication)	3
Extension (decerebrate)	2
None (flaccid)	1
Verbal Response	
Oriented	5
Confused conversation	4
Inappropriate words	3
Incomprehensible sounds	2
None	1

FIGURE 6.8 The Glasgow Coma Scale

Multiple Choice

188. The diabetic nurse educator is teaching a patient who is newly diagnosed with diabetes about site rotation for insulin injections. What is the purpose of site rotation for subcutaneous insulin injections?

1. To decrease the risk for development of lipodystrophy.
2. To ensure that insulin is delivered to all areas of the body.
3. To reduce the risk of infection associated with injection.
4. To minimize the pain associated with insulin injections.

SECTION I
SECTION II
SECTION III
SECTION IV
SECTION V
SECTION VI
SECTION VII
SECTION VIII
SECTION IX
SECTION X

189. Which nursing intervention is appropriate for a patient with a platelet count of 34,000/μL?

1. Pad sharp surfaces to avoid trauma.
2. Assess for a decrease in petechiae.
3. Keep the room darkened.
4. Check for the presence of white blood cells in the urine.

190. The nurse is caring for a patient with thrombocytopenia. For which finding would it be most appropriate for the nurse to monitor the patient?

1. Jaundice.
2. Fatigue.
3. Ecchymosis.
4. Fever.

191. A patient is admitted with chronic obstructive pulmonary disease (COPD). The patient has dyspnea and a low PaO_2 level. The nurse plans to administer oxygen as ordered. Which statement is true concerning oxygen administration to a COPD patient?

1. Elevated oxygen concentrations will cause coughing.
2. High oxygen concentrations may inhibit the hypoxic stimulus for breathing.
3. Increased oxygen use will promote oxygen dependency.
4. Oxygen administration is contraindicated.

192. A postoperative patient is receiving the opioid morphine 2 mg IV every 2–4 hours prn for pain. Based on the nurse's knowledge of the effects of opioids on the gastrointestinal system, for which potential problem should the nurse monitor the patient?

1. Diarrhea.
2. Heartburn.
3. Flatulence.
4. Constipation.

PHYSIOLOGICAL ADAPTATION

Multiple Choice

193. A patient is hospitalized for an acute exacerbation of ulcerative colitis. The patient is experiencing 14 to 16 bloody stools per day as well as cramping and abdominal pain. The physician orders the patient to have nothing by mouth (NPO) on admission. What is the rationale for the NPO order?

1. To prevent nausea and vomiting.
2. To decrease abdominal distention.
3. To promote bowel rest and healing.
4. To prepare the patient for diagnostic testing.

194. Which intervention should the nurse anticipate implementing during the emergency care of a patient with diabetic ketoacidosis?

1. Administer NPH insulin by subcutaneous injection.
2. Administer regular insulin by intramuscular injection.
3. Administer regular insulin by the intravenous route.
4. Administer glargine insulin by inhalation.

195. A patient reports having clay-colored stools. What is the pathophysiologic basis for the finding?

1. Bile is not being broken down by the bacterial flora of the intestine.
2. There is a lack of bilirubin in the intestine to color the feces.
3. A decrease in the amount of cholecystokinin prevents the release of lipase.
4. There is too much bilirubin in the intestine, causing discoloration of stools.

196. A 21-year-old female patient is seen in the clinic with complaints of dyspnea, fatigue, and lightheadedness. She reports that her menstrual periods are heavy. Laboratory findings show a low hemoglobin, hematocrit, and red blood cell (RBC) count. The RBC smear revealed microcytic, hypochromic cells. With which type of anemia are these findings consistent?

1. Folic acid-deficiency anemia.
2. Vitamin B_{12} anemia.
3. Iron-deficiency anemia.
4. Acute blood loss.

197. A patient is admitted with a diagnosis of ruptured cerebral aneurysm. The condition is most often manifested by which patient finding?

1. "I was unable to speak for about 30 minutes."
2. "This is the worst headache I have ever had."
3. "I lost control of my bowels and bladder."
4. "I am unable to move my left side."

Fill in the Blank

198. Fill in the blanks of the statement with the appropriate terms regarding the pathophysiology of a patient who has Alzheimer's disease: Researchers have identified two microscopic changes, _____ and _____, that occur in the brain of a patient with Alzheimer's disease. These changes result in cortical atrophy.

> *Words*
>
> Neuritic plaques
>
> Neurofibrillary tangles
>
> Nerve demyelination
>
> Sclerotic plaques
>
> Dysplasia

Multiple Choice

199. Given four CD4 T-cell values for patients diagnosed with an HIV infection, identify the patient who is at greatest risk for the development of an opportunistic infection?

1. 100 cells/mm^3.
2. 400 cells/mm^3.
3. 800 cells/mm^3.
4. 1,200 cells/mm^3.

200. A meat cutter lacerates a finger. The healthcare provider sutures the wound closed. Wound healing will occur by which process?

1. Primary intention.
2. Secondary intention.
3. Granulation.
4. Proliferation.

201. Which skin disorder develops on sun-exposed areas, is seen in elderly patients, and would be considered a pre-malignant skin lesion?

1. Solar lentigines.
2. Actinic keratoses.
3. Nevocellular nevi.
4. Seborrheic keratoses.

202. Identify a clinical manifestation of the early or first stage of Alzheimer's disease?

1. Difficulty with problem solving.
2. Inability to recognize family or friends.
3. Short-term memory loss.
4. Wandering.

203. Which finding is characteristic of diabetes insipidus?

1. Delayed development.
2. Hyperglycemia.
3. Virilization of females.
4. Copious, dilute urine.

204. The nurse is assessing an adult male patient with no significant past medical history who was admitted to the Emergency Department. The assessment findings include a decrease in level of consciousness; rapid, shallow respirations; nasal flaring; sternal and intercostal retractions; and cyanosis around the lips and oral mucosa. The ABG reveals pH 7.24, pCO$_2$ 55, and PaO$_2$ 50. Which statement best describes these findings?

1. Acute respiratory distress with respiratory acidosis and hypoxemia.
2. Mild respiratory distress with acidosis and hypoxemia.
3. Acute respiratory distress with respiratory alkalosis and hypoxemia.
4. No distress; ABG is normal.

205. Upon assessment of a burn victim, the nurse finds reddened skin with mild edema. Thin-walled blisters are present, and the patient complains of pain. These assessment findings are indicative of which type of burn injury?

1. Superficial.
2. Superficial partial thickness.
3. Deep partial thickness.
4. Full thickness.

206. A patient has swelling in the ankles and feet associated with prolonged standing. Which physiologic description best explains the reason for the swelling?

1. Increased hydrostatic pressure.
2. Decreased osmotic pressure.
3. Increased capillary permeability.
4. Altered lymph channels.

207. The nurse is developing a case study about Graves' disease. When explaining the pathophysiology, what should be discussed as the cause of Graves' disease?

1. Hypersecretion of thyroid hormone.
2. Hyposecretion of thyroid hormone.
3. Hyposecretion of thyroid-stimulating hormone.
4. Hypersecretion of adrenocorticotrophic hormone (ACTH).

SECTION I

SECTION II

SECTION III

SECTION IV

SECTION V

SECTION VI

SECTION VII

SECTION VIII

SECTION IX

SECTION X

Identification

Identify whether the descriptions apply to hemodialysis or peritoneal dialysis.

208. Provides the most rapid clearance of waste products. _____

209. Requires extracorporeal circulation. _____

210. Provides for more independence, such as greater flexibility when traveling and increased mobility. _____

211. Requires inflow, dwell, and drain times. _____

Multiple Choice

212. Because of hypoxia, a patient's cells have converted to anaerobic metabolism. Which substance accumulates in the cells as a result of anaerobic metabolism?

  1. Free radicals.
  2. Lactic acid.
  3. Myoglobin.
  4. Lipofuscin.

213. The nurse in the newborn nursery is discussing the genotype of Down syndrome with a nursing student. Which statement should the nurse include in the discussion?

  1. "Down syndrome is caused by a missing X chromosome."
  2. "Down syndrome is caused by the trisomy of chromosome 21."
  3. "A characteristic of Down syndrome is mental retardation."
  4. "Microencephaly is associated with Down syndrome."

214. The nurse is preparing a staff conference on the care of patients with head injuries. When discussing interventions used to minimize or treat increased intracranial pressure, which intervention should the nurse include in the presentation?

  1. Administration of beta blockers to decrease the buildup of excitatory amino acids.
  2. Induction of a coma state using barbiturates to reduce the patient's neuronal metabolic rate.
  3. Administration of furosemide (Lasix) to reduce cerebral edema.
  4. Increasing the $PaCO_2$ level to promote cerebral vasodilation.

215. Cullen's sign may be indicative of which condition?

  1. Basilar skull fracture.
  2. Hemothorax.
  3. Pelvic fracture.
  4. Hemorrhagic pancreatitis.

216. What clinical manifestation would the nurse expect to find in a patient diagnosed with heat stroke?

  1. Hot, dry, ashen skin.
  2. Profuse perspiration.
  3. Muscle cramps.
  4. Thirst.

217. With asthma, what is the primary cause of airway constriction?

  1. Thick mucus produced by hypertrophied glands.
  2. Viral infection that produces a toxin.
  3. Bronchospasm secondary to the inflammatory response.
  4. Thinning of the smooth muscle in the bronchioles.

218. A teenage patient presents to the outpatient clinic with complaints of pharyngitis, fever, and fatigue. The physical examination reveals splenomegaly and swollen anterior and posterior cervical lymph nodes. The history reveals a recent exposure to a virus. Which clinical condition should the nurse suspect?

  1. Non-Hodgkin's lymphoma.
  2. Acute myelocytic leukemia.
  3. Mononucleosis.
  4. Agranulocytosis.

219. Which agent of bioterrorism has no established treatment?

  1. *Bacillus anthracis* (anthrax).
  2. *Clostridium botulinum* (botulism).
  3. *Francisella tularensis* (tularemia).
  4. Ebola virus (hemorrhagic fever).

220. A patient presents to the emergency room with a productive cough, elevated white blood cell (WBC) count, and fever. A chest x-ray reveals consolidation in the left lower lobe. Pneumonia is diagnosed. Which term most accurately describes this type of infection?

1. Community-acquired infection.
2. Prodromal infection.
3. Atypical infection.
4. Nosocomial infection.

221. Upon review of the interdisciplinary progress notes, the nurse finds that a patient is neutropenic. The nurse understands that the patient care plan should reflect observations for what problem?

1. Gastrointestinal bleeding.
2. Pulmonary emboli.
3. Respiratory infections.
4. Venous thrombosis.

222. A patient had a respiratory arrest and required endotracheal intubation. Which auscultory findings would indicate correct placement of the tube?

1. Auscultate bilateral breath sounds, and observe the chest wall rising and falling.
2. Auscultate stomach gurgling when ventilating the patient, and observe no rise or fall of the chest wall.
3. Auscultate breath sounds only on the right, and observe rise and fall of the chest wall on the right.
4. Auscultate stomach gurgling when ventilating the patient, and observe chest rise only on the left side of the chest.

SECTION I

SECTION II

SECTION III

SECTION IV

SECTION V

SECTION VI

SECTION VII

SECTION VIII

SECTION IX

SECTION X

MANAGEMENT OF CARE

1. Correct Answers: 2, 3, and 6

Rationale: The Health Insurance Portability and Accountability Act (HIPAA) is federal legislation that was passed in 1996 and is intended to promote a national framework for health information. HIPAA comprises three standards, dealing with privacy, security, and transaction and code sets. Privacy relates to the patient's rights over the use and disclosure of his or her own personal health information. Security relates to the specific steps a healthcare organization must take to protect personal health information from being viewed by unauthorized people, stolen, lost, or destroyed accidentally. All healthcare organizations that use electronic transactions and code sets, such as healthcare claims and claim payments, must comply with HIPAA standards. Protected health information is that information, whether oral or recorded in any form, that relates to the physical or mental health of an individual, the provision of health care to that individual, or the payment of healthcare services delivered to an individual. Identifiers for the information include a patient's name, address, phone number, driver's license number, and so forth.

2. Correct Answers: 2 and 10

3. Correct Answers: 1 and 5

4. Correct Answers: 6 and 9

5. Correct Answers: 3 and 11

6. Correct Answers: 4 and 8

7. Correct Answers: 7 and 12

Rationale: Nurses work collaboratively with other members of the healthcare team to ensure that desired patient outcomes are achieved. A dietician will work with the patient to evaluate nutritional status and determine dietary and caloric needs. The home health aide will come into a patient's home and assist the patient with personal care and hygiene as well as perform light housekeeping and meal preparation. A speech therapist will work with a patient to assess and treat swallowing problems and to improve a patient's expressive abilities. The physician has responsibility for the diagnosis, treatment, and follow-up of the disease and its associated complications. The physical therapist works to restore function and to prevent further disability through activities intended to improve musculoskeletal strength and gait training.

8. Correct Answer: 3

Rationale: Functional nursing is a type of care delivery model where nurses are assigned to complete patient care tasks. In the question, the nurse is functionally assigned the task of medication administration to all patients.

9. Correct Answer: 2

Rationale: Team nursing is a patient care delivery model where care providers are organized into groups. The members of the group include staff with different educational backgrounds. The group is lead by a registered nurse (RN). In the question, the RN is the team leader who assesses the patients and then determines the most appropriate patient care assignments for the members of her team based on patient needs.

10. Correct Answer: 3

Rationale: A variance is a deviation from the expected outcome established for a critical pathway. Variance analysis is one method for assessing whether the expected patient outcomes were achieved and the effectiveness of meeting the established outcomes of the critical pathway.

11. Correct Answer: 3

Rationale: Effective discharge planning must begin upon admission of the patient to the acute care facility.

12. Correct Answer: 4

Rationale: In the postoperative period, respirations will be shallow because of pain associated with the surgical procedure. The priority teaching intervention would be to teach the patient to splint the abdominal incision and to cough and deep breathe.

13. Correct Answer: 4

Rationale: The nurse should care for the patient who is complaining of shortness of breath first. Airway, breathing and circulation would be the framework used to determine the priority of the scenarios presented.

14. Correct Answer: 2

Rationale: Each individual nurse should purchase professional liability insurance to ensure that the nurse's individual interests are represented in liability issues.

15. Correct Answer: 2

Rationale: Morphine is a controlled substance and should be secured at all times. The nurse should immediately remove the vial from the patient's bedside and notify the supervisor that an unsecured vial of morphine was found. The supervisor should then proceed to intervene and follow organizational policy.

16. Correct Answer: 2

Rationale: The nurse should document only the facts of the situation. Based on the scenario, the cause of the fall was not identified. Thus the facts for documentation are that the patient was found lying on the floor upon entering the room.

17. Correct Answer: 2

Rationale: A patient has the right to withdraw informed consent at any time. The nurse must first inform the surgeon of the patient's wishes to withdraw consent.

18. Correct Answer: 2

Rationale: The confidentiality of computerized medical records must be maintained. The nurse should never share computer access passwords with other colleagues, as another person could then use the nurse's personal identifier to compromise a patient's confidentiality.

19. Correct Answer: 3

Rationale: The patient is exhibiting the clinical manifestations of a stroke, including slurred speech, facial drooping, and unilateral weakness of extremities. The patient also has high blood pressure, a known risk factor for stroke. Emergency management services should be contacted immediately for screening, assessment, intervention, and transport to a facility that provides care for stroke patients.

20. Correct Answer: 1

Rationale: The nurse should include all of the information in the report, but the finding that will best promote continuity of care and a positive outcome is the neurological assessment. The nurse can use the assessment information as a baseline to identify any changes in the patient's neurological assessment during the next shift.

21. Correct Answer: 4

Rationale: The best practice for a nurse who is unable to read a written medication order is to directly contact the prescriber to seek clarification of the order. Attempts to clarify the order that do not involve the prescriber could result in a medication error.

22. Correct Answer: 2

Rationale: The diagnosis with the highest priority for the patient during the acute phase of care is the risk for infection posed by an open wound. An open wound represents a break in the normal defense provided by the skin and a potential route of entry for microorganisms. The development of an infection could result in increased length of stay and treatment time for the patient.

23. Correct Answer: 2

Rationale: The patient who is dying should be given the private room. A private room will allow privacy for the patient and family. The family could stay with the patient or come and go as needed.

24. Correct Answer: 3

Rationale: A hypothesis is the statement of the predicted relationships between variables that are being studied.

25. Correct Answer: 3

Rationale: The state licensing board or state board of nursing is responsible for overseeing the competency of the state's nurse workforce. The board of nursing has the authority to discipline nurses through licensure revocation if, after due process, it determines that a nurse exhibited unprofessional conduct or failed to adhere to the standards of safe practice.

26. Correct Answer: 1

Rationale: The diabetic patient who had a recent hypoglycemic episode should be assessed first to determine the effectiveness of the intervention.

SECTION I

SECTION II

SECTION III

SECTION IV

SECTION V

SECTION VI

SECTION VII

SECTION VIII

SECTION IX

SECTION X

27. Correct Answer: **1**

Rationale: The most appropriate resource for the nurse to consult regarding the ethical dilemma would be the hospital ethics committee. The scope of an ethics committee's responsibilities may vary from organization to organization. Common functions of such a committee include evaluation of institutional policies, provision of educational programs, and consultation on cases with ethical issues.

28. Correct Answer: **1**

Rationale: Abandonment occurs when there is a unilateral severance of the professional relationship with the patient without adequate notice and while the care requirement still exists. In this scenario, the nurse is at risk for patient abandonment, as adequate notice to find coverage for the shift was not given and the patient's care requirement remains.

29. Correct Answer: **4**

Rationale: The charge nurse used an accommodating or smoothing style of conflict management. The style is characterized by actions that involve eliminating expressions of differences, or giving in without addressing the cause of the problem.

30. Correct Answer: **2**

Rationale: A process standard is a statement of the standardized processes used to accomplish a desired outcome. It can be used to evaluate performance and achievement of goals. Competent performance of the procedure by the catheterization lab staff to achieve catheter site hemostasis should prevent the complication of groin hematomas.

31. Correct Answer: **1**

Rationale: An FTE position is equivalent to 40 hours of work per week for 52 weeks. The total annual hours is 2,080 (40 hours × 52 weeks).

32. Correct Answer: **3**

Rationale: Sleep apnea is characterized by partial or complete upper airway obstruction during sleep that results in apnea or hypopnea. BiPAP is one intervention for the problem. A respiratory therapist would be a resource for assisting the patient with education about the use of the equipment.

33. Correct Answer: **2**

Rationale: A convenience sample is the selection of the most readily available persons for participation in a study. Posting a notice that asks for volunteers would generate study participants who are part of a convenience sample.

34. Correct Answer: **2**

Rationale: The nurse should follow the chain of command and discuss the patient's request with the charge nurse.

35. Correct Answer: **1**

Rationale: In-service education and training are provided by an organization in an effort to increase the knowledge and skills of the organization's employees and staff. Instruction on a new piece of equipment would be an example of one type of in-service training a nurse might receive.

36. Correct Answer: **1**

Rationale: The nurse used assessment to determine the level of pain the patient was experiencing and, based on those findings, chose to intervene by administering medication.

37. Correct Answer: **3**

Rationale: An intrapersonal conflict occurs within an individual when he or she must choose between two alternatives. Nurse Jones experienced an intrapersonal conflict when, as an individual, she could not decide which alternative to select.

38. Correct Answer: **3**

Rationale: The opening of an entire dressing change kit to obtain a sterile gauze would contribute to the cost of care, as the nurse is not demonstrating efficient use of the available supplies.

39. Correct Answer: **2**

Rationale: The primary problem with type 1 diabetes is a deficiency of insulin owing to the destruction of beta cells in the pancreas. The disease management plan for a patient with type 1 diabetes would include glycemic control through the use of insulin therapy, nutrition management, and blood glucose monitoring.

40. Correct Answer: **4**

Rationale: Patients who could benefit from advocacy include those who lack knowledge,

Answers and Rationales **201**

SECTION I
SECTION II
SECTION III
SECTION IV
SECTION V
SECTION VI
SECTION VII
SECTION VIII
SECTION IX
SECTION X

have little power, need to make decisions, and currently receive inadequate care. The geriatric patient who has no family members and must make a decision about care would benefit most from a nurse advocate in the scenarios identified in this question.

41. Correct Answer: 1

Rationale: The randomized controlled trial research study would provide the highest level of evidence. A randomized controlled trial is an experimental test of an intervention or treatment that involves the assignment of individuals to a treatment group in a manner determined by chance only. This design ensures that a study can attribute any differences found between groups to the intervention/treatment and has a low susceptibility to bias.

42. Correct Answer: 2

Rationale: Prior to resigning from a position, the nurse should familiarize himself or herself with the policies of the organization. Organizational policy should address the notification time frame for resignation, whether a resignation letter is required, how accrued benefits are managed, and whether an exit interview is performed. When resigning from a position, the nurse should consider that future employers will be contacting the employer for references and handle the dissatisfaction in a constructive manner.

43. Correct Answer: 4

Rationale: The charge nurse should discuss with the physician the inappropriate manner in which he communicated with the nurse, all the while ensuring that the patient receives proper care.

44. Correct Answer: 4

Rationale: The use of an open-ended response to validate the patient's understanding of the DNR designation should be addressed first.

SAFETY AND INFECTION CONTROL

45. Correct Answer: 2

Rationale: For overdoses of morphine, an opioid receptor antagonist such as naloxone (Narcan) is given. Naloxone acts by competing with morphine at the opioid receptor sites. The competitive antagonist action of Naloxone prevents morphine from acting at receptor sites and thereby blocks the actions of morphine.

46. Correct Answer: 3

Rationale: For insulin overdoses, glucagon is given. Glucagon is a hormone that is normally produced in the alpha cells of the pancreas and acts to increase plasma levels of glucose by promoting the breakdown of glycogen.

47. Correct Answer: 1

Rationale: For an overdose of acetaminophen, acetylcysteine is given. Acetaminophen is metabolized by two pathways in the liver, minor and major. In the minor pathway, the drug is broken down to a toxic substance and then converted to a nontoxic form. Glutathione is needed to convert the toxic metabolite, created from the metabolism of acetaminophen in the minor pathway, to a nontoxic substance. Acetylcysteine acts by substituting for glutathione in a reaction that removes the toxic metabolite of acetaminophen.

48. Correct Answer: 4

Rationale: For an overdose of a benzodiazepine, flumazenil is administered. Flumazenil acts as a competitive benzodiazepine receptor antagonist and prevents the action of the benzodiazepine at the receptor site.

49. Correct Answer: 1

Rationale: The Centers for Disease Control and Prevention (CDC) have issued guidelines for healthcare workers regarding hand hygiene practices. These guidelines incorporate the use of alcohol-based hand rubs for routine hand antisepsis. It would be inappropriate for the nurse to use an alcohol-based hand rub when hands are visibly dirty or contaminated with blood or body fluid. If visibly soiled, the hands should be washed with soap and water or an antimicrobial soap and water.

50. Correct Answer: 1

Rationale: The triage classifications in a four-tier system include emergent, urgent, delayed or non-urgent, and expectant. A patient with hemorrhagic shock from an arterial puncture has a life-threatening injury that requires immediate care and continuous reassessment. The most appropriate triage classification for this patient is emergent.

51. Correct Answer: 4

Rationale: Most needlestick injuries occur during recapping of the needle. To prevent the possibility of a needlestick injury, the safest action by the nurse would be to place the uncapped needle in a puncture-resistant container.

52. Correct Answer: **4**

Rationale: Charcoal acts to adsorb drugs and other chemicals in the gastrointestinal tract. The substances bind with the charcoal, which prevents their absorption into the bloodstream. The charcoal-bound substance can then be eliminated via the gastrointestinal tract.

53. Correct Answer: **2**

Rationale: The feeding bag and tubing should be changed every 24 hours to minimize the potential for bacterial growth.

54. Correct Answer: **2**

Rationale: Body position can affect blood pressure measurement. If the person is prone, the pressure measurement may be lower; if the person is standing, the pressure measurement may be higher. The patient should be placed in a sitting position with the arm at the level of the heart to ensure accurate readings.

55. Correct Answer: **4**

Rationale: The National Institute for Occupational Health and Safety has identified risk factors for hospital violence. Examples include overcrowded, uncomfortable waiting areas; long waits for services; working alone; poorly lit corridors and parking areas; and unrestricted movement of the public in and out of the facility. Hospital workers and employers should be aware of the risk factors for violence and work to create safe environments.

56. Correct Answer: **1**

Rationale: The resolution of symptoms does not mean that the disease can no longer be transmitted. The herpes simplex type 2 virus remains in a latent state and results in recurrence of symptoms. At this time, there is no cure for genital herpes.

57. Correct Answer: **4**

Rationale: The patient with an undetermined cause of pneumonia who has AIDS should receive the airborne precautions room. Patients with AIDS are at risk for opportunistic infections such as tuberculosis but may not present with classic symptoms of the disease, owing to their immunocompromised state. Until a causative organism can be identified,

prevention and control for tuberculosis should be implemented.

58. Correct Answer: **1**

Rationale: Aspiration of oral or gastric fluids is a contributing factor to the development of a ventilator-associated pneumonia. A patient in the supine position has an increased potential for pulmonary aspiration. Elevating the head of the bed 30 to 45 degrees can reduce this risk.

59. Correct Answer: **2**

Rationale: Handwritten medication orders can often be misinterpreted and lead to actual medication errors. The use of the abbreviation q.d. (or Q.D.) has been interpreted as q.i.d. and led to medication errors in some cases. The Joint Commission on Accreditation of Healthcare Organizations and the Institute for Safe Medication Practice recommend writing the word "daily" instead.

60. Correct Answer: **4**

Rationale: When a nurse cannot read a written order, safe practice would dictate that the nurse clarify the order with the original author of the order. Therefore the nurse should contact the prescriber who wrote the order to clarify it.

61. Correct Answer: **4**

Rationale: Emergence of antibiotic resistance is a major concern with the use of antimicrobial therapy. Culture and sensitivity testing will promote the goal of prescribing medications that target the pathogen and source of infection.

62. Correct Answer: **3**

Rationale: HIV may be transmitted by blood-to-blood contact, through sexual contact, from infected mothers to their offspring in utero, during delivery, or with breastfeeding. The individual who is at greatest risk for transmission would be the phlebotomist who collects blood and would be working with needles. The phlebotomist would be at risk for a needlestick injury and the possibility of blood-to-blood transmission.

63. Correct Answer: **4**

Rationale: According to the American Heart Association's journal *Circulation*, the lower-energy, biphasic defibrillator waveform shocks have an equivalent or higher success rate for the termination of ventricular fibrillation. The optimal energy level for the first biphasic shock has not yet been determined, so a range is recommended for defibrillation until research can support selection of a specific energy level.

64. Correct Answer: **1**

Rationale: A neuromuscular blocking agent interferes with nicotinic receptor activation, resulting in skeletal muscle relaxation. An adverse effect of all neuromuscular blockers is relaxation of the respiratory muscles to the point of respiratory arrest. When using neuromuscular blocking agents, the nurse should always have a bag-valve mask device and oxygen at hand.

65. Correct Answer: **3**

Rationale: A seizure is a type of epileptic event characterized by abnormal excitability of the neurons in the central nervous system. A tonic-clonic seizure is characterized by periods of muscle rigidity followed by muscle jerks and impairment in the patient's level of consciousness. A patient who is at risk for seizures should not have oral temperatures assessed using a glass thermometer. Should a seizure occur, the glass could break and result in patient injury.

66. Correct Answer: **3**

Rationale: The patient is a vital part of ensuring the safe administration of medications. The nurse should listen to the patient and double-check the medication order to ensure its accuracy. If the order was correct, the nurse has identified an opportunity for patient teaching.

HEALTH PROMOTION AND MAINTENANCE

67. Correct Answer: **1**

Rationale: The National Network of Libraries of Medicine defines health literacy as the ability to obtain, process, and understand basic health information and services needed to make appropriate health decisions. The Institute of Medicine reports that 90 million people in the United States have difficulty understanding and using health information. Research indicates that well-educated people who are fully literate may nevertheless have problems understanding health-related terms.

68. Correct Answer: **1**

Rationale: The nurse should instruct a patient who is diagnosed with latex allergies to avoid the application of elastic bandages. The

elasticity of the bandage oftentimes is associated with the use of the natural rubber, latex.

69. Correct Answer: **inspection → auscultation → percussion → palpation**

Rationale: The order for an abdominal physical examination differs from the usual physical assessment guidelines, which call for inspection → palpation → percussion → auscultation. With an abdominal examination, auscultation is done prior to percussion and palpation because manipulation of the abdomen using palpation or percussion could alter the frequency and intensity of bowel sounds and lead to inaccurate exam results.

70. Correct Answer: **1**

Rationale: The transmission of West Nile virus occurs through the bite of an infected mosquito. Prevention efforts should focus on reduction of the mosquito population and prevention of bites.

71. Correct Answer: **1**

Rationale: Cranial nerve II is the optic nerve and is responsible for the transmission of visual impulses. A patient who has a problem with cranial nerve II would be assessed using a Snellen chart. This chart, which is used to test visual acuity, is composed of letters, numbers, or symbols arranged in decreasing size from top to bottom.

72. Correct Answer: **2**

Rationale: African American men in a low socioeconomic class have a higher mortality rate due to prostate cancer. In this population, the cancer has been found to be more advanced at the time of diagnosis. Members of this group often do not use screening services, or are unable to use or access such services because of their socioeconomic status.

73. Correct Answer: **1–6**

Rationale: A total of 10 indicators have been identified by *Healthy People 2010* for use in measuring the nation's health over a 10-year period. All of the factors listed in the question, plus substance abuse, immunization, injury and violence, and mental health, will serve as indicators of population health.

SECTION I
SECTION II
SECTION III
SECTION IV
SECTION V
SECTION VI
SECTION VII
SECTION VIII
SECTION IX
SECTION X

74. Correct Answer: **1**

Rationale: A lemon-lime soda such as Sprite would contain no caffeine.

75. Correct Answer: **1**

Rationale: Encasing pillows, mattresses, and box springs in covers that are impermeable to the dust mite allergens can reduce exposure and decrease triggers for an asthma exacerbation.

76. Correct Answer: **3**

Rationale: The nurse should further assess the patient to determine the source of frustration. Once the source of the problem is identified, the nurse can establish a teaching plan that will address the patient's needs.

77. Correct Answers: **1, 2, and 6**

Rationale: Avoidance of pulling, pushing, or lifting objects greater than 10 to 15 pounds will prevent an increase in intraocular pressure, which could damage the eye. A protective eye shield prevents rubbing or damage to the surgical site from foreign objects. The physician should be contacted when pain is not relieved by the prescribed analgesics, as pain could be a sign of a complication.

78. Correct Answer: **2**

Rationale: The major risk factor for development of hepatitis C infection is percutaneous exposure. Practices such as intravenous drug abuse, transfusion of infected blood products, and occupational exposure to blood and blood products could result in transmission of the infection.

79. Correct Answer: **2**

Rationale: Patients with upper body obesity have been found to be at a greater risk for health problems than those with lower body obesity. Upper body obesity is associated with an increased risk of insulin resistance, diabetes, hypertension, coronary artery disease, and stroke.

80. Correct Answer: **3**

Rationale: Body mass index (BMI) and waist circumference can be used as indicators for disease risk. As BMI rises and waist circumference increase, the disease risk increases. A female patient with a body mass index of 31 is considered obese. A waist circumference greater than 35 inches in a female indicates increased abdominal fat. The female with a BMI of 32 and a waist circumference of 40 demonstrates an increased health risk.

81. Correct Answer: **2**

Rationale: An intervention at the secondary level of prevention is used to detect disease early in its course, when the problem is asymptomatic and treatment may be able to promote a cure. A Pap test is an example of a secondary prevention measure.

82. Correct Answer: **2**

Rationale: Menactra is recommended for the prevention of invasive meningococcal disease in people 11 to 55 years of age.

83. Correct Answer: **1, right upper quadrant**

Rationale: The liver is found in the right upper quadrant of the abdomen. The nurse would palpate the liver in the right upper abdominal quadrant.

84. Correct Answer: **3**

Rationale: The use of monthly testicular exams is an important health promotion intervention for the early detection of testicular cancer. The self-exam includes palpation of the scrotum, epididymis, and spermatic cord. The testicles should be smooth and uniform in consistency with palpation. Lumps, soreness, swelling, and irregularities of the scrotum should be reported to the physician.

85. Correct Answer: **3**

Rationale: Health promotion activities increase patients' health awareness and are a component of preventing illness. A presentation to a class of fifth-graders on the risks of tobacco use is an example of a health promotion activity. By providing information to the class on the risks of smoking, the nurse hopes to promote health and wellness.

86. Correct Answer: **2**

Rationale: Protection against solar radiation is most effective when adequate time is allowed for a sunscreen product to penetrate the skin. To allow for penetration, the application of sunscreens should occur between 30 minutes and 2 hours prior to sun exposure.

PSYCHOSOCIAL INTEGRITY

87. Correct Answer: 1

Rationale: Anorexia nervosa is characterized by self-starvation and a distorted body image.

88. Correct Answer: 2

Rationale: Bulimia nervosa is characterized by binge eating and inappropriate compensatory mechanisms for the binge eating, such as self-induced vomiting or excessive exercise.

89. Correct Answer: 2

Rationale: Adaptation is the ability to successfully create a balance between stressors and the ability to cope with the stressor. Factors that affect the ability to cope include age, nutrition, hardiness, physiologic and anatomical reserves, sleep–wake cycles, and psychosocial factors. Patient B is more likely to adapt to the respiratory infection because of age and physiologic and anatomical reserves.

90. Correct Answer: 1

Rationale: Adaptation is the ability of a patient to successfully create a balance between a stressor and the ability to cope with the stressor. Factors that affect the ability to cope include age, nutrition, hardiness, physiologic and anatomical reserves, sleep–wake cycles, and psychosocial factors. Patient A is more likely to adapt to the diagnosis of liver cancer because of the psychosocial factor of a supportive family.

91. Correct Answer: 3

Rationale: Confusion is a mental state characterized by disorientation to person, place, time, or situation. Confusion in a patient can be diminished by keeping items familiar to the patient at the bedside.

92. Correct Answer: 1

Rationale: When a healthcare provider goes through a resuscitation experience for the first time, it is normal to experience an unsettling reaction to the stressful event. The most therapeutic response that the colleague can provide is to offer the nurse the opportunity to talk about the situation. The sharing of thoughts and feelings is a healthy intervention when experiencing a reaction to a stressful event.

93. Correct Answer: 4

Rationale: Denial is a common defense mechanism used by patients who are abusing alcohol. This defense mechanism is used to avoid dealing with the problems and responsibilities associated with the substance abuse behavior.

94. Correct Answer: 2

Rationale: A desirable short-term outcome for this patient is participation in the treatment plan. Victims of physical violence often feel trapped, dependent, and helpless. A short-term goal is, therefore, to ensure that the patient keeps appointments and works with a counselor on recommended interventions to prevent further violence.

95. Correct Answer: 3

Rationale: Presbycusis is the term used to describe hearing loss associated with normal aging. This problem is often characterized by a loss of hearing sensitivity and a reduction in the clarity of speech. When speaking with a patient with presbycusis, the nurse should speak directly to the patient in a normal and clear voice.

96. Correct Answer: 2

Rationale: This patient has experienced a loss (job) that is contributing to his feelings of uselessness to his family. The diagnosis of situational low self-esteem is the most appropriate diagnosis for this patient. The North American Nursing Diagnosis Association (NANDA) definition for the nursing diagnosis is the development of a negative perception of self-worth in response to a current situation.

97. Correct Answer: 2

Rationale: A goal when caring for patients with spinal cord injuries is to promote their adjustment to the injury and their independence. A patient who is using modified feeding utensils at every meal is demonstrating an attempt at independence for the functional activity of eating. The patient's statement recognizes that the activity is one that requires continued work, but progress is being made toward the goal of developing as much independence as possible with eating.

SECTION I
SECTION II
SECTION III
SECTION IV
SECTION V
SECTION VI
SECTION VII
SECTION VIII
SECTION IX
SECTION X

98. Correct Answer: **2**

Rationale: Autism is a mental disorder that is often diagnosed during the toddler years. Clinical manifestations such as impairment in social interaction, verbal, and nonverbal communication skills are often identified during the toddler period of development.

99. Correct Answer: **1**

Rationale: Twelve-step programs are built on the premise that support and encouragement from others can aid in a person's recovery from alcohol abuse. According to Alcoholics Anonymous, the first step in a 12-step program is the admission that a problem exists. The person admits that he or she is powerless over alcohol and that life has become unmanageable.

100. Correct Answer: **4**

Rationale: The characteristic clinical manifestations of attention deficit hyperactivity disorder are inattention, hyperactivity, and impulsivity. The disorder can be subclassified as predominately inattentive, hyperactive-impulsive, or combined.

101. Correct Answer: **1**

Rationale: The statement "You've been upset about your blood pressure" is a reflective comment that describes the patient's feelings. A reflective comment repeats what a patient has said or describes the person's feelings. It is used by the nurse to encourage the patient to elaborate on the topic.

102. Correct Answer: **1**

Rationale: One component of a smoking cessation program is the identification of triggers that promoted the smoking habit. Once they are identified, the patient should avoid exposure and return to those triggers.

103. Correct Answer: **4**

Rationale: A chronic, intermittent stressor is one to which a person is chronically exposed. A genital herpes infection would be an example of a chronic, intermittent stressor. The virus can be latent or manifest itself in intermittently reoccurring symptoms once acquired.

104. Correct Answer: **4**

Rationale: Grief can be classified as acute, anticipatory, or pathologic. Anticipatory grief is associated with the anticipation of a death or loss that has yet to take place. A patient who is newly diagnosed with liver cancer is most likely to experience anticipatory grieving when anticipating death.

105. Correct Answer: **2**

Rationale: Three types of symptoms of post-traumatic stress syndrome are distinguished: intrusion, or reexperiencing the event; avoidance, or the emotional numbing and disruption of personal relationships; and hyperarousal. The symptoms exhibited by this patient include all three types: nightmares (intrusion), survivor guilt (avoidance), and difficulty concentrating (hyperarousal).

106. Correct Answer: **4**

Rationale: Self-esteem is the need to feel good about oneself and to believe that others hold one in high regard. Patients who have been the victims of domestic violence are at risk for a disturbance in self-esteem. One desirable outcome of counseling when working with victims of domestic violence is for the patient to develop increased self-esteem.

BASIC CARE AND COMFORT

107. Correct Answer: **2**

Rationale: Saw palmetto is used for the relief of symptoms associated with benign prostatic hypertrophy. The herb's mechanism of action is unknown, but it is thought that saw palmetto may contain substances that prevent the growth of prostate epithelial cells.

108. Correct Answer: **3**

Rationale: Gingko biloba is used to improve memory, sharpen concentration, and promote clear thinking. These effects are thought to be related to vasodilation and increased blood flow and the stimulation of prostaglandin synthesis in the brain.

109. Correct Answer: **1**

Rationale: St. John's wort is used to relieve depression. Its action is thought be associated with the herb's active ingredients, which may act on neurotransmitters such as serotonin, norepinephrine, dopamine, and gamma-aminobutyric acid.

110. Correct Answer: **4**

Rationale: Black cohosh is used as a treatment for the symptoms of menopause. The supplement's mechanism of action is unknown.

111. Correct Answer: 4

Rationale: A mild soap and water should be used to cleanse the perianal area for a patient who is experiencing frequent diarrheal stools. The area should then be dried thoroughly. Maintaining clean, dry skin will help to prevent an alteration in skin integrity.

112. Correct Answer: 4

Rationale: Oliguria is defined as a decreased capacity to form and pass urine. Urine output of less than 500 mL but more than 100 mL is described as oliguria.

113. Correct Answer: 1

Rationale: A clear liquid diet consists of fluids and foods that are clear liquids at room temperature. Ice cream is composed of milk, which is not clear at room temperature, so it would be an inappropriate choice for a clear liquid diet.

114. Correct Answer: 4

Rationale: Aspiration pneumonitis is a serious complication associated with patients who receive enteral feedings. The nurse should establish a plan of care that includes a nursing diagnosis of risk of aspiration for the patient who is receiving enteral feedings.

115. Correct Answer: 2

Rationale: Dysphagia is the medical term for difficulty swallowing. The head of the bed should be elevated, and the patient observed for signs of aspiration.

116. Correct Answer: 1

Rationale: Urea is a nitrogenous waste product and a by-product of protein metabolism. The kidneys are responsible for the excretion of urea. When the kidneys are not functioning, urea accumulates in the blood [blood urea nitrogen (BUN)]. A decrease in the amount of protein ingested will result in a decrease in the amount of nitrogenous wastes in the blood.

117. Correct Answer: 3

Rationale: A more accurate assessment of weight is obtained when the weight is measured at the same time each day.

118. Correct Answer: 1

Rationale: Ingestion of ice will artificially lower the patient's oral temperature reading. The nurse should instruct the patient not to take any additional cold fluids or ice by mouth, wait 15 to 30 minutes, and then take the oral temperature. Waiting 15 to 30 minutes will allow the oral cavity tissues to return to the patient's basal temperature.

119. Correct Answer: 3

Rationale: The use of restraints should be a last choice as an intervention because of issues associated with patient safety. An alternative that the nurse might incorporate into care is the use of familiar family members to reorient a confused patient.

120. Correct Answer: 1

Rationale: The best method for assessment of fluid volume increases is a daily weight measurement.

121. Correct Answer: 1

Rationale: The oral mucosa would be the most appropriate site to assess for central cyanosis.

122. Correct Answer: 3

Rationale: It is often difficult for a nurse to assess for jaundice by inspecting the skin of a dark-skinned patient. The nurse should check the sclera for this finding in dark-skinned patients.

123. Correct Answer: 2

Rationale: The patient with a complete bowel obstruction would be unable to take anything by the oral or enteral route. The most likely choice for nutritional support for such a patient would be parenteral therapy.

124. Correct Answer: 1

Rationale: A typical daily urine volume is 1 to 2 L. The normal hourly urine output is approximately 1 mL of urine per kilogram of body weight per hour. The nurse should report the urine output of 20 mL in 1 hour.

125. Correct Answer: 2

Rationale: Hair loss associated with alkylating chemotherapy is caused by injury to the hair follicles from the alkylation of DNA in the cells. Hair loss can also include loss of eyebrows and eyelashes. Hair loss occurs approximately 7 to 10 days after treatment has begun. Once treatment has completed, hair regeneration occurs in 1 to 2 months.

SECTION I
SECTION II
SECTION III
SECTION IV
SECTION V
SECTION VI
SECTION VII
SECTION VIII
SECTION IX
X

126. Correct Answer: 3

Rationale: The female urethra is approximately 1.5 to 2.5 inches in length. The urinary catheter should be inserted 2 to 3 inches into the urinary meatus or until urine flow is observed.

PHARMACOLOGICAL AND PARENTERAL THERAPIES

127. Correct Answer: 2

Rationale: Hypoalbuminemia contributes to the development of ascites. Albumin is administered to maintain plasma colloid osmotic pressure and reduce the formation of ascites.

128. Correct Answer: 3

Rationale: Cephulac reduces ammonia formation by enhancing intestinal excretion.

129. Correct Answer: 1

Rationale: Inderal decreases portal venous pressure and reduces the potential for bleeding from esophageal varices.

130. Correct Answer: 4

Rationale: Aldactone is a diuretic that acts to block the action of aldosterone. It promotes the reabsorption of sodium in the kidney. Aldactone, often in combination with a loop diuretic, reduces the likelihood that ascites will occur.

131. Correct Answer: 3

Rationale: Xigris is a derivative of activated protein C, an endogenous compound that has anticoagulant and anti-inflammatory actions. This drug is used to regulate the systemic inflammatory response associated with severe sepsis. Bleeding is the most common serious adverse effect associated with the administration of Xigris.

132. Correct Answer: 2

Rationale: The use of an anabolic steroid for the purpose of athletic enhancement is illegal. Because of the potential for abuse, most anabolic steroids are Schedule 3 substances and are controlled under the Anabolic Steroids Control Act of 2004.

133. Correct Answer: 4

Rationale: A nebulized beta$_2$ agonist, such as albuterol, is the treatment of choice for a patient with an acute asthma exacerbation. Albuterol acts to relieve bronchospasm by activating beta$_2$ receptors that promote bronchodilation.

134. Correct Answer: 1

Rationale: Vasopressin is used in the treatment of ventricular fibrillation. The Advanced Cardiac Life Support recommendations call for a one-time use of vasopressin 40 units IV as an alternative to epinephrine in the ventricular fibrillation/ventricular tachycardia algorithm. This medication promotes vasoconstriction of vascular smooth muscle and raises the blood pressure.

135. Correct Answer: 3

Rationale: Orlistat acts to promote weight loss by decreasing the absorption of dietary fat from the gastrointestinal tract. This drug inhibits release of the gastric and pancreatic enzymes responsible for fat breakdown. When fats are not broken down in the gastrointestinal system by gastric and pancreatic enzymes, fat cannot be absorbed.

136. Correct Answer: 3

Rationale: Recombinant DNA technology is a type of genetic engineering that recombines genes into hybrid molecules. These molecules are inserted into one-celled organisms, which then reproduce. The technology allows for large quantities of substances to be produced. Humolog insulin is one example of a substance that is produced by recombinant DNA technology.

137. Correct Answer: 2

Rationale: Botox Cosmetic blocks transmission at the neuromuscular junction and cholinergic synapses. Neuronal function is restored after several months, once new terminals develop. Thus the effect of Botox Cosmetic on the elimination of glabellar ("frown") lines is only temporary.

138. Correct Answer: 3

Rationale: An iatrogenic effect of drug therapy is defined as a disease produced by use of the drug. For example, a side effect of taking antipsychotic medications is the development of clinical manifestations that mimic the symptoms of Parkinson's disease.

139. Correct Answer: 2

Rationale: Avastin, is the first angiogenesis inhibitor to become available in the United States. It is a monoclonal antibody that binds with vascular endothelial growth factor and prevents the formation of new blood vessels. Without an adequate blood supply, solid tumor growth is inhibited. Avastin does not destroy existing tumor cells. This drug is approved for use in combination with other chemotherapeutic agents for colon or rectal cancer.

140. Correct Answer: 4

Rationale: The Controlled Substances Act established five categories for drugs. Drugs in Schedule 1 have no acceptable medical use. Drugs in Schedules 2–5 have at least some accepted medical uses. The abuse potential of the drug lessens as you move from Schedule 1 to 5, such that a Schedule 5 drug would have an accepted medical use and the least potential for abuse.

141. Correct Answer: 4 units

Rationale: Sliding-scale insulin coverage is used to promote glycemic control in patients whose blood glucose levels have not yet been regulated. The prescriber will identify the frequency of capillary blood glucose monitoring to be done (e.g., capillary blood glucose before meals [AC] and at bedtime [HS]) and provide a scale of regular insulin coverage to be administered based on the glucose monitoring results. In this way, sliding-scale insulin coverage is individualized for each patient.

142. Correct Answer: 2

Rationale: The administration technique used for smallpox vaccination is termed scarification. The vaccine is given through multiple, superficial skin punctures.

143. Correct Answer: 2

Rationale: A reduction in the respiratory rate is an adverse effect of the central nervous system depression caused by an opioid analgesic.

144. Correct Answer: 2

Rationale: Nesiritide is the synthetic form of endogenous human B-type natriuretic peptide, a substance released by the ventricles in response to fluid overload and increased ventricular pressure. This drug acts to decrease the preload to the heart.

145. Correct Answer: 3

Rationale: Drug metabolism is the pharmacokinetic process that would be altered in a patient with chronic alcoholism. Chronic exposure of the liver to alcohol would result in cellular damage that would affect drug metabolism.

146. Correct Answer: 4

Rationale: Anaphylaxis is a severe allergic response characterized by hypotension, bronchoconstriction, and edema of the glottis. Epinephrine is the treatment of choice for anaphylactic shock. Epinephrine acts to stimulate alpha- and beta-adrenergic receptors and to reverse the action of mediators released in the allergic response. The expected outcome from the administration of epinephrine would be an increase in blood pressure and bronchodilation.

147. Correct Answer: 4

Rationale: Cyclosporin acts by inhibiting calineurin, a substance that is needed to produce interleukin-2. Interleukin-2 is needed for the production of T cells. Cyclosporin suppresses the immune system response by inhibiting the production of interleukin-2.

148. Correct Answer: 2 tablets

Rationale: There is 1,000 micrograms in 1 milligram. The first step of the problem is to convert milligrams to micrograms: 0.1 mg × 1,000 mcg = 100 mcg. The nurse needs to administer 100 mcg. The drug is supplied in 50-mcg tablets. A proportion is set up where 50 mcg/1 tablet = 100 mcg/x tablets; x = 2 tablets.

149. Correct Answer: 2

Rationale: Levothyroxine is a synthetic preparation of the thyroid hormone thyroxine (T_4). Tremors, nervousness, and insomnia may indicate an overdose of the medication. The patient should be instructed to contact the prescriber if he or she experiences these symptoms.

150. Correct Answer: 1

Rationale: There currently is no evidence to support the use of estrogen to prevent heart disease. Evidence does, however, indicate that the drug may have adverse cardiovascular effects such as an increased risk for myocardial infarction.

SECTION I

SECTION II

SECTION III

SECTION IV

SECTION V

SECTION VI

SECTION VII

SECTION VIII

SECTION IX

SECTION X

151. Correct Answer: **2**

Rationale: Both sildenafil and nitrates can result in hypotension from action on the enzyme cyclic guanosine monophosphate. Taking the drugs in combination can result in life-threatening hypotension. The use of sildenafil in combination with nitrates is, therefore, contraindicated.

152. Correct Answer: **4**

Rationale: Vancomycin, linezolid, and dalfopristin/quinupristin are used for the treatment of methicillin-resistant *Staphylococcus aureus*.

153. Correct Answer: **4**

Rationale: A drug that is an agonist acts by binding with and activating a receptor site.

154. Correct Answer: **4**

Rationale: Oral hypoglycemic agents are used in patients with type 2 diabetes that is uncontrolled by dietary and/or activity modifications.

155. Correct Answer: **1**

Rationale: Degeneration of cholinergic neurons and the presence of neuritic plaques and neurofibrillary tangles are findings associated with Alzheimer's disease. Donepezil acts to prevent the breakdown of acetylcholine by acetylcholinesterase, thereby increasing the availability of acetylcholine at the cholinergic junction. Because of this increased acetylcholine availability, cholinergic transmission is enhanced.

156. Correct Answer: **2**

Rationale: A nephrotoxic agent is a substance that destroys the kidneys. An adverse effect of the administration of amphotericin, a drug used to treat systemic mycoses, is damage to the kidneys.

157. Correct Answer: **1**

Rationale: Fever is not always a clinical manifestation of infection. The treatment of fever of unknown origin with an antibiotic would be a potential misuse of the drug.

158. Correct Answer: **4**

Rationale: Oropharyngeal candidiasis and dysphonia result from the local deposit of inhaled glucocorticoids. These local deposits of medication suppress the immune response,

promote the development of candidiasis, and cause local edema in the oropharyngeal area, resulting in hoarseness and difficulty speaking.

159. Correct Answer: **1**

Rationale: Intravenous Cipro or Vibramycin is recommended as the initial treatment of a patient who has been infected with anthrax. Because of the potential for resistance noted with these organisms, one or two additional IV antibiotics should be included in the regimen.

REDUCTION OF RISK POTENTIAL

160. Correct Answer: **2**

Rationale: Metabolic syndrome X is a group of abnormalities characterized by abdominal obesity, elevated triglyceride levels, decreased high-density lipoprotein levels, elevated blood pressure, and elevated fasting glucose. The lab tests most likely to aid in the diagnosis of this syndrome are a fasting glucose and lipid profile.

161. Correct Answer: **1**

Rationale: A teratogen is any agent or factor that increases the potential for developmental abnormalities in a fetus. A patient in the first trimester of pregnancy would be at greatest risk for the development of a teratogenic effect of drug therapy. The first trimester is the period when internal organs and structures are established.

162. Correct Answer: **1**

Rationale: Continuous renal replacement therapy is a type of dialysis that is used when hemodialysis is not tolerated and peritoneal dialysis is not an option. Less extracorporeal circulation is needed with CRRT than with hemodialysis. The various forms of CRRT include continuous arteriovenous hemofiltration (CAVH) and continuous venoveno hemofiltration–dialysis (CVVH-D).

163. Correct Answer: **decerebrate posturing**

Rationale: Decerebrate posturing is a type of abnormal response associated with interruption of the motor tracts of the spinal cord at certain levels. It is characterized by rigid arms with the palms of the hands turned away from the body. There is plantar flexion of the feet, with the legs being stiffly extended.

164. Correct Answer: 3

Rationale: Early identification and treatment of a possible cause of pulseless electrical activity will promote the best outcome for the patient. Hyperkalemia can result in this dysrhythmia. Treatment with insulin will cause a shift of potassium into the cells and result in a temporary decrease in the potassium level. The administration of calcium will decrease the cardiac effects of a high serum potassium level.

165. Correct Answer: 2

Rationale: The priority intervention when a patient loses an artificial airway is to ensure that the airway is open and patent. Once the airway is maintained, supportive ventilation and oxygenation can be provided and preparation for reintubation done, if needed.

166. Correct Answer: 4

Rationale: The cerebral perfusion pressure (CPP) is the difference between the mean arterial blood pressure (MAP) and the intracranial pressure (ICP). It is calculated by subtracting the mean arterial pressure from the intracranial pressure: CPP = MAP – ICP. A normal CPP is in the range of 70 to 100 mm Hg. Brain ischemia can occur with a CPP between 50 to 70 mm Hg. A CPP of 39 mm Hg represents a significant decrease in cerebral perfusion and, if not treated promptly, can result in brain injury from ischemia.

167. Correct Answer: 2

Rationale: An ischemic, embolic stroke is the result of an embolus, from which there is an interruption of blood flow to an artery of the brain. Clot formation that occurs with atrial fibrillation is a factor associated with ischemic, embolic strokes. That is, a clot forms on the wall of the atria because of the disruption of blood flow caused by the dysrhythmia. If the clot breaks loose, it can travel to the brain, where it can lodge and disrupt blood flow. A 68-year-old patient with atrial fibrillation is the most likely candidate for the development of an ischemic, embolic stroke.

168. Correct Answer: 4

Rationale: A normal potassium level is 3.5 to 5.0 mEq/L. A patient with a potassium level of 6.2 mEq/L is hyperkalemic. Sodium polystyrene sulfonate (Kayexalate) is an exchange resin that is administered via an enteral route for patients with hyperkalemia. It promotes the absorption and removal of potassium from the body via the gastrointestinal tract.

169. Correct Answer: 25%

Rationale: Autosomal recessive disorders are manifested only when both members of the gene pair are affected (CC and cc are homozygous pairings of traits). In the example, both parents are carriers. The risk that they will have a child with sickle cell disease (cc) is 25% (1 in 4 chance).

170. Correct Answer: 50%

Rationale: The risk that their child will be a carrier of the disease (Cc) is 50% (2 in 4).

171. Correct Answer: 25%

Rationale: The chance that they will have a normal child (CC) is 25% (1 in 4).

172. Correct Answer: 2

Rationale: The development of amenorrhea, decreased breast size, and the loss of pubic hair in patients with anorexia nervosa are associated with a decreasing level of estrogen production associated with malnutrition.

173. Correct Answer: 2

Rationale: The Agency for Health Care Policy and Research identified the most reliable indicator of the existence and intensity of acute pain to be the patient's self-report.

174. Correct Answer: 3

Rationale: According to the NIH Consensus Development Panel on Impotence, erectile dysfunction is the inability to achieve and maintain an erection sufficient to permit satisfactory sexual intercourse. Risk factors for the development of erectile dysfunction include advancing age, hypertension, hyperlipidemia, cigarette smoking, diabetes mellitus, and pelvic irradiation. The 60-year-old patient with a 15-year history of uncontrolled diabetes is at the highest risk for the development of erectile dysfunction.

175. Correct Answer: 1

Rationale: Maintenance of muscle strength requires movement against resistance. The wasting away of muscle or a decrease in the size of muscle from prolonged bed rest would

SECTION I

SECTION II

SECTION III

SECTION IV

SECTION V

SECTION VI

SECTION VII

SECTION VIII

SECTION IX

SECTION X

be described as atrophy of a muscle. In conjunction with prolonged bed rest, skeletal muscles would undergo atrophy from lack of use.

176. Correct Answer: 3

Rationale: A contusion is an injury that does not result in the tearing of the skin, and may or may not produce a bruise.

177. Correct Answer: 3

Rationale: The electrolyte and acid–base imbalances associated with renal failure are hyperkalemia, hypocalcemia, and metabolic acidosis. Functions of a normal kidney include the elimination of potassium; the activation of vitamin D, which leads to the absorption of calcium from the gastrointestinal tract; and the elimination of hydrogen ions through a buffer system and the regeneration of bicarbonate. When the kidney is no longer able to perform these functions, the person experiences an accumulation of potassium in the blood (hyperkalemia), a reduction in serum calcium (hypocalcemia), and acidosis (metabolic acidosis) as a result of the increase in hydrogen ions and decreased buffer production.

178. Correct Answer: 3

Rationale: Type 2 diabetes results in hyperglycemia from a combination of insulin resistance and impaired insulin secretion by pancreatic beta cells. Type 2 diabetes has a slower onset than type 1 diabetes and is often asymptomatic owing to the gradual increase in blood sugar levels. This problem is often detected during routine medical visits. Because type 2 diabetes can result from insulin resistance as well as impaired insulin secretion, one of the best ways to manage glucose is to monitor blood sugar at home via the use of a glucometer.

179. Correct Answer: 33 mm Hg

Rationale: Mean arterial pressure = diastolic blood pressure – (pulse pressure/3).

CPP = MAP – ICP.

MAP = 60 + 40/3

MAP = 60 + 13 = 73

CPP = 73 – 40 = 33

180. Correct Answer: Abnormal

Rationale: The normal CPP range is 70 to 100 mm Hg. The finding of 33 mm Hg is abnormal. A CPP of 33 reflects a significant decrease in the perfusion pressure of the brain.

181. Correct Answer: 2

Rationale: A normal potassium level is in the range of 3.5 to 5.0 mEq/L. A patient with a potassium of 3.0 mEq/L is hypokalemic. Hypokalemia can result in excitability of cardiovascular, neuromuscular, and gastrointestinal function. The physician should be notified, and the need for potassium replacement discussed.

182. Correct Answer: 2

Rationale: The malnutrition associated with anorexia nervosa results in a decreased level of estrogen. Estrogens have an effect on bone mass and block the process of bone resorption. In patients with low estrogen levels, the rate of bone resorption may exceed the rate of bone deposition. Thus the anorectic patient is at risk for the development of osteoporosis, a problem characterized by low bone mass.

183. Correct Answer: 1

Rationale: Risk factors for the development of tuberculosis include being homeless, as these individuals often lack adequate health care, and immigration from regions (Southeast Asia, Africa, Latin America) where there is a high prevalence of the disease. Tuberculosis is spread by airborne transmission, after which the bacteria migrate to the alveoli. Clinical manifestations include fatigue, anorexia, fever, night sweats, and cough.

184. Correct Answer: 2

Rationale: The parathyroid glands are found on the posterior aspect of the thyroid gland. The parathyroid glands secrete parathyroid hormone in response to low serum calcium levels. A complication sometimes associated with thyroid surgery is injury to the parathyroid glands and a resulting disturbance in calcium metabolism, including a decreased response to low calcium levels and subsequent hypocalcemia. The clinical manifestations of hypocalcemia include facial spasm and hyperreflexia.

185. Correct Answer: **1**

Rationale: Pre-renal failure is caused by an alteration in renal blood flow that results in hypoperfusion. Excessive fluid loss caused by dehydration could result in decreased vascular volume, and a decrease in cardiac output, thereby decreasing renal perfusion and placing the patient at risk for pre-renal failure.

186. Correct Answer: **2**

Rationale: The findings of weight gain, peripheral edema, hypertension, and jugular neck vein distention are clinical manifestations associated with hypervolemia. Fluid retention and overload are complications associated with renal failure that result from the retention of sodium and water and disruption of the renin–angiotensin–aldosterone system.

187. Correct Answer: **Glasgow Coma Scale score = 11**

Rationale: The patient opens his eyes to noxious stimuli (score 2), localizes pain by attempting to remove the offending stimulus (score 5), and has confused conversation (score 4).

188. Correct Answer: **1**

Rationale: Typical sites for insulin injection include the upper arm, thigh, and abdomen. The injection site should be rotated to prevent lipodystrophy, an alteration in the deposition of subcutaneous fat that can occur at a site of insulin injection.

189. Correct Answer: **1**

Rationale: A normal platelet count is in the range of 150,000 to 400,000 µL. A patient whose platelet count is 34,000 µL is at risk for bleeding. To prevent this complication, sharp surfaces should be padded to avoid inadvertent trauma.

190. Correct Answer: **3**

Rationale: Thrombocytopenia is a decrease in the number of circulating platelets to a level less than 100,000 µL. This bleeding disorder is caused by the decreased ability to form a platelet plug due to decreased numbers of circulating platelets when a vessel is injured. Bleeding under the skin (ecchymosis) is a common clinical manifestation of thrombocytopenia.

191. Correct Answer: **2**

Rationale: Chemoreceptors monitor blood levels of oxygen and carbon dioxide. Central chemoreceptors in the medulla sense changes in carbon dioxide levels; peripheral chemoreceptors found in the carotid and aortic bodies sense arterial oxygen levels. Because of the chronically high levels of carbon dioxide found in the blood of patients with COPD, hypoxic stimulation of the peripheral chemoreceptors becomes the primary stimulus for ventilation in these patients. A sudden increase in serum oxygen levels can result in stimulation of the peripheral chemoreceptors and a decrease in respirations to the point of respiratory arrest.

192. Correct Answer: **4**

Rationale: A patient taking opioids should be monitored for a decrease in gastrointestinal motility and the development of constipation. Opioids act on the gastrointestinal tract by decreasing the muscle contractions that would otherwise propel the food bolus and inhibit the secretion of fluids into the intestinal lumen. Inhibition of these actions promotes the development of constipation.

PHYSIOLOGICAL ADAPTATION

193. Correct Answer: **3**

Rationale: Ulcerative colitis is a type of inflammatory bowel disease that affects primarily the rectum and colon. Diarrhea is a characteristic clinical manifestation of this disorder. The rationale for the NPO order for a patient with an acute exacerbation of ulcerative colitis is to promote the rest and healing of the bowel.

194. Correct Answer: **3**

Rationale: Diabetic ketoacidosis results from altered glucose and fat metabolism. It is characterized by hyperglycemia, production of ketoacids, hemoconcentration, acidosis, and coma. Diabetic ketoacidosis is an emergency condition that requires normalization of glucose and potassium levels, correction of acidosis, and replacement of fluids and sodium. The normalization of glucose levels is accomplished by the administration of intravenous regular insulin.

SECTION I
SECTION II
SECTION III
SECTION IV
SECTION V
SECTION VI
SECTION VII
SECTION VIII
SECTION IX
SECTION X

195. Correct Answer: 2

Rationale: Biliverdin is a component of red blood cell breakdown. In plasma, biliverdin is acted on to become free bilirubin. Hepatocytes in the liver conjugate bilirubin, which is then secreted from the liver as a component of bile. In fact, bilirubin gives bile its color. Bilirubin moves through the bile duct into the small intestine and is converted to urobilinogen by the normal intestinal microbes. Urobilinogen is then excreted in the feces or reabsorbed and returned to the liver. A clay-colored appearance of stool is indicative of a lack of bilirubin in the intestines.

196. Correct Answer: 3

Rationale: Microcytic, hypochromic cells are associated with iron-deficiency anemia. A patient with heavy menstrual cycles is at risk for an increased loss of iron. Normally, iron is recycled from old red blood cells. With heavy menstrual cycles, however, iron cannot be recycled and must be replenished via dietary means. If the iron is not replenished, the shortfall results in iron-deficiency anemia.

197. Correct Answer: 2

Rationale: The clinical manifestations of a ruptured cerebral aneurysm often present with the patient describing "the worst headache of my life." The headache is caused by meningeal irritation and the presence of blood in the cerebral spinal fluid.

198. Correct Answers: <u>neuritic plaques, neurofibrillary tangles</u>

Rationale: Neuritic plaques consist of a beta-amyloid core and remnants of dendrites and axons. Neurofibrillary tangles are twisted nerve cell fibers that form due to the presence of a faulty protein that normally maintains an orderly arrangement of the neural tubules. The two microscopic findings of neuritic plaques and neurofibrillary tangles are found on autopsy in patients with Alzheimer's disease. The changes associated with these findings result in cortical atrophy.

199. Correct Answer: 1

Rationale: A CD4 T-cell count is an indicator of immunodeficiency. Prophylaxis for opportunistic infections is recommended for any patient whose CD4 T-cell count is less than 200 cells/mm³. A patient with a CD4 T-cell count of 100 cells/mm³ would be at greatest risk for the development of an opportunistic infection.

200. Correct Answer: 1

Rationale: A sutured wound heals by primary intention. The primary intention of the intervention is the union of the edges of the wound, which is accomplished by suturing the wound. The wound heals without granulation.

201. Correct Answer: 2

Rationale: Actinic keratoses are pre-malignant skin lesions that develop on sun-exposed areas. These lesions appear as dry, brown, thickened, scaly areas on the outer layer of skin.

202. Correct Answer: 3

Rationale: Alzheimer's disease is a progressive disease characterized by three stages: early (first), confusional (second), and terminal (third). Short-term memory loss is a characteristic of the first (early) stage of the disease.

203. Correct Answer: 4

Rationale: Diabetes insipidus is a disorder caused by a deficiency or a decreased response to antidiuretic hormone. The affected individual is unable to concentrate urine during periods of water restriction. Clinical manifestations of the disorder include the excretion of copious amounts of dilute urine and excessive thirst. Urine output can be anywhere from 3 to 20 L in 24 hours.

204. Correct Answer: 1

Rationale: A normal serum pH is in the range of 7.35 to 7.45. This patient's blood gas pH is low and represents acidosis. The pCO_2 is elevated (normal pCO_2 is 35–45 mm Hg) and demonstrates hypercapnea. A normal PaO_2 is in the range of 75 to 100 mm Hg, so this patient's PaO_2 is considered low. The analysis of the blood gas information in conjunction with the clinical manifestations indicates acute respiratory distress with respiratory acidosis and hypoxemia.

205. Correct Answer: 2

Rationale: A superficial partial-thickness burn is characterized by reddened skin and a blistering wound that blanches with pressure. These wounds are also typically moist and weeping. Pain is associated with a superficial partial-thickness burn because the nerve endings within the skin are exposed and irritated by the loss of skin.

206. Correct Answer: **1**

Rationale: Edema (swelling of the ankles and feet) occurs with prolonged standing because of increased capillary filtration pressure. Prolonged standing results in an increase in venous hydrostatic pressure (the pushing force of fluid inside the capillaries).

207. Correct Answer: **1**

Rationale: Graves' disease is an autoimmune disorder that is caused by the stimulation and hypersecretion of thyroid hormone. Thyroid-stimulating immunoglobulins act on thyroid-stimulating hormone receptors to promote increased stimulation of the thyroid gland and hypersecretion of thyroid hormone.

208. Correct Answer: **Hemodialysis**

Rationale: Hemodialysis can provide the most rapid clearance of waste products from the blood as compared to other forms of dialysis.

209. Correct Answer: **Hemodialysis**

Rationale: Hemodialysis requires extracorporeal circulation of the blood. That is, blood is removed from the body, run through a filtering process, and then returned to the body. A hemodialysis access device such as an arteriovenous fistula or shunt is needed for blood removal and return in hemodialysis.

210. Correct Answer: **Peritoneal dialysis**

Rationale: Peritoneal dialysis can allow for more independence, such as greater flexibility when traveling and increased mobility, because it does not require use of a dialysis machine.

211. Correct Answer: **Peritoneal dialysis**

Rationale: Peritoneal dialysis requires monitoring of inflow, dwell, and drain times. That is, the dialysate solution is infused through a surgically implanted peritoneal catheter, allowed to dwell in the body for a prescribed period of time, and then drained.

212. Correct Answer: **2**

Rationale: Lactic acid is a product of the conversion of the cells to anaerobic metabolism. The accumulation of this acid reduces the body's pH and results in cellular damage.

213. Correct Answer: **2**

Rationale: A genotype is the genetic composition of an organism, which is determined by the combination and location of genes on the chromosome. Normally, humans have 22 pairs of autosomal chromosomes and 2 pairs of sex chromosomes, for a total of 24 chromosomal pairs. Down syndrome is a genetic problem characterized by an alteration in the number of chromosomes—namely, trisomy (the presence of three chromosomes rather than two) of chromosome 21.

214. Correct Answer: **2**

Rationale: Barbiturates act either by mimicking the action of the neurotransmitter gamma-aminobutyric acid (GABA) or by enhancing the inhibitory action of GABA. The outcome of their administration is central nervous system depression. The goal for the use of barbiturates is to induce coma in the management of increased intracranial pressure, thereby reducing the cellular metabolic rate. The induction of a comatose state through the administration of barbiturates is thought to reduce the metabolic requirements of the brain.

215. Correct Answer: **4**

Rationale: Cullen's sign is a bluish discoloration of the skin around the umbilicus. It is indicative of intraperitoneal or intra-abdominal hemorrhage, ectopic pregnancy that has ruptured, or acute hemorrhagic pancreatitis.

216. Correct Answer: **1**

Rationale: Heat stroke is the most serious form of heat-related emergency. It is characterized by failure of the body's thermoregulatory mechanisms. Hot, dry, ashen skin indicates that the sweat glands are not functioning and circulatory compromise is in process.

217. Correct Answer: **3**

Rationale: Bronchospasm and inflammation, which oftentimes occur in response to exposure to an allergen, result in an inflamed, constricted airway that obstructs air flow and ventilation.

218. Correct Answer: **3**

Rationale: Mononucleosis is a disorder caused by infection with the Epstein-Barr virus. The highest incidence of this disease is found in adolescents and young adults. The incubation

SECTION I

SECTION II

SECTION III

SECTION IV

SECTION V

SECTION VI

SECTION VII

SECTION VIII

SECTION IX

SECTION X

period for the virus is 4 to 8 weeks, after which the patient experiences a prodromal period characterized by fever, fatigue, and anorexia. The prodromal period is followed with pharyngitis and enlargement of the spleen and cervical, axillary, and groin lymph nodes.

219. Correct Answer: **4**

Rationale: Treatment modalities such as antibiotics and vaccines are available for many of the agents of bioterrorism. Ebola virus (hemorrhagic fever) has no known treatment.

220. Correct Answer: **1**

Rationale: A community-acquired infection begins outside the hospital, in the community. It can also be defined as an infection that is diagnosed within 48 hours of admission to the hospital in a person who has not resided in a long-term care facility for 14 or more days prior to the hospital admission.

221. Correct Answer: **3**

Rationale: Neutropenia is an abnormal decrease in the number of neutrophils. Neutrophils act to maintain normal host defenses against pathogens. A decrease in the number of neutrophils would predispose a patient to infection.

222. Correct Answer: **1**

Rationale: An endotracheal tube has been correctly placed when it is located approximately 3 to 4 centimeters above the carina. Verification of correct placement is done by auscultating the chest for equal bilateral breath sounds and observing for the symmetrical rise and fall of the chest with ventilation.

Math, Dosage Calculations, and Related Problems

MANAGEMENT OF CARE

Multiple Choice

1. To best manage care, you need to know when an intravenous fluid is scheduled to be completed and how long its infusion is supposed to last. Based on the following information, determine the infusion time in hours and the completion time in clock time: 1000 mL NS at 50 mL/h was hung at 0845 hours (8:45 A.M.).

1. Infusion time in hours = 50; completion time = 1045 (10:45 A.M.).
2. Infusion time in hours = 5; completion time = 1345 (1:45 P.M.).
3. Infusion time in hours = 10; completion time = 1845 (6:45 P.M.).
4. Infusion time in hours = 20; completion time = 0445 (4:45 A.M.).

2. Mr. Cooper is in the critical care unit and requires sedation for an emergency procedure. The prescription reads midazolam (Versed) 10 mcg/kg intravenous now. The patient weighs 220 pounds. How many micrograms of Versed do you give Mr. Cooper?

1. 22 mcg.
2. 1,000 mcg.
3. 100 mcg.
4. 2,200 mcg.

3. You are preparing to give Mr. Hamptou his Lopressor (metoprolol tartrate) 100 mg PO daily as prescribed. The pharmacy sends up Lipitor 50-mg tablets. How many tablets do you give to Mr. Hamptou?

1. 2 tablets.
2. ½ tablet.
3. None; the pharmacy sent up the wrong medication.
4. None; the prescription is for capsules and the pharmacy sent up tablets.

4. Prescription: Synthroid, generic name levothyroxine, 100 mcg PO daily.

50 mcg = 0.05 mg. The pharmacy sends up a 0.1-mg tablet of Synthroid. Is this the correct dose?

1. No, it should be 0.5 mg.
2. Yes, this is the correct dose.
3. Yes, but you should give one-half of the tablet daily.
4. No, you cannot convert micrograms to milligrams.

5. Prescription: Lamivudine 30 mg by mouth. Have: Lamivudine oral solution = 10 mg/mL. How much will you give?

1. 300 mL.
2. 30 mL.

3. 3.33 mL.

4. 3 mL.

Short Answer

6. Mrs. Wallace is scheduled to be discharged, and you need to teach her daughter about fluid replacement for her PEG tube. The prescription for fluid replacement is as follows: For every 100 mL of urine output, you replace it with 25 mL water through the NG tube every 4 hours. The patient's output over the last 4 hours was 500 mL. How much fluid replacement should Mrs. Wallace have now if her daughter calculated the replacement amount correctly?

Multiple Choice

7. Prescription: Indomethacin 20 mg by mouth every morning. Have: Indomethacin oral suspension = 25 mg/5 mL. How much Indomethacin will you give each morning?

1. 3 mL.

2. 4 mL.

3. 5 mL.

4. 100 mL.

8. Prescription: Valproic acid 400 mg by mouth now. Have: Valproic acid oral syrup = 250 mg/5 mL. How much valproic acid will you give?

1. 8 mL.

2. 3.125 mL.

3. 20 mL.

4. 5 mL.

9. Prescription: Albuterol 1.6 mg by mouth. Have: Albuterol oral syrup = 2 mg/5 mL. How much will you give?

1. 6 mL.

2. 5 mL.

3. 4 mL.

4. 3 mL.

Short Answer

10. To manage Mr. Urzan's care, you need to replace fluids via his PEG tube based on the prescription. The prescription is as follows: For every 100 mL of urine output, you replace it with 40 mL water through the PEG tube every 4 hours. The patient's output over the last 4 hours was 250 mL. How much fluid do you replace now?

Multiple Choice

11. Prescription: Amprenivir 450 mg by mouth. Have: Amprenivir 150-mg capsules. How many capsules of Amprenivir will you give?

1. 2 capsules.

2. 3 capsules.

3. 4 capsules.

4. 5 capsules.

12. Nine-year-old Peter is diagnosed with otitis media and receives the following prescription: Cefprozil oral suspension 350 mg by mouth. Have: Cefprozil oral suspension = 250 mg/5 mL. How much Cefprozil will you give?

1. 7 mL.

2. 5 mL.

3. 3.57 mL.

4. 120 mL.

13. Mrs. Jennings has herpes zoster due to immunosuppression as a result of chemotherapy given to treat her breast cancer. She receives the following prescription: Acyclovir 200 mg IV. Have: Acyclovir solution for IV infusion = 500 mg/10 mL. How much will you give?

1. 25 mL.

2. 4 mL.

3. 6 mL.

4. 70 mL.

Short Answer

14. You have received an order to give heparin 15,000 units subcutaneously. The computer screen indicates that you have three prefilled cartridges, each of which contains 10,000 units/mL. How many prefilled syringes should you take from the draw to be able to administer 15,000 units of heparin?

Multiple Choice

15. Mr. Markwood is diagnosed with severe adrenocortical insufficiency and is prescribed hydrocortisone sodium succinate (Solu-Cortef) 250 mg IV now. The pharmacy sends up multiple vials of Solu-Cortef intravenous solution 125 mg/2 mL. How much Solu-Cortef will you give?

1. 75 mL.

2. 187.5 mL.

3. 4 mL.

4. 2 mL.

Short Answer

16. Thioridazine (Mellaril) 100 mg is prescribed for your patient. Thioridazine 25-mg tablets are available. How many tablets will you administer?

Multiple Choice

17. Erica is seven years old and needs to be premedicated to prevent nausea from the chemotherapy that she is set to receive in 1 hour. The standing order reads as follows: Metaclopramide syrup 8 mg by mouth 1 hour prior to chemotherapy. The pharmacy sends up multiple containers of metaclopramide syrup 5 mg/5 mL. How much metaclopramide will you give 1 hour prior to chemotherapy?

   1. 40 mL.

   2. 8 mL.

   3. 3.125 mL.

   4. 5 mL.

18. Mr. Walberg has a history of seizures, and his laboratory work indicates that he has a therapeutic blood level of phenytoin. Therefore, the nurse practitioner prescribes the usual dose of phenytoin Mr. Walberg takes at home: phenytoin 75 mg orally by suspension every evening. The pharmacy sends up phenytoin 125 mg/5 mL. How much phenytoin will you give Mr. Walberg this evening?

   1. 7 mL.

   2. 8.33 mL.

   3. 2.5 mL.

   4. 3 mL.

19. Mrs. Corliss was in Mexico for vacation 3 months ago and has stomach complaints. She has just been diagnosed with intestinal amebiasis. The physician prescribes the following: erythromycin (Estolate suspension) 400 mg by mouth now. The pharmacy sends up Estolate suspension 250 mg/5 mL. How much Estolate suspension do you give now?

   1. 8 mL.

   2. 3.125 mL.

   3. 1.6 mL.

   4. 200 mL.

Short Answer

20. Clonazepam (Klonopin) 1.5 mg is prescribed for your patient. Clonazepam 0.5-mg tablets are available. How many tablets will you administer?

Multiple Choice

21. Mr. Johanson just arrived on the unit and is prescribed loracarbef (Lorabid) 400 mg orally now. The pharmacy dispenses Lorabid 200 mg/5 mL suspension. How much Lorabid do you give Mr. Johanson?

   1. 2.5 mL.

   2. 5 mL.

   3. 10 mL.

   4. 20 mL.

22. Mrs. Bailey says she cannot sleep without her sleeping pill. The nurse practitioner prescribes what Mrs. Bailey has been taking at home, which is lorazepam (Ativan) 1 mg orally every evening at bedtime. The pharmacy sends up scored 2-mg tablets of lorazepam. How much lorazepam do you give Mrs. Bailey tonight?

   1. 0.5 tablet.

   2. 1 tablet.

   3. 2 tablets.

   4. 4 tablets.

23. Mr. Doe comes into your clinic with an extreme case of poison ivy. He says the last time he had this problem, you gave him a "shot" that worked miracles. His medical records show that he received dexamethasone (Decadron) 10 mg IM, so you prescribe the same medication and dose. The pharmacy dispenses dexamethasone 4 mg/mL per vial. How many milliliters of Decadron do you draw up?

   1. 0.4 mL.

   2. 1.5 mL.

   3. 2 mL.

   4. 2.5 mL.

Short Answer

24. Potassium chloride 60 mEq is prescribed. You have potassium chloride in the form of 15 mEq/3 cc. How many milliliters of potassium chloride will you need to administer?

Multiple Choice

25. Ms. Turner is prescribed fluoxetine hydrochloride (Prozac) oral solution 10 mg orally daily in the morning by her psychiatric Clinical Nurse Specialist. The pharmacy sends up Prozac liquid 20 mg/5 mL. How much Prozac do you draw up to give Ms. Turner?

1. 4 mL.
2. 2 mL.
3. 2.5 mL.
4. 10 mL.

26. The physician prescribes phenobarbital elixir 60 mg PO now for the patient. The pharmacy dispenses a 120-mL bottle of phenobarbital elixir labeled 20 mg/5 mL. How much of the elixir should you administer to this patient?

1. 5 mL.
2. 15 mL.
3. 30 mL.
4. 1.2 mL.

27. Randy has an infection in his foot from a cut he received at the beach. His nurse practitioner prescribes cephalothin (Keflin) 0.5 g orally every 8 hours × 10 days. The pharmacist has dispensed Keflin in 250-mg capsules. How many capsules should you educate Randy to take every 8 hours?

1. 1 capsule.
2. 2 capsules.
3. 4 capsules.
4. 5 capsules.

28. Mr. Klingon is prescribed Demerol 150 mg intramuscularly as a preoperative medication. The pharmacy dispenses meperidine hydrochloride (Demerol) 100 mg/mL for IM use. How much Demerol do you draw up to administer?

1. 1.5 mL.
2. 2 mL.
3. 2.5 mL.
4. 0.66 mL.

29. Your patient in the intensive care unit has an infection that the culture and sensitivity indicate is sensitive to fluconazole (Diflucan). The physician prescribes 4 mg of fluconazole intravenously now. The pharmacy sends up multiple vials of fluconazole 2 mg/mL for IV infusion. How much Diflucan do you draw up in preparation for mixing the medication with the proper intravenous fluids per policy?

1. 0.5 mL.
2. 2 mL.
3. 3 mL.
4. 4 mL.

30. Ten-year-old Seraphima ate some peanuts about 5 minutes ago; she is allergic to nuts. She comes to the Emergency Department with hives. The nurse practitioner prescribes diphenhydramine hydrochloride (Benadryl) 25 mg intravenously now. The pharmacy dispenses a vial of Benadryl at 50 mg/mL for IM or IV use. How much Benadryl do you draw up to administer to Seraphima?

1. 0.5 mL.
2. 1 mL.
3. 0.75 mL.
4. 2 mL.

Short Answer

31. Haloperidol (Haldol) 1.5 mg orally is prescribed for your patient. Haloperidol 0.5 mg is available in tablet form. How many tablets of Haldol will you administer?

Multiple Choice

32. Daniel is a 9-year-old patient who has broken his ankle while playing football. He is prescribed atropine sulfate 0.2 mg IV as a preoperative medication. The pharmacy dispenses a vial of atropine sulfate 0.4 mg/mL. How much atropine do you draw up to give Daniel preoperatively?

1. 0.25 mL.
2. 0.5 mL.
3. 2 mL.
4. 0.8 mL.

33. Mr. Cooper is prescribed midazolam HCl (Versed) 3 mg intramuscularly 30 minutes prior to colonoscopy. The pharmacy dispenses a multidose vial of Versed 1 mg/mL. How many milliliters do you draw up to give Mr. Cooper?

1. 1 mL.
2. 2 mL.
3. 3 mL.
4. 4 mL.

Short Answer

34. Thioridazine (Mellaril) 75 mg is prescribed for your patient. Thioridazine 25-mg tablets are available. How many tablets of Mellaril will you administer?

Multiple Choice

35. Mrs. Skiba has developed heart failure and is prescribed Lanoxin (digoxin) 250 mcg IV push now. The pharmacy dispenses digoxin 500 mcg/2 mL. How much digoxin do you administer?

1. 0.25 mL.
2. 0.5 mL.
3. 1 mL.
4. 4 mL.

36. Ms. Calugar has severe nausea related to a stomach virus. The physician in the Emergency Department prescribes cimetidine (Tagamet) 300 mg IM now. The pharmacy sends up vials of Tagamet 300 mg/2 mL for IM use. How much Tagamet do you draw up to give Ms. Calugar?

1. 0.75 mL.
2. 0.5 mL.
3. 1 mL.
4. 2 mL.

Short Answer

37. Mr. Ellis comes to the Emergency Department in heart failure, and his physician prescribes furosemide (Lasix) IV 40 mg now. The pharmacy sends up a multidose vial of Lasix 10 mg/mL. How many milliliters of furosemide do you draw up?

Multiple Choice

38. Mr. Holden is prescribed Fragmin (dalteparin sodium) 7,500 units SC daily for 5 days. The pharmacy dispenses Fragmin 5,000 units/0.2 mL. How much Fragmin do you draw up per day?

1. 0.2 mL.
2. 0.3 mL.
3. 0.75 mL.
4. 1.5 mL.

39. Mrs. Fowler is prescribed Kenalog (triamcinolone) 60 mg IM × 1. The pharmacy dispenses Kenalog 40 mg/mL for intramuscular use. How much Kenalog do you draw up to administer?

1. 1.5 mL.
2. 0.75 mL.
3. 2 mL.
4. 3.5 mL.

Short Answer

40. Mr. Prohorik comes into the Emergency Department with a broken tibia that is a compound fracture. He is in extreme pain, and his blood pressure is somewhat high. The physician prescribes meperidine hydrochloride (Demerol) 150 mg IM now for pain. The pharmacy sends up a multidose vial of Demerol 75 mg/mL. How much Demerol do you draw up now to give Mr. Prohorik?

Multiple Choice

41. Mr. Havens comes to the Emergency Department with intractable hiccups lasting for 2 days. The physician prescribes chlorpromazine (Thorazine) 50 mg IM now. The pharmacy dispenses vials of Thorazine 25 mg/mL for IM use. How much medication do you draw up?

1. 1 mL.
2. 2 mL.
3. 3 mL.
4. 4 mL.

42. Your patient needs anticoagulation therapy, and the physician prescribes heparin sodium injection of 12,500 units SC now. The pharmacy sends up vials of heparin sodium 5,000 units/mL for subcutaneous injection. How much heparin sodium do you draw up?

1. 0.4 mL.
2. 2 mL.
3. 2.5 mL.
4. 5 mL.

43. Your patient is 10 days post-chemotherapy and is prescribed epoetin alfa (Procrit) 12,000 units SC three times per week. The pharmacy dispenses a vial of Procrit 20,000 units/mL. How much epoetin alfa do you draw up for each dose?

1. 1.66 mL.
2. 0.6 mL.
3. 2 mL.
4. 0.8 mL.

44. To keep Ms. Grimmitt's cardiac output within normal range, she must receive Lanoxin (digoxin) 750 mcg intravenously daily. The medication strength received from pharmacy is Lanoxin 500 mcg/2 mL. How much Lanoxin do you draw up daily to give Ms. Grimmitt?

1. 5 mL.
2. 0.33 mL.
3. 1.33 mL.
4. 3 mL.

SAFETY AND INFECTION CONTROL

Multiple Choice

45. You must administer 1 unit of regular insulin for every 8 g of carbohydrates consumed. Carbohydrates consumed = 10 g + 7 g + 17 g + 6 g. What is the total amount of insulin you will administer?

1. 4 units.
2. 5 units.
3. 3 units.
4. 50 units.

46. Allowing an IV solution to run dry may result in loss of IV access due to catheter occlusion. Therefore, you need to determine when an intravenous infusion should be totally complete. Based on the information below, what time should the infusion be completed?

> Prescription: Infuse D_5 ½ NS 1,000 mL IV at 125 mL until taking PO fluids.
>
> You have a 1,000-mL bag of D_5 ½ NS and you hang the bag at 0800 hours (8 A.M.).

1. 2400 hours (12:00 midnight).
2. 1600 hours (4:00 P.M.).
3. 1400 hours (2:00 P.M.).
4. 1200 hours (12:00 noon).

47. Based on safety as a rationale, 1 unit of packed red blood cells should run in completely between 2 and 4 hours according to your hospital policy. The nurse from whom you are receiving report states that she set the 1 unit of packed cells (250 mL) to run at 80 mL/h and hung it at 1400 hours (2:00 P.M.). Based on your calculations, how long should it take the complete unit to be administered and is this time frame according to hospital policy time frame?

1. Complete infusion time should be 3.1 hours, which is within the 2- to 4-hour time range.
2. Complete infusion time should be 6 hours, which is not within the 2- to 4-hour time range.
3. Complete infusion time should be 2.4 hours, which is within the 2- to 4-hour time range.
4. Complete infusion time should be 4.1 hours, which is within the 2- to 4-hour time range.

True or False

48. A prescription of 11 units regular and 20 units NPH insulin SC every A.M. can be mixed so that both insulins are contained in one insulin syringe.

Multiple Choice

49. Your patient, Mrs. Sullivan, needs a bolus of heparin at 80 units/kg intravenously. You ask your colleague to determine the dose based on the patient's weight of 94 kg, as you want to compare your calculation result to that made by your colleague. How many units of heparin should you administer?

1. 752 units.
2. 7,520 units.
3. 7,220 units.
4. 3,442 units.

Short Answer

Reading a medication label correctly is essential to safety in patient care. Read the label below and answer the two questions that follow:

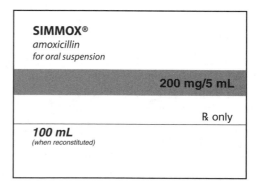

50. What is the generic name of this medication?

51. What is the dose strength of this medication?

52. Determine the total number of units of insulin to be drawn up from the following prescription: 4 units of regular insulin plus 32 units NPH insulin.

Multiple Choice

53. Five-year-old Johnny has an order for Tylenol (acetaminophen) liquid 128 mg for fever of more than 100°F. His temperature is currently 100.4°F. The pharmacy sends up Tylenol oral solution at a dose strength of 160 mg/5 mL. How much Tylenol do you give Johnny?

1. 6.25 mL.
2. 4096 mL.
3. 4 mL.
4. 31.25 mL.

54. Karen is a 9-year-old patient with a diagnosis of fever who has been prescribed Cleocin (clindamycin palmitrate hydrochloride) 150 mg orally daily. The pharmacy sends up Cleocin oral solution at a dose strength of 75 mg/5 mL. How much medication do you give Karen?

1. 2 mL.
2. 150 mL.
3. 2.5 mL.
4. 10 mL.

55. Your patient has a discharge prescription for methotrexate 2.5 mg orally twice a day × 20 tablets. Your patient asks you how many days in total she should take her medication. What do you tell her?

1. 10 days.
2. 20 days.
3. 8 days.
4. 50 days.

56. Medication labels often indicate that two medications are mixed into one tablet. If the medication label reads "amoxicillin and clavulanate potassium tablets 500 mg/125 mg," how many milligrams of amoxicillin would be in 2 tablets?

1. 4 mg.
2. 8 mg.
3. 1,000 mg.
4. 250 mg.

Short Answer

57. To be cost-effective and more accurate, you need to use the correct unit size of insulin syringe. Which syringe would be ideal to administer a dose of 18 units of regular insulin plus 14 units of NPH if your three choices of syringe sizes are 100 units, 50 units, and 30 units?

Multiple Choice

58. The nurse practitioner prescribes 10 mg ondansetron hydrochloride dehydrate every 12 hours orally. The pharmacy sends up Zofran (ondansetron hydrochloride) 8 mg. The package insert from the pharmaceutical company states that each tablet contains 10 mg of ondansetron hydrochloride dehydrate, which is equivalent to 8 mg of Zofran. It is time to give your patient the first dose of the prescribed medication. How many Zofran tablets do you give?

1. None.
2. 1 tablet.
3. 1.25 tablets.
4. 2 tablets.

59. Twelve-year-old Jonathon has an infection. He is prescribed 75 mg of Vibramycin (doxycycline monohydrate) orally daily. The bottle from the local pharmacy reads "raspberry-flavored Vibramycin 25 mg/5 mL." Jonathon's mother, who is a nurse, left to go to work early and forgot to give Jonathon his medication. When she called home, her husband said, "Don't worry. I gave Jonathon 10 mL of his medicine." What should the mother instruct the husband to do?

1. Thank him for giving Jonathon his medicine.
2. Tell him to give Jonathon another 10 mL of the medicine.
3. Tell him to give Jonathon another 5 mL of the medicine.
4. Tell him to call 9-1-1 as he has overdosed Jonathon.

60. Six-year-old Helen comes into the pediatric nurse clinic complaining of ear pain. According to her mother, she keeps pulling on her ear. The nurse practitioner diagnoses otitis media and prescribes an antibiotic for Helen's ear infection. Which of the following words would you find written on this prescription?

1. Optic.
2. Topical.
3. Otic.
4. Intradermal.

61. Prior to administering a vaginal suppository to a female patient, you should have the patient

1. Void.
2. Defecate.
3. Do 3 sit-ups.
4. Lie on her stomach.

Short Answer

62. Based on the anatomy of the sigmoid colon, which body position is best for a patient to receive an enema?

63. After the administration of a vaginal cream, the patient should remain in which body position for 5 to 10 minutes to aid in absorption and to prevent gravity drainage?

64. Prior to administering a medication, what should you do first: check the prescription or wash your hands?

65. Why should you not shave the area where you plan to place a transdermal patch?

66. To safely administer intravenous medications, you need to be able to determine the rate of infusion. Mr. Holiday is prescribed 500 mg Vancomycin IV every 12 hours. The pharmacy sends up the medication mixed in 500 mL of normal saline with a total infusion time of 2 hours. What is the infusion rate in milliliters per hour?

HEALTH PROMOTION AND MAINTENANCE

Short Answer

67. Determine the total number of units of insulin to be drawn up from the following prescription, which Mr. Cruz receives every morning: 17 units regular plus 24 units NPH insulin.

Multiple Choice

68. Mr. Rolliou needs to have his heparin adjusted daily based on the results of his PTT lab test to maintain proper coagulation. The physician writes the following prescription: Adjust IV heparin daily based on PTT results and use the sliding scale below:

> PTT < 35: Give 80 units/kg bolus.
>
> PTT 35–45: Give 40 units/kg bolus.
>
> PTT 46–70: No change.
>
> PTT > 70: Call the physician immediately.

Mr. Rolliou's PTT result came back as 44. What is your intervention?

1. Do nothing; give him no heparin.
2. Call the physician immediately.
3. Give an 80 units/kg bolus now.
4. Give a 40 units/kg bolus now.

69. Prior to her hospital discharge, your patient brings you the prescription the nurse practitioner has written out, which reads, "Tolterodine tartrate (Detrol) extended release 4 mg PO QD in A.M." The patient asks you how many pills per day she should take and how often should she take them. You call the pharmacy, and the pharmacist states that the Detrol will be dispensed in 4-mg tablets. What is your response to the patient?

1. Take 1 tablet every morning.
2. Take 2 tablets every morning.
3. Take 1 tablet in the morning and 1 tablet in the evening every day.
4. Take 1 tablet every other day.

70. Your patient, Mr. Lawrence, has been prescribed Mucinex (guaifenesin) 300 mg orally daily as part of his treatment for bronchitis. The pharmacy sends up Mucinex 600-mg extended-release tablets. How many tablets do you give Mr. Lawrence?

1. None.
2. 0.5 tablet.
3. 1 tablet.
4. 2 tablets.

71. For Mrs. Kolanowski to keep her serum potassium within normal limits, she needs to take KCl (potassium chloride) 40 mEq orally daily. Her pharmacist has dispensed KCl tablets, each of which contains 10 mEq of KCl medication. How many tablets per day should Mrs. Kolanowski take?

1. 2 tablets.
2. 3 tablets.
3. 4 tablets.
4. 5 tablets.

Short Answer

72. To maintain adequate hydration for Mrs. Collins, you need to replace fluids through her PEG tube based on the following prescription: For every 300 mL of urine output, replace 50 mL of water through the PEG tube every 4 hours. The patient's output over the last 4 hours was 1,800 mL. How many milliliters of fluid do you replace now?

Multiple Choice

73. Mr. Whitney takes Captopril 12.5 mg orally daily to maintain his blood pressure around 120/80 mm Hg. He tells you that he has a new pharmacist and the pills "look different." The pill bottle states that it contains "Captopril 25 mg tablets." How many tablets should Mr. Whitney take per day?

1. 0.5 tablet.
2. 1 tablet.
3. 2 tablets.
4. 4 tablets.

74. Mrs. Flanceski is prescribed digoxin 0.25 mg orally daily. The pharmacy dispenses her prescription using digoxin 0.125-mg tablets. How many tablets should Mrs. Flanceski take per day?

1. 0.5 tablet.
2. 1 tablet.
3. 2 tablets.
4. 4 tablets.

75. Mrs. Hopi keeps her type 2 diabetes under control by taking metformin (Glucophage) 1 g orally daily. Her pharmacist dispenses metformin in 250-mg tablets because they are easier to swallow. How many tablets should Mrs. Hopi take per day?

1. 1 tablet.
2. 2 tablets.
3. 3 tablets.
4. 4 tablets.

Short Answer

76. To prevent aspiration from surgery, Ms. Cates may have up to 1,000 mL oral fluids until 0000 (12 midnight); then she is to be NPO. It is 1600 (4:00 P.M.), and she has already consumed 500 mL. How many more milliliters can she have before she has to be NPO?

Multiple Choice

77. Ms. Oglethorpe is post-cholecystectomy and has gas and bloating. You contact the nurse practitioner on call and receive a prescription for simethicone 100 mg now. The pharmacy sends up a simethicone suspension that is labeled 40 mg/2 mL. How much suspension do you pour to administer to Ms. Oglethorpe?

1. 1.25 mL.
2. 5 mL.

3. 2,000 mL.
4. 0.2 mL.

78. Mr. Smith's blood sugar has not stabilized, so the physician decides to add glyburide to his medication regimen to control the blood sugar. The new medication comes as a combination of glyburide and metformin (2.5 mg/500 mg). The physician states that you should give Mr. Smith the amount of glyburide that matches his 1 g of metformin per day. How many milligrams per day of glyburide will he receive in this new combination medication?

1. 2.5 mg.
2. 5 mg.
3. 7.5 mg.
4. 1,000 mg.

79. Mrs. Raphael is scheduled to begin her maintenance dose of an antidepressant, specifically, a selective serotonin reuptake inhibitor. She prefers a liquid to a pill. Paroxetine 30 mg orally every morning is prescribed. The paroxetine suspension is packaged as 10 mg/5 mL. How many milliliters will you administer every morning?

1. 3 mL.
2. 5 mL.
3. 60 mL.
4. 15 mL.

80. Ms. Thompson has Graves' disease and is prescribed methimazole 7.5 mg orally every morning. Her pharmacist fills the prescription with methimazole 5-mg tablets. How many tablets do you tell Ms. Thompson to take every morning?

1. 1.5 tablets.
2. 3 tablets.
3. 0.75 tablet.
4. 0.66 tablet.

81. Mr. Rollins is a known alcoholic who is brought to the Emergency Department by the police. He has severe ascites from his chronic alcoholism, and the physician prescribes spironolactone 50 mg orally now. The pharmacy dispenses spironolactone 25-mg tablets. How many tablets do you give Mr. Rollins?

1. 0.5 tablet.
2. 1 tablet.
3. 2 tablets.
4. 4 tablets.

SECTION I

SECTION II

SECTION III

SECTION IV

SECTION V

SECTION VI

SECTION VII

SECTION VIII

SECTION IX

SECTION X

Short Answer

82. To maintain adequate hydration, Mrs. Wallace is receiving NS (0.9% normal saline) intravenously at 200 mL/h after her surgery. How many hours will it take for 1,000 mL of NS to infuse at this rate?

Multiple Choice

83. To relieve Mrs. Bailey's bilateral leg edema due to heart failure, the physician prescribes furosemide (Lasix) 80 mg intravenously now. The pharmacy sends up multiple vials of furosemide 40 mg/mL for intravenous use. How many milliliters of furosemide do you draw up now?

1. 1 mL.
2. 2 mL.
3. 0.5 mL.
4. 20 mL.

84. To maintain adequate kidney function, your renal failure patient, Mr. Borick, is on fluid restriction. Specifically, his oral fluid intake is restricted to 1,200 mL/day. You note that Mr. Borick has ingested 300 mL over the 11:00 to 7:00 shift. How much oral intake can he have over the next 16 hours?

1. 600 mL.
2. 1,500 mL.
3. 900 mL.
4. 400 mL.

85. Mr. Boyle is postoperative day 2 from repair of a compound leg fracture. On nurse-to-nurse report, you are told he is 56 years old, has a low pain tolerance, is demanding, and is allergic to Tylenol (acetaminophen). His patient-controlled analgesia (PCA) medication has just been discontinued, and he has been prescribed oxycodone with acetaminophen (Percocet 5/325) 1–2 tablets orally every 4 to 6 hours as needed for pain. Mr. Boyle calls the nurses' desk and asks, "Can my new nurse give me whatever I can have the most of for pain? I am really hurting." What is your next action?

1. Give Mr. Boyle 2 oxycodone tablets.
2. Give Mr. Boyle 1 oxycodone tablet and reevaluate his pain in 30 minutes.
3. Call the physician for a new prescription for pain control.
4. Share with Mr. Boyle that he should try watching television as distraction and to call back in 15 minutes if he is still having pain.

86. To maintain adequate hydration initially in your patient who is burned, you need to use a formula like the following:

Parkland formula = 4 mL/kg × %BSA burn for milliliters of fluid over 24 hours

Your patient weighs 77 kg and the % BSA (percent body surface area) burned is 35. How many milliliters of fluid should you give the patient over the next 24 hours?

1. 1.8 mL.
2. 108 mL.
3. 10,780 mL.
4. 23,716 mL.

PSYCHOSOCIAL INTEGRITY

Multiple Choice

87. Smoking cigarettes often increases the metabolism of some psychiatric medications. If this is true, then how should the medication dose be adjusted?

1. Decrease the dose.
2. Increase the dose.
3. Administer the entire dose of medication in the morning.
4. Administer the entire dose of medication at bedtime.

88. Mr. Yeh is manic depressive and is being treated with lithium carbonate (Eskalith) for this condition. He is also anxious and has been prescribed diazepam (Valium). These two medications can interact and cause hypothermia as a side effect. To assess for this potential side effect, what would you ask the patient?

1. "Have you been feeling dizzy?"
2. "Do you have a skin rash anywhere on your body?"
3. "Have you been going to the bathroom a lot?"
4. "Have you been feeling cold?"

89. Mrs. Allison is being treated with olanzapine (Zyprexa) 7.5 mg daily orally for her schizophrenia. The pharmacy dispenses Zyprexa 2.5-mg tablets. How many tablets do you give Mrs. Allison daily?

1. 2 tablets.
2. 3 tablets.
3. 4 tablets.
4. 6 tablets.

90. Mr. Collins is receiving aripiprazole 15 mg orally daily. The pharmacy dispenses aripiprazole 15-mg tablets. How many tablets do you give Mr. Collins daily?

1. 0.5 tablet.
2. 1 tablet.
3. 2 tablets.
4. 3 tablets.

Identification

91. Mr. Williamson is being treated for depression with imipramine hydrochloride (Tofranil) 200 mg orally as a total daily dose; half of the dose is taken in the morning and half of the dose is taken in the evening. The pharmacist dispenses Tofranil in 25-mg tablets. How many tablets do you give Mr. Williamson in the morning?

Multiple Choice

92. Ms. Fluoski is prescribed fluoxetine hydrochloride (Prozac) 30 mg orally daily. The pharmacy dispenses 10-mg capsules of Prozac. How many capsules do you educate Ms. Fluoski to take daily?

1. 1 capsule.
2. 2 capsules.
3. 3 capsules.
4. 5 capsules.

93. Mr. Mohammed is being treated with buspirone hydrochloride (BuSpar) for anxiety. He is prescribed BuSpar 5 mg twice a day, once in the morning and once in the evening. The pharmacy dispenses 10-mg scored tablets. How many tablets of BuSpar do you administer to Mr. Muhammed in the morning?

1. 0.5 tablet.
2. 1 tablet.
3. 2 tablets.
4. 4 tablets.

94. Mr. Lordin is prescribed valproic acid (Depakene) 750 mg orally every morning for treatment of his bipolar disorder. The pharmacy dispenses valproic acid 250-mg capsules. How many capsules do you give Mr. Lordin every morning?

1. 2 capsules.
2. 3 capsules.
3. 6 capsules.

4. 8 capsules.

Fill in the Blank

95. Mrs. Peabody has been taking a tricyclic antidepressant for the last few days and experiences dizziness upon getting out of a chair or bed. When her physician assesses her blood pressure while Mrs. Peabody is standing and sitting, her blood pressure is much lower when she stands up. This medication side effect on blood pressure is called _____ hypotension.

Multiple Choice

96. Mrs. Washington is prescribed chlordiazepoxide (Librium) 200 mg orally now for treatment of alcohol withdrawal. The pharmacy dispenses Librium 25-mg tablets. How many tablets of Librium do you give Mrs. Washington now?

1. 2 tablets.
2. 3 tablets.
3. 4 tablets.
4. 8 tablets.

97. Mrs. McCormick has acute psychosis and is being treated with chlorpromazine hydrochloride (Thorazine) 10 mg four times per day. What is her total daily dose of Thorazine?

1. 20 mg.
2. 30 mg.
3. 40 mg.
4. 60 mg.

98. Mr. White has been taking risperidone (Risperdal) for treatment of his schizophrenia. He receives 2 mg of Risperdal in the morning and 3 mg in the evening. What is the total dose of Risperdal that Mr. White receives daily?

1. 1.5 mg.
2. 4 mg.
3. 7 mg.
4. 5 mg.

Short Answer

99. Your patient has a tendency to experience gastric irritation from taking medications. What might you suggest that the patient take with the medication so that it will cause less gastric irritation?

 SECTION I
 SECTION II
 SECTION III
 SECTION IV
 SECTION V
 SECTION VI
 SECTION VII
 SECTION VIII
 SECTION IX

Multiple Choice

100. Mr. Merriweather has his psychosis treated with trifluoperazine (Stelazine) 2-mg tablets orally daily. Pharmacy dispenses trifluridine (Viroptic 1%). How many tablets do you administer daily?

1. None.
2. 1 tablet.
3. 0.5 tablet.
4. 2 tablets.

101. Charlie Eagle is a 38-year-old Native American who is being treated with haloperidol (Haldol) 1.5 mg orally twice per day for schizophrenia. His pharmacist dispenses Haldol as 1-mg tablets. How many tablets should Mr. Eagle take in the morning?

1. 0.5 tablet.
2. 1.5 tablets.
3. 3 tablets.
4. 6 tablets.

102. Ms. Gszewski is prescribed amitriptyline hydrochloride (Elavil) 150 mg orally at bedtime daily to treat her depression. The pharmacist dispenses 75-mg tablets of Elavil. How many tablets should Ms. Gszewski take at bedtime?

1. 2 tablets.
2. 3 tablets.
3. 4 tablets.
4. 0.5 tablet.

103. Mr. Lazarus is being treated for anxiety with clorazepate dipotassium (Tranxene) 22.5 mg orally every morning. The pharmacy dispenses Tranxene 7.5-mg tablets. How many tablets should Mr. Lazarus take every morning?

1. 2 tablets.
2. 3 tablets.
3. 5 tablets.
4. 6 tablets.

104. Mr. Johnson is prescribed 200 mg daily of desipramine hydrochloride (Norpramin) for treatment of cocaine withdrawal. The pharmacy dispenses 100-mg Norpramin tablets. How many tablets do you administer to Mr. Johnson daily?

1. None.
2. 0.5 tablet.
3. 1 tablet.
4. 2 tablets.

Short Answer

105. Your patient complains of insomnia as a side effect of his medication. When would be a good time to administer the medication to try to prevent this side effect?

Multiple Choice

106. Mr. Alfred is clinically depressed, and his physician has recently prescribed nefazodone hydrochloride (Serzone) 300 mg daily orally for his depression. The pharmacy dispenses 150-mg tablets. How many tablets of Serzone should Mr. Alfred take daily?

1. 0.5 tablet.
2. 2 tablets.
3. 4 tablets.
4. 10 tablets.

BASIC CARE AND COMFORT

Multiple Choice

107. It is 10 o'clock in the morning. Mrs. Hoppi has a STAT blood sugar drawn, and the results are 272 mg/dL. The advanced nurse practitioner prescribes 5 units regular plus 8 units NPH insulin now. What is the total number of units of insulin you need to draw up?

1. 12 units.
2. 19 units.
3. 13 units.
4. 14 units.

108. Mrs. Carrolowitz has the following prescription for pain: Tylenol 650 mg PO every 4 hours for pain. What is the maximum dose in milligrams that the patient can receive in a 24-hour period of time?

1. 1,300 mg.
2. 2,600 mg.
3. 1,950 mg.
4. 3,900 mg.

109. When Mr. Frances visits your clinic, his blood pressure is 168/102 mm Hg. He says he has not taken his pills in days because he ran out of them. You look at his medication bottle, which is empty, and see that the physician prescribed atenolol (Tenormin) 50 mg by mouth each morning. The nurse has samples of atenolol 25-mg tablets to dispense to the patient. How many tablets should the patient be instructed to take each morning?

1. 0.5 tablet.
2. 1 tablet.
3. 2 tablets.
4. 4 tablets.

110. Mr. Cortez is seen in the clinic post myocardial infarction and has slight pitting edema of the legs bilaterally. The physician prescribes hydrochloro-thiazide (HydroDiurel) 12.5 mg to be given orally now. The clinic stocks hydrochlorothiazide 25-mg tablets. How many tablets should the nurse give?

1. 0.05 tablet.
2. 0.5 tablet.
3. 1 tablet.
4. 1.5 tablets.

111. Mrs. Harrington arrives in the Emergency Room with shortness of breath and edema. The physician prescribes a bolus of furosemide (Lasix) 100 mg IV push to be given STAT. The available vials are labeled "Furosemide 40 mg/2 mL." How many milliliters of Lasix will the nurse give?

1. 2 mL.
2. 3 mL.
3. 5 mL.
4. 10 mL.

112. Tony Giampitruzzi broke his right tibia playing football and is now postoperative day 1. He is prescribed morphine sulfate 6 mg slow IV push for moderate to severe pain every 6 hours. Tony says his pain is "8" on a 1–10 scale. The nurse has available morphine sulfate 2 mg/mL for intra-venous use. How many milliliters of morphine should the nurse administer?

1. 2 mL.
2. 3 mL.
3. 4 mL.
4. 0.33 mL.

113. Ms. Wallace complains of nausea after receiving her pain tablets. The physician prescribes promethazine hydrochloride (Phenergan) 12.5 mg to be given intramuscularly for nausea now. The pharmacy sends up a vial of Phenergan 25 mg/mL for IM use.

How many milliliters of Phenergan should the nurse administer?

1. 0.5 mL.
2. 1 mL.
3. 2 mL.
4. 4 mL.

Identification

114. To make 5-year-old Jonathon comfortable, the physician has prescribed furosemide (Lasix) 140 mg now IV. You know the maximum dosing for this drug is 6 mg/kg/day. Jonathon weighs 22 kg. Is the dosage prescribed lower than the maximum dose allowed?

Multiple Choice

115. Mrs. Smith has taken twice the recommended dose of her blood pressure pills by mistake. She comes into the Emergency Department with a blood pressure of 70/40 mm Hg. To treat the hypotension, the advanced practice nurse prescribes a 500-mL NS bolus to run in over 30 minutes. How many milliliters per hour should the pump be programmed to deliver?

1. 500 mL/h.
2. 1,000 mL/h.
3. 16.66 mL/h.
4. 250 mL/h.

Short Answer

116. Ellie is 10 years old and having pain associated with her broken leg. The physician prescribes meperidine (Demerol) 40 mg IM now. The pharmacy sends up Demerol in one tube labeled 50 mg/mL for intramuscular use. How much Demerol will you give?

Multiple Choice

117. When Mr. Skiba's serum electrolytes come back, the results indicate he is becoming hypo-kalemic. The physician orders KCl elixir 40 mEq orally twice a day, to be given with his breakfast and evening meals. The concentration pharmacy dispenses is 20 mEq KCl/10 mL. How many milliliters of KCl elixir will the patient receive in the morning?

1. 2 mL.
2. 5 mL.
3. 10 mL.
4. 20 mL.

118. After surgery, Mr. Collins requires a bolus of heparin. The nurse receives a written prescription from the surgeon for a heparin 5,000-unit bolus subcutaneously now. The heparin is dispensed in a vial with a concentration of 5,000 units/mL. How many milliliters should the nurse administer for the bolus?

1. 0.1 mL.
2. 0.5 mL.
3. 0.8 mL.
4. 1 mL.

Short Answer

119. Six-year-old Nancy has a fever and is prescribed acetaminophen (Tylenol) 150 mg orally every 6 hours. The maximum medication dosing for this drug is 10 mg/kg every 6 hours. Nancy weighs 25 kg. Is the prescribed amount less than the maximum dose?

Multiple Choice

120. A 36-year-old patient, who is postoperative from a colectomy related to a gunshot wound, reports feeling anxious and asks the nurse if he is having a heart attack. The nurse reports the patient's increasing anxiety level to the physician, who prescribes alprazolam (Xanax) 0.25 mg to be given by mouth. The alprazolam is available in tablets each labeled 0.5 mg. How many tablets should the nurse administer?

1. 0.5 tablet.
2. 1 tablet.
3. 2 tablets.
4. 4 tablets.

121. Mr. Williamson has just converted back to NSR (normal sinus rhythm) after being on a nitroglycerin drip. The physician prescribes diltiazem hydrochloride (Cardizem) 180 mg by mouth daily, with the first dose to be given now. The diltiazem hydrochloride is available in 60-mg tablets. How many tablets should the nurse give?

1. 2 tablets.
2. 3 tablets.
3. 4 tablets.
4. 6 tablets.

122. Mr. Juswishin complains of severe headache (9 out of 10 on a pain scale). The nurse obtains the following vital signs: BP 126/76, NSR at 82, RR 18.

Patient denies shortness of breath. The physician orders morphine sulfate 2 mg slow IV push now. The nurse has available morphine sulfate 4 mg/mL for intravenous use. How many milliliters of morphine sulfate should the nurse administer?

1. 0.2 mL.
2. 0.5 mL.
3. 1 mL.
4. 2 mL.

Short Answer

123. The laboratory reported a K^+ (potassium) value of 6 mEq for your patient in the intensive care unit. The physician prescribes lactulose 20 mg by mouth now. The medication is available as lactulose 10 mg/15 mL. How many milliliters of lactulose should the nurse give now?

Multiple Choice

124. Mrs. Ramsey has pulmonary edema, so the physician prescribes furosemide (Lasix) 60 mg slow IV push now. You have furosemide available as a 100 mg/10 mL vial. How many milliliters of Lasix should you administer?

1. 0.6 mL.
2. 1.66 mL.
3. 6 mL.
4. 60 mL.

125. To control Mr. Anderson's blood pressure, the physician prescribes metoprolol tartrate (Lopressor, Toprol XL) 75 mg by mouth now. The pharmacy dispenses Lopressor as 50 mg per scored tablet. How many tablets should the nurse give?

1. 0.75 tablet.
2. 1.25 tablets.
3. 1.5 tablets.
4. 2.5 tablets.

126. For the prevention of postoperative thromboembolism, the surgeon prescribes heparin 4,000 units subcutaneously now. The dosage available is heparin 5,000 units/mL. How many milliliters should the nurse administer?

1. 0.2 mL.
2. 0.8 mL.
3. 1.25 mL.
4. 1.8 mL.

PHARMACOLOGICAL AND PARENTERAL THERAPIES

Identification

127. Your diabetic patient, Mrs. Lucy, normally receives 30 units of NPH subcutaneously every morning. She is also on hyperalimentation and needs to be covered by sliding-scale regular insulin. Her blood sugar is 467, and she is prescribed to receive 12 units of regular insulin and 30 units of NPH. Draw an arrow next to the syringe to indicate where the total dose of insulin would be drawn up to.

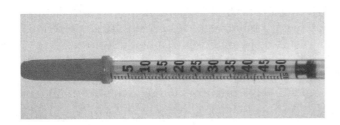

Multiple Choice

128. Mrs. Sullens has chronic bronchitis with an infection. To treat the infection, the physician prescribes gatifloxacin (Tequin) 400 mg to infuse in over 2 hours. The pharmacy delivers gatifloxacin 400 mg in a 200-mL bag of NS. What should be the rate of the infusion, in milliliters per hour, to complete the Tequin infusion?

1. 25 mL/h.
2. 50 mL/h.
3. 100 mL/h.
4. 200 mL/h.

129. The physician prescribes meperidine (Demerol) 50 mg IM now for a patient's acute pain. Meperidine 100 mg/mL for intramuscular injection is available in a prefilled syringe. How much Demerol do you give the patient?

1. 0.5 mL.
2. 1 mL.
3. 2 mL.
4. 10 mL.

Short Answer

130. Your patient complains of sharp inspirational pain near his fifth rib on the left side. You inform the physician, who prescribes morphine sulfate 1 mg IM now. You have available morphine sulfate in the form of 2 mg/mL for IM use. How many milliliters should you administer?

Multiple Choice

131. Mrs. Slater has a migraine headache. The physician prescribes promethazine 12.5 mg intramuscularly now. The pharmacy dispenses a prefilled syringe of promethazine 25 mg/mL. How much promethazine do you administer?

1. 0.4 mL.
2. 0.5 mL.
3. 1 mL.
4. 2 mL.

132. Mrs. Zegin has a gram-negative bacterial infection. The physician prescribes Amikin (amikacin sulfate) 250 mg intramuscularly now. The pharmacy dispenses Amikin 500 mg/2 mL. How many milliliters do you administer?

1. 0.5 mL.
2. 1 mL.
3. 2 mL.
4. 4 mL.

133. Mr. Heinz has been bitten by a spider and has an infection. The physician prescribes Rocephen (ceftriaxone sodium) 250 mg intramuscularly now. The pharmacy dispenses ceftriaxone sodium 1 g/10 mL. How much of the medication do you administer now?

1. 1 mL.
2. 2.5 mL.
3. 5 mL.
4. 20 mL.

True or False

134. You should inject air into ampules before withdrawing the desired amount of medication.

Multiple Choice

135. Mr. Horner has been diagnosed with syphilis, and the physician has prescribed penicillin G benzathine 600,000 units intramuscularly now. The pharmacy dispenses the penicillin G in 300,000 units/mL. How many milliliters do you give Mr. Horner?

1. 0.5 mL.
2. 0.75 mL.
3. 1 mL.
4. 2 mL.

136. Jane Doe is admitted with severe psychotic disorder and prescribed prochlorperazine edisylate (Compazine) 20 mg intramuscularly STAT. The pharmacy dispenses prochlorperazine edisylate as 5 mg/mL. How many milliliters should you prepare to give to Jane Doe?

   1. 1 mL.

   2. 2 mL.

   3. 4 mL.

   4. 0.25 mL.

137. Jared Brown has been diagnosed with male hypogonadism. He comes to the clinic every 4 weeks to receive an intramuscular injection of 400 mg of testosterone enanthate. On this visit, the pharmacy dispenses testosterone enanthate 200 mg/mL. How much medication do you draw up to give Jared?

   1. 2 mL.

   2. 3 mL.

   3. 4 mL.

   4. 0.5 mL.

Short Answer

138. The physician prescribes 1,000 mL of D_5 NS to infuse at a rate of 200 mL/h. How many hours will it take for infusion of the entire bag of fluid?

Multiple Choice

139. Ms. Chambers has isoniazid-induced vitamin B_6 deficiency and is prescribed pyridoxine hydrochloride (vitamin B_6) 200 mg intramuscularly now. The pharmacy dispenses pyridoxine hydrochloride as 100 mg/mL. How many milliliters do you give Ms. Chambers?

   1. 1 mL.

   2. 2 mL.

   3. 4 mL.

   4. 0.5 mL.

140. Mrs. Gutierrez is 88 years old and has a fever of 101.4°F (taken orally). She is prescribed acetaminophen (Tylenol) 320 mg orally now. The pharmacy dispenses the medication as 160 mg/5 mL. How much acetaminophen do you administer?

   1. 0.5 mL.

   2. 5 mL.

   3. 8 mL.

   4. 10 mL.

141. Six-year-old Ursula has a fever, and the nurse practitioner has prescribed acetaminophen (Tylenol) 160 mg orally every 6 hours × 24 hours. The pharmacy dispenses acetaminophen 80 mg per $^1/_2$ teaspoon. How much Tylenol do you tell Ursula's mother to give her child every 6 hours?

   1. $^1/_4$ teaspoon.

   2. $^1/_2$ teaspoon.

   3. 1 teaspoon.

   4. 2 teaspoons.

Short Answer

142. Mr. Cushman has just had his jaw wired shut following a motor vehicle accident. He is prescribed his usual daily medication in liquid form: fluoxetine hydrochloride (Prozac) Oral solution 40 mg orally daily. The pharmacy dispenses Prozac liquid 20 mg/5 mL. How many milliliters should Mr. Cushman take each day?

Multiple Choice

143. Mrs. Derrick has congestion due to bronchitis, and her nurse practitioner has prescribed guaifenesin (Mucinex) 1,200 mg now, in the form of extended-release tablets, then one tablet every 8 hours. The pharmacy dispenses Mucinex as 600-mg ER tablets. How many tablets do you give Mrs. Derrick for her initial dose?

   1. $^1/_2$ tablet.

   2. 1 tablet.

   3. 2 tablets.

   4. 4 tablets.

144. After Mr. Wallace went hunting, he was diagnosed with Lyme disease as the result of a tick bite. He is prescribed a single dose of doxycycline monohydrate (Vibramycin) 200 mg orally within 72 hours of removing the tick. The tick was removed 14 hours ago. The pharmacy dispenses Vibramycin as a 25 mg/5 mL oral suspension. How much do you administer to Mr. Wallace?

   1. 20 mL.

   2. 40 mL.

   3. 8 mL.

   4. 25 mL.

Short Answer

145. One of the potential sites in which to give an intramuscular injection—particularly in an infant— is the vastus lateralis. Where on the body is this site located?

Multiple Choice

146. Mr. Jennings has developed oropharyngeal candidiasis as a result of his radiation therapy. The radioatononcologist prescribes fluconazole (Diflucan) 100 mg orally daily. The pharmacy dispenses fluconazole 10 mg/mL. How much of this medication do you administer to Mr. Jennings daily?

1. 1 mL.
2. 5 mL.
3. 10 mL.
4. 0.1 mL.

147. Bobby Smart is diagnosed with tonsillitis and is prescribed clarithromycin (Biaxin) 750 mg orally, once daily for 7 days. The pharmacy dispenses clarithromycin as 250-mg tablets. How many tablets do you give daily?

1. 2 tablets.
2. 3 tablets.
3. 4 tablets.
4. 6 tablets.

Short Answer

148. What is the appropriate angle at which to insert the needle into the skin for an intramuscular injection?

Multiple Choice

149. Mrs. Sharpe has had breast cancer and is prescribed tamoxifen citrate (Nolvadex) 20 mg orally every day. Her pharmacy dispenses a 30-day supply of the medication as 10-mg tablets. How many total tablets should the pharmacist dispense for a 30-day supply of the Nolvadex?

1. 15 tablets.
2. 30 tablets.
3. 45 tablets.
4. 60 tablets.

True or False

150. The deltoid site in adults should only be used for intramuscular injections of 3 mL or less of total medication.

Multiple Choice

151. Mr. Roland has type 2 diabetes and is prescribed Glucophage (metformin) 500 mg orally twice a day, once in the morning and once in the evening. The pharmacy dispenses metformin as 500-mg tablets. How many tablets should Mr. Roland take every morning?

1. 0.5 tablet.
2. 1 tablet.
3. 2 tablets.
4. 4 tablets.

True or False

152. The deltoid injection site is found midway between the clavicle and the elbow of each arm.

Multiple Choice

153. Mrs. Sorensino's blood pressure is not being well controlled on her current medication, so her physician prescribes an angiotensin-converting enzyme (ACE) inhibitor, captopril (Capoten) 50 mg orally daily. The pharmacy dispenses carbamazepine as 100-mg tablets. How much medication do you give Mrs. Sorensino?

1. None.
2. 0.5 tablet.
3. 1 tablet.
4. 2 tablets.

154. Mrs. Taritis has an overactive bladder and is prescribed tolterodine tartrate (Detrol) extended-release capsules 4 mg orally daily. The pharmacy dispenses Detrol immediate-release tablets 2 mg per tablet. How many tablets do you give?

1. None.
2. 0.5 tablet.
3. 2 tablets.
4. 4 tablets.

True or False

155. Vigorous massage of the injection site after an intramuscular injection may damage tissue.

Multiple Choice

156. Mr. Gustufson has hypertension and has been prescribed metoprolol tartrate (Lopressor) 100 mg orally daily. The pharmacy dispenses Lopressor as 50-mg tablets. How many tablets should Mr. Gustufson take daily?

SECTION
I

SECTION
II

SECTION
III

SECTION
IV

SECTION
V

SECTION
VI

SECTION
VII

SECTION
VIII

SECTION
IX

SECTION
X

1. 0.5 tablet.
2. 1 tablet.
3. 2 tablets.
4. 3 tablets.

Short Answer

157. The dorsogluteal site (upper, outer quadrant of the buttock) is a traditional site for intramuscular injections. This site has been associated with injuries to which nerve?

Multiple Choice

158. Mrs. Yelenovsky had a total thyroidectomy due to goiter and is prescribed Synthroid 50 mcg orally daily. The pharmacy dispenses Synthroid as 50-mcg tablets. How many tablets should Mrs. Yelenovsky take daily?

1. $^{1}/_{2}$ tablet.
2. 1 tablet.
3. 5 tablets.
4. 10 tablets.

159. Mr. Koo has just been diagnosed with hypertension, and his physician has prescribed the angiotensin-converting enzyme (ACE) inhibitor lisinopril (Zestril) 20 mg orally daily. The physician has office samples of this medication that he can give Mr. Koo for today until Mr. Koo can get his prescription filled tomorrow. The office samples are 5-mg tablets. How many tablets should Mr. Koo take now?

1. 1 tablet.
2. 2 tablets.
3. 3 tablets.
4. 4 tablets.

REDUCTION OF RISK POTENTIAL

Multiple Choice

160. Prescription: Measure blood glucose levels before every meal and at bedtime.

If the blood glucose exceeds 150 mg/dL, administer 1 unit of insulin for every 30 mg/dL increase in the blood glucose above 150 mg/dL. Your patient's blood sugar is currently 240 mg/dL. How many units of insulin should he receive?

1. 90 units.
2. 8 units.
3. 35 units.

4. 3 units.

Identification

161. The patient is to receive insulin as follows to help control the risk of developing retinopathy and neuropathy: Administer 1 unit of insulin for every 15 g of carbohydrates consumed. For lunch, your patient ate the following items:

Item	Carbohydrate Content
1 apple	15 g
8 ounces of milk	12 g
3-ounce ground beef patty	0 g
1 hamburger bun	23 g
4 ounces of french fries	25 g

Mark the syringe with the amount of insulin that you should administer.

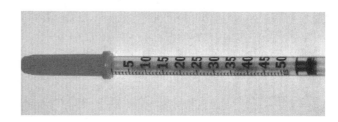

Multiple Choice

162. Your patient has been prescribed furosemide (Lasix) 120 mg orally now. To reduce the patient's risk of cardiac dysrhythmias, which electrolyte should you monitor?

1. Magnesium.
2. Theophylline.
3. Potassium.
4. Epinephrine.

Short Answer

163. You are asked to administer 2 g of a medication that is dispensed in the form of 500-mg tablets. How many tablets should you administer?

Multiple Choice

164. Your patient is on morphine for pain control following orthopedic surgery. To prevent constipation, the physician prescribes Colace (docusate sodium) elixir 60 mg PO daily. Each teaspoon (5 mL) of liquid contains 20 mg of docusate sodium. How much medication do you give your patient?

1. 300 mL.
2. 40 mL.

3. 240 mL.

4. 15 mL.

165. Your patient is in the hospital as part of a palliative care program. He is prescribed Dilaudid (hydromorphone HCl) 4 mg orally, every 4 hours around the clock. The pharmacy sends up 2-mg tablets of morphine. How many tablets do you give your patient?

1. None.

2. 0.5 tablet.

3. 2 tablets.

4. 8 tablets.

166. As part of his treatment for chronic hepatitis C, Mr. Gregory is receiving interferon alfacon-1 (Infergen) 9 mcg subcutaneously three times a week (on Mondays, Wednesdays, and Fridays). The pharmacy dispenses prefilled syringes of Infergen 9 mcg. How many syringes do you need to give Mr. Gregory for one of his doses on Monday?

1. One syringe.

2. Two syringes.

3. Three syringes.

4. Four syringes.

167. Mr. Barrios has an AIDS-related opportunistic infection, cytomegalovirus, for which he is being treated with foscarnet sodium (Foscavir) 90 mg/kg given as an intravenous infusion. He weighs 70 kg. How many milligrams of Foscavir should Mr. Barrios receive?

1. 129 mg.

2. 630 mg.

3. 6,300 mg.

4. 5,600 mg.

Fill in the Blank

168. Some doses of medications are based on body surface area. The two most important values in determining body surface area are height and

_____.

Multiple Choice

169. Mrs. Ellis is prescribed ethacrynic acid (Edecrin) 75 mg × 1 for lymphedema following a mastectomy. The pharmacy has dispensed 50-mg scored tablets of ethacrynic acid. How many tablets do you administer to Mrs. Ellis?

1. 0.5 tablet.

2. 1 tablet.

3. 1.5 tablets.

4. 2 tablets.

170. Mr. Belske has open-angle glaucoma and is prescribed pilocarpine hydrochloride ophthalmic solution 0.25%, one drop in each eye every morning and evening. The pharmacy dispenses pilocarpine hydrochloride ophthalmic solution 0.5%. How many drops do you give Mr. Belske in the morning?

1. None.

2. 1 drop.

3. 2 drops.

4. 4 drops.

171. Mr. Hawkins has bronchial asthma and is prescribed a total dose of 800 mg theophylline (Elixophyllin) per day, to be given in equal doses every 6 hours around the clock. The pharmacy dispenses theophylline (Elixophyllin) as an 80 mg/15 mL liquid. How many milliliters should Mr. Hawkins receive every 6 hours?

1. 37.5 mL.

2. 90 mL.

3. 32 mL.

4. 6 mL.

172. Katherine Nottingham is a nurse who has been diagnosed with an active duodenal ulcer. Her nurse practitioner has prescribed omeprazole (Prilosec) 40 mg orally daily. The pharmacy dispenses Prilosec 20-mg enteric-coated capsules. How many capsules should Katherine take daily?

1. None.

2. 1 capsule.

3. 2 capsules.

4. 4 capsules.

Short Answer

173. How much atropine do you give a patient preoperatively if the physician prescribes 0.3 mg of atropine for every 100 lbs the patient weighs, and the patient weighs 200 lbs?

Multiple Choice

174. Mrs. Vishton is receiving her second round of chemotherapy for ovarian cancer. She experienced severe nausea and vomiting with her first chemotherapy treatment, so her oncologist has prescribed 24 mg ondansetron hydrochloride (Zofran) orally 1 hour prior to chemotherapy. The pharmacy dispenses

Zofran 8-mg tablets. How many tablets of Zofran should Mrs. Vishton receive?

1. 3 tablets.
2. 4 tablets.
3. 6 tablets.
4. 9 tablets.

175. Steven Porter is a 32-year-old man who wants to quit smoking. He has been prescribed a nicotine transdermal (Habitrol) patch 21 mg daily for the first 4 weeks. He wants to quit smoking today, but cannot get to the pharmacy because it will be closed by the time he leaves the physician's office, so the nurse offers him pharmaceutical samples. The samples include nicotine transdermal patches in strengths of 14 mg and 7 mg. What should the nurse give the patient for today's dose?

1. One 14-mg patch.
2. One 14-mg patch and one 7-mg patch.
3. One 14-mg patch and two 7-mg patches.
4. Two 14-mg patches.

176. Mrs. Gloria Smith has been diagnosed with ankylosing spondylitis and prescribed naproxen (Apo-Naproxen) 750 mg orally daily. The pharmacy dispenses naproxen 250-mg tablets. How many tablets should Mrs. Smith receive daily?

1. 1 tablet.
2. 2 tablets.
3. 3 tablets.
4. 5 tablets.

177. Michael Morris is diagnosed with allergic rhinitis and is prescribed mometasone furoate monohydrate (Nasonex) nasal spray, with a total daily dose of 200 mcg. Each spray releases 50 mcg of medication. What is the maximum number of sprays per day?

1. 1 spray.
2. 2 sprays.
3. 3 sprays.
4. 4 sprays.

True or False

178. A 1% solution is more potent (stronger) than a 5% solution.

Multiple Choice

179. Jenny Montgomery is diagnosed with vulvovaginal candidiasis and is prescribed miconazole (Monostat) vaginal suppositories 200 mg per day × 3 days. What is the total amount of Monostat Jenny should be dispensed for use for all 3 days?

1. 200 mg.
2. 600 mg.
3. 800 mg.
4. 66.7 mg.

180. Mr. Cox has acquired immune deficiency syndrome (AIDS) and is prescribed megestrol acetate (Megace) as an appetite stimulant, 800 mg orally per day. Megace is dispensed as 40 mg/mL. How many milliliters of Megace should Mr. Cox take per day?

1. 20 mL.
2. 40 mL.
3. 80 mL.
4. 160 mL.

Short Answer

181. Zantac or ranitidine hydrochloride comes in a syrup form consisting of 15 mg/1 mL. Your patient is prescribed to receive 4 mL. How many milligrams of Zantac will the patient receive?

Multiple Choice

182. Mrs. Heffernan is diagnosed with secondary amenorrhea and is prescribed medroxyprogesterone acetate (Provera) 5 mg per day, to be taken for 7 days during her menstrual cycle every month. The pharmacy dispenses Provera 5-mg tablets. How many tablets, in total, should Mrs. Heffernan take each month?

1. 5 tablets.
2. 7 tablets.
3. 25 tablets.
4. 35 tablets.

183. The physician prescribes 0.875 g of Augmentin orally for Ms. Battles every 12 hours (BID) to assist in healing her ear infection. The pharmacist dispenses Augmentin as 875-mg tablets. How many tablets should Ms. Battles take every 24 hours?

1. ½ tablet.
2. 1 tablet.

3. 2 tablets.

4. 4 tablets.

184. Mrs. Wolinski is prescribed Cardizem (diltiazem hydrochloride) 60 mg orally every morning. The pharmacy dispenses Cardizem 30-mg tablets. How many tablets should Mrs. Wolinski take every morning?

   1. ½ tablet.

   2. 1 tablet.

   3. 2 tablets.

   4. 3 tablets.

185. Mr. Vasques is prescribed Lopid (gemfibrozil) 300 mg orally daily. You receive a medication from the pharmacy labeled "Lopid 0.3 g per tablet." How many tablets do you give Mr. Vasques daily?

   1. None.

   2. 1 tablet.

   3. 9 tablets.

   4. 10 tablets.

186. Mr. Pollard is having atrial fibrillation and is prescribed digoxin (Digitek) 0.375 mg orally STAT. The pharmacy dispenses digoxin 0.125-mg tablets. How many tablets do you give Mr. Pollard now?

   1. 1 tablet.

   2. 2 tablets.

   3. 3 tablets.

   4. 6 tablets.

Short Answer

187. Your patient is in pain and has a prescription for codeine 60 mg orally every 6 hours. It has been 8 hours since his last pain pill. The pharmacy dispenses codeine 30-mg tablets. How many tablets do you give the patient?

Multiple Choice

188. Mrs. Greene has had an allergic reaction to laundry detergent. Her physician prescribes 1 mg dexamethasone orally now. The pharmacy dispenses dexamethasone 0.5-mg tablets. How many tablets do you give Mrs. Greene now?

   1. 0.25 tablet.

   2. 0.5 tablet.

   3. 1 tablet.

   4. 2 tablets.

189. Prior to Annie's surgery, the surgeon prescribes a skeletal muscle relaxant for her: dantrolene sodium (Dantrium) 0.5 mg/kg. Annie weighs 40 kg. How much Dantrium should Annie receive?

   1. 10 mL.

   2. 20 mL.

   3. 40 mL.

   4. 80 mL.

190. Seven-year-old Eleanor is prescribed erythromycin stearate 20 mg/kg daily. She weighs 30 kg. How much erythromycin stearate do you give Eleanor?

   1. 600 mg.

   2. 1.5 mg.

   3. 0.67 mg.

   4. 300 mg.

191. Mrs. Anderson is prescribed heparin sodium 5,000 units subcutaneously now. The pharmacy dispenses heparin sodium as 10,000 units/mL. How much heparin sodium do you give Mrs. Anderson?

   1. 0.25 mL.

   2. 0.5 mL.

   3. 2 mL.

   4. 5 mL.

192. Your patient is prescribed codeine 45 mg orally every 8 hours. It has been 8 hours since his last pain pill and he is asking for more. The pharmacy dispenses codeine 15-mg tablets. How many tablets do you give the patient?

   1. 0.33 tablet.

   2. 1 tablet.

   3. 2 tablets.

   4. 3 tablets.

PHYSIOLOGICAL ADAPTATION

Multiple Choice

193. Your patient's blood sugars have been consistently high in the morning, so the physician has increased the patient's prescription to read "Metformin 500 mg PO twice a day." The pharmacy sends up 250-mg metformin tablets. How many tablets do you give the patient in the morning?

   1. 1 tablet.

   2. 2 tablets.

   3. 3 tablets.

   4. 4 tablets.

194. Your patient is prescribed Capoten 25 mg PO twice a day, if her systolic blood pressure is greater than 150 mm Hg. When you take the patient's blood pressure, it is 165/54 mm Hg. What action should you take?

1. Do not give the medication; 54 mm Hg is below the parameter prescribed.

2. Do not give the medication, as the pulse pressure is 111.

3. Give the medication, as 165 mm Hg is above the parameter prescribed.

4. Give the medication twice now, as the patient's blood pressure is extremely elevated.

195. Mr. Hill has the following prescription: Ativan (lorazepam) 4 mg PO daily; divide the total dose so that equal amounts are given every 6 hours. You mark the times on the medication sheet according to hospital policy to be 0600, 1200, 1800, and 2400 hours. What is the dose of Ativan to be given at each of those times?

1. 4 mg.

2. 2 mg.

3. 6.66 mg.

4. 1 mg.

196. Mr. Lolitto requires daily doses of phenobarbital to prevent seizures by maintaining a consistent blood level of the medication. He is prescribed phenobarbital elixir 80 mg orally at bedtime. The pharmacy sends up an elixir consisting of 20 mg phenobarbital per 5 mL. What volume do you administer to Mr. Lolitto at bedtime?

1. 20 mL.

2. 16 mL.

3. 360 mL.

4. 0.8 mL.

197. Eleanor Solana is prescribed penicillin V potassium oral solution 375 mg every 8 hours for her infection. The pharmacy sends up penicillin V potassium oral solution 200,000 units (125 mg) per 5 mL. How much medication do you pour every 8 hours?

1. 40,000 units.

2. 15 mL.

3. 4.26 mL.

4. 75 mL.

198. Your patient, Mrs. Wollenstein, needs her blood pressure maintained below 110/70 mm Hg due to increased intracranial pressure. She is alert and oriented and able to take oral medications. Her physician prescribes 50 mg metoprolol tartrate (Lopressor) if her systolic blood pressure is between 111 and 125 mm Hg, 75 mg if her systolic blood pressure is between 126 and 150 mm Hg, and 100 mg if her systolic blood pressure is more than 151 mm Hg. Mrs. Wollenstein's blood pressure is currently 226/128 mm Hg. How much Lopressor do you administer?

1. None.

2. 75 mg.

3. 100 mg.

4. 50 mg.

True or False

199. After adding an additive to a bag of intravenous fluid, you should invert the bag several times so the additive is distributed evenly.

Multiple Choice

200. Mrs. Zollinski is prescribed levothyroxine sodium (Synthroid) 0.1 mg orally every morning. The pharmacy sends up Synthroid 50-mcg tablets. How many tablets do you give Mrs. Zollinski each morning?

1. 0.5 tablet.

2. 1 tablet.

3. 2 tablets.

4. 5 tablets.

201. Mr. Coles is scheduled to take Mellaril (thioridazine hydrochloride) once a day. He is prescribed 75 mg orally daily of Mellaril. How much do you pour if the pharmacy sends up liquid Mellaril in the form of 30 mg/mL?

1. 2 mL.

2. 2.5 mL.

3. 1.5 mL.

4. 0.4 mL.

202. José is allergic to bees, and he was just stung by one. You have liquid diphenhydramine hydrochloride (Benadryl) on hand in the form of 12.5 mg/5 mL. Josés's mother gives you a note from his doctor that she carries with her, stating that you should give 25 mg Benadryl within 5 minutes of bee stings. How much Benadryl do you give José?

1. 2.5 mL.
2. 25 mL.
3. 50 mL.
4. 10 mL.

True or False

203. Liquid medications are calibrated in grains.

Multiple Choice

204. Six-year-old Olga has an infection, and her nurse practitioner has prescribed clindamycin oral solution 125 mg orally now, then 50 mg every 8 hours. The pharmacy dispenses clindamycin (Cleocin) as 75 mg/5 mL. How much medication do you give Olga for her initial dose?

1. 12 mL.
2. 10 mL.
3. 3.33 mL.
4. 8.33 mL.

205. Mrs. Helena is beginning dexamethasone (Decadron) for treatment of leukemia. She is to receive a dose of 1 mg orally now. The pharmacy dispenses Decadron 0.25-mg tablets. How many tablets do you give Mrs. Helena for the current dose?

1. 2 tablets.
2. 4 tablets.
3. 8 tablets.
4. 10 tablets.

206. Mr. Budnik's serum potassium came back very low. The physician prescribes potassium chloride ER 2,250 mg orally now. The pharmacy dispenses potassium chloride ER (Klor-Con) 10 mEq tablets, which contain 750 mg of medication in each tablet. How many tablets do you give Mr. Budnik?

1. 3 tablets.
2. 5 tablets.
3. 6 tablets.
4. 7.5 tablets.

207. Mrs. Maiorino is to begin chemotherapy treatment with methotrexate. She is prescribed 7.5 mg orally of methotrexate as her initial treatment. The pharmacy dispenses methotrexate 2.5-mg tablets. How many tablets do you give to Mrs. Maiorino?

1. 2 tablets.
2. 3 tablets.

3. 4 tablets.
4. 6 tablets.

208. Mr. Gordon is to begin antiviral therapy and is prescribed CellCept 1.25 g orally twice a day. The pharmacy dispenses mycophenolate mofetil (CellCept) 250-mg capsules. How many capsules per dose should Mr. Gordon receive?

1. 2 capsules.
2. 3 capsules.
3. 4 capsules.
4. 5 capsules.

True or False

209. Heparin sodium given intravenously is compatible with all known medications.

Multiple Choice

210. Mr. Hall is newly prescribed ziprasidone HCl (Geodon) 60 mg orally daily as part of his mental health care. The pharmacy dispenses Geodon 20-mg capsules. How many capsules do you give Mr. Hall daily?

1. None.
2. 3 capsules.
3. 4 capsules.
4. 6 capsules.

211. Mr. Cook is in pain and is prescribed fentanyl citrate 50 mcg intravenously for pain that rates more than 7 on a 1–10 scale. Mr. Cook reports his pain is a 9 and asks for his medicine. How much medication do you draw up if the pharmacy dispenses fentanyl citrate as 250 mcg/5 mL for intravenous injection?

1. 1 mL.
2. 2 mL.
3. 5 mL.
4. 25 mL.

212. Mr. Cortez has just been admitted to your floor with onset of disruptive behavior due to unknown cause. He is prescribed haloperidol 2.5 mg intramuscularly now. The pharmacy dispenses haloperidol for injection in the form of 5 mg/mL. How much medication do you draw up to give to Mr. Cortez?

1. 2 mL.
2. 5 mL.
3. 0.5 mL.
4. 12.5 mL.

True or False

213. One of the side effects of nitroglycerin is severe headache.

Multiple Choice

214. Mrs. Smart was working in her garden and was bitten by a spider. She comes to the Emergency Department with a swollen hand that is infected. The physician prescribes Rocephen 2 g intramuscularly now. The pharmacy dispenses four vials, each of which contains Rocephen (ciftriaxone sodium) 1 g as a single dose for intramuscular or intravenous use. What is your next step?

1. Call the pharmacy and ask the pharmacist to send up the correct medication.
2. Draw up two vials of the medication that the pharmacy sent up.
3. Draw up four vials of the medication that the pharmacy sent up.
4. Send back the medication and ask for Rocephen tablets.

215. Mrs. Childs comes in for her Neupogen injection because her white blood cell count is low due to her chemotherapy. She is prescribed Neupogen 450 mcg subcutaneously today. The pharmacy dispenses filgrastim (Neupogen) 300 mcg/mL for subcutaneous or intravenous use only. How much medication do you draw up?

1. 1 mL.
2. 1.5 mL.
3. 2 mL.
4. 3 mL.

216. Your patient needs an emergency bronchoscopy, and you are asked to assist the physician. The physician prescribes midazolam HCl (Versed) 3 mg intravenously now. The pharmacy sends up midazolam HCl for injection in the form of 5 mg/5 mL. How much Versed to you give the patient?

1. 2.5 mL.
2. 3 mL.
3. 1.6 mL.
4. 15 mL.

217. Mrs. Rahnned has been diagnosed with herpes zoster and is prescribed acyclovir (Zovirax) 800 mg, 5 times per day × 7 days. The pharmacy has acyclovir (Zovirax) available as 200-mg capsules. What is the total number of capsules Mrs. Rahnned should receive in her 7-day prescription?

1. 35 capsules.
2. 100 capsules.
3. 105 capsules.
4. 140 capsules.

Short Answer

218. The ingestion of which fat-soluble vitamin can interfere with clotting?

Multiple Choice

219. For angina pain, your patient is prescribed nitroglycerin grain 1/150, one tablet sublingually every 5 minutes × 3. What is the least amount of time that can pass by if the patient has taken all 3 tablets correctly?

1. 5 minutes.
2. 10 minutes.
3. 15 minutes.
4. 30 minutes.

220. Mrs. Eckroyd has been diagnosed with uterine fibroids and is prescribed leuprolide acetate (Lupron) 3.75 mg intramuscularly once a month. The pharmacy dispenses 3.75 mg Lupron per milliliter. How much Lupron do you give Mrs. Eckroyd monthly?

1. 0.25 mL.
2. 0.5 mL.
3. 0.75 mL.
4. 1 mL.

Fill in the Blank

221. A person on nitroglycerin who also drinks alcohol can expect his blood pressure to _____ (increase or decrease).

Multiple Choice

222. Mr. Roswell comes to the Emergency Department because he had a seizure at home. The physician has just prescribed phenobarbital 240 mg now intravenously. You call pharmacy and the pharmacist asks, "How many vials do you need? We have phenobarbital as 130 mg/mL vials." How many vials do you tell the pharmacist you need?

1. 1 vial.
2. 2 vials.
3. 4 vials.
4. 10 vials.

ANSWERS AND RATIONALES

MANAGEMENT OF CARE

1. Correct Answer: <u>**Completion time 0445 hours (4:45 A.M.)**</u>
   Rationale:

   $$\frac{50 \text{ mL (hourly infusion volume)}}{1 \text{ h}}$$

   $$= \frac{1,000 \text{ mL (total volume)}}{x \text{ (total infusion time)}}$$

   $$= \frac{1,000}{50x}$$

   $$x = 20 \text{ h}$$

   $$\frac{1,000 \text{ mL (total volume)}}{0 \text{ mL (hourly infusion volume)}}$$

   $$= 20 \text{ (total number of hourly rate increments)}$$

   $$= \text{ total infusion time}$$

2. Correct Answer: <u>**2**</u>
   Rationale: 220 lb/2.2 kg/lb = 100 kg;
   $100 \times 10 = 1,000$ mcg.

3. Correct Answer: <u>**3**</u>
   Rationale: Lipitor is not Lopressor. The pharmacy sent up the wrong medication.

4. Correct Answer: <u>**2**</u>
   Rationale: 50 mcg = 0.05; x mcg = 0.1 mg;
   $x = 0.1$.

5. Correct Answer: <u>**4**</u>
   Rationale: The ratio is 10:1 = 30:x; $x = 30/10 = 3$.

6. Correct Answer: <u>**125 mL**</u>
   Rationale: $25 \times 500/100 = 25 \times 5 = 125$ mL.

7. Correct Answer: <u>**2**</u>
   Rationale: The ratio is 25:5 = 20:x;
   $x = 100/25 = 4$.

8. Correct Answer: <u>**1**</u>
   Rationale: The ratio is 250:5 = 400:x;
   $x = 2,000/250 = 8$ mL.

9. Correct Answer: <u>**3**</u>
   Rationale: The ratio is 2:5 = 1.6:x; $x = 1.6 \times 5/2$
   $= 8/2 = 4$.

10. Correct Answer: <u>**100 mL**</u>
    Rationale: $250/100 \times 40 = 2.5 \times 40 = 100$ mL.

11. Correct Answer: <u>**2**</u>
    Rationale: The ratio is 150:1 = 450:x;
    $x = 450/150 = 3$.

12. Correct Answer: <u>**1**</u>
    Rationale: The ratio is 250:5 = 350:x;
    $x = 1750/250 = 7$.

13. Correct Answer: <u>**2**</u>
    Rationale: The ratio is 500:10 = 200:x;
    $2,000/500 = 4$.

14. Correct Answer: <u>**2 prefilled syringes; you will administer 1.5 of them.**</u>

15. Correct Answer: <u>**3**</u>
    Rationale: The ratio is 125:2 = 250:x;
    $x = 500/125 = 4$.

16. Correct Answer: <u>**4 tablets**</u>
    Rationale: $100/25 = 4$.

17. Correct Answer: <u>**2**</u>
    Rationale: The ratio is 5:5 = 8:x; $40/5 = x = 8$.

18. Correct Answer: <u>**4**</u>
    Rationale: The ratio is 125:5 = 75:x;
    $x = 375/125 = 3$.

19. Correct Answer: <u>**1**</u>
    Rationale: The ratio is 250:5 = 400:x;
    $x = 2,000/250 = 8$.

20. Correct Answer: <u>**3 tablets**</u>
    Rationale: $1.5/0.5 = 3$.

21. Correct Answer: <u>**3**</u>
    Rationale: The ratio is 200:5 = 400:x;
    $x = 2,000/200 = 10$.

22. Correct Answer: <u>**1**</u>
    Rationale: The ratio is 2:1 = 1:x; $x = \frac{1}{2} = 0.5$.

23. Correct Answer: <u>**4**</u>
    Rationale: The ratio is 4:1 = 10:x; $x = 10/4 = 2.5$.

24. Correct Answer: <u>**2 mL**</u>
    Rationale: The ratio is 15:3 = 60:x; $x = 180/15$.

25. Correct Answer: **3**
    Rationale: The ratio is 20:5 = 10:x; x = 2.5.

26. Correct Answer: **2**
    Rationale: The ratio is 20:5 = 60:x;
    x = 300/20 = 15.

27. Correct Answer: **2**
    Rationale: 1,000 mg = 1 g; 500/250 = 2.

28. Correct Answer: **1**
    Rationale: The ratio is 100:1 = 150:x;
    x = 150/100 = 1.5.

29. Correct Answer: **2**
    Rationale: The ratio is 2:1 = 4:x; x = 4/2 = 2.

30. Correct Answer: **1**
    Rationale: The ratio is 50:1 = 25:x;
    x = 25/50 = 0.5.

31. Correct Answer: **3 tablets**
    Rationale: 1.5/0.5 = 3.

32. Correct Answer: **2**
    Rationale: The ratio is 0.4:1 = 0.2:x;
    x = 0.2/0.4 = 0.5.

33. Correct Answer: **3**
    Rationale: The ratio is 1:1 = 3:x; x = 3/1 = 3.

34. Correct Answer: **3 tablets**
    Rationale: 75/25 = 3.

35. Correct Answer: **3**
    Rationale: The ratio is 500:2 = 250:x;
    x = 500/500 = 1.

36. Correct Answer: **4**
    Rationale:

    $$\frac{300\text{ mg}}{2\text{ mL}} = \frac{300\text{ mg}}{x\text{ mL}}$$
    $$300x = 600$$
    $$x = 2\text{ mL}$$

37. Correct Answer: **4 mL**
    Rationale:

    $$\frac{10\text{ mg}}{1\text{ mL}} = \frac{40\text{ mg}}{x\text{ mL}}$$
    $$10x = 40$$
    $$x = 4\text{ mL}$$

38. Correct Answer: **3**
    Rationale:

    $$\frac{5,000\text{ units}}{0.2\text{ mL}} = \frac{7,500\text{ units}}{x\text{ mL}}$$
    $$5,000x = 1,500$$
    $$x = 0.3\text{ mL}$$

39. Correct Answer: **1**
    Rationale:

    $$\frac{40\text{ mg}}{1\text{ mL}} = \frac{60\text{ mg}}{x\text{ mL}}$$
    $$40x = 60$$
    $$x = 1.5\text{ mL}$$

40. Correct Answer: **2 mL**
    Rationale:

    $$\frac{150\text{ mg}}{1\text{ mL}} = \frac{75\text{ mg}}{x\text{ mL}}$$
    $$150x = 75$$
    $$x = 2\text{ mL}$$

41. Correct Answer: **2**
    Rationale:

    $$\frac{25\text{ mg}}{1\text{ mL}} = \frac{50\text{ mg}}{x\text{ mL}}$$
    $$25x = 50$$
    $$x = 2\text{ mL}$$

42. Correct Answer: **3**
    Rationale: The ratio is 5,000:1 = 12,500:x;
    x = 12,500/5,000 = 2.5 mL.

43. Correct Answer: **2**
    Rationale: The ratio is 20,000:1 = 12,000:x;
    x = 12,000/20,000 = 0.6 mL.

44. Correct Answer: **4**
    Rationale: The ratio is 500:2 = 750:x;
    x = 1,500/500 = 3.

SAFETY AND INFECTION CONTROL

45. Correct Answer: **5**
    Rationale: 10 + 7 + 17 + 6 = 40; 40/8 = 5.

46. Correct Answer: **2**
    Rationale: 1,000/125 = 8 h; 0800 + 8 h = 1600 hours (4 P.M.).

47. Correct Answer: **1**
    Rationale:

    $$\frac{80\text{ mL (hourly infusion volume)}}{1\text{ h}}$$

    $$= \frac{250\text{ mL (total volume)}}{x\text{ (total infusion time)}}$$

    $$= \frac{250}{80x}$$

    $x = 3.1\text{ h}$

    $$\frac{250\text{ mL (total volume)}}{80\text{ mL (hourly infusion volume)}}$$

    $= 3.1\text{ (total number of hourly rate increments)}$

    $=$ total infusion time

    Completion time $= 1700$ hours (4 P.M.)

48. Correct Answer: **True.**

49. Correct Answer: **2**
    Rationale: $94 \times 80 = 7,520$.

50. Correct Answer: **Amoxicillin**

51. Correct Answer: **200 mg/5 mL**

52. Correct Answer: **4 + 32 = 36 units of insulin**

53. Correct Answer: **3**
    Rationale: The ratio is $160:5 = 128:x$; $640 = 160x$; $x = 4$.

54. Correct Answer: **4**
    Rationale: The ratio is $75:5 = 150:x$; $750 = 75x$; $x = 10$.

55. Correct Answer: **1**
    Rationale: 20 total tablets divided by 2 tablets per day = 10 days total for tablets.

56. Correct Answer: **3**
    Rationale: $500 \times 2 = 1,000$.

57. Correct Answer: **50-unit syringe**
    Rationale: $18 + 14 = 32$.

58. Correct Answer: **1**
    Rationale: 10 mg ondansetron hydrochloride dehydrate is equal to one 8-mg tablet of Zofran.

59. Correct Answer: **3**
    Rationale: The ratio is $25:5 = 75:x$; $x = 15$ mL; $15 - 10 = 5$ mL.

60. Correct Answer: **3**
    Rationale: *Otic* means "ear."

61. Correct Answer: **1**
    Rationale: Voiding or urinating prior to this procedure prevents urination and possible infection during the procedure.

62. Correct Answer: **Lying down on the left side facilitates absorption/retention.**

63. Correct Answer: **Supine or lying flat.**

64. Correct Answer: **Check the patient-specific prescription for the medication ordered and its time, dose, and route of administration. Next, gather supplies, explain care, and finally wash your hands.**

65. Correct Answer: **Shaving can cause irritation, lead to infection, or affect the medication's absorption.**

66. Correct Answer: **250 mL/h**
    Rationale: $500/2 = 250$.

HEALTH PROMOTION AND MAINTENANCE

67. Correct Answer: **24 + 17 = 41 units**

68. Correct Answer: **4**
    Rationale: The PTT result was 44, so you give a 40 unit/kg bolus now.

69. Correct Answer: **1**
    Rationale: 4/4 is 1 tablet; A.M. means "morning."

70. Correct Answer: **1**
    Rationale: You should not cut extended-release tablets in half.

71. Correct Answer: **3**
    Rationale: The ratio is $10:1 = 40:x$; $x = 40/10 = 4$.

72. Correct Answer: **350 mL**
    Rationale: $1,800/300 \times 50 = 7 \times 50 = 350$ mL.

73. Correct Answer: **1**
    Rationale: The ratio is $25:1 = 12.5:x$; $x = 12.5/25 = 0.5$.

74. Correct Answer: **3**
    Rationale: The ratio is $0.125:1 = 0.25:x$; $x = 0.25/0.125 = 2$.

75. Correct Answer: **4**
    Rationale: $1,000$ mg $= 1$ g, so the ratio is $250:1 = 1,000:x$; $x = 1,000/250 = 4$.

SECTION I
SECTION II
SECTION III
SECTION IV
SECTION V
SECTION VI
SECTION VII
SECTION VIII
SECTION IX
SECTION X

76. Correct Answer: **1,100 mL**
    Rationale: 1,600 − 500 = 1,100 mL.

77. Correct Answer: **2**
    Rationale: The ratio is 40:2 = 100:x;
    $x = 200/40 = 5$.

78. Correct Answer: **2**
    Rationale: 1,000 mg = 1 g; 1 g/500 mg = 2;
    $2 \times 2.5 = 5$.

79. Correct Answer: **4**
    Rationale: The ratio is 10:5 = 30:x;
    $x = 150/10 = 15$.

80. Correct Answer: **1**
    Rationale: The ratio is 5:1 = 7.5:x; $x = 7.5/5 = 1.5$.

81. Correct Answer: **3**
    Rationale: The ratio is 25:1 = 50:x; $x = 50/25 = 2$.

82. Correct Answer: **5 hours**
    Rationale: 1,000/200 = 5.

83. Correct Answer: **2**
    Rationale: The ratio is 40:1 = 80:x; $x = 80/40 = 2$.

84. Correct Answer: **3**
    Rationale: 1,200 − 300 = 900.

85. Correct Answer: **3**
    Rationale: Call the physician. Mr. Boyle is allergic to acetaminophen, which is present in his pain medication.

86. Correct Answer: **3**
    Rationale: $4 \times 77 = 308$; $308 \times 35 =$ 10,780 mL/24 h.

PSYCHOSOCIAL INTEGRITY

87. Correct Answer: **2**
    Rationale: Increasing the dose will help maintain blood levels based on increased metabolism.

88. Correct Answer: **4**
    Rationale: Hypothermia is feeling cold from low body temperature.

89. Correct Answer: **2**
    Rationale: The ratio is 2.5:1 = 7.5:x; $x = 7.5/2.5 = 3$.

90. Correct Answer: **2**
    Rationale: The ratio is 15:1 = 15:x; $x = 15/15 = 1$.

91. Correct Answer: **4 tablets**
    Rationale: $25 \times 4 = 100$.

92. Correct Answer: **3**
    Rationale: The ratio is 10:1 = 30:x; $x = 30/10 = 3$.

93. Correct Answer: **1**
    Rationale: The ratio is 10:1 = 5:x; $x = 5/10 = 0.5$.

94. Correct Answer: **2**
    Rationale: The ratio is 250:1 = 750:x;
    $x = 750/250 = 3$.

95. Correct Answer: **Orthostatic**

96. Correct Answer: **4**
    Rationale: The ratio is 25:1 = 200:x;
    $x = 200/25 = 8$.

97. Correct Answer: **3**
    Rationale: $10 \times 4 = 40$.

98. Correct Answer: **4**
    Rationale: 2 + 3 = 5.

99. Correct Answer: **Food**

100. Correct Answer: **1**
    Rationale: You do not administer any tablets; the pharmacy has dispensed the wrong medication in the wrong form.

101. Correct Answer: **2**
    Rationale: The ratio is 1:1 = 1.5:x; $x = 1.5/1 = 1.5$.

102. Correct Answer: **1**
    Rationale: The ratio is 75:1 = 150:x;
    $x = 150/75 = 2$.

103. Correct Answer: **2**
    Rationale: The ratio is 7.5:1 = 22.5:x;
    $x = 22.5/7.5 = 3$.

104. Correct Answer: **4**
    Rationale: The ratio is 100:1 = 200:x;
    $x = 200/100 = 2$.

105. Correct Answer: **Administer the medication during the waking hours, usually the morning.**

106. Correct Answer: **2**
    Rationale: The ratio is 150:1 = 300:x;
    $x = 300/150 = 2$.

BASIC CARE AND COMFORT

107. Correct Answer: **3**

Rationale: $5 + 8 = 13$.

108. Correct Answer: **4**

Rationale: $650 \times 24/4 = 650 \times 6 = 3{,}900$ mg.

109. Correct Answer: **3**

Rationale: The ratio is $25:1 = 50:x$; $x = 50/25 = 2$.

110. Correct Answer: **2**

Rationale: The ratio is $25:1 = 12.5:x$; $x = 12.5/25 = 0.5$.

111. Correct Answer: **3**

Rationale: The ratio is $40:2 = 100:x$; $x = 200/40 = 5$.

112. Correct Answer: **2**

Rationale: The ratio is $2:1 = 6:x$; $x = 6/2 = 3$.

113. Correct Answer: **1**

Rationale: The ratio is $25:1 = 12.5:x$; $x = 12.5/25 = 0.5$.

114. Correct Answer: **No**

Rationale: $6 \times 22 = 132$; the dose prescribed is too large.

115. Correct Answer: **2**

Rationale: The ratio is $500:0.5$ h $= x:1$ h; $x = 500/0.5 = 1{,}000$.

116. Correct Answer: **0.8 mL**

Rationale: The ratio is $50:1 = 40:x$; $x = 40/50 = 0.8$ mL.

117. Correct Answer: **4**

Rationale: The ratio is $20:10 = 40:x$; $x = 400/20 = 20$.

118. Correct Answer: **4**

Rationale: The ratio is $5{,}000:1 = 5{,}000:x$; $x = 5{,}000/5{,}000 = 1$.

119. Correct Answer: **Yes**

Rationale: $25 \times 10 = 250$ mg every 6 hours; only 150 mg is prescribed.

120. Correct Answer: **1**

Rationale: The ratio is $0.5:1 = 0.25:x$; $x = 0.25/0.5 = 0.5$.

121. Correct Answer: **2**

Rationale: The ratio is $60:1 = 180:x$; $x = 180/60 = 3$.

122. Correct Answer: **2**

Rationale: The ratio is $4:1 = 2:x$; $x = 2/4 = 0.5$.

123. Correct Answer: **30 mL**

Rationale: The ratio is $10:15 = 20:x$; $x = 300/10 = 30$.

124. Correct Answer: **3**

Rationale: The ratio is $100:10 = 60:x$; $x = 600/100 = 6$.

125. Correct Answer: **3**

Rationale: The ratio is $50:1 = 75:x$; $x = 75/50 = 1.5$.

126. Correct Answer: **2**

Rationale: The ratio is $5{,}000:1 = 4{,}000:x$; $x = 4{,}000/5{,}000 = 0.8$.

PHARMACOLOGICAL AND PARENTERAL THERAPIES

127. Correct Answer:

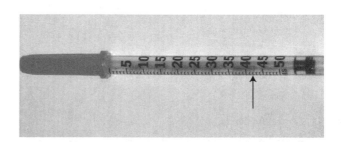

Rationale: $30 + 12 = 42$ units.

128. Correct Answer: **3**

Rationale: The ratio is 200 mL$:2$ h $= x$ mL$:1$ h; $x = 200/2 = 100$ mL/h.

129. Correct Answer: **1**

Rationale: The ratio is $100:1 = 50:x$; $x = 50/100 = 0.5$.

130. Correct Answer: **0.5 mL**

Rationale: The ratio is $2:1 = 1:x$; $x = 1/2 = 0.5$.

131. Correct Answer: **2**

Rationale: The ratio is $25:1 = 12.5:x$; $x = 12.5/25 = 0.5$.

132. Correct Answer: **2**

Rationale: The ratio is $500:2 = 250:x$; $x = 500/500 = 1$.

SECTION I
SECTION II
SECTION III
SECTION IV
SECTION V
SECTION VI
SECTION VII
SECTION VIII
SECTION IX
SECTION X

133. Correct Answer: <u>2</u>

Rationale: The ratio is 1,000 mg:10 mL = 250:x; x = 2,500/1,000 = 2.5.

134. Correct Answer: **False**

Rationale: Injecting air will cause bubbles and possibly overflow of the medication from the ampule.

135. Correct Answer: <u>4</u>

Rationale: The ratio is 300,000:1 = 600,000:x; x = 600,000/300,000 = 2.

136. Correct Answer: <u>3</u>

Rationale: The ratio is 5:1 = 20:x; x = 20/5 = 4.

137. Correct Answer: <u>1</u>

Rationale: The ratio is 200:1 = 400:x; x = 400/200 = 2.

138. Correct Answer: <u>5 hours</u>

Rationale: 1,000/200 = 5.

139. Correct Answer: <u>2</u>

Rationale: The ratio is 100:1 = 200:x; x = 200/100 = 2.

140. Correct Answer: <u>4</u>

Rationale: The ratio is 160:5 = 320:x; x = 1,600/160 = 10.

141. Correct Answer: <u>3</u>

Rationale: The ratio is 80:0.5 = 160:x; x = 80/80 = 1.

142. Correct Answer: <u>10 mL</u>

Rationale:

$$\frac{20\,\text{mg}}{5\,\text{mL}} = \frac{40\,\text{mg}}{x\,\text{mL}}$$
$$= \frac{200}{20}$$
$$= 10\,\text{mL}$$

143. Correct Answer: <u>3</u>

Rationale: The ratio is 300:1 = 600:x; x = 600/300 = 2.

144. Correct Answer: <u>2</u>

Rationale: The ratio is 25:5 = 200:x; so x = 1,000/25 = 40.

145. Correct Answer: **Anterior lateral thigh**

146. Correct Answer: <u>3</u>

Rationale: The ratio is 10:1 = 100:x; x = 100/10 = 10.

147. Correct Answer: <u>2</u>

Rationale: The ratio is 250:1 = 750:x; x = 750/250 = 3.

148. Correct Answer: **90-degree angle**

149. Correct Answer: <u>4</u>

Rationale: The ratio is 10:1 = 20:x; x = 20/10 = 2; then multiply 2 × 30 days = 60.

150. Correct Answer: **False**

Rationale: The deltoid should be used for injections of fluid equal to or less than 1 mL.

151. Correct Answer: <u>2</u>

Rationale: The ratio is 500:1 = 500:x; x = 500/500 = 1.

152. Correct Answer: **False**

Rationale: The deltoid injection site is found three fingers below the acromion process.

153. Correct Answer: <u>1</u>

Rationale: Do not give any tablets because the pharmacy has dispensed the wrong medication.

154. Correct Answer: <u>1</u>

Rationale: Do not give any medication, as the patient has been prescribed extended-release capsules and the pharmacy has dispensed immediate-release tablets.

155. Correct Answer: **True**

156. Correct Answer: <u>3</u>

Rationale: The ratio is 50:1 = 100:x; x = 100/50 = 2.

157. Correct Answer: **Sciatic nerve**

158. Correct Answer: <u>2</u>

Rationale: The ratio is 50:1 = 50:x; x = 50/50 = 1.

159. Correct Answer: <u>4</u>

Rationale: The ratio is 5:1 = 20:x; x = 20/5 = 4.

REDUCTION OF RISK POTENTIAL

160. Correct Answer: <u>4</u>

Rationale: $240 - 150 = 90$; $90/30 = 3$.

161. Correct Answer:

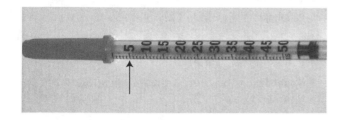

Rationale: $75/15 = 5$ units.

162. Correct Answer: <u>3</u>

Rationale: Potassium needs to be monitored when the patient is receiving a diuretic, such as Lasix, because potassium affects the electrical activity of the heart.

163. Correct Answer: <u>4 tablets</u>

Rationale: $2,000$ mg $= 2$ g; $2,000/500 = 4$.

164. Correct Answer: <u>4</u>

Rationale: The ratio is $5:20 = x: 60$; $20x = 300$; $x = 15$.

165. Correct Answer: <u>1</u>

Rationale: The pharmacy has sent up the wrong medication. Hydromorphone can easily be mistaken for morphine.

166. Correct Answer: <u>1</u>

Rationale: One syringe contains 9 mcg.

167. Correct Answer: <u>3</u>

Rationale: $90 \times 70 = 6,300$.

168. Correct Answer: <u>Weight</u>

169. Correct Answer: <u>3</u>

Rationale: The ratio is $50:1 = 75:x$; $x = 75/50 = 1.5$.

170. Correct Answer: <u>1</u>

Rationale: None; the pharmacy has dispensed the medication in the wrong strength.

171. Correct Answer: <u>1</u>

Rationale: There are four 6-hour time periods in 24 hours, so $800/4$ equals 200 mg every 6 hours. The ratio is $80:15 = 200:x$; $x = 3,000/80 = 37.5$.

172. Correct Answer: <u>3</u>

Rationale: The ratio is $20:1 = 40:x$; $x = 40/20 = 2$.

173. Correct Answer: <u>0.6 mg</u>

Rationale: $0.3 \times 200/100 = 0.6$.

174. Correct Answer: <u>1</u>

Rationale: The ratio is $8:1 = 24:x$; $x = 24/8 = 3$.

175. Correct Answer: <u>2</u>

Rationale: $14 + 7 = 21$.

176. Correct Answer: <u>3</u>

Rationale: The ratio is $250:1 = 750:x$; $x = 750/250 = 3$.

177. Correct Answer: <u>4</u>

Rationale: The ratio is $50:1 = 200:x$; $x = 200/50 = 4$.

178. Correct Answer: <u>False</u>

Rationale: $5/100$ is larger than $1/100$.

179. Correct Answer: <u>2</u>

Rationale: $200 \times 3 = 600$.

180. Correct Answer: <u>1</u>

Rationale: The ratio is $40:1 = 800:x$; $x = 800/40 = 20$.

181. Correct Answer: <u>60 mg</u>

Rationale: The ratio is $15:1 = x:4$; $x = 60/1 = 60$.

182. Correct Answer: <u>2</u>

Rationale: One 5-mg tablet daily $\times 7$ days per month $= 7$ tablets.

183. Correct Answer: <u>3</u>

Rationale: $1,000$ mg $= 1$ g; 0.875 g $= 875$ mg. 1 tablet $\times 2$ per day $= 2$ tablets.

184. Correct Answer: <u>2</u>

Rationale: The ratio is $30:1 = 60:x$; $x = 60/30 = 2$.

SECTION I
SECTION II
SECTION III
SECTION IV
SECTION V
SECTION VI
SECTION VII
SECTION VIII
SECTION IX
SECTION X

185. Correct Answer: **2**

Rationale: 1,000 mg = 1 g; 300 mg = 0.3 g.

186. Correct Answer: **3**

Rationale: The ratio is 0.125:1 = 0.375:x;
x = 0.375/0.125 = 3.

187. Correct Answer: **2 tablets**

Rationale: The ratio is 30:1 = 60:x; x = 60/30 = 2;
30 × 2 = 60.

188. Correct Answer: **4**

Rationale: The ratio is 0.5:1 = 1:x; x = 1/0.5 = 2.

189. Correct Answer: **2**

Rationale: 40 × 0.5 = 20.

190. Correct Answer: **1**

Rationale: 20 × 30 = 600.

191. Correct Answer: **2**

Rationale: The ratio is 10,000:1 = 5,000:x.
x = 5,000/10,000 = 0.5.

192. Correct Answer: **4**

Rationale: The ratio is 15:1 = 45:x and x = 45/15
= 3 tablets.

PHYSIOLOGICAL ADAPTATION

193. Correct Answer: **2**

Rationale: 500/250 = 2 tablets.

194. Correct Answer: **3**

Rationale: 165 is the systolic blood pressure.

195. Correct Answer: **4**

Rationale: 4 mg/4 times per day = 1 mg.

196. Correct Answer: **1**

Rationale: The ratio is 20:5 = 80:x;
x = 400/20 = 20.

197. Correct Answer: **2**

Rationale: The ratio is 125:5 = 375:x;
x = 1,875/125 = 15.

198. Correct Answer: **3**

Rationale: The systolic blood pressure is 226 mm
Hg, which is greater than 151 mm Hg.

199. Correct Answer: **True**

200. Correct Answer: **3**

Rationale: The ratio is 50:0.05 = x:0.1; x = 5/.05 =
100 mcg. Also, 50:1 = 100:x; x = 2 tablets.

201. Correct Answer: **2**

Rationale: 75/30 = 2.5.

202. Correct Answer: **4**

Rationale: The ratio is 12.5:5 = 25:x;
x = 125/12.5 = 10.

203. Correct Answer: **False**

Rationale: Liquid medications are calibrated in
milliliters.

204. Correct Answer: **4**

Rationale: The ratio is 75:5 = 125:x;
x = 625/75 = 8.33

205. Correct Answer: **2**

Rationale: The ratio is 1:0.25 = x:1.0;
x = 1/0.25 = 4.

206. Correct Answer: **1**

Rationale: The ratio is 1:750 = x:2,250;
x = 2,250/750 = 3.

207. Correct Answer: **2**

Rationale: The ratio is 1:2.5 = x:7.5;
x = 7.5/2.5 = 3.

208. Correct Answer: **4**

Rationale: 1,000 mg = 1 g; 1,250/250 = 5.

209. Correct Answer: **False**

Rationale: Heparin is incompatible with many
medications.

210. Correct Answer: **2**

Rationale: The ratio is 1:20 = x:60; x = 60/20 = 3.

211. Correct Answer: **1**

Rationale: The ratio is 250:5 = 50:x;
x = 250/250 = 1.

212. Correct Answer: **3**

Rationale: The ratio is 5:1 = 2.5:x; x = 2.5/5 = 0.5.

213. Correct Answer: **True**

Rationale: Other effects include flushing,
dizziness, and postural hypotension.

214. Correct Answer: **2**

Rationale: The ratio is 1:1 = 2:x; x = 2 vials.

215. Correct Answer: **2**

Rationale: The ratio is 300:1 = 450:*x*;
x = 450/300 = 1.5.

216. Correct Answer: **2**

Rationale: The ratio is 5:5 = 3:*x*; *x* = 3 (there is 1 mg/1 mL).

217. Correct Answer: **4**

Rationale: 800/200 = 4 capsules × 5 times/day = 20 capsules/day × 7 days = 140 capsules.

218. Correct Answer: **Vitamin K**

Rationale: Vitamin K is the fat soluble vitamin that interferes with clotting because Vitamin K is necessary for the synthesis of clotting factors VII, IX, X and prothrombin by the liver.

219. Correct Answer: **3**

Rationale: 5 × 3 = 15.

220. Correct Answer: **4**

Rationale: The ratio is 3.75:1 = 3.75:*x*;
x = 3.75/3.75 = 1.

221. Correct Answer: **Decrease**

222. Correct Answer: **2**

Rationale: The ratio is 130:1 = 240:*x* ;
x = 240/130 = 1.8 = 2 vials.

Care of Patients with Diabetes

MANAGEMENT OF CARE

Multiple Choice

1. Based on the sliding-scale prescription below, what is your intervention if the patient's blood sugar is 224?

> Blood glucose < 150 mg/dL: Administer 0 units of insulin.
>
> Blood glucose 150–200 mg/dL: Administer 2 units of regular insulin.
>
> Blood glucose 201–250 mg/dL: Administer 3 units of regular insulin.
>
> Blood glucose 251–300 mg/dL: Administer 5 units of regular insulin.
>
> Blood glucose > 300 mg/dL: Administer 6 units of regular insulin and contact the physician immediately.

1. Administer 2 units of regular insulin.
2. Administer 3 units of regular insulin.
3. Administer 3 units NPH insulin.
4. Contact the physician immediately.

2. Based on the sliding-scale prescription below, what is your intervention if the patient's blood sugar is 136?

> Blood glucose < 150 mg/dL: Administer 0 units of insulin.
>
> Blood glucose 150–200 mg/dL: Administer 2 units of regular insulin.
>
> Blood glucose 201–250 mg/dL: Administer 3 units of regular insulin.
>
> Blood glucose 251–300 mg/dL: Administer 5 units of regular insulin.
>
> Blood glucose > 300 mg/dL: Administer 6 units of regular insulin and contact the physician immediately.

1. Administer 0 units of insulin.
2. Administer 2 units of regular insulin.
3. Administer 3 units of regular insulin.
4. Administer 6 units of regular insulin and contact the physician immediately.

3. Mrs. Kitchens has the following sliding-scale insulin prescription: Measure blood glucose levels at bedtime. When insulin is given before bedtime, the blood glucose must be checked in 2 hours.

> Blood glucose < 130 mg/dL: Administer 0 units of insulin.
>
> Blood glucose 130–160 mg/dL: Administer 2 units of regular insulin.
>
> Blood glucose 161–190 mg/dL: Administer 4 units of regular insulin.
>
> Blood glucose 191–220 mg/dL: Administer 6 units of regular insulin.
>
> Blood glucose 221–250 mg/dL: Administer 8 units of regular insulin.
>
> Blood glucose > 250 mg/dL: Administer 10 units of regular insulin and contact the physician immediately.

Mrs. Kitchens' bedtime blood sugar is 222. How much regular insulin should she administer?

1. Administer 2 units of regular insulin.
2. Administer 4 units of regular insulin.
3. Administer 6 units of regular insulin.
4. Administer 8 units of regular insulin.

4. Mr. Bolton has the following sliding-scale insulin prescription: Measure blood glucose levels at bedtime. When insulin is given before bedtime, the blood glucose must be checked in 2 hours.

> Blood glucose < 130 mg/dL: Administer 0 units of insulin.
>
> Blood glucose 130–190 mg/dL: Administer 3 units of regular insulin.
>
> Blood glucose 191–250 mg/dL: Administer 6 units of regular insulin.
>
> Blood glucose > 250 mg/dL: Administer 10 units of regular insulin and contact the physician immediately.

Mr. Bolton's bedtime blood sugar is 128. How much regular insulin should he administer?

1. Administer no insulin.
2. Administer 3 units of regular insulin.
3. Administer 6 units of regular insulin.
4. Administer 10 units of regular insulin and contact the physician.

5. Kevin is a 15-year-old diabetic who plays sports and eats fast food. He keeps his blood sugars under control by using the following sliding-scale insulin prescription after he checks his blood sugar.

> Blood glucose < 150 mg/dL: Give 0 units of lispro insulin.
>
> Blood glucose 150–199 mg/dL: Give 1 unit of lispro insulin.
>
> Blood glucose 200–249 mg/dL: Give 2 units of lispro insulin.
>
> Blood glucose 250–300 mg/dL: Give 3 units of lispro insulin.
>
> Blood glucose > 300 mg/dL: Call the physician immediately.

Kevin's blood sugar is 300 mg/dL. How much lispro insulin should he administer to himself?

1. Administer no insulin.
2. Administer 2 units of lispro insulin.
3. Administer 3 units of lispro insulin.
4. Call the physician immediately.

6. The pancreas contains cells that act as endocrine glands and are the source of pancreatic hormones. What are these cells called?

1. Glomerular filtration cells.
2. Purkinje fibers.
3. Kupfer cells.
4. Islets of Langerhans.

True or False

7. The major cause of death among older people with diabetes is cardiovascular disease.

Multiple Choice

8. Which of the following situations will affect blood sugar levels?

1. Physical activity and stress.
2. Illness and playing a fun card game.
3. Surgery and reading a book.
4. Travel and talking on the phone to a friend.

9. Which of the following laboratory tests is also known as glycosylated hemoglobin?

1. Hemoglobin A_{1C}.
2. Hematocrit.
3. Complete blood count (CBC).
4. Mean corpuscular hemoglobin.

10. Which of the following conditions is a complication of diabetes that is associated with the kidneys?

1. Diabetic retinopathy.
2. Atherosclerosis.
3. Diabetic nephropathy.
4. Glaucoma.

True or False

11. In addition to retinopathy, the person with diabetes mellitus is at increased risk for cataract formation.

Multiple Choice

12. Which of the following is the leading cause of blindness in diabetics?

1. Smoking cigarettes.
2. Retinopathy.
3. Hypotension.
4. Low serum triglycerides.

13. A normal blood glucose level in a nondiabetic person is maintained between

1. 70 and 100 mg/dL.
2. 120 and 240 mg/dL.
3. 100 and 180 mg/dL.
4. 200 and 400 mg/dL.

14. Polydipsia, polyphagia, polyuria, weight loss, and fatigue are classic signs of

1. Stroke.
2. Heart failure.
3. Hyperglycemia.
4. Hypoglycemia.

True or False

15. Hypolipidemia and hypotension are comorbidities often found in persons with diabetes mellitus.

Multiple Choice

16. Mr. Coggins receives 3 units of regular insulin and 5 units of NPH insulin every morning to control his diabetes. How many total units should Mr. Coggins draw up in one syringe?

1. 3 units.
2. 5 units.
3. 8 units.
4. 13 units.

17. Mrs. Chandler gives herself regular insulin only when her blood sugar exceeds 160 mg/dL. In the past 3 months, this has happened only four times. Based on these data, how would you tell Mrs. Chandler to store her vial of regular insulin?

1. Store it in the refrigerator.
2. Freeze it.
3. Keep it warm, at a temperature of 90°F.
4. Keep it at room temperature.

18. Mr. Krech has trouble remembering to rotate his sites for insulin injections. In the past week he has self-injected into the right abdomen, left abdomen, right upper arm, left thigh, and right thigh. Into which site should he self-inject his insulin next?

1. Left ankle.
2. Right abdomen.
3. Left midback.
4. Left upper arm.

Fill in the Blank

19. Symmetrical peripheral polyneuropathy is first seen as bilateral sensory loss in the _____ (lower, upper) extremities.

Multiple Choice

20. Mr. Muska has diabetes and is under extreme stress at work. How would you expect his work situation to affect his blood sugar?

1. Increase his blood sugar.
2. Decrease his blood sugar.
3. Have no effect on his blood sugar.
4. Elevate only his antidiuretic hormone production.

Fill in the Blank

21. Mrs. Sanchez is to receive 3 units of NPH insulin every morning to control her diabetes. She should use a _____ (low-dose, high-dose) syringe for best care.

Multiple Choice

22. Mr. Chernecky has been diagnosed with atherosclerosis. One of the risk factors for this condition is diabetes, with which he has also been diagnosed. What is another risk factor for atherosclerosis?

1. Low total cholesterol values.
2. High values of high-density lipoproteins (HDL).
3. High iron values.
4. High triglyceride values.

23. Mrs. Sullivan has type 2 diabetes mellitus and is trying to determine how she can change her lifestyle so as to decrease her serum glucose levels. Which of the following measures would you suggest as an appropriate intervention?

1. Get 10 to 12 hours of sleep per day.
2. Exercise.
3. Undergo gastric bypass surgery.
4. Smoke less than 1 pack of cigarettes per day.

24. Which of the following signs of diabetes mellitus might a dentist be likely to discover?

1. High serum glucose.
2. Vulvovaginitis.
3. Periodontal disease.
4. Pneumonia.

True or False

25. Coronary artery disease occurs in persons who have diabetes at a higher rate than in the general population.

Multiple Choice

26. You are reading the box that a vial of insulin comes in and need to know the origin of the insulin. Which of the following indicates the insulin's source?

1. Novolin.
2. 70/30.
3. Recombinant DNA.
4. 100 units/mL.

27. What is the usual standardization of insulin in vials?

1. 1 unit/mL.
2. 100 units/mL.
3. 50 mg/dL.
4. 70 units/30 mL.

28. Which of the following insulins should not be mixed with other kinds of insulin?

1. NPH insulin.
2. Regular insulin.
3. Lantus insulin.
4. 70/30 insulin.

29. Your hospital provides you with three types of insulin syringes: 30 units, 50 units, and 100 units. If your patient is to receive 10 units of regular insulin plus 28 units of NPH insulin in one syringe, which syringe should you choose?

1. A 30-unit syringe.
2. A 50-unit syringe.
3. A 100-unit syringe.
4. A 3-mL syringe.

30. What does it mean when a prescription for insulin is written for Novolin 70/30?

1. 70% regular insulin and 30% NPH insulin.
2. 70% NPH insulin and 30% regular insulin.
3. 70% regular insulin and 30% Lente insulin.
4. 70% NPH insulin and 30% Lantus insulin.

True or False

31. Insulin can be delivered through an insulin syringe, an insulin pen, or an insulin pump.

Multiple Choice

32. Lispro is designated as a "fast-acting" insulin. How quickly does its onset of action begin?

1. In less than 5 seconds.
2. In less than 15 minutes.
3. Within 1 to 4 hours.
4. Within 4 to 6 hours.

33. Insulins are defined by how quickly their onset begins, when this action peaks, and how long this action lasts. What is the term associated with how long the action lasts?

1. Standardization.
2. Origin.
3. Route.
4. Duration.

True or False

34. It is not harmful to leave a vial of insulin in the glove box of your car.

Multiple Choice

35. Which type of diabetes is usually diagnosed in children and young adults and occurs because the body does not produce insulin?

1. Gestational diabetes.
2. Type 1 diabetes.
3. Type 2 diabetes.
4. Gerontological diabetes.

36. What is the most common classification of diabetes mellitus?

1. GDM.
2. ITT.
3. IDDM, type 1.
4. NIDDM, type 2.

37. Which of the following conditions results when a person suffers a deficiency of insulin?

1. Insipidus.
2. Hyperglycemia.
3. Hypoglycemia.
4. Ketoacidosis.

SECTION I

SECTION II

SECTION III

SECTION IV

SECTION V

SECTION VI

SECTION VII

SECTION VIII

SECTION IX

SECTION X

Fill in the Blank

38. Fresh foods are better than canned or frozen foods because canned and frozen foods contain large amounts of _____ (potassium, chloride, sodium).

Multiple Choice

39. Which of the following organizations establishes the dietary recommendations for persons with diabetes?

1. American Dietary Association.
2. American Diabetes Association.
3. American Medical Association.
4. American Renal Association.

40. Which of the following findings would be a positive assessment indicating dehydration in a person with diabetes insipidus?

1. High urine specific gravity.
2. Hypotension.
3. Fever.
4. Complaints of thirst.

41. Which of the following laboratory tests might indicate diabetes insipidus?

1. High serum sodium and decreased ADH levels.
2. Low serum sodium and high ADH levels.
3. High urine specific gravity and low serum iron.
4. High urine osmolality and serum chloride.

42. Which type of diet should the nurse instruct a patient with diabetes insipidus to follow?

1. High sodium and low potassium.
2. High iron and high protein.
3. Low sodium and low caffeine.
4. High carbohydrate and high sodium.

43. Mrs. Wallace is a 72-year-old widow who is on a fixed income. She says she cannot afford to care for her newly diagnosed diabetes because she cannot pay for the blood glucose monitor. What would be your best response to Mrs. Wallace?

1. "Well, you need to get the money to buy what you need or bad things might happen."
2. "Medicare covers the expense of diabetes products and supplies."
3. "Maybe the doctor will ask you to check your sugar only twice a day."
4. "You might ask your doctor for a free machine; he might have one."

44. What is the name of the equipment that pokes the finger to obtain a drop of blood that is to be used in the glucose monitoring machine?

1. Pump.
2. Glucowatch.
3. Syringe.
4. Lancet.

SAFETY AND INFECTION CONTROL

Multiple Choice

45. Based on the sliding-scale prescription below, what is your intervention if the patient's blood sugar is 251?

> Blood glucose < 150 mg/dL: Administer 0 units of insulin.
> Blood glucose 150–200 mg/dL: Administer 2 units of regular insulin.
> Blood glucose 201–250 mg/dL: Administer 3 units of regular insulin.
> Blood glucose 251–300 mg/dL: Administer 5 units of regular insulin.
> Blood glucose > 300 mg/dL: Administer 6 units of regular insulin and contact the physician immediately.

1. Administer 2 units of regular insulin.
2. Administer 3 units of regular insulin.
3. Administer 5 units of regular insulin.
4. Administer 6 units of regular insulin and contact the physician immediately.

46. Based on the sliding-scale prescription below, what is your intervention if the patient's blood sugar is 312?

> Blood glucose < 150 mg/dL: Administer 0 units of insulin.
> Blood glucose 150–200 mg/dL: Administer 2 units of regular insulin.
> Blood glucose 201–250 mg/dL: Administer 3 units of regular insulin.
> Blood glucose 251–300 mg/dL: Administer 5 units of regular insulin.
> Blood glucose > 300 mg/dL: Administer 6 units of regular insulin and contact the physician immediately.

1. Administer 3 units of regular insulin.
2. Administer 6 units of NPH insulin.
3. Administer 5 units of regular insulin.
4. Administer 6 units of regular insulin and contact the physician immediately.

47. Mr. Herrod has the following sliding-scale insulin prescription:

> Blood glucose < 150 mg/dL: Administer 0 units of insulin.
>
> Blood glucose 150–200 mg/dL: Administer 4 units of regular insulin.
>
> Blood glucose 201–250 mg/dL: Administer 7 units of regular insulin.
>
> Blood glucose 251–300 mg/dL: Administer 10 units of regular insulin.
>
> Blood glucose > 300 mg/dL: Administer 13 units of regular insulin and contact the physician immediately.

Mr. Herrod's blood glucose was 181. What is your intervention?

1. Administer no insulin.
2. Administer 4 units of regular insulin.
3. Administer 7 units of regular insulin.
4. Administer 10 units of NPH insulin.

48. Mrs. Flowers has the following sliding-scale insulin prescription:

> Blood glucose < 150 mg/dL: Administer 0 units of insulin.
>
> Blood glucose 150–200 mg/dL: Administer 4 units of regular insulin.
>
> Blood glucose 201–250 mg/dL: Administer 7 units of regular insulin.
>
> Blood glucose 251–300 mg/dL: Administer 10 units of regular insulin.
>
> Blood glucose > 300 mg/dL: Administer 13 units of regular insulin and contact the physician immediately.

Mrs. Flowers' blood glucose was 316. What is your intervention?

1. Administer 7 units of regular insulin.
2. Administer 10 units of NPH insulin.
3. Administer 10 units of regular insulin and call the physician immediately.
4. Administer 13 units of regular insulin and call the physician immediately.

49. Which common diuretic medication can induce hyperglycemia?

1. Furosemide (Lasix).
2. Imipramine (Thorazine).
3. Simvastatin (Zocor).
4. Doxazosin mesylate (Cardura).

50. Which of the following insulins is considered to be "short acting"?

1. NPH insulin.
2. Lente insulin.
3. Regular insulin.
4. Novolin 70/30 insulin.

51. What is the best way to store an insulin vial that will be used within 30 days?

1. Keep it at room temperature.
2. Keep it in freezer.
3. Keep it heated to more than 160°F.
4. Keep it wrapped in a heating blanket.

True or False

52. You should never use insulin that is past its expiration date.

Multiple Choice

53. Mrs. Golson is newly diagnosed with insulin-dependent diabetes. She has been prescribed both NPH and regular insulin mixed in one syringe to help control her diabetes. You are teaching her to give insulin injections. Which insulin do you tell her to draw up first in the insulin syringe?

1. Draw up the NPH insulin first.
2. Draw up the regular insulin first.
3. It does not matter which insulin you draw up first.
4. Alternate which insulin you draw up first for each injection.

54. Common sites to teach patients to give insulin injections into include the buttocks, upper arms, abdomen, and

1. Calf of the leg.
2. Dorsal aspect of either hand.
3. Thighs.
4. Forehead.

55. You are teaching a patient with insulin-dependent diabetes about the importance of absorption of insulin to controlling his diabetes. To best avoid absorption problems, you will teach him to

1. Shake the insulin vial prior to drawing up insulin.
2. Rotate insulin injection sites.
3. Inject the insulin while it is still cold from refrigeration.
4. Use an 18-gauge needle for injection.

56. Individuals who have diabetes mellitus are susceptible to infection. For this reason, which organ should the nurse concentrate on during the assessment of a patient with diabetes?

　1. Skin.
　2. Lungs.
　3. Adrenal glands.
　4. Liver.

True or False

57. Safe disposal of used syringes includes disposal of the syringe with needle in a special container.

Multiple Choice

58. How long before you give an injection of insulin should you remove the vial of insulin from the refrigerator?

　1. 5 minutes prior to injection.
　2. 30 minutes prior to injection.
　3. 2 hours prior to injection.
　4. 4 to 6 hours prior to injection.

59. When Mr. Holland looks at his vial of insulin, he sees that it is cloudy and tan in color and contains some large chunks. What should he do regarding his insulin injection?

　1. Shake the vial vigorously to break up the protein.
　2. Give his insulin injection as prescribed.
　3. Inject extra air into the vial to disengage the chunks.
　4. Open and inspect a new vial of insulin.

60. Which of the following laboratory values would indicate infection?

　1. Increased red blood cell count.
　2. Decreased platelet count.
　3. Increased leukocyte count.
　4. Decreased mean corpuscular hemoglobin.

Fill in the Blank

61. Diabetics have to be concerned about two main effects of diabetes: high blood sugar, which is known as hyperglycemia, and low blood sugar, which is known as _____.

Multiple Choice

62. Assessment of foot ulcers, poor wound healing, and atrophy includes assessing which of the following body systems?

　1. Cardiovascular system.
　2. Gastrointestinal system.
　3. Renal system.
　4. Integumentary system.

63. You are assessing your patient who has diabetes for an impaired immune system. Which response by the patient would indicate impairment?

　1. "I see halos when I look at something far away."
　2. "I have vaginitis, and I need some medication for it."
　3. "I am constipated. Can I have something for that?"
　4. My knees make cracking sounds when I bend down low sometimes."

64. Your patient is in the waiting room for her usual clinic visit to the diabetic educator. A few minutes ago, she was rude and inappropriate to the secretary. Now she tells you that she has a headache, is weak, and has slight tremors. You recognize these as signs of which condition?

　1. Hypoglycemia.
　2. Hyperglycemia.
　3. Hyperlipidemia.
　4. Hypertension.

65. Your patient takes both regular and NPH insulin in the morning and afternoon according to a sliding-scale prescription. You ask her to show you the bottle of insulin she uses for covering the sliding scale. Which bottle should she choose to be correct?

　1. NPH insulin.
　2. Lente insulin.
　3. Regular insulin.
　4. Glucophage (Metformin).

Short Answer

66. Mrs. Christopher was first diagnosed with insulin-dependent diabetes at age 15. When she came into your clinic for a follow-up visit, you noticed that she had massive scratches on her right ankle and a resulting infection. When you question

her about this problem, she states, "Oh, my cat Morris must have been using my leg as a scratching post and I did not even feel it." Which diabetic complication does Mrs. Christopher have?

HEALTH PROMOTION AND MAINTENANCE

Multiple Choice

67. To maintain normalized blood sugars, Mrs. Johnson has the following sliding-scale insulin prescription:

> Blood glucose < 130 mg/dL: Administer 0 units of insulin.
>
> Blood glucose 130–160 mg/dL: Administer 2 units of regular insulin.
>
> Blood glucose 161–190 mg/dL: Administer 4 units of regular insulin.
>
> Blood glucose 191–220 mg/dL: Administer 6 units of regular insulin.
>
> Blood glucose 221–250 mg/dL: Administer 8 units of regular insulin.
>
> Blood glucose > 250 mg/dL: Administer 10 units of regular insulin and contact the physician immediately.

Mrs. Johnson's blood sugar is 186. What is your intervention?

1. Administer 4 units of regular insulin.
2. Administer 6 units of regular insulin.
3. Administer 8 units of regular insulin.
4. Administer 10 units of regular insulin and contact the physician immediately.

68. To maintain normalized blood sugars, Mr. Hernandez has the following sliding-scale insulin prescription:

> Blood glucose < 130 mg/dL: Administer 0 units of insulin.
>
> Blood glucose 130–160 mg/dL: Administer 2 units of regular insulin.
>
> Blood glucose 161–190 mg/dL: Administer 4 units of regular insulin.
>
> Blood glucose 191–220 mg/dL: Administer 6 units of regular insulin.
>
> Blood glucose 221–250 mg/dL: Administer 8 units of regular insulin.
>
> Blood glucose > 250 mg/dL: Administer 10 units of regular insulin and contact the physician immediately.

Mr. Hernandez's blood sugar is 122. What is your intervention?

1. Administer no insulin.
2. Administer 2 units of regular insulin.
3. Administer 4 units of regular insulin.
4. Administer no regular insulin and contact the physician immediately.

69. To maintain blood glucose levels within normal limits, 16-year-old Matthew must inject himself with lispro insulin after determining his blood sugar level several times per day. Based on the following sliding-scale prescription, how much lispro insulin should Matthew administer if his blood sugar was 198?

> Blood glucose < 150 mg/dL: Administer 0 units of lispro insulin.
>
> Blood glucose 150–199 mg/dL: Administer 1 unit of lispro insulin.
>
> Blood glucose 200–249 mg/dL: Administer 2 units of lispro insulin.
>
> Blood glucose 250–300 mg/dL: Administer 3 units of lispro insulin.
>
> Blood glucose > 300 mg/dL: Call the physician immediately.

1. Administer no insulin.
2. Administer 1 unit of lispro insulin.
3. Administer 2 units of lispro insulin.
4. Administer 3 units of regular insulin.

Identification

70. Draw a line on the insulin syringe to indicate how much regular insulin you should administer if your patient is on the following sliding-scale insulin and her blood glucose level before lunch is 181 mg/dL.

> Blood glucose < 150 mg/dL: Administer 0 units of insulin.
>
> Blood glucose 150–200 mg/dL: Administer 2 units of regular insulin.
>
> Blood glucose 201–250 mg/dL: Administer 3 units of regular insulin.
>
> Blood glucose 251–300 mg/dL: Administer 5 units of regular insulin.
>
> Blood glucose > 300 mg/dL: Administer 6 units of regular insulin and contact the physician immediately.

SECTION I
SECTION II
SECTION III
SECTION IV
SECTION V
SECTION VI
SECTION VII
SECTION VIII
SECTION IX
SECTION X

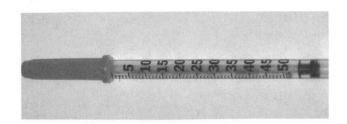

Multiple Choice

71. Often individuals who have diabetes mellitus also have high triglyceride and cholesterol values. Elevated levels of these lipids increase a patient's mortality risk due to

1. Kidney failure.
2. Pancreatic neoplasm.
3. Peripheral vascular disease.
4. Atherosclerosis.

72. In females who develop diabetes, a common symptom that leads them to seek medical care is skin irritation of the vulva. This irritation occurs due to large amounts of

1. Protein in the urine.
2. Glucose in the urine.
3. Magnesium in the serum.
4. Ketones in the feces.

73. You need to teach a group of newly diagnosed diabetics about nutrition. On which three areas of dietary management should you concentrate?

1. Saturated and nonsaturated fats and vitamin A.
2. Iron, vitamin A, and protein.
3. Carbohydrates, minerals, and essential elements such as zinc.
4. Carbohydrates, fats, and protein.

Identification

74. Draw a line on the insulin syringe to indicate how much regular insulin you should administer if your patient is on the following sliding-scale insulin and his blood glucose level before lunch is 181 mg/dL.

Blood glucose < 150 mg/dL: Administer 0 units of insulin.

Blood glucose 150–200 mg/dL: Administer 2 units of regular insulin.

Blood glucose 201–299 mg/dL: Administer 4 units of regular insulin.

Blood glucose 300–399 mg/dL: Administer 5 units of regular insulin.

Blood glucose > 400 mg/dL: Administer 8 units of regular insulin and contact the physician immediately.

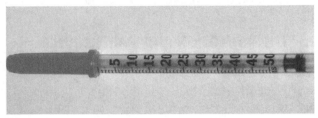

Multiple Choice

75. Which of the following laboratory blood tests is useful in monitoring the average blood glucose levels over a 3-month period?

1. Hematocrit.
2. Total albumin.
3. Hemoglobin A_{1C}.
4. Fasting blood sugar.

76. To understand maintenance care, a diabetic should know that insulin pens contain

1. Prefilled insulin cartridges.
2. An infusion set that is inserted into the skin for 48 to 72 hours.
3. No needles but rather use pressure to deliver insulin.
4. A 5-mL syringe.

77. Which of the following is a symptom associated with diabetes' effects on the integumentary system?

1. Blurred vision.
2. Dry skin.
3. Fatigue.
4. Anorexia.

Short Answer

78. Your patient is to administer regular insulin based on the following formula: (blood sugar – 100)/30 = number of units regular insulin. Your patient's blood sugar is 190 mg/dL. How many units of regular insulin should she administer?

Multiple Choice

79. A blood test is usually performed to diagnose diabetes. Which unit is used to measure the amount of glucose in blood?

1. mg/mcg.
2. mcg/mg.

3. mg/dL.

4. L/min.

80. What is the normal range of a fasting glucose?

1. 70–100 mg/dL.

2. 100–140 mg/dL.

3. 140–160 mg/dL.

4. 160–180 mg/dL.

Short Answer

81. Your patient is to administer regular insulin based on the following formula: (blood sugar − 100)/30 = number of units regular insulin. Your patient's blood sugar is 250 mg/dL. How many units of regular insulin should he administer?

Multiple Choice

82. In which test do patients take an oral glucose solution and have blood drawn several times over 3 hours?

1. Fasting plasma glucose.

2. Urine test for ketones.

3. Random plasma glucose.

4. Oral glucose tolerance test.

83. A random blood glucose test finding that is greater than which of the following values indicates diabetes?

1. 100 mg/dL.

2. 120 mg/dL.

3. 200 mg/dL.

4. 250 mg/dL.

84. Impaired glucose tolerance (IGT) is an indicator that a person is at increased risk for developing

1. Type 1 diabetes.

2. Type 2 diabetes.

3. Renal neoplasm.

4. Prostatitis.

85. Which of the following conditions are associated with impaired glucose tolerance (IGT)?

1. Hypotension and hyperlipidemia.

2. Hypoglycemia and prostatitis.

3. Obesity and hypotension.

4. Obesity and syndrome X.

86. Some women develop a condition that includes insulin resistance, hyperinsulinemia, and impaired glucose tolerance (IGT). What is this condition called?

1. Proctitis.

2. Polycystic ovary syndrome (PCOS).

3. Uterine glucose dysplasia (UGD).

4. Duodenal ulcer.

PSYCHOSOCIAL INTEGRITY

Multiple Choice

87. Mr. Whitfield is at a party when he begins to feel nauseated and have blurred vision. To maintain normalized blood sugars, Mr. Whitfield has the following sliding-scale insulin prescription:

Blood glucose < 130 mg/dL: Administer 0 units of insulin.

Blood glucose 130–160 mg/dL: Administer 2 units of regular insulin.

Blood glucose 161–190 mg/dL: Administer 4 units of regular insulin.

Blood glucose 191–220 mg/dL: Administer 6 units of regular insulin.

Blood glucose 221–250 mg/dL: Administer 8 units of regular insulin.

Blood glucose > 250 mg/dL: Administer 10 units of regular insulin and contact the physician immediately.

Mr. Whitfield's blood sugar is 241. What should he do?

1. Administer 4 units of regular insulin.

2. Administer 6 units of regular insulin.

3. Administer 8 units of regular insulin.

4. Administer 10 units of regular insulin and contact the nurse practitioner on call immediately.

True or False

88. Directions: Sugar-free foods are also carbohydrate-free foods.

Multiple Choice

89. Ms. Eglin is walking in the mall doing some shopping when she begins to feel nauseated yet hungry, and has blurred vision. To maintain

SECTION I

SECTION II

SECTION III

SECTION IV

SECTION V

SECTION VI

SECTION VII

SECTION VIII

SECTION IX

SECTION X

normalized blood sugars, Ms. Eglin has the following sliding-scale insulin prescription:

> Blood glucose < 130 mg/dL: Administer 0 units of insulin.
>
> Blood glucose 130–160 mg/dL: Administer 2 units of regular insulin.
>
> Blood glucose 161–190 mg/dL: Administer 4 units of regular insulin.
>
> Blood glucose 191–220 mg/dL: Administer 6 units of regular insulin.
>
> Blood glucose 221–250 mg/dL: Administer 8 units of regular insulin.
>
> Blood glucose > 250 mg/dL: Administer 10 units of regular insulin and contact the physician immediately.

Ms. Eglin's blood sugar is 156. What should she do?

1. Administer no insulin.
2. Administer 2 units of regular insulin.
3. Administer 4 units of regular insulin.
4. Administer 6 units of regular insulin.

90. Thirty minutes after lunch, your patient is to administer regular insulin based on the following formula: (blood sugar – 100)/30 = number of units regular insulin. Your patient's blood sugar 30 minutes after lunch is 310 mg/dL. How many units of regular insulin should she administer?

1. 14 units.
2. 10 units.
3. 8 units.
4. 7 units.

91. Thirty minutes after lunch, your patient is to administer regular insulin based on the following formula: (blood sugar – 100)/30 = number of units regular insulin. Your patient's blood sugar 30 minutes after lunch is 110 mg/dL. How many units of regular insulin should he administer?

1. No insulin.
2. 2 units.
3. 4 units.
4. 7 units.

True or False

92. Triglycerides are fats that are carried through the bloodstream in packages known as lipoproteins.

Multiple Choice

93. You are trying to teach a patient who has diabetes mellitus how to shop for foods. Your patient is single and prefers frozen food. What is your best advice to her?

1. Avoid foods that are high in fiber.
2. Avoid foods that are low in sodium.
3. Avoid foods that are high in fat and cholesterol.
4. Avoid foods that are high in vegetable content.

94. Your diabetic patient asks you which of the following ingredients is best to use in a recipe. How should you respond?

1. Vegetable oil.
2. Shortening.
3. Lard.
4. Butter.

95. Which of the following foods will increase the amount of fiber in your diet?

1. Oatmeal.
2. Chocolate chip cookies.
3. Yogurt.
4. White bread.

96. Which of the following milk products contain the least amount of fat?

1. Half-and-half.
2. 1% milk.
3. 2% milk.
4. Whole milk.

97. Which of the following foods is considered a free food/drink for diabetics?

1. Sugar-free cookies.
2. Milkshake.
3. Slice of wheat bread.
4. Diet soft drink.

Short Answer

98. You have diabetes and are 2 hours into a great party with your friends. You begin to feel sleepy, your vision becomes blurred, and you are hungry and thirsty. What is probably wrong?

Multiple Choice

99. Which of the following foods is a good source of protein?

1. Cooked oatmeal.
2. Honey.
3. Apricots.
4. Nuts.

100. You are a nurse who is discussing treatment involving insulin with Julie Johnson, a woman who is newly diagnosed with type 1 diabetes mellitus. Julie asks, "Why can't I just take the pill like my friend who has diabetes?" After you give your explanation, which of the following responses by the patient would indicate that she understood your explanation?

1. "After I am on insulin for some time, then I can wean myself off insulin and take pills."
2. "With exercise twice a day and a 1,200-calorie diet, I should be able to avoid having to take insulin."
3. "Because my body does not produce insulin, I will need to take insulin by injection for the rest of my life."
4. "When my body starts to make insulin again, then I can stop the insulin injections and try the pills."

Short Answer

101. To be prepared for emergencies, it is best if patients wear a bracelet stating that they have diabetes. What is this type of bracelet called?

Multiple Choice

102. Members of which of the following ethnic groups are more likely to develop impaired glucose tolerance (IGT)?

1. Caucasians and African Americans.
2. Native Americans and African Americans.
3. Hispanic Americans and Caucasians.
4. Scandinavians and Asian Americans.

103. Which of the following is necessary if an overweight person is to lose weight?

1. Calories consumed must be greater than calories burned.
2. Calories burned must be greater than calories consumed.

3. Calories burned must be equal to calories consumed.
4. Calories play no part in weight reduction.

104. What specific dietary change will help maintain good health in diabetics?

1. Limiting consumption of protein and water.
2. Limiting consumption fats and carbohydrates.
3. Limiting consumption of water and alcohol.
4. Limiting exercise to 15 minutes per day.

105. Which of the following foods are high in omega-3 fatty acids, which have been shown to decrease triglyceride, lipoprotein, and cholesterol levels without affecting blood glucose?

1. Salmon and herring.
2. Apples and kiwi fruits.
3. Oranges and cranberries.
4. Tuna and broccoli.

106. You are going to a restaurant and know you should eat fish high in omega-3 fatty acids. Which fish should you choose for your dinner?

1. Farm-raised salmon.
2. Non-farm-raised (wild) salmon.
3. Pufferfish.
4. Lobster.

BASIC CARE AND COMFORT

Multiple Choice

107. The nurse has a very important role in teaching patients about diet, exercise, and medication in terms of living with diabetes mellitus. Ultimately, however, what does the outcome of the disease process for each person depend on?

1. Diet and exercise.
2. Medication and diet.
3. Self-medication.
4. Self-management.

108. You are teaching a patient who is newly diagnosed with diabetes how to choose healthy snacks. Of the following foods, which is the best choice for your patient?

1. Buttered popcorn.
2. Baked chips and salsa.
3. Ice cream.
4. Chocolate chip cookies with nuts.

SECTION I

SECTION II

SECTION III

SECTION IV

SECTION V

SECTION VI

SECTION VII

SECTION VIII

SECTION IX

SECTION X

Identification

109. Draw a line on the insulin syringe to indicate how much regular insulin you should administer if your patient has the following sliding-scale prescription and her blood glucose level before lunch is 250 mg/dL:

> Blood glucose < 150 mg/dL: Administer 0 units of insulin.
>
> Blood glucose 150–250 mg/dL: Administer 4 units of regular insulin.
>
> Blood glucose 251–300 mg/dL: Administer 6 units of regular insulin.
>
> Blood glucose > 300 mg/dL: Administer 8 units of regular insulin and contact the physician immediately.

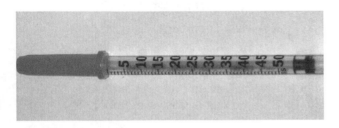

Multiple Choice

110. The best way for a patient with diabetes to protect against diabetic ketoacidosis is to monitor the blood sugar how many times per day?

1. Once per day.
2. Twice per day.
3. Four times per day.
4. Twenty-four times per day.

111. One symptom of hypoglycemia is that the heartbeat is

1. Rapid.
2. Slow.
3. Between 68 and 78 beats per minute.
4. Normal.

112. Which of the following symptoms is a sign of diabetes associated with the gastrointestinal system?

1. Contractures.
2. Peripheral vascular disease.
3. Cataracts.
4. Constipation.

Identification

113. Draw a line on the insulin syringe to indicate how much lispro insulin you should administer if your patient has the following sliding-scale prescription and his blood glucose level before lunch is 279 mg/dL:

> Blood glucose < 150 mg/dL: Administer 0 units of lispro insulin.
>
> Blood glucose 150–250 mg/dL: Administer 2 units of lispro insulin.
>
> Blood glucose 251–350 mg/dL: Administer 4 units of lispro insulin.
>
> Blood glucose > 350 mg/dL: Administer 6 units of lispro insulin and call the physician immediately.

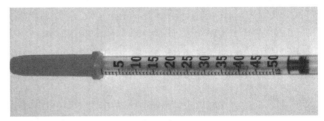

Multiple Choice

114. Which body system would you assess if you are looking for edema, albuminuria, and urinary tract infections?

1. Integumentary system.
2. Renal system.
3. Metabolic system.
4. Sensory system.

115. When assessing for diabetic retinopathy, what body system do you examine?

1. Cardiovascular system.
2. Reproductive system.
3. Metabolic system.
4. Neurological system.

116. Which of the following types of diabetes is usually treated with only oral hypoglycemic medications?

1. Type 1 diabetes.
2. Type 2 diabetes.
3. Type 3 diabetes.
4. Diabetic ketoacidosis.

117. In a patient who is hospitalized for diabetes, the nurse should monitor intake and output, serum glucose, and

1. Urinary iron.
2. Serum electrolytes.
3. Urine fructose.
4. Dysrhythmias through electrocardiography (ECG).

118. Which of the following terms is used to describe the time at which insulin has its greatest effect?

1. Onset.
2. Peak.
3. Duration.
4. Action potential.

True or False

119. During periods when he or she has a viral or other infection, the diabetic patient may require more insulin.

Multiple Choice

120. Which of the following nursing diagnoses would be the most appropriate for a patient with diabetes mellitus?

1. Actual suicide, related to hypoglycemia.
2. Altered nutrition and risk for self-care deficit.
3. Impaired cognition related to constipation.
4. Risk for fluid volume excess.

121. Your patient is newly diagnosed with type 1 diabetes. Which statement by the patient tells you that further teaching is required?

1. "I have to test my blood sugar 4 times per day—30 minutes before meals and bedtime."
2. "If I am sick and don't eat much, I do not have to take my insulin."
3. "I need to take my insulin as it has been prescribed."
4. "I need to tell my healthcare professional if my blood glucose is out of the target ranges."

122. Which of the following snack choices indicates the patient understands that a snack containing starches and protein is appropriate for a diabetic?

1. Fruit in sugar-free gelatin.
2. Fried potato chips with sour cream dip.
3. Low-fat peanut butter on a Graham cracker with a slice of banana.
4. Half of a club sandwich with bacon and mayonnaise.

123. Diabetes mellitus is a disorder of

1. The intestines.
2. Carbon dioxide and gas exchange.
3. The adrenal glands.
4. Metabolism.

True or False

124. Individuals with type 2 diabetes mellitus usually have high triglycerides and low high-density lipoprotein (HDL) cholesterol levels.

Multiple Choice

125. Frequent hunger is a sign of diabetes mellitus. What is another name for this sign?

1. Polyuria.
2. Polyphagia.
3. Polydipsia.
4. Dysphagia.

126. Which of the following statements is true about persons with type 1 diabetes?

1. They have high triglyceride levels.
2. They have hypertension.
3. They are thin.
4. They need to take small doses of insulin, usually less than 10 units per day.

PHARMACOLOGICAL AND PARENTERAL THERAPIES

Multiple Choice

127. Mr. Timms's insulin drip rate is set at 10 mL/h. The insulin drip protocol states, "For blood sugar between 100 and 150, reduce the insulin drip by 50%." When you check Mr. Timms's blood sugar, you find that it is 146. How should you set the rate of the insulin drip now?

1. 5 mL/h.
2. 8 mL/h.
3. 10 mL/h.
4. 15 mL/h.

128. Mr. Sztuka's insulin drip rate is set at 20 mL/hr. The insulin drip protocol states, "For blood sugar between 100 and 150, reduce the insulin drip by 70%." When you check Mr. Sztuka's blood sugar, you find that it is 133. How should you set the rate of the insulin drip now?

1. 18 mL/h.
2. 14 mL/h.
3. 6 mL/h.
4. 3 mL/h.

129. Your patient's blood sugar is 244. The protocol states that if the blood sugar is more than 200, you should increase the insulin drip by 0.6 units/h. Currently, the drip is set at 9.5 units/h. To which setting should you adjust the insulin drip now?

1. 8.9 units/h.
2. 9.1 units/h.
3. 15.8 units/h.
4. 10.1 units/h.

True or False

130. Immediate conversion from insulin injections to oral hypoglycemic agents is possible if the patient is taking less than 100 units of insulin per day.

Multiple Choice

131. Your patient's blood sugar is 269. The protocol states that if the blood sugar is more than 200, you should increase the insulin drip by 3 mL/h. Currently, the drip is set at 13.2 mL/h. To which setting should you adjust the insulin drip now?

1. 13.5 mL/h.
2. 16.2 mL/h.
3. 17.6 mL/h.
4. 10.2 mL/h.

132. Your patient is on an insulin drip at 9.8 mL/h. When you make rounds at 3 A.M. (0300 hours), you find the patient to be lethargic and diaphoretic with a blood sugar of 62. You, as the nurse, should call the physician and take which other action?

1. Make no change in the insulin drip.
2. Turn the insulin drip off.
3. Decrease the insulin drip rate by one-half.
4. Increase the insulin drop rate by one-half.

133. Your patient was hypoglycemic 4 hours ago, but you administered a fast-acting carbohydrate × 2. Now the patient's blood sugar is 150. The physician writes the following prescription: "Resume insulin drip at 50% of previous rate." Previously, the insulin drip was set at 11.4 mL/h. At what rate should you set the drip?

1. 5.7 mL/h.
2. 6.7 mL/h.
3. 17.1 mL/h.
4. 22.8 mL/h.

134. Individuals who use insulin pumps often receive a dose of insulin continuously through the pump. What is this dose called?

1. Bolus dose.
2. Basal dose.
3. Normalized target dose.
4. Divided dose.

135. Which of the following substances is a carbohydrate?

1. C_6H_4.
2. $C_6H_2O_6$.
3. $C_6H_{10}OH$.
4. CH_2NH_2.

Fill in the Blank

136. Glipizide (Glucotrol), an oral hypoglycemic agent, should be taken _____ minutes before a meal.

Multiple Choice

137. To be used by cells, carbohydrates must be changed to

1. Glucose.
2. Glucogen.
3. Gladmium.
4. Glycerin.

138. Which of the following medications is used for the treatment of neurogenic diabetes insipidus?

1. Docusate sodium (Colace).
2. Epinephrine.
3. Vasopressin (Pitressin, Pressyn).
4. Furosemide (Lasix).

139. Which of the following classes of drugs include oral hypoglycemic agents?

1. Diuretics.
2. Biguanides.
3. Angiotensin-converting enzyme (ACE) inhibitors.
4. Antihypertensives.

True or False

140. Elderly patients might need a decrease in oral hypoglycemic agent dosages due to the changes in renal function that often occur in the elderly.

Multiple Choice

141. How do sulfonylureas (SFUs) work when they are prescribed as oral hypoglycemic agents?

1. They delay the absorption of glucose from the intestine.
2. They lower cell resistance to insulin.
3. They act on the pancreatic tissue to produce insulin.
4. They utilize sulfur compounds to combine with glucose for excretion.

142. The effectiveness of oral hypoglycemic agents may be decreased with concurrent use of

1. Diuretics.
2. Acetaminophen (Tylenol).
3. Iron.
4. Vitamin D.

143. What is the normal adult dose of glyburide (Diabeta, Micronase) per day?

1. 0.125 to 1.25 mg/day.
2. 2.5 to 5 mg/day.
3. 25 to 50 mg/day.
4. 250 to 500 mg/day.

Short Answer

144. Metformin (Glucophage) has the potential to cause renal dysfunction. Which serum laboratory test, besides blood urea nitrogen (BUN), would you monitor to assess for renal dysfunction?

Multiple Choice

145. One of the potential side effects of oral hypoglycemics is photosensitivity. What should you teach your patient with diabetes in this regard?

1. Take one aspirin daily.
2. Use sunscreen.
3. Always carry candy or sugar with you.
4. Do not have a photograph taken of yourself.

146. A diabetic patient who is taking an oral hypoglycemic calls you, complaining of abdominal cramps, nausea, flushing, headache, and hypoglycemia. Which of the following questions should you ask to determine if a disulfiram-like reaction is occurring?

1. Are you pregnant?
2. Are you still smoking cigarettes?
3. Have you had any alcohol recently?
4. Are you spitting up any blood?

147. Which of the following is a treatment for severe hypoglycemia?

1. Oral hypoglycemic agents.
2. $D_{50}W$ given intravenously.
3. Oral prepackaged glucose paste.
4. D_5LR given intravenously.

Short Answer

148. Metformin (glucophage) also comes in the form designated as XR. What does XR stand for?

Multiple Choice

149. Your patient is taking an oral hypoglycemic agent. Based on how the body metabolizes this medication, which laboratory value would you want to monitor?

1. Aspartate aminotransferase (AST).
2. Creatinine.
3. Blood urea nitrogen (BUN).
4. Total protein.

150. Which of the following complications is a possible hematological side effect from oral hypoglycemic agents?

1. Hyponatremia.
2. Agranulocytosis.
3. Photosensitivity.
4. Drowsiness.

151. Oral hypoglycemic agents are usually stopped prior to utilization of iodinated contrast media due to these drugs' potential to cause

1. Cardiac standstill.
2. Ulcerated stomach ulcer.
3. Hemorrhage.
4. Lactic acidosis.

True or False

152. One technique for making insulin relies on recombinant DNA.

SECTION I
SECTION II
SECTION III
SECTION IV
SECTION V
SECTION VI
SECTION VII
SECTION VIII
SECTION IX
SECTION X

Multiple Choice

153. Glucophage (Metformin) is a common oral hypoglycemic agent that is classified as a biguanide. With which organ is this drug's main mechanism of action associated?

1. Pancreas.
2. Stomach.
3. Liver.
4. Thyroid gland.

154. If hypoglycemia occurs, which of the following should you advise your patient to take?

1. A glass of diet soda.
2. A glass of orange juice.
3. A glass of skim milk.
4. Two bites of an apple.

155. To minimize gastrointestinal side effects, at what time should you advise your patient to administer Metformin (glucophage)?

1. Two hours prior to breakfast.
2. During a meal.
3. At bedtime.
4. After fasting.

Short Answer

156. As a patient's weight increases, does his or her dose of insulin usually increase or decrease?

Multiple Choice

157. Your patient who has type 2 diabetes is NPO for surgery tomorrow. He has been NPO for 8 hours, and surgery is scheduled 3 hours from now. The patient is prescribed Metformin (glucophage) for a morning dose of 500 mg. The physician's order reads, "Give all meds as was taking at home." What should be your nursing intervention?

1. Give the patient his usual dose of metformin, which the pharmacy has sent up, in the morning.
2. Call the physician to clarify the prescription for metformin, as the patient is NPO.
3. Call the physician and ask which type of breakfast food should be prescribed so that the patient can take his medication.
4. Give half the prescribed dose of metformin because the patient is scheduled for surgery.

158. Prior to the administration of $D_{50}W$ to treat severe hypoglycemia, for which intervention do you need to assess the patient?

1. Patent intravenous line.
2. Patent chest tube.
3. Electrocardiogram (ECG) monitor attached to patient.
4. Availability of an electronic intravenous pump.

159. Which of the following would be an appropriate reason *not* to give your patient insulin?

1. The patient is pregnant.
2. The patient is under extreme stress.
3. The patient has an allergy to insulin.
4. The patient has an infection.

REDUCTION OF RISK POTENTIAL

Multiple Choice

160. The patient has decided to proceed with having an insulin pump implanted to better control her diabetes and decrease her risk for stroke. For breakfast, she eats 4 carbohydrates (60 g). She is supposed to supplement her meal with 1 unit of regular insulin/carbohydrate. How many units of regular insulin should the patient pump in?

1. 2 units.
2. 3 units.
3. 4 units.
4. 15 units.

161. Mrs. Livingston has decided to try out an insulin pump to help decrease her risk factors for heart attack and stroke, as both comorbidities run in her family. Her nurse practitioner prescribed 2 units of regular insulin for every 20 g of carbohydrates Mrs. Livingston consumes in a meal. For breakfast, she ate 80 g of carbohydrates. How many units of regular insulin should the patient pump in?

1. 2 units.
2. 4 units.
3. 8 units.
4. 40 units.

162. Your patient has been diagnosed with diabetic ketoacidosis (DKA) and is receiving potassium replacement by intravenous drip. Which type of monitoring is required based on the intravenous drip?

1. Blood pressure monitoring.
2. Mean arterial pressure monitoring.
3. Temperature monitoring.
4. Electrocardiogram (ECG) monitoring.

163. Which of the following clinical finding indicates the presence of diabetes?

1. Ingrown toenail.
2. Fruity odor on the patient's breath.
3. Hypotension.
4. Fasting blood sugar of 85 mg/dL.

164. You know that individuals with diabetes are at risk for developing cataracts. Which of the following patient complaints would indicate cataracts of the eyes?

1. Night blindness.
2. Halos.
3. Decreased sense of smell.
4. Headaches.

165. You know that individuals with diabetes are at risk for developing glaucoma. Which of the following patient complaints would indicate glaucoma of the eyes?

1. Loss of hearing.
2. Halos.
3. Yellow conjunctiva.
4. Night blindness.

Fill in the Blank

166. Anxiety, chills, cold sweats, and difficulty concentrating are signs of _____ (hypoglycemia, hyperglycemia).

Multiple Choice

167. Which of the following is a risk factor for non-insulin-dependent diabetes mellitus (NIDDM) type 2?

1. Obesity.
2. Young age (less than 20 years old).
3. Having more than five live births.
4. Smoking cigarettes.

168. To reduce his risk of hyperglycemia, Mr. Edwards is to inject himself with 1 unit of regular insulin for every 15 g of carbohydrates he consumes at mealtime. For breakfast, he has eaten cereal (34 g of carbohydrates), 8 ounces of milk

(12 g), and 1 piece of toast (14 g). How much insulin should Mr. Edwards inject based on this breakfast?

1. 2 units.
2. 4 units.
3. 7 units.
4. 10 units.

True or False

169. Antiretrovirals may increase the need for insulin.

Multiple Choice

170. To reduce her risk of hyperglycemia, Mrs. Gottleib is to inject herself with 2 units of regular insulin for every 45 g of carbohydrates she consumes at mealtime. For breakfast, she has eaten a muffin (48 g of carbohydrates), 8 ounces of milk (12 g), and a banana (30 g). How much insulin should Mrs. Gottleib inject based on this breakfast?

1. 4 units.
2. 6 units.
3. 8 units.
4. 12 units.

171. Which of the following individuals is at the highest risk for developing type 2 diabetes mellitus?

1. A 6-year-old girl whose father has diabetes.
2. A 22-year-old man whose mother has type 2 diabetes.
3. A 42-year-old woman who is 40 pounds overweight.
4. A 65-year-old man who is 8 pounds overweight.

172. What is the leading cause of blindness in persons with diabetes?

1. Diabetic neuropathy.
2. Diabetic retinopathy.
3. Diabetic nephropathy.
4. Diabetic renal dysplasia.

True or False

173. Itching and redness can be local skin reactions to insulin injections.

Multiple Choice

174. Which of the following is a potential cause of diabetes insipidus?

1. Pregnancy.
2. Acute liver failure.
3. Head trauma.
4. Schizophrenia.

175. Which of the following endocrine disorders places a person at risk for developing diabetes?

1. Down syndrome.
2. Hyperthyroidism.
3. Iron deficiency.
4. Hypomagnesemia.

176. Which of the following medical conditions places a person at risk for developing diabetes?

1. Kidney stones.
2. Paranoid schizophrenia.
3. Obesity.
4. Hypotension.

True or False

177. Smoking is a risk factor in the development of hypertension and peripheral vascular disease.

Multiple Choice

178. Your patient has type 2 diabetes and wants to get off his oral hypoglycemic agent. What would you recommend as one solution?

1. Increase the amount of carbohydrates in the diet.
2. Increase the amount of fat in the diet.
3. Increase daily exercise.
4. Play less golf and watch more television.

179. Your patient is taking lispro insulin and asks you when he should administer the insulin. What is your best answer?

1. Within 1 hour prior to eating.
2. Either 1 hour before or 1 hour after eating.
3. About 15 minutes before eating.
4. 2 hours before eating.

180. Which of the following syringes is an appropriate choice for accurately drawing up insulin?

1. Low-dose insulin syringe.
2. 3-mL syringe.
3. 5-mL syringe.
4. 2-mL glass syringe.

True or False

181. The management of adolescents with diabetes can be difficult and demanding.

Multiple Choice

182. Which of the following activities will help decrease hyperglycemia?

1. Watching television.
2. Playing cards.
3. Traveling in the car.
4. Walking.

183. To reduce his or her risk of complications from diabetes, a patient's hemoglobin A_{1C} level should be less than

1. 2%.
2. 7%.
3. 15%.
4. 40%.

184. Which of the following measures is a basic cardiac test to assess for macrovascular disease?

1. Chest x-ray.
2. Bone scan.
3. Exercise stress test.
4. Serum myoglobin.

True or False

185. The majority of persons with non-insulin-dependent diabetes mellitus (NIDDM) type 2 are underweight at the time when the disease is discovered.

Multiple Choice

186. Which of the following assessments will help the nurse evaluate a patient for ocular complications from diabetes?

1. Ear cerumen.
2. Visual acuity.
3. Microalbuminemia.
4. Sensory neuropathy.

187. Mr. Ezzone has type 2 diabetes. When he visits your clinic, he complains that he feels as if bees are biting his feet. Which complication from diabetes does this sign indicate that Mr. Ezzone is experiencing?

1. Hypertension.
2. Hyperlipidemia.
3. Neuropathy.
4. Maculopathy.

188. Mr. Johannson has diabetes and hyperlipidemia. Which of the following medications could help him improve his serum lipid profile?

1. Docusate sodium (Colace).
2. Oxycodone and acetaminophen (Percocet).
3. Ezetimibe and simvastatin (Vytorin).
4. Furosemide (Lasix).

189. Mr. Cortez is obese and unable to look directly at the bottoms of his feet to assess for skin problems related to his diabetes. What could you, as a nurse, suggest that might help Mr. Cortez complete his foot assessment?

1. Soaking the feet in water enlarges them and will make them easier to see.
2. Use a mirror for better visualization.
3. Foot assessment will be necessary only at his every-12-week diabetic clinic appointments.
4. Wear 100% cotton socks and he won't have any foot problems.

190. Which of the following statements is true regarding insulin resistance and diabetes?

1. The exact mechanism of insulin resistance is known.
2. These conditions are more common in underweight people.
3. Exercise can not help restore insulin sensitivity.
4. A genetic predisposition to insulin resistance/diabetes exists.

191. Impaired glucose tolerance (IGT) is one of a number of conditions collectively known as

1. Nephrogenic hypothalamic dysfunction (NHD).
2. Cytogenic glucose impairment (CGI).
3. Syndrome X.
4. Obsessive destructive syndrome (ODS).

True or False

192. Insulin pens contain prefilled syringes of insulin, so they do not need to be placed in a cool environment when patients are traveling.

PHYSIOLOGICAL ADAPTATION

Multiple Choice

193. Which of the following is primarily a disorder of type 1 diabetes?

1. Alzheimer's disease.
2. Diabetic ketoacidosis.
3. Migraine headaches.
4. Coronary artery disease.

194. Which of the following properties associated with smoking is particularly bad for patients with diabetes?

1. Vasoconstriction.
2. Vasodilatation.
3. Excessive cerumen.
4. Increased renal glomerular filtration rates.

195. To detect diabetic ketoacidosis (DKA), which of the following would you test for ketones?

1. Feces.
2. Sputum.
3. Plasma.
4. Urine.

196. Glucose intolerance whose onset occurs during pregnancy is known as

1. Insulin-dependent type 1 diabetes.
2. Pancreatic neoplasm.
3. Gestational diabetes.
4. Non-insulin-dependent type 2 diabetes.

197. The major pathophysiological alteration associated with hyperglycemia is increased blood osmolality, which leads to

1. Overhydration.
2. Dehydration.
3. Headaches.
4. Hyponatremia.

True or False

198. Insulin is a hormone produced by the pituitary gland.

Multiple Choice

199. Mrs. Wolberg is a 72-year-old Caucasian female who is admitted to your hospital with uncontrolled diabetes mellitus and altered skin integrity. The third and fourth toes on her left foot are black, are cold, and have no feeling. Which condition does Mrs. Wolberg most likely have?

1. Gangrene of the toes.
2. Renal failure.
3. Peripheral vascular disease.
4. Left femoral thrombus.

200. A patient is admitted to your hospital unit with a diagnosis of chronic diabetes mellitus. The patient also has the following symptoms: fatigue, nausea, loss of appetite, peripheral edema, hypertension, and flank pain. Based on these symptoms, what is this patient's most likely diagnosis?

1. Retinopathy.
2. Myocardial infarction.
3. Renal failure.
4. Intestinal obstruction.

201. Individuals with diabetes mellitus can have a chronic complication in which there is pain in the lower extremities due to lack of blood supply. What is this complication called?

1. Claudication.
2. Stroke.
3. Angina.
4. Retinopathy.

True or False

202. Acetone in the urine of a person with diabetes usually indicates that the diabetes is poorly controlled.

Multiple Choice

203. Which of the following complaints by Mr. Gladden would indicate that he has nerve damage from his diabetes?

1. Hearing loss.
2. Erectile dysfunction.
3. Stuffy nose.
4. Fever.

204. What is the physiological reason for increased infection in patients with hyperglycemia?

1. Increased blood sugar impairs tissue reperfusion.
2. Increased blood sugar damages the autonomic nervous system.
3. Increased blood sugar hinders osmotic diuresis.

4. Increased blood sugar impairs leukocyte function.

205. Contiguous spread of an infection from a skin ulcer to adjacent bone is a common complaint of persons with diabetes mellitus. What is this condition called?

1. Cystitis.
2. Cholecystitis.
3. Osteomyelitis.
4. Vascular occlusion.

Fill in the Blank

206. The pancreas is a glandular organ of the digestive system that is connected to the _____ (small, large) intestine at the duodenum.

Multiple Choice

207. Individuals with diabetes mellitus may suffer a variety of acute-onset mononeuropathies. Which of the following is a sign of third cranial nerve (oculomotor) damage?

1. Diplopia.
2. Loss of smell.
3. Loss of use of lower legs.
4. Gastric gas.

208. Where does most of the work of the kidney take place?

1. Neurons.
2. Ureter.
3. Nephrons.
4. Islets of Langerhans.

209. Which of the following substances is the end product of protein digestion?

1. Lipids.
2. Cholesterol.
3. Amino acids.
4. Fats.

210. Individuals with type 2 NIDDM tend to be resistant to ketoacidosis. If it does occur, however, ketoacidosis will most likely arise during

1. Fasting.
2. Times of excessive stress.
3. Consumption of carbohydrate-filled meals.
4. The menstrual cycle.

True or False

211. Insulin is produced by beta cells in the islets of Langerhans.

Multiple Choice

212. What is the cause of blindness due to diabetic retinopathy?

   1. Tiny lesions in the tear ducts.

   2. Scar tissue.

   3. Hemorrhage.

   4. Acidosis.

213. Diabetes insipidus (DI) is a disorder of the posterior pituitary gland in which the affected individual suffers an insufficiency of which hormone?

   1. Beta-cell hormone (BCH).

   2. Dopamine.

   3. Antidiuretic hormone (ADH).

   4. Thyroid-stimulating hormone (TSH).

214. Diabetes insipidus leads to large amounts of urine excretion. What is this condition called?

   1. Polydipsia.

   2. Polyphagia.

   3. Polyuria.

   4. Hyponatremia.

215. Persons with diabetes mellitus who have hyperosmolar nonketotic coma (HNKC) or diabetic ketoacidosis (DKA) also have dehydration as a result of a decrease in which electrolyte?

   1. Potassium.

   2. Bicarbonate.

   3. Magnesium.

   4. Sodium.

True or False

216. A positive test for glucose in the urine may be indicative of diabetes mellitus.

Multiple Choice

217. In which circumstance does diabetic ketoacidosis occur?

   1. Severe insulin deficiency.

   2. Increased carbohydrate intake.

   3. Severe dehydration.

   4. Blood glucose more than 190 mg/dL.

218. Mrs. Infortuna is hospitalized with hyperosmolar nonketotic coma. For which potential complication should you monitor her?

   1. Infection.

   2. Pancreatitis.

   3. Dehydration.

   4. Hypotension.

219. Mrs. Langley has hyperosmolar nonketotic coma with hyperglycemia. She begins to experience CNS dysfunction. What is the most likely source of this dysfunction?

   1. Cellular fluid loss.

   2. Hypoxia.

   3. Adrenal gland tumor.

   4. Fever.

True or False

220. Ketones are chemical compounds that result from the breakdown of proteins.

Multiple Choice

221. When the renal tubules are not sensitive to antidiuretic hormone (ADH) in a person with diabetes insipidus (DI), what is this condition called?

   1. Neurogenic DI.

   2. Nephrogenic DI.

   3. Inappropriate sodium DI.

   4. Myxedema.

222. Fasting prompts the body to release which hormone that acts to raise normal blood glucose levels?

   1. Fructose.

   2. Growth hormone.

   3. Glucagon.

   4. Sodium.

SECTION I

SECTION II

SECTION III

SECTION IV

SECTION V

SECTION VI

SECTION VII

SECTION VIII

SECTION IX

SECTION X

ANSWERS AND RATIONALES

MANAGEMENT OF CARE

1. Correct Answer: **2**

   Rationale: A blood sugar of 224 requires 3 units of regular insulin.

2. Correct Answer: **1**

   Rationale: The patient's blood sugar of 136 is less than 150, so you do not administer any insulin.

3. Correct Answer: **4**

   Rationale: The patient's blood sugar of 222 is between 221 and 250.

4. Correct Answer: **1**

   Rationale: The patient's blood sugar of 128 is less than 130.

5. Correct Answer: **3**

   Rationale: Blood glucose of 300 mg/dL is the upper limit for administering 3 units of lispro insulin.

6. Correct Answer: **4**

   Rationale: The islets of Langerhans are cells of endocrine glands that are found in the pancreas.

7. Correct Answer: **True**

   Rationale: Most of these deaths are due to atherosclerosis.

8. Correct Answer: **1**

   Rationale: Physical activity, stress, illness, surgery, and travel are all factors that affect blood sugar levels.

9. Correct Answer: **1**

   Rationale: Hemoglobin A_{1C} is glycosylated hemoglobin.

10. Correct Answer: **3**

    Rationale: The kidneys are associated with the nephrons and hence with nephropathy.

11. Correct Answer: **True**

    Rationale: Patients with diabetes mellitus are also at risk for open-angle glaucoma.

12. Correct Answer: **2**

    Rationale: Diabetic retinopathy is the leading cause of blindness.

13. Correct Answer: **1**

    Rationale: The normal range is 70–110 mg/dL for nondiabetic blood glucose.

14. Correct Answer: **3**

    Rationale: Hyperglycemia (increased blood glucose) causes fatigue, hunger, excessive oral intake, excessive urination, and weight loss.

15. Correct Answer: **False**

    Rationale: Hyperlipidemia and hypertension are commonly found as comorbid conditions in individuals with diabetes.

16. Correct Answer: **3**

    Rationale: $3 + 5 = 8$.

17. Correct Answer: **1**

    Rationale: Vials of insulin that are not used within a few months should be refrigerated.

18. Correct Answer: **4**

    Rationale: He is due for an injection in the left upper arm owing to the site rotation.

19. Correct Answer: **Lower**

    Rationale: Neuropathy appears first in the lower extremities, then progresses to the upper extremities.

20. Correct Answer: **1**

    Rationale: Stress is one cause of hyperglycemia.

21. Correct Answer: **Low-dose**

    Rationale: Low-dose syringes are more accurate when drawing up small amounts of insulin.

22. Correct Answer: **4**

    Rationale: High triglycerides and high total cholesterol are also risk factors for atherosclerosis in diabetics.

23. Correct Answer: **2**

    Rationale: Exercise can decrease blood sugar levels.

24. Correct Answer: **3**

    Rationale: Periodontal disease of the oral cavity is common sign of diabetes mellitus.

25. Correct Answer: **True**

    Rationale: Nurses should assess patients with diabetes for coronary artery disease (CAD) and intervene as necessary to prevent CAD.

26. Correct Answer: **3**

    Rationale: Recombinant DNA is one technique used to produce insulin.

27. Correct Answer: **2**

    Rationale: The common standard for insulin is 100 units per milliliter.

28. Correct Answer: **3**

    Rationale: Lantus, although clear, should not be mixed with other kinds of insulin.

29. Correct Answer: **2**

    Rationale: $10 + 28 = 38$.

30. Correct Answer: **2**

    Rationale: Novolin 70/30 contains 70% NPH insulin and 30% regular insulin.

31. Correct Answer: **True**

    Rationale: These are all valid methods of delivery, as is the insulin jet injector.

32. Correct Answer: **2**

    Rationale: Fast-acting insulin generally takes effect in less than 15 minutes.

33. Correct Answer: **4**

    Rationale: Its duration describes how long insulin continues to affect the body.

34. Correct Answer: **False**

    Rationale: Subjecting insulin to temperature extremes will degrade the insulin and cause it to spoil.

35. Correct Answer: **2**

    Rationale: Type 1 diabetes is often called juvenile diabetes.

36. Correct Answer: **4**

    Rationale: Non-insulin-dependent diabetes mellitus (NIDDM), type 2, is much more common in young people. Its incidence in this group is currently increasing.

37. Correct Answer: **2**

    Rationale: Lack of insulin leads to large amounts of insulin in the bloodstream.

38. Correct Answer: **Sodium**

    Rationale: Consuming excess amounts of sodium elevates blood pressure and increases fluid retention.

39. Correct Answer: **2**

    Rationale: The American Diabetes Association publishes dietary recommendations for diabetes.

40. Correct Answer: **4**

    Rationale: Dehydration signs include complaints of thirst, poor skin turgor, dry skin, weakness, decreased urine output, and dry mucous membranes.

41. Correct Answer: **1**

    Rationale: Hypernatremia and low ADH levels are classic signs of diabetes insipidus.

42. Correct Answer: **3**

    Rationale: Consuming a low-sodium diet will help decrease the individual's serum sodium. Consuming a low-caffeine diet is recommended because caffeine increases urine output.

43. Correct Answer: **2**

    Rationale: Medicare covers all expenses for diabetes products and the supplies.

44. Correct Answer: **4**

    Rationale: The lancet is the equipment that pokes the finger to obtain blood. The Glucowatch is a noninvasive monitor, a syringe is a needle with a body, and a pump is a machine that injects insulin.

SAFETY AND INFECTION CONTROL

45. Correct Answer: **3**

    Rationale: For a blood sugar of 251, you would administer 5 units of regular insulin.

46. Correct Answer: **4**

    Rationale: The patient's blood sugar of 312 is greater than 300.

47. Correct Answer: **2**

    Rationale: The patient's blood sugar of 181 is between 150 and 200.

SECTION I
SECTION II
SECTION III
SECTION IV
SECTION V
SECTION VI
SECTION VII
SECTION VIII
SECTION IX
SECTION X

48. Correct Answer: **4**

    Rationale: The patient's blood sugar of 315 is greater than 300.

49. Correct Answer: **1**

    Rationale: Furosemide is a diuretic that commonly causes hyperglycemia owing to its dehydration effects.

50. Correct Answer: **3**

    Rationale: Regular insulin is short acting.

51. Correct Answer: **1**

    Rationale: Insulin can be properly stored at room temperature for at least 30 days.

52. Correct Answer: **True**

    Rationale: Expiration dates are based on product potency, among other values.

53. Correct Answer: **2**

    Rationale: Always draw regular insulin up first. Remember: Clear before cloudy.

54. Correct Answer: **3**

    Rationale: The thighs also contain subcutaneous tissue and are less sensitive to injections.

55. Correct Answer: **2**

    Rationale: Rotation of injection sites aids in absorption and gives used sites needed rest.

56. Correct Answer: **1**

    Rationale: The skin is the largest organ and needs to be assessed daily—especially the feet—for broken areas and infection.

57. Correct Answer: **True**

    Rationale: Your local health department can help out in terms of proper disposal. In the meantime an empty laundry bottle or peanut butter plastic jar can be used for syringe disposal as long as it is labeled and kept out of the reach of children.

58. Correct Answer: **2**

    Rationale: Thirty minutes is enough time for the insulin to reach room temperature.

59. Correct Answer: **4**

    Rationale: A tan color and the presence of chunks are abnormal. They mean that the insulin is not good.

60. Correct Answer: **3**

    Rationale: An increased white blood cell count indicates the presence of an infection. Red blood cells play roles in oxygenation and anemia. Platelets affect the blood's clotting ability.

61. Correct Answer: **Hypoglycemia**

62. Correct Answer: **4**

    Rationale: Skin assessment is also known as integumentary system assessment.

63. Correct Answer: **2**

    Rationale: Vaginitis, skin infections, urinary tract infections, and lung infections are all signs of a weakened immune system.

64. Correct Answer: **1**

    Rationale: Irritability, weakness, fatigue, tremors, and headache are all signs of hypoglycemia.

65. Correct Answer: **3**

    Rationale: Regular insulin is used to cover the sliding scale because it is fast acting.

66. Correct Answer: **Neuropathy includes loss of sensation, particularly in the lower extremities.**

HEALTH PROMOTION AND MAINTENANCE

67. Correct Answer: **1**

    Rationale: The patient's blood sugar of 186 is between 161 and 190.

68. Correct Answer: **1**

    Rationale: The patient's blood sugar of 122 is less than 130 and is not an emergency value.

69. Correct Answer: **2**

    Rationale: The patient's blood sugar of 198 is between 150 and 199.

70. Correct Answer: **2 units**

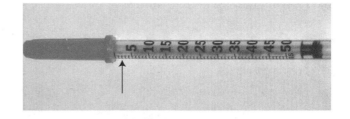

71. Correct Answer: <u>4</u>

Rationale: Atherosclerosis is a major cause of mortality in individuals with diabetes.

72. Correct Answer: <u>2</u>

Rationale: Glucose in the urine irritates the vulva and causes bacterial growth.

73. Correct Answer: <u>4</u>

Rationale: Nutrient ratios and types to be included in patient education should include management of carbohydrates, fats, and protein.

74. Correct Answer: <u>**5 units**</u>

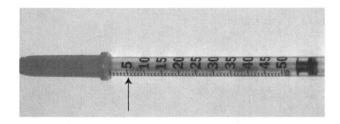

75. Correct Answer: <u>3</u>

Rationale: The HgbA$_{1C}$ monitors glucose over a 3-month period and should be less than 7%.

76. Correct Answer: <u>1</u>

Rationale: Insulin pens are prefilled, jet injectors work by pressure, and pumps contain small infusion sets.

77. Correct Answer: <u>2</u>

Rationale: Dry skin is a common symptom of diabetes associated with the skin/integumentary system. Blurred vision and fatigue are also signs of diabetes.

78. Correct Answer: <u>**3 units**</u>

Rationale: 190 − 100 = 90; 90/30 = 3.

79. Correct Answer: <u>3</u>

Rationale: Blood glucose is measured in milligrams per deciliter (mg/dL).

80. Correct Answer: <u>1</u>

Rationale: Fasting glucose should be in the range of 70–100 mg/dL.

81. Correct Answer: <u>**5 units**</u>

Rationale: 250 − 100 = 150; and 150/30 = 5.

82. Correct Answer: <u>4</u>

Rationale: The oral glucose tolerance test includes drinking a glucose solution and having blood drawn over the next 3 hours. When blood is drawn in 2 hours, a glucose reading of less than 140 mg/dL is normal.

83. Correct Answer: <u>3</u>

Rationale: Any random glucose test finding greater than 200 mg/dL indicates diabetes.

84. Correct Answer: <u>2</u>

Rationale: IGT is an indicator of type 2 diabetes, a condition in which the body does not properly utilize insulin.

85. Correct Answer: <u>4</u>

Rationale: Obesity and syndrome X are associated with IGT. Syndrome X includes four conditions: insulin resistance, hyperinsulinemia, hypertension, and dyslipidemia.

86. Correct Answer: <u>2</u>

Rationale: Polycystic ovary syndrome includes IGT, insulin resistance, and hyperinsulinemia. Proctitis is a rectal inflammation. Duodenal ulcers affect the intestine. Uterine glucose dysplasia is a made-up condition.

PSYCHOSOCIAL INTEGRITY

87. Correct Answer: <u>3</u>

Rationale: The patient's blood sugar of 241 is between 221 and 250.

88. Correct Answer: <u>**False**</u>

Rationale: Sugar-free foods sometimes contain as many (or more) carbohydrates than the non-sugar-free versions.

89. Correct Answer: <u>2</u>

Rationale: The patient's blood sugar of 156 is between 130 and 160.

90. Correct Answer: <u>4</u>

Rationale: 310 − 100 = 210; 210/30 = 7.

91. Correct Answer: <u>1</u>

Rationale: 110 − 100 = 10; 10/30 = 0.33, which is less than 1, so no insulin is necessary.

92. Correct Answer: <u>**True**</u>

Rationale: A high triglyceride level is a risk factor for diabetes.

SECTION I

SECTION II

SECTION III

SECTION IV

SECTION V

SECTION VI

SECTION VII

SECTION VIII

SECTION IX

SECTION X

93. Correct Answer: **3**

Rationale: Consumption of foods that are high in fat and cholesterol will not aid in controlling diabetes.

94. Correct Answer: **1**

Rationale: Vegetable oil is the best option.

95. Correct Answer: **1**

Rationale: Oatmeal, which contains oats, will increase the amount of fiber.

96. Correct Answer: **2**

Rationale: 1% milk contains the least amount of fat.

97. Correct Answer: **4**

Rationale: The diet soft drink has very few (if any) calories.

98. Correct Answer: **Signs of hyperglycemia (high blood sugar) include hunger, thirst, frequent urination, dry itchy skin, sleepiness, and blurred vision.**

99. Correct Answer: **4**

Rationale: Nuts are the only source of protein listed. The other options are carbohydrate- or fiber-containing foods.

100. Correct Answer: **3**

Rationale: In diabetes, the beta cells do not produce insulin, so the patient needs lifelong insulin therapy.

101. Correct Answer: **Medic alert bracelet or medical alert bracelet.**

102. Correct Answer: **2**

Rationale: Groups considered to be at high risk for developing IGT include Native Americans, African Americans, Hispanic Americans, Asian Americans, and Pacific Islanders.

103. Correct Answer: **2**

Rationale: To lose weight, you must burn more calories than you ingest.

104. Correct Answer: **2**

Rationale: Limiting intake of fats, carbohydrates, and alcohol and getting 30 minutes of aerobic exercise 3 to 5 times per week will help maintain good health.

105. Correct Answer: **1**

Rationale: Fatty, cold-water fish are rich in omega-3 fatty acids. These fish include salmon, tuna, mackerel, halibut, and herring.

106. Correct Answer: **2**

Rationale: Wild fish, including salmon, have more omega-3 fatty acids than farm-raised fish.

BASIC CARE AND COMFORT

107. Correct Answer: **4**

Rationale: Self-management of one's diet, exercise, medication, and lifestyle affects an individual's outcome.

108. Correct Answer: **2**

Rationale: Baked chips contain carbohydrates, but salsa has no fat or calories. All of the other snack options are high in fat.

109. Correct Answer: **4 units**

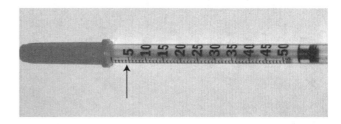

110. Correct Answer: **3**

Rationale: Monitoring before meals and before bedtime is adequate.

111. Correct Answer: **1**

Rationale: A rapid heartbeat is associated with hypoglycemia. It arises when the heart tries to shunt more blood (which carries glucose) through the body.

112. Correct Answer: **4**

Rationale: Constipation and diarrhea are two signs of gastrointestinal dysfunction in diabetes.

113. Correct Answer: **4 units**

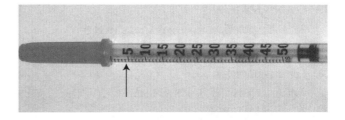

114. Correct Answer: **2**

Rationale: Renal assessment includes checking for edema, albuminuria, and urinary tract infections as well as assessing for chronic renal failure.

115. Correct Answer: <u>4</u>

Rationale: Disorders of the neurological system include retinopathy, cataracts, glaucoma, paresthesias, and neuropathies.

116. Correct Answer: <u>2</u>

Rationale: Type 2 (non-insulin-dependent) diabetes is usually treated with oral medications. Type 1 (insulin-dependent) diabetes is treated with insulin. There is no such thing as type 3 diabetes. Ketoacidosis is an emergency, not a type of diabetes.

117. Correct Answer: <u>2</u>

Rationale: Monitoring of serum electrolytes is imperative due to the potential for changes in sodium, chloride, and potassium in particular.

118. Correct Answer: <u>2</u>

Rationale: The peak is when a drug has its greatest effect, the onset is when the drug begins to work, and the duration is length of time for which it affects the body.

119. Correct Answer: <u>**True**</u>

Rationale: Periods of sickness may lead to hyperglycemia.

120. Correct Answer: <u>2</u>

Rationale: Given that diet is a major contribution to diabetes, altered nutrition is a major diagnosis.

121. Correct Answer: <u>2</u>

Rationale: Sickness usually produces greater hyperglycemia, so more insulin is usually needed during periods of ill health.

122. Correct Answer: <u>3</u>

Rationale: Low-fat peanut butter is a protein, Graham crackers are a starch, and banana is a fruit.

123. Correct Answer: <u>4</u>

Rationale: Diabetes mellitus is a metabolic disorder that results in persistent hyperglycemia.

124. Correct Answer: <u>**True**</u>

Rationale: Individuals with type 2 diabetes have increased triglycerides and decreased HDL (good cholesterol) and also have hypertension and are obese.

125. Correct Answer: <u>2</u>

Rationale: Polyphagia is excessive hunger, polyuria is excessive urination, polydipsia is excessive liquid intake, and dysphagia is difficulty swallowing.

126. Correct Answer: <u>3</u>

Rationale: Individuals with type 1 diabetes are thin, have no history of diabetes mellitus, do not have high cholesterol or high triglyceride levels, do not have hypertension, and usually require doses of 50 units or more of insulin per day.

PHARMACOLOGICAL AND PARENTERAL THERAPIES

127. Correct Answer: <u>1</u>

Rationale: 10

128. Correct Answer: <u>3</u>

Rationale: 20

129. Correct Answer: <u>4</u>

Rationale: $9.5 + 0.6 = 10.1$.

130. Correct Answer: <u>**False**</u>

Rationale: Immediate conversion is possible if the individual is taking less than 20 units of insulin per day. Otherwise, conversion needs to take place gradually.

131. Correct Answer: <u>2</u>

Rationale: $13.2 + 3 = 16.2$.

132. Correct Answer: <u>2</u>

Rationale: The patient is hypoglycemic, so giving this individual more insulin will do the patient harm.

133. Correct Answer: <u>1</u>

Rationale: 11.4

134. Correct Answer: <u>2</u>

Rationale: Basal dose is another name for continuous dose.

135. Correct Answer: <u>2</u>

Rationale: Carbohydrates contain carbon, hydrogen, and oxygen, with a 2:1 ratio of hydrogen to oxygen.

136. Correct Answer: <u>30</u>

Rationale: Glipizide has an onset of 15 to 30 minutes.

137. Correct Answer: <u>1</u>

Rationale: Carbohydrates must be changed into glucose so they can pass through cell membranes and be utilized within the cell body.

SECTION I
SECTION II
SECTION III
SECTION IV
SECTION V
SECTION VI
SECTION VII
SECTION VIII
SECTION IX
X

138. Correct Answer: **3**

Rationale: Vasopressin decreases urine output and increases urine osmolality.

139. Correct Answer: **2**

Rationale: Biguanides act by lowering cell resistance to insulin. These agents include drugs such as glucophage (Metformin). Diuretics are used for fluid overload. ACE inhibitors and antihypertensives are prescribed to treat high blood pressure.

140. Correct Answer: **True**

Rationale: As a person ages, renal function decreases. Hence dosages of many medications may need to be lowered in elderly patients.

141. Correct Answer: **3**

Rationale: SFUs act on the pancreas to make it produce more insulin. Biguanides lower cell resistance to insulin. Alpha-glucosidase inhibitors delay absorption of glucose from the intestines.

142. Correct Answer: **1**

Rationale: Diuretics, steroids, estrogens, phenytoin, and phenothiazines may all decrease the effectiveness of oral hypoglycemic agents.

143. Correct Answer: **2**

Rationale: Glyberide is a sulfonylurea whose normal dose for adults is 2.5 to 5 mg once daily. The maximum dose is 20 mg.

144. Correct Answer: **Creatinine**

Rationale: A creatinine value of more than 1.4 mg/dL indicates an underlying renal dysfunction.

145. Correct Answer: **2**

Rationale: Photosensitivity requires the use of sunscreen to avoid skin damage.

146. Correct Answer: **3**

Rationale: Concurrent use of alcohol can cause a disulfiram-like reaction, including cramps, nausea, flushing, headache, and hypoglycemia.

147. Correct Answer: **2**

Rationale: The treatment of choice for severe hypoglycemia is 50% dextrose given intravenously.

148. Correct Answer: **Extended release capsules have prolonged drug action.**

149. Correct Answer: **1**

Rationale: The AST is reflective of liver function; the liver is where medications are metabolized. Creatinine and BUN are renal function tests. Total protein indicates the amount of protein in the body.

150. Correct Answer: **2**

Rationale: Agranulocytosis, thrombocytopenia, leukopenia, and pancytopenia are all potential hematological side effects.

151. Correct Answer: **4**

Rationale: Lactic acidosis can occur as the iodinated contrast media increases the accumulation of acidic ketones, leading to an alteration in the body's acid–base equilibrium.

152. Correct Answer: **True**

Rationale: Other sources are biosynthetic, semisynthetic, and bovine (cattle) and/or porcine (pigs) origins.

153. Correct Answer: **3**

Rationale: Glucophage decreases hepatic (liver) production of glucose.

154. Correct Answer: **2**

Rationale: A glass of orange juice or 2 to 3 teaspoons of sugar, honey, or corn syrup dissolved in water will help counteract hypoglycemia.

155. Correct Answer: **2**

Rationale: The patient can minimize any gastrointestinal effects by taking the medication with food.

156. Correct Answer: **Increase**

Rationale: More weight means more carbohydrates and more fat, which increases the person's need for insulin.

157. Correct Answer: **2**

Rationale: Given that the patient is designated as NPO, the Metformin should probably be temporarily discontinued.

158. Correct Answer: **1**

Rationale: Since $D_{50}W$ can be given as an IV push, you need a patent intravenous line.

159. Correct Answer: **3**

Rationale: An allergy to insulins and their preservatives is a reason not to give the patient insulin.

REDUCTION OF RISK POTENTIAL

160. Correct Answer: **3**

Rationale: 4

161. Correct Answer: **3**

Rationale: 80/20 = 4; 4.

162. Correct Answer: **4**

Rationale: ECG monitoring is needed to assess for cardiac dysrhythmias due to potassium replacement.

163. Correct Answer: **2**

Rationale: Breath with a fruity odor is a sign of diabetes.

164. Correct Answer: **1**

Rationale: Night blindness is a common sign of cataracts.

165. Correct Answer: **2**

Rationale: Halos are a common sign of glaucoma.

166. Correct Answer: **Hypoglycemia**

Rationale: Other signs of hypoglycemia (decreased blood sugar) include drowsiness, nausea, headache, and shakiness.

167. Correct Answer: **1**

Rationale: Obesity is a risk factor for NIDDM.

168. Correct Answer: **2**

Rationale: 34 + 12 + 14 = 60; 60/15 = 4; 4.

169. Correct Answer: **True**

Rationale: Antiretroviral medications increase serum glucose.

170. Correct Answer: **1**

Rationale: 48 + 12 + 30 = 90; 90/45 = 2; 2.

171. Correct Answer: **3**

Rationale: Women who are older than age 40 and are obese are at the highest risk of developing type 2 diabetes.

172. Correct Answer: **2**

Rationale: Retinopathy of the eye is the leading cause of blindness. Neuropathy is nerve sensation dysfunction. Neuropathy and renal dysfunction relate to the kidneys.

173. Correct Answer: **True**

Rationale: Other skin reactions may include lipodystrophy, lipohypertrophy, and swelling.

174. Correct Answer: **3**

Rationale: Head trauma with damage to the pituitary and the presence of a tumor are possible causes; otherwise, this disease is considered to have an unknown etiology.

175. Correct Answer: **2**

Rationale: Hyperthyroidism and Cushing's disease are two endocrine disorders that place a person at risk for developing diabetes. Down syndrome is also a risk factor, but is genetic in nature.

176. Correct Answer: **3**

Rationale: Obesity, cirrhosis, end-stage renal disease, Cushing's disease, hyperthyroidism, cystic fibrosis, and Down and Turner syndromes are all risk factors for diabetes.

177. Correct Answer: **True**

Rationale: Smoking causes vasoconstriction, which does not help hypertension or peripheral vascular disease.

178. Correct Answer: **3**

Rationale: Increasing his or her amount of exercise will help a person lose weight as long as the individual does not increase the amount of calories consumed. Weight loss, in turn, decreases the need for oral hypoglycemics.

179. Correct Answer: **3**

Rationale: Lispro is short acting, so it should be administered within 15 minutes prior to eating.

180. Correct Answer: **1**

Rationale: Insulin syringes are accurate for drawing up insulin. They come in two versions: low-dose and high-dose types. Glass syringes cause insulin to adhere to the glass, thereby affecting the dose.

181. Correct Answer: **True**

Rationale: Often regular involvement in care is necessary for younger patients. Including a stay at a children's camp can also be a plus.

182. Correct Answer: **4**

Rationale: Any form of physical activity—even walking—can help lower serum glucose.

SECTION I

SECTION II

SECTION III

SECTION IV

SECTION V

SECTION VI

SECTION VII

SECTION VIII

SECTION IX

SECTION X

183. Correct Answer: **2**

Rationale: $HgbA_{1c}$ should be less than 7%.

184. Correct Answer: **3**

Rationale: An exercise stress test will help assess for cardiac function and, when combined with an echocardiogram, can give even more information about the patient's cardiovascular health. A chest x-ray gives information mostly on the lungs but provides very little information about macrovascular disease. A bone scan is usually performed to detect cancer in the bone or other bone abnormalities. A serum myoglobin is a blood test, not a cardiac test.

185. Correct Answer: **False**

Rationale: Most persons with type 2 diabetes are obese at the time of their diagnosis.

186. Correct Answer: **2**

Rationale: Visual acuity is an assessment of the eyes or for ocular complications. The ear, protein in urine, and sensory function are not associated with assessment of the eye.

187. Correct Answer: **3**

Rationale: This patient has neuropathy, which may include not just numbness but often a stinging sensation.

188. Correct Answer: **3**

Rationale: Vytorin is a combination of two medications; its simvastatin component is a statin, which is intended to help improve the patient's lipid profiles. Colace is a stool softener, Percocet is an analgesic, and Lasix is a diuretic.

189. Correct Answer: **2**

Rationale: Using a mirror can help a person look at the underside as well as sides of his or her feet.

190. Correct Answer: **4**

Rationale: Individuals may have a genetic predisposition to insulin resistance/diabetes. The exact mechanism by which this condition arises is not known, but it is common in obese persons. Engaging in exercise and eating a well-balanced diet can help restore insulin sensitivity.

191. Correct Answer: **3**

Rationale: Syndrome X includes IGT, polycystic ovary syndrome (PCOS), hyperthyroidism, and Cushing's disease as well as some other conditions. The other answers are all made-up words.

192. Correct Answer: **False**

Rationale: All insulin should be kept cool while the person is traveling, even if the insulin is in a prefilled syringe.

PHYSIOLOGICAL ADAPTATION

193. Correct Answer: **2**

Rationale: DKA is primarily a disorder of type 1 diabetes and is characterized by the presence of ketones in the urine.

194. Correct Answer: **1**

Rationale: Vasoconstriction impairs circulation and makes the heart work harder.

195. Correct Answer: **4**

Rationale: To detect DKA, you would test for ketones in the urine.

196. Correct Answer: **3**

Rationale: "Gestational" refers to pregnancy.

197. Correct Answer: **2**

Rationale: Increased osmolality increases urine output, leading to dehydration.

198. Correct Answer: **False**

Rationale: Insulin is produced in the pancreas.

199. Correct Answer: **1**

Rationale: Gangrene includes black toes that are cold. It usually occurs in the lower extremities.

200. Correct Answer: **3**

Rationale: All of this patient's symptoms are signs of renal failure.

201. Correct Answer: **1**

Rationale: Claudication is pain—sometimes described as cramps—in the lower extremities.

202. Correct Answer: **True**

203. Correct Answer: **2**

Rationale: Erectile dysfunction is common in diabetic males.

204. Correct Answer: **4**

Rationale: Impaired white blood cells allow infection to thrive in the body.

205. Correct Answer: 3

Rationale: Osteomyelitis is an infection of the bone.

206. Correct Answer: **Small**

Rationale: The small intestine is anatomically located at the duodenum.

207. Correct Answer: 1

Rationale: Diplopia is a common complaint following damage to the third cranial nerve.

208. Correct Answer: 3

Rationale: Nephrons are found in the kidney, neurons are found in cells, a ureter connects to the bladder, and islets of Langerhans are cells found in the pancreas.

209. Correct Answer: 3

Rationale: Amino acids are the result of protein breakdown. Lipids, cholesterol, and fats are all types of fats.

210. Correct Answer: 2

Rationale: Stress causes the breakdown of protein to acids and increases blood osmolality.

211. Correct Answer: **True**

Rationale: Beta cells produce insulin. Alpha-2 cells produce glucagon.

212. Correct Answer: 3

Rationale: Hemorrhage causes retinal damage.

213. Correct Answer: 3

Rationale: ADH insufficiency occurs in diabetes insipidus and causes excessive fluid excretion.

214. Correct Answer: 3

Rationale: Polyuria is excessive urination, polydipsia is excessive thirst, and polyphagia is excessive hunger.

215. Correct Answer: 4

Rationale: Low sodium results from dehydration.

216. Correct Answer: **True**

Rationale: Glucose in the urine can indicate diabetes, although it is not a precise measure.

217. Correct Answer: 1

Rationale: Ketoacidosis occurs when there is no insulin, so blood osmolality increases.

218. Correct Answer: 3

Rationale: HNKC can lead to dehydration owing to diuresis and consequent loss of sodium.

219. Correct Answer: 1

Rationale: Cellular fluid loss resulting in dehydration causes CNS dysfunction.

220. Correct Answer: **False**

Rationale: Ketones result from the breakdown of fat. It is the acid end-product of fat metabolism.

221. Correct Answer: 2

Rationale: "Nephrogenic" means nephrons; these cells are found in the kidneys (the renal system).

222. Correct Answer: 3

Rationale: Glucagon is the hormone that the body releases after 12 to 14 hours of fasting. In people who do not have diabetes, the body releases insulin to bring the high blood glucose back down to normal.

Care of Patients with Orthopedic Problems

MANAGEMENT OF CARE

Multiple Choice

1. What are the immediate care priorities for a patient who has experienced a sprain of the lower extremity? (Select all that apply.)

1. Rest.
2. Encouraging movement.
3. Ice application.
4. Heat application.
5. Compression.
6. Elevation.

2. A patient with acute low back pain is seen in the clinic. One desired patient outcome was to use proper body mechanics at all times. Which finding would indicate that this goal was met?

1. The patient slides an object across the floor rather than lifting.
2. To pick up an object off the floor, the patient bends at the waist and tightens the abdominal muscles.
3. The patient twists at the waist while reaching for an object.
4. The patient stands using a slouched position to reduce strain.

3. A goal for a patient with the nursing diagnosis of a self-care deficit in feeding is to assist the patient with the use of adaptive devices to enhance his or her capabilities. Which member of the collaborative healthcare team would be the most appropriate choice to consult to achieve the desired goal?

1. Occupational therapist.
2. Social worker.
3. Respiratory therapist.
4. Physician's assistant.

4. A pressure ulcer is identified after a patient underwent a long, extensive recovery following a surgical procedure. An incident/occurrence report is completed upon identification of the ulcer. Which statement about an incident/occurrence report is true?

1. A nurse manager must always complete the report.
2. Only the name of the person completing the report should be listed.
3. A notation should be made in the medical record that the report was completed.
4. Trending of incident report data helps to identify quality improvement issues.

5. Which actions should the nurse take to ensure the accuracy of a telephone order? (Select all that apply.)

1. Limit the use of telephone orders to emergency situations or when it is impossible for the healthcare provider to actually write the order.

2. Repeat the order back to the physician after it is written in the medical record for confirmation.

3. Implement the order, and then write it in the medical orders.

4. Record the name of prescriber, the date and time of the order, and the nurse's signature and title.

5. The co-signature of the ordering healthcare provider must be obtained within 8 hours of the original order.

6. The nurse should ask the unlicensed clerical staff to write the order, but the licensed nurse must implement the order.

6. When planning for a home discharge, a nurse suggests that respite care may be needed for the family of a quadriplegic patient. A family member asks, "How can respite care help us?" What is the nurse's best response?

1. "The primary caregiver is provided with time away from day-to-day care responsibilities."

2. "Respite care is a program that provides holistic support and care for a terminally ill patient."

3. "Respite care is provided to relieve or reduce the intensity of uncomfortable symptoms."

4. "Respite care is continuation of care that is provided after a family member dies."

7. An elderly patient has fallen and experienced a hip fracture. The patient is admitted to an acute care setting and will require rehabilitative care. Which statement about the rehabilitation process is true?

1. Rehabilitation should begin on admission to the hospital.

2. The focus of rehabilitative care is on the physical injuries.

3. No more than one rehabilitation facility at a time should be contacted when planning for patient placement.

4. All components of rehabilitation are covered by commercial insurance providers.

8. Which action by the nurse would demonstrate a lack of concern for a patient's privacy?

1. The nurse knocks on the door before entering the patient's room.

2. The healthcare provider takes a patient from a semi-private room to a small conference room to discuss the results of a biopsy.

3. The nurse forgets to cover up a patient when transporting the individual in the hallway.

4. A curtain is drawn and the door to the room is shut when a patient's wound dressing is changed.

9. While on duty, a nurse sustains a back injury when trying to prevent a patient injury from a fall. Which law would allow the nurse to obtain compensation for illness and injuries suffered during employment?

1. Fair Labor Standards Act.

2. Worker's compensation laws.

3. Americans with Disabilities Act.

4. Family Medical Leave Act.

True or False

10. Reimbursement for DRG 209, major joint replacement, is approximately $10,000. The hospital has established a case management system and is able to deliver care for a total of $9,500. The hospital will profit from performing the procedure.

Multiple Choice

11. A nurse makes a medication error. The patient was immediately assessed and no untoward effects of the error were identified. The nurse decides not to report the error because the patient did not experience any injury from it. Which ethical principle did the nurse violate?

1. Autonomy.

2. Justice.

3. Veracity.

4. Confidentiality.

12. A nurse educator is preparing an in-service education class for a group of graduate nurses about organ donation. Which statement about organ donation is appropriate for the nurse to include in the class?

1. Consent for organ donation is required in the United States.

2. Donation costs are the responsibility of the donor's family and estate.

3. A transplant waiting list is maintained by the for-profit organization, United Network for Organ Sharing (UNOS).

4. The organ donor's family may choose who receives the organ.

13. A registered nurse believes that the patient care assignment made by the charge nurse is unfair. What is the most appropriate response by the registered nurse?

1. Contact the nursing supervisor and ask him or her to intervene on the registered nurse's behalf.
2. Ask another registered nurse to review the equity of the assignment.
3. Talk with the charge nurse about the assignment and the registered nurse's concerns.
4. Accept the assignment and talk with the nurse manager at a later time.

14. A nurse applies for a charge nurse position at a local hospital and asks to see the job description. Which information would the nurse expect to find in the job description?

1. A summary of the training, experience, and special skills needed for the job.
2. Information on the rate of pay and differentials the applicant will receive.
3. A philosophy statement about the nursing unit where the applicant will work.
4. A chart identifying the organizational structure for the entire hospital.

True or False

15. A patient who experienced a debilitating stroke after hip replacement surgery is being transferred to a long-term care facility. To ensure continuity of care, the nurse will transfer the original chart along with the patient to the facility.

Multiple Choice

16. A quality indicator for the orthopedic nursing unit is "The patient exhibits no signs or symptoms of wound infection on discharge." Which type of standard is this indicator?

1. Structure.
2. Process.
3. Outcome.
4. Practice.

17. Which statement about the use of restraints is true?

1. Assessment of a restrained patient is required every 8 hours.
2. A restraint should be the first choice for management of confused patients.
3. Restraints promote patient safety and prevent injuries.

4. Alternatives to restraint should be considered prior to the application of restraints.

18. A nurse educator is preparing a class for staff nurses on a new infusion pump that is to be implemented on the orthopedic unit during the next week. Which teaching strategy best demonstrates the application of an adult learning principle?

1. Provide a written procedure for the use of the device for the staff to review.
2. Demonstrate the device use and allow the staff hands-on time to practice with it.
3. Place the new infusion pumps on the unit and allow the staff to self-instruct on its use.
4. Identify all the differences and new features of the device in a written brochure.

19. Upon assessment of the temporomandibular joint, a nurse identifies pain, crepitus, and a popping sound. Based on the findings, to which healthcare provider would the patient mostly likely be referred?

1. Occupational therapist.
2. Oral surgeon.
3. Physical therapist.
4. Ear, nose, and throat physician.

True or False

20. Nurses who maintain continuity of care across healthcare settings to enhance positive outcomes, effectively utilize resources, and contain costs are called team nurses.

Multiple Choice

21. Which nursing diagnosis would have the highest priority for a patient who is diagnosed with a disorder of musculoskeletal function?

1. Impaired physical mobility.
2. Risk for ineffective health maintenance.
3. Risk for activity intolerance.
4. Impaired skin integrity.

22. The nurse is caring for a patient with an open fracture of the radius. The nursing diagnosis for the patient is risk for peripheral neurovascular dysfunction. Which intervention would be the most important to perform?

1. Observe the condition of the fracture site for signs of infection.
2. Assess the involved extremity for pain, pallor, paresthesia, pulse, and temperature.

3. Perform range of motion on the bilateral extremities.

4. Check the bilateral radial and brachial pulses.

23. A staff member is observed taking medical supplies from the unit for personal use. Who is the most appropriate person for the nurse to communicate with about this observation?

1. The nurse manager.

2. The hospital administrator responsible for equipment and supplies.

3. Another nurse on the unit.

4. The chief nursing officer.

True or False

24. Each state establishes a nurse practice act that protects the public by defining the legal scope of nursing practice within the state.

Multiple Choice

25. The nurse is completing a patient history and physical examination. Which pieces of information are considered subjective data?

1. Blood pressure and pulse rate.

2. Complaints of fatigue and pain.

3. Nausea and vomiting.

4. Cyanosis and cool, clammy skin.

26. The discharge plan for a patient with a ligamentous injury to the knee will include the use of axillary crutches. Which healthcare team member would be most helpful in teaching the patient safe, effective use of the crutches?

1. Nursing assistant.

2. Physical therapist.

3. Physician's assistant.

4. Home health nurse.

27. A patient signs the informed consent paperwork for the surgical repair of a fractured femur. In which situation would informed consent be valid?

1. A 50-year-old patient who is alert but confused.

2. A 35-year-old patient with a blood alcohol level of 150 mg/dL.

3. A 16-year-old patient who is alert and oriented and whose family is not present.

4. An 88-year-old patient who is alert and oriented.

28. Identify a rehabilitation go[...] a spinal fracture and complete [...] transection at the level of C5.

1. Ability to achieve independe[...] bed to wheelchair.

2. Independent control of bowel [...] function.

3. Use of a wheelchair with a chin or mouth stick.

4. Feeds self with the use of adaptive equipment.

29. Which action by a nurse would demonstrate a violation of confidentiality?

1. Discussing a patient's surgical procedure with the nurse manager.

2. Reporting laboratory findings to a patient's friend who asks about the results.

3. Notifying the physician of physical assessment findings.

4. Identifying the patient by name when making a referral for home health services.

30. Identify the nursing care priority in the immediate postoperative period for a patient who has undergone surgical repair of a mandibular fracture.

1. Pain control.

2. Airway management.

3. Oral hygiene.

4. Nutritional support.

31. The charge nurse is assigning care responsibilities for the upcoming shift. A postoperative patient who underwent hip replacement surgery is to be admitted from the post-anesthesia care unit. Which staff member would be the best person for the nurse to assign to this patient?

1. Certified nursing assistant.

2. Licensed practical nurse.

3. Registered nurse.

4. Student nurse.

True or False

32. A nurse would consult the American Nurses Association's Code of Ethics to identify violations that can result in disciplinary actions against the nurse and his/her professional license.

Multiple Choice

33. A patient has suffered a hip fracture that requires surgical repair. Which healthcare professional is responsible for obtaining informed consent for the procedure?

SECTION III · SECTION IV · SECTION V · SECTION VI · SECTION VII · SECTION VIII · SECTION IX · SECTION X

1. Nurse.

2. Anesthesiologist.

3. Surgeon.

4. Operating room nurse.

34. Eight hours following a femur fracture, a patient complains of a sudden onset of dyspnea and severe chest pain. Which action should the nurse take first?

1. Administer oxygen and assess vital signs.

2. Notify the physician and prepare to transfer the patient to an ICU.

3. Increase intravenous infusion and medicate for pain.

4. Complete and document a head-to-toe assessment.

35. A nurse arrives at the scene of a motor vehicle accident. The patient is not breathing and there is a high index of suspicion for a cervical vertebrae fracture. What is the priority of care for this patient?

1. Place the patient in a hard cervical collar.

2. Open the airway using the jaw-thrust maneuver.

3. Assess the patient for other injuries.

4. Complete a neurological assessment.

36. A patient has a short leg cast that has been newly applied to the lower extremity. Which finding would require immediate notification of the physician?

1. Patient report of a moderate pain level.

2. Presence of dependent edema distal to the cast.

3. Inability to flex or extend toes on the casted foot.

4. Increased temperature of the affected extremity.

True or False

37. A competent, adult patient has refused an injection, but the nurse administers the injection against the patient's will. The nurse has committed battery.

Multiple Choice

38. What is the initial assessment priority for a patient who is admitted to the emergency room with suspected multiple facial fractures?

1. Vital signs.

2. Patent airway.

3. Breath sounds.

4. Skin color.

39. Which treatment priority would the nurse expect to implement for a patient with acute osteomyelitis?

1. Alternating heat and cold to the affected area.

2. Administration of antibiotics.

3. Active and passive range-of-motion exercises.

4. Surgical fusion of the bone with internal fixation.

40. The nurse notices another healthcare worker entering the room of a patient who is on transmission-based precautions without the appropriate protective equipment. What initial action should a nurse take?

1. Provide the appropriate protective equipment to the healthcare worker while he or she is in the room.

2. Notify the charge nurse and complete an incident report.

3. Contact the organization's epidemiology staff to address the problem.

4. Speak with the healthcare worker after he or she has left the patient's room about the problem.

41. The Patient's Bill of Rights, which was established by the American Hospital Association in 1972 and revised in 1992 and 2003, addresses the expectations, rights, and responsibilities of the patient when receiving care in the hospital. Which are examples of patient's rights? (Select all that apply.)

1. Clean and safe environment.

2. Involvement in care.

3. Error-free care.

4. The provision of care without concern for payment.

5. Help with the bill and filing insurance claims.

6. Protection of privacy.

42. Immunization for tetanus would be an example of which type of community-based preventive care?

1. Primary.

2. Secondary.

3. Tertiary.

4. Quaternary.

43. The nurse is preparing a 65-year-old female patient for knee replacement surgery. The presurgical, screening, lab results are returned. Which finding should the nurse notify the surgeon about before proceeding with surgical preparation?

1. WBC count 20,000/mm³.
2. Hematocrit 40 mL/dL.
3. Creatinine 1.1 mg/dL.
4. Potassium 3.8 mEq/L.

44. Which situation is an example of nursing negligence?

1. Upon neurovascular assessment of a fractured extremity at 1:00 A.M., the nurse identified the absence of a peripheral pulse. A code is called on another patient and the nurse became busy. The physician is notified of the absent pulse at 7:00 A.M.

2. A competent patient refuses an antidepressant medication. The nurse dissolves the medication and administers it to the patient without the patient's knowledge.

3. A patient who is alert and oriented makes an informed decision to leave the hospital against medical advice. The nurse physically restrains the patient to prevent him from leaving.

4. A nurse identifies an incorrect narcotic count. The nurse makes a false entry into the narcotic record to correct the count.

SAFETY AND INFECTION CONTROL

Multiple Choice

45. The nurse needs to insert a peripheral intravenous catheter. The patient is allergic to iodine. Which solution would be best to use for asepsis and site preparation?

1. Betadine.
2. Soap and water.
3. 70% isopropyl alcohol.
4. 5% sodium hypochlorite.

46. A person presents to a blood donation center and completes a donor history. Which finding would prevent this person from becoming a blood donor?

1. A 24-year-old individual who had new tattoo placed in the past week.
2. An 18-year-old with a pulse rate between 60 and 100 beats per minute.
3. A 32-year-old with a body weight of 60 kg.
4. A 38-year-old with a hemoglobin of 10 g/dL.

47. Which feature of a patient-controlled analgesia device will most likely prevent an overdose of pain medication?

1. Bolus dose.
2. Patient-controlled dose.
3. Timing control/lockout.
4. Locked drug depository.

48. The nurse is developing an in-service program on the prevention of medication errors. Identify the example that demonstrates the safest way to write an order for a medication with a decimal point.

1. 0.2 mg.
2. .2 mg.
3. 2.0 mg.
4. 02.0 mg.

49. A patient is diagnosed with osteomyelitis. What is the most common infectious organism associated with the disease?

1. *Escherichia coli.*
2. *Candida albicans.*
3. *Staphylococcus aureus.*
4. *Mycobacterium tuberculosis.*

Identification

50. Identify the correct sequence for the removal of personal protective equipment when a nurse is preparing to leave the room of a patient on airborne precautions.

_____ Gloves.
_____ Mask/respirator.
_____ Gown.
_____ Hand hygiene.

Multiple Choice

51. The nurse removes a dressing from an infected wound site that is saturated with blood and has purulent drainage. What is the best means of disposal of the dressing material?

1. Discard the dressing in the bedside trash receptacle.
2. Dispose of the dressing in a biohazardous waste container.
3. Place the dressing in a clear plastic bag and discard in the bedside trash receptacle.
4. Double-bag the dressing in a bag labeled "biohazard" and send it for sterilization.

52. Prior to surgery, a patient had a urinary catheter inserted. Three days postoperatively, a urinary tract infection is identified. Which term most accurately describes this type of infection?

1. Community-acquired infection.

2. Prodromal infection.

3. Exogenous infection.

4. Nosocomial infection.

53. Identify the nursing action that would increase the risk of an intravascular device-related infection.

1. Washing the hands before and after device dressing changes.

2. Reinforcing a damp, loosened, or soiled dressing.

3. Prepping the skin prior to device insertion with povidone iodine solution.

4. Changing fluids and tubing as per hospital policy.

54. What interventions might the nurse consider prior to the application of restraints? (Select all that apply.)

1. Involve the family in the patient's care.

2. Increase the noise in the area.

3. Avoid the use of a nightlight.

4. Assist with toileting at frequent intervals.

5. Use an electronic position-sensitive device.

6. Use diversionary activities.

55. A nosocomial wound infection with vancomycin-resistant enterococcus is identified. What type of transmission-based precautions should the healthcare team implement?

1. Droplet precautions.

2. Contact precautions.

3. Airborne precautions.

4. Wound precautions.

56. Which action is contraindicated when caring for a patient with continuous skeletal traction of the lower extremity?

1. Inspect the skin for signs of breakdown.

2. Remove the traction weights for 30 minutes to 1 hour every 8 hours.

3. Ensure that the traction weights are unobstructed and hanging freely.

4. Perform neurovascular assessments of the injured extremity.

57. After experiencing a mandible fracture, a patient has had her jaws wired. What is the best position for a patient to be placed in during the immediate postoperative period to protect the airway and prevent aspiration?

1. Supine.

2. Lateral with the head of bed elevated 15 to 30 degrees.

3. Trendelenburg position.

4. Dorsal recumbent position.

Identification

58. Which picture demonstrates the effective use of body mechanics when picking up an object?

1.

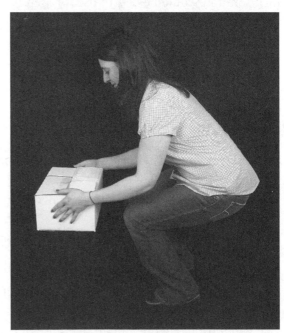

2.

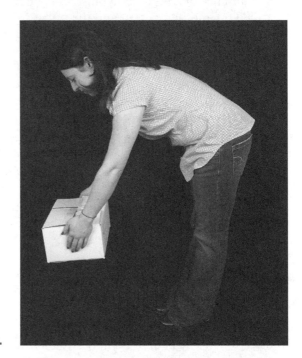

Multiple Choice

59. To promote the safe use of a cane as an assistive device for a patient who is recovering from a musculoskeletal injury to the left lower extremity, which instruction should the nurse provide?

1. Hold the cane on the right side to provide support for the injured left leg.
2. Rubber tips should not be used on the end of a cane.
3. Support the weight on the injured left leg and the cane, and then advance the right leg.
4. Place the cane approximately 24 inches in front of the feet before advancing.

60. The nurse is caring for a patient who is experiencing severe symptoms of alcohol withdrawal. To ensure safe care, which nursing action would be contraindicated?

1. Monitoring vital signs.
2. Assessing intake and output.
3. Ambulating in the hallway.
4. Decreasing unnecessary stimuli.

61. A nurse is teaching a class on fall prevention to a group of assisted-living residents. Which statement by a resident best indicates an understanding of the teaching?

1. "It is a good idea to have handrails or grab bars installed in the bathroom."
2. "I should use chairs without armrests."
3. "I should place throw rugs throughout the living area."
4. "Bathroom doors should have locks that can be opened only from the inside."

Identification

62. A patient is found smoking in the hospital room. The ashes from the cigarette have ignited trash in the wastebasket and now smoke is filling the room. Identify the actions the nurse should take in the order of priority.

_____ Rescue the patient from immediate danger.

_____ Activate the fire alarm system.

_____ Confine the fire by closing doors and windows.

_____ Extinguish the fire if possible.

Multiple Choice

63. To promote the safe care of a patient with multiple facial fractures, which type of equipment should the nurse have at the bedside?

1. Suction equipment.
2. Central venous catheter.
3. Chest tube and drainage unit.
4. Intravenous infusion pump.

64. Which hospitalized patient is at the highest risk for a fall?

1. An elderly, confused patient with urinary incontinence whose bed is left in a high position.
2. An adult patient with visual impairment whose call light is within reach.
3. A patient who is getting out of bed for the first time with the assistance of two physical therapists.
4. An adolescent patient who has been using crutches for only the past 3 days.

65. Which equipment should be readily available at the bedside of a patient who is about to receive a neuromuscular blocking agent?

1. Bag-valve-mask device and oxygen.
2. Defibrillator and pacemaker.
3. Ventricular catheter and transducer.
4. Central venous catheterization equipment and IV fluids.

66. A central venous catheter has been placed in the patient, and the nurse is disposing of the equipment used in the procedure when an accidental needlestick occurs. What is the initial action the nurse should take?

1. Initiate post-exposure pharmacological prophylaxis.
2. Flush and wash the exposed area with warm water and soap.
3. Obtain a blood sample from the patient to determine the presence of any transmittable diseases.
4. Complete an accident and injury report.

HEALTH PROMOTION AND MAINTENANCE

Multiple Choice

67. The nurse is completing a neurovascular assessment of a fractured lower extremity after a surgical intervention to reduce the fracture. Which parameters are included as a part of a neurovascular assessment? (Select all that apply.)

1. Color.
2. Temperature.
3. Capillary refill time.
4. Pulse.
5. Pain.
6. Sensation.
7. Movement.

68. Which finding would indicate that the patient is experiencing normal, physiologic musculoskeletal changes associated with pregnancy?

1. Gradual lordosis with trimester progression.
2. Leans forward for balance.
3. Decreased joint mobility.
4. 3 to 4 + deep tendon reflexes.

69. Which health promotion advice would a nurse give to a patient who has a history of low back pain?

1. Lift only items that are located below the level of the elbows.
2. Sleep lying flat with the legs extended straight.
3. Continue exercising even if there is associated pain.
4. Maintain your recommended body weight.

70. A nurse is teaching an adult patient with a low literacy level about the subcutaneous administration of dalteparin (Fragmin). Which strategies could the nurse use to promote the patient's understanding?

1. Use technical words and short sentences.
2. Ask the patient to demonstrate the skill.
3. Provide the patient with written, large-print materials.
4. Plan for a longer session than normal.

True or False

71. The use of stretching and warm-up exercises is a health promotion activity that helps to reduce ligamentous sprains and muscular strains.

Multiple Choice

72. A patient with osteomalacia has been advised to increase vitamin D intake as a part of the treatment plan. Which recommendations could be made to the patient to ensure an adequate intake of vitamin D?

1. Increase the daily amount of sunlight exposure.
2. Reduce the amount of dairy products and cereals consumed.
3. Promote the intake of calcium, as vitamin D is a by-product of calcium metabolism.
4. Add a regular exercise routine to promote the release of vitamin D from muscle.

73. To reduce the risk of osteoporosis, an adequate intake of calcium is recommended. Which recommendation for calcium intake should be provided to a 55-year-old patient?

1. 500 mg/day.
2. 800 mg/day.
3. 1,000 mg/day.
4. 1,200 mg/day.

74. A ballottement test is performed during the physical examination of a patient's knee. What is the purpose of this test?

1. Detection of the presence of air in the joint capsule.
2. Assessment for fluid and effusion.
3. Examination for inflammation of the nerve roots.
4. Evaluation of a torn meniscus.

75. Which statement about the administration of tetanus toxoid to a 22-year-old patient who was fully immunized as a child is correct?

1. This patient should receive tetanus immune globulin.
2. Tetanus toxoid provides an active, immediate immunity to the patient.
3. One dose of the vaccine should be administered to this patient.
4. A three-dose series of tetanus toxoid injections is required for this patient.

76. What intervention would be contraindicated when planning activities to prevent musculoskeletal problems in an elderly patient?

1. Maintain weight.
2. Avoid the use of ramps in buildings and at street corners.

3. Wear supportive shoes with non-skid surfaces.

4. Participate in weight-bearing activities daily.

77. Which joint protection measure might a nurse communicate to a patient with osteoarthritis?

1. Increase dietary intake of phosphorus.

2. Decrease the use of caffeine.

3. Maintain an ideal body weight.

4. Reduce the amount of purine in the diet.

78. The nurse is preparing a teaching plan for a patient who is visually impaired. Which teaching strategy should be included in the plan?

1. Use of a slow, deliberate speech pattern.

2. Use of auditory or tactile materials.

3. Provision of written information.

4. Use of captioned video materials.

79. Which occupations would place a person at risk for the development of carpal tunnel syndrome? (Select all that apply.)

1. Hair stylist.

2. Truck driver.

3. Computer operator.

4. Seamstress who does handwork.

5. Elementary school teacher.

6. Waitress.

80. What type of physical activity would be the best choice for a 75-year-old, female patient who has been diagnosed with osteoporosis?

1. High-impact aerobics.

2. Walking.

3. Riding a bicycle.

4. Stretching exercises of the arms and shoulders.

81. The nurse is conducting a class on musculo-skeletal changes associated with aging for a group of retired schoolteachers. Which aging-related change should the nurse include in the class?

1. Muscles decrease in elasticity and tone.

2. Closure of the epiphyseal plates occurs.

3. Height slightly increases for men.

4. Calcium levels increase.

82. Which factor might contribute to the develop-ment of osteoarthritis? (Select all that apply.)

1. Obesity.

2. Family history of osteoarthritis.

3. 20 to 30 years of age.

4. Excessive use of alcohol.

5. Caucasian or Asian ethnicity.

6. Regular, strenuous exercise.

83. The nurse is teaching a class on injury prevention to a group of young athletes. Which joint is most susceptible to a sports-related injury?

1. Wrist.

2. Shoulder.

3. Hip.

4. Knee.

84. At which developmental stage would a nurse expect scoliosis screening to occur?

1. Pre-adolescence/adolescence.

2. Toddler.

3. Post menopause.

4. Young adult.

85. A patient diagnosed with gout asks, "Is there anything that I can do to decrease my uric acid levels?" What is the nurse's most appropriate response?

1. Decrease the amount of liver, sardines, and shrimp in your diet.

2. Increase the amount of citrus fruits in your diet.

3. Drink at least 1 to 1.5 liters of fluid each day.

4. Avoid strenuous activity, as it will cause muscle breakdown.

86. Which health promotion activity might reduce the incidence of osteoporosis?

1. Maintaining an average daily intake of 300 to 500 mg of calcium.

2. Annual testing for bone mineral density for women age 20 and older.

3. Regular weight-bearing exercise.

4. Increasing the intake of carbonated beverages.

PSYCHOSOCIAL INTEGRITY

Multiple Choice

87. A patient who is scheduled to undergo hip arthroplasty expresses fear of not being adequately anesthetized during the procedure. What is the nurse's most appropriate response?

1. "I will call the anesthesiologist about your concern."

2. "Can you tell me more about why you have this concern?"

3. "You have nothing to be concerned about. You have a competent anesthesiologist."

4. "You will be constantly monitored when you undergo the procedure. If there are any problems, the healthcare providers will be right there."

88. A patient with metastatic bone cancer has expressed the desire to go home to die. The family is concerned about meeting the patient's care needs at home. Which action by the nurse would be the most appropriate to implement?

1. Discuss a referral to home health and hospice care with the patient and family.

2. Contact the social worker to assist with nursing home placement.

3. Talk with the nurse manager about the possibility of an extended hospital stay.

4. Teach the family how to care for the terminally ill patient.

89. One nurse accuses another nurse of not providing adequate care for a patient who underwent hip replacement surgery. Which statement would represent an assertive response by the nurse?

1. "I feel as though I met the standard of care. Would you tell me more about your concerns?"

2. "You shouldn't talk. You always leave your patients in a mess and in need of care."

3. "I am at a loss for words. I always give good care to my patients."

4. "What do you have against me? You are always complaining about my nursing care."

90. A 48-year-old housewife and mother of three teenage children is hospitalized with a pelvic fracture. Treatment will require bed rest and traction for approximately 4 to 6 weeks. What effect will hospitalization most likely have on the patient's family?

1. Loss of privacy.

2. Decrease in income.

3. Alteration in family members' roles and tasks.

4. Loss of autonomy for the children.

91. A patient experienced a traumatic amputation of the left arm in an industrial accident. Upon the patient's admission to the emergency room, in which initial stage of loss and grieving would the nurse expect to find the patient?

1. Bargaining.

2. Depression.

3. Denial.

4. Acceptance.

92. A patient with a femur fracture states, "I can't stay in this bed any longer. I need to get home so I can take care of my family." The nurse responds by saying, "You have talked about your family. Can you tell me more about your specific concerns?" Which type of therapeutic response communication is the nurse using?

1. Summarizing.

2. Empathizing.

3. Focusing.

4. Confronting.

93. Which group is at the greatest risk for developing systemic lupus erythematosus?

1. Caucasian men.

2. European women.

3. Native American men.

4. African American women.

Matching

Match the situation with the coping mechanism that the patient is using in questions 94–96.

Coping Mechanisms

1. Denial.

2. Displacement.

3. Rationalization.

94. A 28-year-old patient diagnosed with rheumatoid arthritis states, "The pain in my joints has worsened over the past year. I can no longer do my yard work. It is hard to get old."

95. A football player with an anterior cruciate ligament tear is told that he will be unable to play football for the remainder of the season. The patient yells that the healthcare provider doesn't know what he is talking about and kicks a chair.

96. A patient experiences an adverse medication event and states, "The nurse told me not to drink when taking the medication. I am just a social drinker. I didn't realize that having just one drink with my friends would cause such a problem."

Multiple Choice

97. Which patient statement provides support for the nursing diagnosis of disturbed body image?

1. "When I look in the mirror, all I see is a person without a leg."
2. "I have not always made good choices in life. I deserve to lose my leg."
3. "I don't think I will ever be able to play golf again with my friends."
4. "No matter how hard I work in physical therapy, I can't seem to make any progress."

98. Which cultural group would be more likely to consider the use of acupressure or acupuncture as a treatment modality for the pain associated with osteoarthritis?

1. African Americans.
2. Native Americans.
3. Asian Americans.
4. Hispanic Americans.

99. Which food selections should be incorporated into a Hispanic patient's diet that would represent culturally sensitive care?

1. Beans and tortillas.
2. Cheese and olives.
3. Vegetables and rice.
4. Red meat and potatoes.

100. A patient presents to the outpatient clinic with a history of difficulty sleeping, fatigue, and increased consumption of alcohol; the patient also describes problems with concentration. When asked about the onset of the symptoms, the patient states, "My best friend was killed in a car accident 3 months ago. I just don't know what to do." Identify an appropriate nursing diagnosis for this patient based on these findings.

1. Ineffective denial.
2. Risk for suicide.
3. Ineffective coping.
4. Defensive coping.

Identification

101. The nurse is talking with a patient who was just told about the diagnosis of osteosarcoma.

Which nonverbal expression would be unexpected and should be investigated further by the nurse?

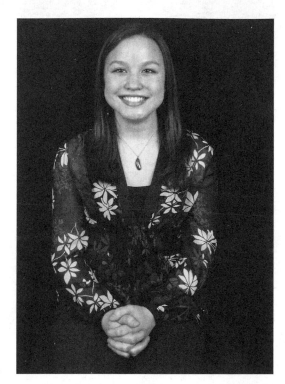

1.

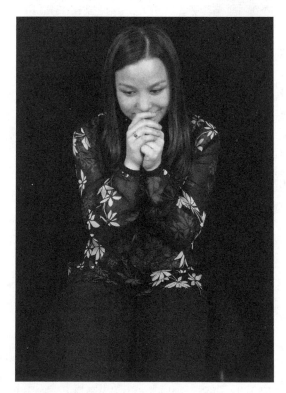

2.

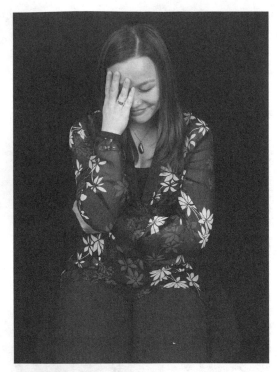

3.

Multiple Choice

102. Based on the nurse's understanding of religious practices, which patient would the nurse expect to exclude pork as a dietary selection?

1. Presbyterian.
2. Catholic.
3. Mormon.
4. Seventh Day Adventist.

103. A patient is experiencing denial over the loss of a limb in a motor vehicle accident. Which intervention by the nurse is most likely to assist the patient in the denial phase of grief and loss?

1. Allow the patient to continue to deny the situation, as this response is a part of recovery.
2. Provide the patient with written information about the phases of loss.
3. Support the patient and slowly intervene to increase the development of awareness.
4. Encourage the continued use of denial as a coping mechanism.

104. The nurse suspects that a paraplegic patient is becoming depressed. Which symptoms would a patient with depression be most likely to exhibit?

1. Flight of ideas, decreased need for sleep and distractibility.
2. Difficulty concentrating, social withdrawal, feeling of sadness.
3. Palpitations, sweating, sensation of shortness of breath.
4. Inability to care for self, paranoia, impaired memory.

105. Which physiologic outcome would the nurse expect to observe in a patient who has been taught relaxation techniques to manage stress?

1. Rhythmic breathing.
2. Elevated pulse rate.
3. Tensed muscles.
4. Perspiration.

106. A patient loses a limb in an accident. The change in body image accompanied by the loss of a body part will affect which type of human need?

1. Self-actualization.
2. Safety.
3. Self-esteem.
4. Physiological.

BASIC CARE AND COMFORT

Multiple Choice

107. Which statements identify the effects of immobility on body systems? (Select all that apply.)

1. Increased metabolic rate.
2. Increased depth and rate of respirations.
3. Muscle atrophy.
4. Venous pooling.
5. Slowed muscular activity in the gastrointestinal tract.
6. Urinary stasis.

108. A patient is scheduled to undergo a closed reduction of a fracture. In addition to the use of medications, the nurse suggests that the patient listen to an audiotape. Which type of non-pharmacologic intervention for pain management is the nurse using?

1. Cutaneous stimulation.
2. Imagery.
3. Biofeedback.
4. Distraction.

109. A postoperative patient is placed on a clear liquid diet. Which food selection would be excluded from this diet?

1. Tea.
2. Fat-free broth.
3. Pudding.
4. Carbonated beverage.

110. The nurse provides a fracture pan for a bedridden female patient with a femur fracture who needs to void. What is the purpose of using a fracture pan versus a regular bedpan?

1. It prevents the malunion of femur fragments.
2. It offers greater ease of patient placement.
3. It reduces the strain on the gluteal muscle groups.
4. It requires minimal patient exertion.

111. What type of crutch gait should be taught to a patient who may bear weight on only one foot?

1. Swing-to gait.
2. Swing-through gait.
3. Two-point gait.
4. Three-point gait.

Matching

Match the range of motion term with the appropriate picture of the movement.

112. Abduction.

113. External rotation.

114. Supination.

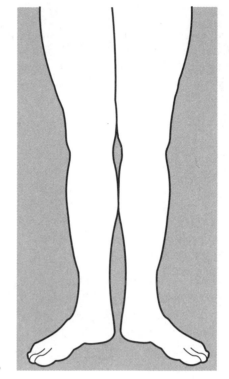

2.

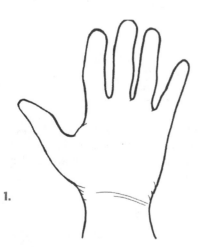

1.

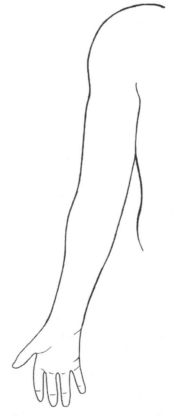

3.

Multiple Choice

115. A treatment goal for a patient with osteoarthritis is relief of symptoms to include pain, stiffness, and inflammation. Which non-pharmacological intervention would promote the achievement of the goal?

1. Increasing the amount of rest by 4 to 5 hours per day.
2. Daily aerobic exercise.
3. Massage therapy.
4. Ice baths.

116. Isometric exercises are prescribed for a patient with a knee injury. What is the expected outcome from completing the exercises?

1. Increased muscle strength, tone, and circulation to the area.
2. Muscle hypertrophy to compensate for decreased joint strength.
3. Promotion of venous stasis to reduce the risk of thrombus formation.
4. Decreased blood flow to the area to promote healing.

117. Which food choice would be most appropriate for a patient with osteoporosis who wants to increase calcium intake?

1. 1 medium apple.
2. 3 ounces of beef.
3. 1 ounce of cream cheese.
4. 1 medium stalk of cooked broccoli.

118. The nurse is caring for a patient with a herniated lumbar disc. The patient is experiencing pain. Which position might the nurse suggest that the patient assume to reduce the pain?

1. Prone with arms raised above head.
2. Side lying with knees flexed.
3. Supine with arms elevated on pillows.
4. Head of the bed elevated 30 degrees.

119. Which outcome is expected when physical rest is included as a part of the treatment plan for a patient with rheumatoid arthritis?

1. Reduced joint stress and pain relief.
2. Maintenance of joint function and muscle strength.
3. Suppression of the inflammatory process and pain relief.
4. Reduced swelling and stiffness.

120. The nursing diagnosis of "sleep pattern disturbance: insomnia related to fear of impending surgery" is formulated for a patient. Which intervention would be most appropriate based on this diagnosis?

1. Maintain the patient's normal sleep times and rituals.
2. Use tactile stimulation to promote relaxation.
3. Provide the patient with a warm, non-caffeinated drink before bedtime.
4. Allow the patient an opportunity to discuss any concerns about the surgery.

121. Which herbal product might a patient report using for the pain associated with osteoarthritis?

1. *Serenoa repens* (saw palmetto).
2. *Echinacea angustifolia* (echinacea).
3. *Cimicifuga racemosa* (black cohosh).
4. Capsicum (cayenne).

122. Following a complete spinal cord transection injury, the patient is described as a paraplegic. The family asks what this term means. What is the best response by the nurse?

1. The lower extremities are without sensation and/or movement.
2. There is decreased sensation in the upper extremities.
3. One side of the body is paralyzed.
4. Both the upper and lower extremities have decreased movement.

123. A nurse is concerned about the amount of sleep that a 25-year-old patient is getting. What is the average amount of sleep recommended for a young adult?

1. 5 hours.
2. 8 hours.
3. 10 hours.
4. 12 hours.

124. When providing care for a patient with facial fractures, the nurse identifies a strong mouth odor. Which term should the nurse use to document the finding?

1. Stomatitis.
2. Otorrhea.
3. Halitosis.
4. Pyorrhea.

125. Which non-pharmacological interventions would a nurse use to promote bowel elimination for a post-operative patient?

1. Increase ambulation.
2. Decrease fluid intake.
3. Administer a laxative.
4. Offer the bedpan every 2 to 4 hours.

126. The nurse is evaluating the 24-hour intake and output record for a hospitalized patient. Which findings would indicate a normal intake and output for a patient who is not on any fluid restrictions?

1. Intake 2,500 cc, output 500 cc.
2. Intake 2,400 cc, output 2,500 cc.
3. Intake 1,200 cc, output 700 cc.
4. Intake 800 cc, output 2,100 cc.

PHARMACOLOGICAL AND PARENTERAL THERAPIES

Multiple Choice

127. A patient has a known history of anaphylaxis to penicillin. The postoperative orders for a patient with an open femur fracture are for cephalosporin 1 g IV. Which action should the nurse take?

1. Administer the medication. Cephalosporins do not pose a risk for someone with a penicillin allergy.
2. Hold the medication until the prescriber can be notified of the patient's penicillin allergy.
3. The medication should not be administered because cephalosporin is a type of penicillin.
4. Administer the medication. There is no association between penicillin and cephalosporin.

128. Which clinical manifestations would the nurse expect to find in a patient with salicylism?

1. Tinnitus, dizziness, and hyperventilation.
2. Jaundice, abdominal discomfort, and enlarged liver.
3. Weight loss, paresthesias, and muscle weakness.
4. Fatigue, insomnia, and irritability.

129. A patient is to receive hydroxychloroquine (Plaquenil) for the treatment of mild symptoms of rheumatoid arthritis. Which baseline examination should be completed prior to the administration of the drug?

1. Hearing exam.
2. Vision exam.
3. Pap smear.
4. Dental exam.

Short Answer

130. The physician orders aspirin 1.3 g BID for a patient with rheumatoid arthritis. The aspirin is supplied in 325-mg tablets. How many tablets would you instruct the patient to take with each dose?

Multiple Choice

131. A patient is receiving morphine via a patient-controlled analgesia (PCA) infusion device after knee replacement surgery. Which patient statement indicates an understanding of appropriate use of the device?

1. "I should not use the device unless absolutely necessary."
2. "I will ask my family to push the PCA dose button when I am asleep."
3. "After pushing the PCA dose button, I will not feel any pain."
4. "I should notify the nurse if my pain is not controlled."

132. The healthcare provider communicates a treatment plan to a patient with osteoarthritis. The plan includes the use of an intra-articular injection of hydrocortisone. What is the purpose of this injection?

1. Systemic pain reduction.
2. Prevention of progressive functional loss.
3. Suppression of local inflammation.
4. Decrease in uric acid crystal production.

133. A patient has been prescribed alendronate (Fosamax) for the treatment of osteoporosis. The nurse instructs the patient to remain sitting or standing for at least 30 minutes after taking the medication. What is the reason for this patient instruction?

1. A sitting or standing position will reduce prolonged contact of the medication with the lining of the esophagus and reduce esophagitis.
2. Orthostatic hypotension may develop after drug administration, and sitting or standing will reduce the potential complication.

3. The drug decreases esophageal muscle contraction and can result in aspiration if not taken when sitting or standing.

4. The risk of musculoskeletal pain associated with drug administration is reduced when the patient is in the sitting or standing position.

134. A patient has been taking high doses of oral glucocorticoids for an extended period of time to treat arthritis. What is the effect of long-term, high-dose, oral glucocorticoids on the skeletal system?

1. Increased bone resorption by osteoblasts.

2. Decreased bone formation by osteoclasts.

3. Increased intestinal absorption of calcium, resulting in chronic hypercalcemia.

4. Decreased bone mineral density and resultant fractures.

135. For which patient would the nurse be most concerned about the ability of the patient to metabolize the drug carisoprodol (Soma)?

1. An 18-year-old patient recovering from hip surgery after a fall.

2. A 45-year-old patient with a history of chronic alcoholism.

3. A 30-year-old patient with a history of gastritis.

4. A 67-year-old patient with renal insufficiency.

Short Answer

136. The nurse is caring for a patient with rhabdomyolysis. The physician orders normal saline to infuse at a rate of 200 mL/h. How many hours will it take for a 1-L bag of normal saline to infuse?

Multiple Choice

137. A patient is taking benztropine mesylate (Cogentin) for Parkinson's disease. The patient presents to the outpatient clinic for follow-up and complains of dry mouth, blurred vision, an inability to urinate, and constipation. The nurse understands that the patient is exhibiting which response to the medication?

1. Desired action.

2. Adverse effects.

3. Drug toxicity.

4. Drug–drug interaction.

138. Which route of drug administration would result in the most rapid absorption of the drug into the bloodstream?

1. Transdermal.

2. Sublingual.

3. Intramuscular.

4. Enteral.

Short Answer

139. The nurse is preparing to administer hydrocortisone to a patient. The physician order reads 80 mg hydrocortisone IV every 12 hours. The medication is supplied in a vial that reads 125 mg/2 mL. How many milliliters of hydrocortisone will the nurse administer for one dose?

Multiple Choice

140. A patient undergoing hip replacement surgery who is at risk for the development of deep vein thrombosis is receiving dalteparin (Fragmin). Which statement correctly describes the administration technique for the medication?

1. Aspirate prior to administering the medication.

2. Use an 18-gauge, $1\frac{1}{2}$-inch needle to administer the drug.

3. Administer the medication by the subcutaneous route.

4. Inject the medication into muscle within 2 inches of the umbilicus.

141. Why is carbidopa–levodopa (Sinemet) preferred over levodopa (L-dopa) alone in the treatment of Parkinson's disease?

1. Absorption of levodopa from the gastrointestinal tract is improved when this drug is combined with carbidopa.

2. The adverse cardiovascular effects of orthostatic hypotension and tachycardia are eliminated with the use of Sinemet.

3. Carbidopa inhibits decarboxylase, allowing more levodopa to reach the brain for conversion to dopamine.

4. There is increased patient compliance with Sinemet as administration is only three times per day.

142. What is the expected outcome from the administration of cyclobenzapine (Flexeril)?

1. Decreased inflammation.

2. Improvement in range of motion.

3. Decreased central nervous system spasticity.

4. Reduced localized swelling.

143. In the postoperative period following a lumbar laminectomy, the nurse administers ondansetron (Zofran) to the patient. What is the expected outcome from this medication?

   1. Incisional pain is decreased.

   2. Nausea and vomiting subside.

   3. Muscle spasms are diminished.

   4. Microorganisms are decreased.

144. A patient develops constipation in association with the use of opioid analgesia after knee replacement surgery. The physician orders one-half (0.5) ounce of magnesium hydroxide (milk of magnesia). How many milliliters of the medication should the patient receive?

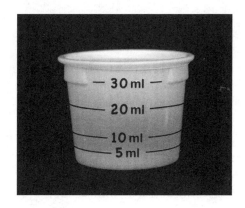

   1. 30 mL.

   2. 20 mL.

   3. 15 mL.

   4. 5 mL.

145. A patient is receiving filgrastim (Neupogen) daily following treatment for osteosarcoma with doxorubicin (Adriamycin) and cisplatin (Platinol-AQ). Which laboratory value would be most appropriate to monitor to determine the effectiveness of the filgrastim?

   1. Red blood cell count.

   2. Neutrophil count.

   3. Alkaline phosphatase.

   4. Serum calcium level.

146. How does aspirin act to promote pain relief in a patient with rheumatoid arthritis?

   1. Inhibits prostaglandins and reduces the sensitivity of pain receptors.

   2. It acts as an antagonist for pain receptors within the spinal cord.

   3. It promotes the increased production of endogenous opioids.

   4. It relieves tension and anxiety through the release of interleukins.

147. Raloxifene (Evista) is classified as being a pregnancy risk category X. How would the nurse interpret this classification to a patient?

   1. The potential for fetal harm outweighs any possible benefits of the drug's use during pregnancy.

   2. There is a remote risk of fetal harm in the first trimester of pregnancy.

   3. There is a risk of fetal harm but the benefits of drug administration may be acceptable.

   4. Animal studies have shown a risk of fetal harm, but no controlled studies have been done in women.

148. Identify the main purpose of using a continuous heparin infusion for a patient who has been diagnosed with a pulmonary embolus.

   1. To dissolve the existing clot and improve blood flow.

   2. To prevent clot enlargement and the formation of new thrombi.

   3. To decrease the formation of a platelet plug and promote circulation.

   4. To promote the formation of a new fibrin clot and decrease bleeding.

Matching

Match the appropriate figure with the name of the intramuscular injection site.

149. Ventrogluteal.

150. Anterolateral.

151. Deltoid.

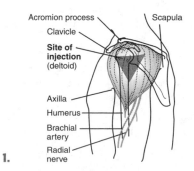

1.

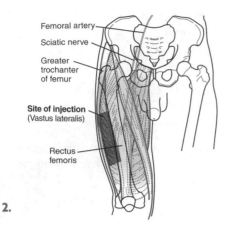

2.

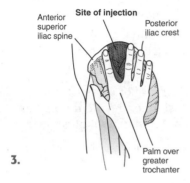

3.

Multiple Choice

152. The nurse is preparing to administer two units of packed red blood cells to a patient who had knee replacement surgery. Which solution is compatible with the blood?

1. 0.9% normal saline.
2. 5% dextrose in water.
3. 3% normal saline.
4. $D_5 \frac{1}{2}$ NS.

153. An elderly patient has been prescribed aspirin for osteoarthritis. What should the nurse teach the patient to ensure safe use of this medication?

1. Enteric-coated tablets should be crushed to make the medication easier to swallow.
2. The medication should be taken on an empty stomach.
3. A prothrombin time should be drawn upon initiation of therapy and every 2 months.
4. The prescriber should be notified if the patient experiences any unusual bruising or bleeding.

154. The nurse determines that the intended outcome from the administration of baclofen (Lioresal) has been achieved when which finding is observed?

1. Muscle spasticity has been relieved.
2. Urinary frequency has been reduced.
3. Heartburn has improved.
4. Inflammation has been suppressed.

155. The patient is taking ibandronate (Boniva) for the prevention of osteoporosis. Which statement should be part of the patient education provided by the nurse?

1. "Take the drug first thing in the morning with a full glass of milk or juice."
2. "Take the medication on a full stomach immediately after a meal."
3. "Take the medication in the morning with a glass of water, and then don't ingest anything for 30 minutes."
4. "Take the medication with a minimal amount of fluid just before bedtime."

156. A patient is started on intravenous tobramycin (Nebcin) for a postoperative infection. To monitor the effectiveness of therapy, a peak level and trough level are ordered. When is the appropriate time for a trough level to be drawn?

1. 30 minutes after the total dose is administered.
2. Immediately prior to the administration of the dose.
3. 4 hours prior to the administration of the dose.
4. 60 minutes after the total dose is administered.

157. Which drug would a nurse anticipate administering for the treatment of inflammation in acute exacerbations of gout?

1. Acetaminophen (Tylenol).
2. Probenecid (Benemid).
3. Colchicine (Novocholchicine).
4. Allopurinol (Zyloprim).

158. A patient with a pelvic fracture is admitted to the emergency room following a motor vehicle accident. Upon admission, the patient is found to be in hypovolemic shock from blood loss associated with the fracture. The emergency room physician orders blood replacement. Which statement is true regarding blood replacement in an emergent situation?

1. Type-specific blood products are immediately available.
2. A full type and cross match takes 5 to 10 minutes to complete.

3. Blood cannot be administered before a complete type and cross match is done.

4. Type O blood can be given until type-specific or fully typed- and cross-matched blood is available.

159. A patient is diagnosed with deep vein thrombosis. A goal for the plan of care is to achieve rapid anticoagulation to prevent the extension of an existing clot. Which drug would be used to achieve the goal?

1. Warfarin (Coumadin).

2. Streptokinase (Streptase).

3. Clopidogrel (Plavix).

4. Heparin.

REDUCTION OF RISK POTENTIAL

Multiple Choice

160. The nurse is caring for a postoperative patient with a Jackson-Pratt drain. Which action should the nurse take to ensure effective drain function?

1. Connect the drain to low intermittent suction.

2. Flush the drain every shift to ensure its patency.

3. Compress and then plug the bulb to establish suction.

4. Connect the drain to gravity drainage.

161. Which patient is at greatest risk for developing a pathological fracture?

1. An 84-year-old female with osteoporosis.

2. A 55-year-old female who fell on the ice.

3. A 19-year-old member of a college gymnastics team.

4. A 28-year-old individual who was involved in a high-impact motor vehicle collision.

162. A patient sprained an ankle after tripping over a step. At what point would it be appropriate to apply heat to the injured area?

1. Immediately after the injury to promote blood flow to the area.

2. 24 to 48 hours after the acute injury to decrease edema.

3. Heat should not be used at any point in the treatment of a sprain.

4. 7 days after the injury to improve ligament flexibility.

Identification

163. Identify the patient who demonstrates assessment findings associated with scoliosis.

1.

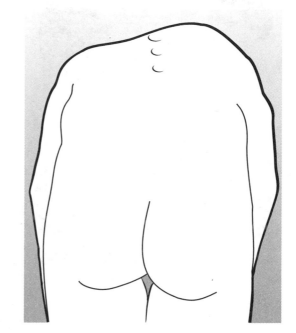

2.

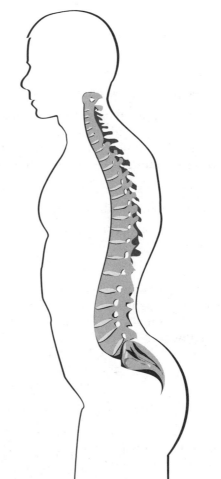

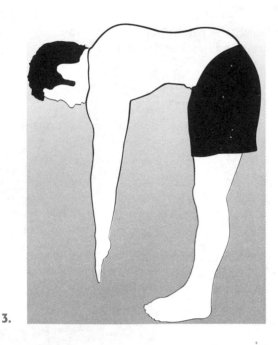

3.

Multiple Choice

164. What are the most serious complications of a femur fracture?

1. Paresthesias and tingling.
2. Hemorrhage and shock.
3. Paralytic ileus and a lacerated urethra.
4. Thrombophlebitis and infection.

165. A patient sustains rib fractures following a fall. A hemothorax is identified on chest x-ray. A chest tube is inserted as an intervention for this condition. What is the main purpose of the chest tube?

1. To decrease pressure on the diaphragm.
2. To remove blood, fluid, and air.
3. To drain lymphatic fluid from the thoracic duct.
4. To improve cardiac output.

166. Upon physical examination, the nurse identifies that the patient is unable to smile or elevate the eyebrows. This finding suggests a problem with which cranial nerve?

1. V.
2. VI.
3. VII.
4. VIII.

167. The nurse wants to assess the motor function of the spinal accessory nerve (cranial nerve XI). Identify the area of the body the nurse would assess.

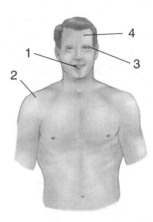

168. A patient is scheduled for an electromyelogram (EMG). Which statement correctly describes the purpose of this procedure?

1. It measures the electrical activity of the brain to assess for connective tissue disease.
2. It records the electrical activity of nerve innervation of skeletal muscles to identify the presence of disease.
3. It involves injection of contrast medium into the subarachnoid space to assess for lesions of the spinal column.
4. It uses sound waves detect blood flow velocity and evaluate for vascular disease.

169. A patient asks, "Why do I still feel pain in my right leg even though it was amputated?" Which response by the nurse would be most helpful?

1. "You must mean you are having pain in your left leg. Your right leg was amputated."
2. "Approximately 70% of patients who undergo an amputation experience phantom limb pain."
3. "The pain is a complication associated with neurovascular damage from the surgery."
4. "This sensation occasionally occurs after amputation. I will report this to your physician."

170. A noncompliant patient with type 2 diabetes presents to the outpatient clinic with a foot ulceration. Which risk factor associated with diabetes might contribute to the development of a foot ulcer?

1. Neuropathy.
2. Polycythemia.
3. Nephropathy.
4. Hyperlipidemia.

171. Which assessments should be made by a nurse prior to implementing pin care for a patient in skeletal traction?

1. Appearance of pin sites.
2. Pulse and blood pressure.
3. Proper setup of traction.
4. Range of motion of extremity.

172. The nurse is reviewing a patient history. Which factors would place the patient at greater risk for the development of osteoporosis? (Select all that apply.)

1. African American ethnicity.
2. Male gender.
3. 55 years of age.
4. A high dietary sodium intake.
5. Fractured wrist that occurred 15 years ago.
6. Postmenopausal female.

173. Which orthopedic injury is considered an emergency due to the potential for the development of avascular necrosis?

1. Meniscus injury.
2. Hip dislocation.
3. Tibial fracture.
4. Rotator cuff tear.

174. An abnormally high compartment pressure is assessed on a patient with a closed tibia fracture. Which procedure would the nurse anticipate preparing for, based on this finding?

1. Embolectomy.
2. Wound debridement.
3. Escharotomy.
4. Fasciotomy.

175. A patient is at risk for the development of foot drop. Which positioning device can be used to prevent this complication?

1. Footboard.
2. Trochanter roll.

3. Trapeze.
4. Bed side rails.

176. Which patient is at highest risk for developing tetanus?

1. A patient with an open wound who is exposed to another patient with tetanus.
2. A farmer with an open ankle fracture who is found lying in a newly plowed field.
3. A food service worker who prepares fresh fish and gets a superficial cut on the finger.
4. A sanitation worker who consistently inhales fumes from degrading trash materials.

177. Which intervention should the nurse implement so as to prevent postoperative respiratory complications in a patient with rib fractures? (Select all that apply.)

1. Repositioning the patient every 2 hours.
2. Maintaining hydration.
3. Use of incentive spirometry every 2 hours.
4. Auscultation of lung sounds.
5. Provision of adequate pain control.
6. Early ambulation.

178. Which statement is true regarding the signs and symptoms of pulmonary emboli resulting from a deep vein thrombosis?

1. Early symptoms of pulmonary emboli include anxiety and sudden dyspnea.
2. The signs and symptoms of deep vein thrombosis may develop if a portion of the pulmonary embolus breaks free and travels into the peripheral circulation.
3. Thick, yellow or gray sputum is commonly associated with a pulmonary embolus.
4. Eupnea and bradycardia are characteristic symptoms of pulmonary emboli.

179. A patient is placed in Crutchfield tongs for a cervical vertebrae fracture. The patient had no neurological deficits after the injury. Which assessment would the nurse use to check for the complication of spinal cord compression?

1. Glasgow Coma Scale.
2. Capillary refill of extremities.
3. Strength of peripheral pulses.
4. Hand strength.

180. Which diagnostic test would be used to determine whether a patient has osteoporosis?

1. Computed tomography scan (CT).
2. Dual-energy x-ray absorptiometry (DEXA).
3. Bone scan.
4. Magnetic resonance imaging (MRI).

181. Which interventions would be contraindicated for a patient who has undergone surgery for the insertion of a femoral head prosthesis after a hip fracture?

1. Use of a toilet-seat elevator.
2. Crossing the legs when seated.
3. Use of an adaptive device to put on shoes.
4. Maintaining the hip in a neutral position when walking, sitting, or standing.

182. Which patient is at the greatest risk for developing a stress fracture?

1. A 70-year-old female with a history of osteoporosis.
2. A 24-year-old marathon runner.
3. A 52-year-old individual with osteoarthritis.
4. A 16-year-old youth who had a broken arm 2 years ago.

Matching

Match the complication of fracture healing with the correct description.

183. Non-union.

184. Delayed union.

185. Malunion.

1. The fracture heals, but angulation or rotation is seen.
2. Fracture healing progresses more slowly than expected, but the healing process eventually occurs.
3. The fracture fails to heal before the bone repair process stops.

Multiple Choice

186. In caring for a client with an open, depressed skull fracture, the nurse should be alert for what complication?

1. Infection.
2. Hypoxia.
3. Hydrocephalus.
4. Herniation.

187. The greatest potential for blood loss and the development of hypovolemic shock is usually associated with fractures of which bones?

1. Tibia and fibula.
2. Ribs and vertebrae.
3. Radius and ulna.
4. Pelvis and femur.

188. A patient with compartment syndrome would exhibit which finding?

1. Increased sensation in the affected extremity.
2. Crepitus with passive stretch.
3. Flaccid compartment on palpation.
4. Pain that is not relieved by narcotics.

189. Following a severe crushing injury to the extremities, a patient develops rhabdomyolysis. Which lab value would be most appropriate for the nurse to monitor to assess for the effectiveness of treatment?

1. Urine myoglobin.
2. Arterial blood gas.
3. White blood cell count.
4. Hemoglobin.

190. A patient is diagnosed with Guillain-Barré syndrome. What is the most serious complication of this syndrome?

1. Acute renal failure.
2. Hepatic coma.
3. Respiratory failure.
4. Neurogenic shock.

191. An adult patient is found on the road after a four-wheeler accident. The lower leg is bleeding and multiple bone fragments are protruding. The skin is avulsed from the knee to the foot. Based on the observations, what type of fracture does this patient have?

1. Closed, spiral.
2. Open, comminuted.
3. Closed, greenstick.
4. Open, depressed.

192. Twenty-four hours following a femoral shaft fracture, a patient suddenly complains of chest pain, tachypnea, and apprehension. The patient has become increasingly confused. Petechiae are noted on the anterior chest wall and in the axilla. Which complication does the nurse suspect?

1. Pneumonia.
2. Pulmonary embolism.
3. Fat embolism.
4. Systemic inflammatory response syndrome.

PHYSIOLOGICAL ADAPTATION

Multiple Choice

193. Immediately following an ankle sprain, ice is applied to the area. What is the purpose of this intervention?

1. To prevent swelling and reduce pain.
2. To decrease deformity and promote vasoconstriction.
3. To increase coagulation and promote hemarthrosis.
4. To improve circulation and promote comfort.

194. Upon assessment of a patient in the emergency room, the nurse notes the internal rotation of the hip. What did the nurse observe?

1. The foot and leg are turned outward away from the other leg.
2. The leg is placed laterally away from the body.
3. The leg is crossed over and on top of the opposite leg.
4. The foot and leg are turned in toward the other leg.

195. A patient with osteoarthritis has had hip replacement surgery. What level of activity would the nurse anticipate for the first postoperative day?

1. Bed rest with turning every 2 hours.
2. Out of bed, weight bearing on the non-operative side.
3. Dangling at the bedside every 4 hours.
4. Non-weight bearing, lifted up to the chair.

Matching

Match the type of fracture with the options in the picture.

196. Comminuted fracture.

197. Oblique fracture.

198. Transverse fracture.

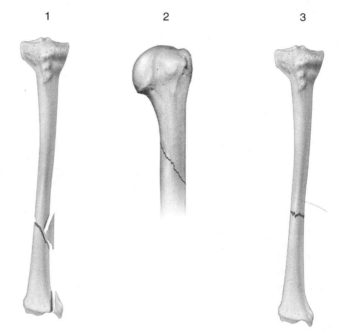

1   2   3

Multiple Choice

199. Which type of pain occurs when a patient sprains an ankle?

1. Cutaneous.
2. Somatic.
3. Visceral.
4. Psychogenic.

200. An autoimmune disorder attacks the myelin sheaths of nerve fibers in the central nervous system and produces lesions called plaques. This statement describes the pathophysiology of which disease?

1. Myasthenia gravis.
2. Amyotrophic lateral sclerosis.
3. Multiple sclerosis.
4. Alzheimer's disease.

SECTION I
SECTION II
SECTION III
SECTION IV
SECTION V
SECTION VI
SECTION VII
SECTION VIII
SECTION IX
SECTION X

201. The nurse in the emergency room is teaching a patient about the care of a cast prior to discharge. Which statement by the patient would indicate the need for further teaching?

1. "I should elevate the extremity above the level of the heart to reduce swelling for the first 48 hours."
2. "It will be important to exercise the joints both above and below the cast regularly."
3. "I should report pain, tingling, burning, or a foul odor to my healthcare provider."
4. "If itching develops under the cast, I can use a thin coat hanger to relieve it."

202. Which clinical manifestations would the nurse expect to find in a patient who has been diagnosed with Parkinson's disease?

1. Tremors, rigidity, bradykinesia.
2. Spasticity, diplopia, paresthesias.
3. Dysarthria, dysphagia, ataxia.
4. Paresthesias, rigidity, aphasia.

203. Battle's sign, facial paralysis, and otorrhea are assessment findings associated with which type of skull fracture?

1. Basilar.
2. Occipital.
3. Orbital.
4. Temporal.

Identification

204. Identify the correct sequence of the four stages of bone healing.

_____ Hematoma formation.

_____ Callus formation.

_____ Ossification.

_____ Remodeling.

Multiple Choice

205. At the scene of a motor vehicle accident, paramedics treat a suspected fracture of the humerus with immobilization. What is the expected outcome of the initial fracture immobilization?

1. Prevention of further damage or complications caused by injury from bone fragments.

2. Realignment of the bone fragments in the correct anatomical position.
3. Reduction in possible skin breakdown from fracture fragments.
4. Stabilization of the bone to prevent contractures.

206. Which is one reason that an adult patient with renal failure is at risk for osteodystrophy?

1. The kidneys are unable to activate vitamin D, so there is a decrease in calcium absorption from the intestine.
2. An elevation in serum creatinine inactivates the parathyroid gland, so the production of parathyroid hormone is diminished.
3. The kidneys are unable to secrete phosphates, so hyperphosphatemia promotes an increase in osteoblast activity.
4. The kidneys are unable to excrete calcitonin in response to low levels of serum calcium.

207. Which statement about an osteosarcoma is true?

1. An osteosarcoma is a benign bone tumor that grows slowly and doesn't invade surrounding tissues.
2. An osteosarcoma originates primarily from cancers of the lung, breast, or prostate.
3. An osteosarcoma is a malignant tumor that moves from the metaphysis to the periosteal surface.
4. An osteosarcoma is a tumor of the cartilage that arises from points of muscle attachment to the bone.

208. An elderly patient is diagnosed with bursitis in the shoulder. The patient asks the nurse, "Just what are bursae?" What is the nurse's best response?

1. "A bursa is a sac filled with synovial fluid that is found in tissues and prevents friction over a tendon."
2. "A bursa is a clear, viscous fluid that acts as a lubricant for joints."
3. "A bursa is the fibrous connective membrane that covers, supports, and separates muscles."
4. "A bursa is a band of fibrous tissue that attaches muscle to bone."

209. Which pathophysiological changes are associated with osteoarthritis? (Select all that apply.)

1. Osteophyte formation.
2. Chronic inflammation of the synovial fluid.
3. Destruction of the articular cartilage from use.
4. Changes in the small ligaments of the hand and feet.
5. Presence of swan-neck deformities.
6. Presence of immune complex.

210. Which clinical manifestations would a patient with a herniated lower lumbar disc experience?

1. Motor paralysis from the waist down.
2. Manifestations of altered sensory and motor functions in the area of the body innervated by the nerve roots.
3. Localized sensory deficits in the area of the body that is supplied by the dorsal root ganglia of that segment.
4. Pain, localized sensory deficits, and hyperactive reflexes along the peripheral distribution of the nerve.

211. Which interventions would the nurse anticipate for a patient who is diagnosed with osteitis deformans (Paget's disease)?

1. A low-phosphorus diet and aerobic exercise.
2. Estrogen and physical therapy.
3. Biphosphonate and recommended doses of calcium and vitamin D.
4. Calcitonin and vitamin A supplements.

212. Which substance is acted on by the kidneys to create a co-factor necessary for calcium absorption from the intestine?

1. Erythropoietin.
2. Aldosterone.
3. Vitamin D.
4. Renin.

213. Coordination of movement and awareness of body position are most closely associated with the function of which part of the brain?

1. Hypothalamus.
2. Medulla.
3. Cerebrum.
4. Cerebellum.

214. While a patient is awaiting surgical repair of a hip fracture, traction is applied to the affected extremity. Which type of traction would be used in this case?

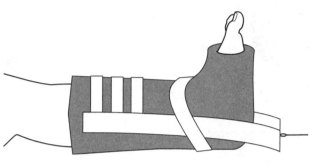

1. Buck's traction.

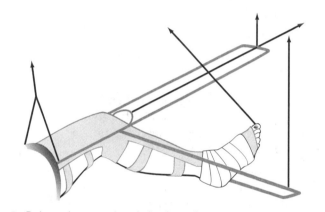

2. Balanced suspension skeletal traction.

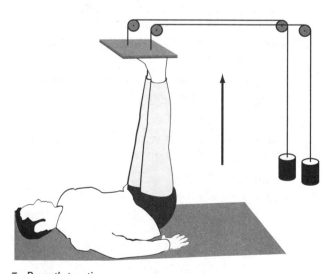

3. Bryant's traction.

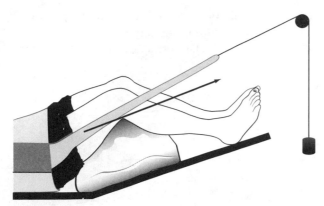

4. Pelvic sling traction.

215. Which cells are responsible for the formation of bone matrix?

1. Osteoclasts.
2. Osteoblasts.
3. Osteocytes.
4. Osteogenic cells.

216. The nurse is caring for a patient with a spinal cord compression associated with a hyperextension injury. Which statements describes how a hyperextension injury occurs ?

1. The patient is thrown forward, causing a tearing of the posterior ligaments and dislocation of the vertebrae.
2. An upward force throws the head back, causing a tear of the anterior ligaments and dislocation of the vertebrae.
3. A crush injury forces bony fragments into the spinal column.
4. The patient is thrown to the side, causing a compression injury and tearing of the lateral ligaments.

217. A patient is diagnosed with carpal tunnel syndrome. Which nerve is involved in this syndrome?

1. Peroneal.
2. Radial.
3. Median.
4. Trigeminal.

218. The nurse is planning an in-service program for the orthopedic outpatient clinic staff on foot disorders. Which information about the diagnosis of hallux valgus should be included?

1. Hallux valgus is a localized thickening of skin that is caused by pressure over bony prominences and is commonly referred to as a corn.
2. Hallux valgus is a wart caused by a virus that occurs on the sole of the foot.
3. Hallux valgus is the loss of the metatarsal arch that results in a flat foot.
4. Hallux valgus is a painful deformity of the great toe and is often referred to as a bunion.

219. A patient is recovering from fractured fourth cervical vertebrae with complete spinal cord transaction. Upon assessment of the patient, which findings would the nurse expect?

1. Head and neck control and some shoulder elevation.
2. Hand and upper extremity strength.
3. Shoulder and scapular movement with elbow and wrist flexion.
4. Full elbow and wrist extension with some finger control.

220. A nurse enters the room of a patient after lunch trays were served and finds the patient alert, hands grasping at his throat, and unable to speak. Which action should the nurse immediately take?

1. Suction the pharyngeal area.
2. Perform the Heimlich maneuver.
3. Assess further for pharyngitis.
4. Administer oxygen.

221. A laminectomy would be performed for a patient with which type of musculoskeletal problem?

1. Herniated disc.
2. Posterior fossa skull fracture.
3. Osteomyelitis.
4. Grade 4 ligamentous injury.

222. Which findings would the nurse expect for a patient who has been diagnosed with rheumatoid arthritis?

1. A negative rheumatoid factor.
2. History of progressive disease course.
3. Osteophytes on radiologic exam.
4. Boutonniere deformity.

MANAGEMENT OF CARE

1. Correct Answers: 1, 3, 5, 6

Rationale: The immediate care of a sprain involves rest, ice application, compression, and elevation. Rest helps to limit the movement of the extremity and prevent further injury. The application of ice causes vasoconstriction and reduces nerve impulse transmission, which provides for both analgesia and reduction of swelling and muscle spasms. Compression and elevation help to decrease swelling.

2. Correct Answer: 1

Rationale: The use of good body mechanics and correct posture are essential when planning care for a patient with acute low back pain to prevent recurrent problems. Sliding an object across the floor rather than lifting it will prevent strain on the lower back muscles.

3. Correct Answer: 1

Rationale: The role of an occupational therapist is to aid and assist physically challenged patients to carry out activities of daily living through the use of adaptive devices and strategies. An occupational therapist could assist someone with a self-care deficit for feeding through the use of adaptive devices.

4. Correct Answer: 4

Rationale: An incident/occurrence report is a document that provides a factual, objective account of an injury or potential for injury of a patient within a healthcare agency. Analysis and trending of incident report data can be used in the process of quality improvement.

5. Correct Answers: 1, 2, 4

Rationale: A telephone order is a form of verbal order. Verbal orders are issued in an emergency or in situations when it is impossible for a healthcare provider to write the order. The order should be given to a licensed nurse and must be repeated back to the healthcare provider after it is written to ensure its accuracy. The order should be written on an order sheet and co-signed by the healthcare provider within a 24-hour period. When documenting the order, the name of the healthcare provider who issued the order, the date and time of the order, and the signature and title of the nurse who accepted the order are written.

6. Correct Answer: 1

Rationale: A quadriplegic patient is dependent and requires support for many activities of daily living and independent activities of daily living. The primary caregiver will need time to meet his or her own personal needs as well. Respite care is provided as a means for primary caregivers to have time away from their day-to-day care responsibilities. Respite care can be provided by professionals or volunteers, depending on the needs of the patient.

7. Correct Answer: 1

Rationale: Rehabilitation is a process that assists an ill person or a person with a disability or impairment to achieve the best possible level of functioning. The rehabilitation process focuses on the patient's physical, mental, social, spiritual, and economic abilities. The process of rehabilitation should begin upon the patient's admission to an acute care hospital.

8. Correct Answer: 3

Rationale: Privacy is a concept that defines the degree of a patient's personal responsibility to others in regulating behavior that is intrusive. Hospitalized patients are vulnerable due to illness, and healthcare providers should be sensitive in facilitating a patient to maintain his or her privacy. Forgetting to cover a patient when transporting him or her would be a violation of the patient's physical privacy.

9. Correct Answer: 2

Rationale: Nurses experience occupational hazards and may become injured on the job. States have implemented worker's compensation laws that allow for compensation for injury and illness when a worker is hurt on the job. The nurse is responsible for following the policies of the workplace in reporting a work-related injury.

10. Correct Answer: **True**

Rationale: The reimbursement for the procedure is $10,000. The actual cost to the hospital is $9,500. The hospital will profit $500 from the procedure by being able to control costs and deliver quality care at a price less than the reimbursed DRG.

11. Correct Answer: **3**

Rationale: Veracity is the duty to tell the truth. The nurse violated the ethical principle of veracity when the nurse chose not to report the error and not to tell the truth.

12. Correct Answer: **1**

Rationale: Prior to his or her death, an organ donor may indicate his or her wishes about organ donation by signing a donor card and discussing the topic with the family. The next of kin will be responsible for giving consent upon the patient's death. Consent is required for organ donation in the United States.

13. Correct Answer: **3**

Rationale: The charge nurse was responsible for making the patient care assignments. When concern arises about the assignment, the nurse should follow the chain of command and appropriate channels of communications. The nurse should discuss any concerns with the party responsible for the assignments, which in this case, was the charge nurse.

14. Correct Answer: **1**

Rationale: Job descriptions are written statements that describe broad general guidelines about the duties and functions of the different jobs in an organization. A job description would provide information on the training, experience, and special skills required for that position. In addition, the duties of the job would be generally defined.

15. Correct Answer: **False**

Rationale: The original chart is a legal document and remains with the organization. A copy of the chart or pertinent aspects of the chart could be sent to the facility where the patient is being transferred. Organizational procedure should be followed when sending medical information to another facility.

16. Correct Answer: **3**

Rationale: An outcome standard is used for evaluation and is a statement of the expected results of care for the patient. A lack of signs and symptoms of wound infection would be an outcome standard for a surgical patient discharged from a healthcare setting.

17. Correct Answer: **4**

Rationale: Restraints physically prevent a patient from moving freely in the environment. Injuries and death have been associated with the use of restraints, so the nurse should consider all other alternatives prior to the implementation of a restraint device.

18. Correct Answer: **2**

Rationale: Malcolm Knowles identified principles for effective adult learning. Using the principles that adults are independent learners and see themselves as doers, a demonstration of device use, followed by time for hands-on practice would be the most effective teaching strategy.

19. Correct Answer: **2**

Rationale: The temporomandibular joint connects the mandible to the temporal bone. The clinical manifestations of pain, crepitus, and a popping sound are abnormal and require further evaluation and assessment. Referral to an oral surgeon for evaluation would be an appropriate intervention.

20. Correct Answer: **False**

Rationale: Team nursing is a type of nursing care delivery in which varying levels of nursing staff are organized into groups to deliver care to the assigned patients. Case management is a type of care delivery in which a patient's health care is monitored for the purpose of maximizing outcomes, effectively utilizing resources, and containing costs.

21. Correct Answer: **1**

Rationale: The nursing diagnosis with the highest priority for a patient with a musculoskeletal disorder would be impaired physical mobility. The diagnosis is defined by NANDA as a limitation in independent, purposeful physical movement of the body or of one or more extremities.

22. Correct Answer: **2**

Rationale: A neurovascular assessment of the involved extremity would be an appropriate intervention for the nursing diagnosis. Peripheral neurological (pain, paresthesia) and vascular (pallor, pulse, and temperature) assessments must be completed to determine whether there has been any compromise in the injured extremity.

SECTION I

SECTION II

SECTION III

SECTION IV

SECTION V

SECTION VI

SECTION VII

SECTION VIII

SECTION IX

SECTION X

23. Correct Answer: **1**

Rationale: The nurse should report the observation through the chain of command. The chain of command is the path of authority and accountability from the nurse to the top administrator. The nurse manager would be the next person in the staff member's chain of command and would be the appropriate person to whom the nurse should report the observations for investigation.

24. Correct Answer: **True**

Rationale: State legal statutes that authorize qualified individuals to perform nursing skills and services are called nurse practice acts. Each state's nurse practice act establishes a board of nursing, whose members have the authority to set and enforce rules and regulations related to nursing practice. The boards of nursing establish licensure requirements.

25. Correct Answer: **2**

Rationale: Subjective data include information that is perceived only by the affected person. No one except the patient would be able to tell the nurse whether fatigue and pain were occurring.

26. Correct Answer: **2**

Rationale: A physical therapist would be the best resource to assist the patient to learn the correct, safe procedure for crutch walking. The role of a physical therapist is to seek to restore function and prevent further patient disability.

27. Correct Answer: **4**

Rationale: Informed consent is a patient's voluntary agreement to proceed with a procedure or treatment. Consent obtained from a patient who is unconscious, a minor, confused, sedated, legally intoxicated, or mentally incompetent would not be valid or considered a legally binding document.

28. Correct Answer: **4**

Rationale: A patient with a spinal cord transection at the level of the fifth cervical vertebrae would be expected to have full neck, partial shoulder, back, biceps, and gross elbow movements. A realistic rehabilitation goal for the patient would be the ability to feed him or herself with the use of adaptive equipment.

29. Correct Answer: **2**

Rationale: Confidentiality is the nondisclosure of information except to an authorized person. Patient information is considered confidential. Reporting laboratory findings to the friend of the patient, without the permission of the patient, would be a violation of confidentiality.

30. Correct Answer: **2**

Rationale: Surgical immobilization often requires the wiring of the jaw to allow the fracture to heal. Potential nursing care problems in the postoperative period for a patient who has undergone surgical repair of a mandibular fracture would include risk for airway obstruction and aspiration. Thus, the nursing care priority would be airway management.

31. Correct Answer: **3**

Rationale: The patient returning from a surgical procedure would require assessment and establishment of a plan of care. The most appropriate person to assign the patient to would be a registered nurse, who is responsible for patient assessment, establishment of an individualized plan of care, and identification of expected patient outcomes.

32. Correct Answer: **False**

Rationale: The nurse should consult the state's nurse practice act to identify violations that could result in disciplinary action against the nurse. The Code of Ethics provides a standard for ethical nursing practice.

33. Correct Answer: **3**

Rationale: The person who is responsible for performing the treatment or procedure is responsible for obtaining informed consent. The surgeon who is performing the hip repair would be responsible for obtaining informed consent.

34. Correct Answer: **1**

Rationale: Based on the symptoms of dyspnea and chest pain, intervention priorities for the nurse would be the administration of supplemental oxygen and assessment of vital signs.

35. Correct Answer: **2**

Rationale: The priorities of care at an accident scene are airway, breathing, and circulation. For a patient who is not breathing and has a suspected cervical spine injury, the jaw-thrust maneuver should be used to open the airway. The jaw-thrust maneuver prevents hyperextension of the neck and reduces the potential for further spinal injury.

36. Correct Answer: **3**

Rationale: The application of a cast can result in compromise of the vascular and/or nerve function of the extremity. The lack of movement of an extremity could indicate a neurovascular compromise and should be immediately reported to the physician.

37. Correct Answer: **True**

Rationale: Assault is a threat or attempt to make bodily contact without the other person's permission. Battery is the impermissible, unprivileged touching of one person by another or assault that is carried out. When a nurse administers an injection to a competent adult who has refused the injection, battery has been committed.

38. Correct Answer: **2**

Rationale: A patient with facial fractures will experience inflammation and swelling. An initial assessment priority would include ensuring a patent airway.

39. Correct Answer: **2**

Rationale: Osteomyelitis is an acute or chronic infection of the bone. The anticipated treatment for the acute infection is the administration of antibiotics.

40. Correct Answer: **1**

Rationale: Due to the potential for the spread of organisms to other patients who are being cared for by the healthcare worker, the nurse should intervene while the worker is in the patient's room by providing the appropriate personal protective equipment.

41. Correct Answers: **1, 2, 5, 6**

Rationale: Patient rights were a part of the 2003 revision of the American Hospital Association's Patient's Bill of Rights, which is entitled "The Patient Care Partnership: Understanding Expectations, Rights, and Responsibilities." Included in this document are expectations the patient should have during the hospital stay. These expectations include high-quality hospital care, a clean and safe environment, involvement in care, protection of privacy, help preparing the patient and family for when the patient leaves the hospital, and help with the bill and filing of insurance claims.

42. Correct Answer: **1**

Rationale: Nurses in a community-based practice setting utilize three levels of preventive care: primary, secondary, and tertiary. The primary level of preventive care focuses on health promotion and the prevention of disease. Immunization is one example of an intervention to prevent disease.

43. Correct Answer: **1**

Rationale: The normal white blood cell or leukocyte count is between 4,500 and $11,000/mm^3$. The presurgical screening labs indicate a significant elevation in the WBC count, which could indicate the presence of an infection. The surgeon should be notified of the abnormal finding prior to surgery.

44. Correct Answer: **1**

Rationale: Negligence is conduct that does not show due care. It can be an act of commission, such as performing an act that a reasonably prudent person, under similar circumstances, would not do; or an act of omission, which is the failure to perform an act that a reasonable prudent person, under similar circumstances, would do. Negligence is a type of unintentional tort. The nurse who completed the neurovascular assessment and identified abnormal findings, but did not report the findings until 6 hours later, committed an act of negligence. The nurse failed to notify the physician of an absent pulse until 6 hours after the assessment. A reasonably prudent nurse would notify the physician immediately.

SAFETY AND INFECTION CONTROL

45. Correct Answer: **3**

Rationale: A 70% isopropyl alcohol solution would be the best choice for site preparation for a patient who is allergic to iodine. The nurse should consult the policies and procedures of the organization for specifics on alternatives for site preparation when an iodine solution cannot be used.

SECTION I
SECTION II
SECTION III
SECTION IV
SECTION V
SECTION VI
SECTION VII
SECTION VIII
SECTION IX
SECTION X

46. Correct Answer: 1

Rationale: Tattoos are created by the injection of a permanent coloration pigment under the skin using needles. Because of the risk of blood-borne infections such as hepatitis or human immunodeficiency virus, a patient who has had a recent tattoo would not be a candidate for a blood donation.

47. Correct Answer: 3

Rationale: A feature of patient-controlled analgesia devices is the timing control or lockout, which provides for a minimum interval of time between medication doses. The safety feature is one means of preventing an overdose. The patient is prevented from administering another dose of medication until the established time interval or lockout period has passed. The time interval or lockout is defined by the healthcare provider who prescribes the use of the device.

48. Correct Answer: 1

Rationale: The use and placement of a decimal point can cause a medication error. A zero should precede a decimal point (0.2 mg), but should not be used after a decimal point (2.0 mg).

49. Correct Answer: 3

Rationale: Osteomyelitis is a local or generalized infection of the bone or bone marrow. The microorganism most commonly associated with the development of osteomyelitis is *Staphylococcus aureus*.

50. Correct Answers: 1, 2, 3, 4

Rationale: Gloves are the first item to be removed when exiting a patient's room, as they are the most contaminated personal protective equipment. Removal of the mask, followed by gown removal, are the next steps in the process. The final action by the nurse is the performance of hand hygiene.

51. Correct Answer: 2

Rationale: Potentially infective material, such as a dressing that is saturated with blood, should be disposed of in a biohazardous materials container and should be separated from the regular trash. A bloody saturated dressing with purulent drainage that is not properly handled and identified could result in transmission of blood-borne pathogens to others.

52. Correct Answer: 4

Rationale: A nosocomial infection is a hospital-acquired infection or an infection that occurs while the patient was receiving health care. In this case, the infection resulted from the use of an invasive procedure (Foley catheterization) for patient treatment.

53. Correct Answer: 2

Rationale: To prevent the occurrence of an intravascular device-related infection, dressing changes should occur as per the hospital policy. Dressings that are damp, loosened, or soiled should be changed. Bacteria can grow in moist, damp environments, and a loosened dressing may allow for more frequent site contamination and organism entry.

54. Correct Answers: 1, 4, 5, 6

Rationale: Restraints are devices used to limit a patient's movement and should be applied as a last resort due to the hazards associated with their use, such as impaired circulation and pressure ulceration. The nurse should assess the reasons for unwanted or disruptive patient movement and intervene based on the assessment. Alternatives to the use of restraint devices might include the involvement of familiar family members in the patient's care, assisting the patient with toileting at regular intervals, use of an electronic position-sensitive device, and/or use of diversionary activities.

55. Correct Answer: 2

Rationale: Transmission-based precautions are used in addition to standard precautions. Contact precautions are a type of transmission-based precaution used for patients who are infected or colonized by an organism such as vancomycin-resistant enterococcus, which may be spread by either direct or indirect contact. A patient with a wound infection caused by a drug-resistant organism should be placed on contact precautions.

56. Correct Answer: 2

Rationale: Traction applies a pulling force to an injured extremity and acts to immobilize and/or reduce the fracture. The traction should be continuously maintained and not disrupted so as to promote alignment and healing.

57. Correct Answer: 2

Rationale: The lateral position with the head of the bed slightly elevated allows for respiratory expansion and the prevention of aspiration should the patient experience nausea and vomiting.

58. Correct Answer: 2

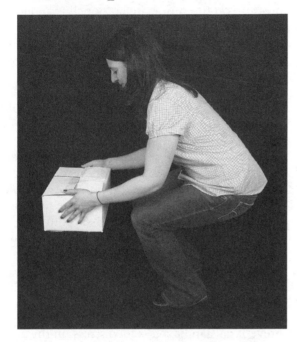

Rationale: The best position for lifting an item from the floor is one where the long and strong muscles of the arms and legs are used. The knees should be flexed and close to the object to be lifted. The line of gravity should fall within the base of support.

59. Correct Answer: 1

Rationale: The patient should be instructed to hold the cane on the right side (the uninjured side). Positioning the cane on the uninjured side provides additional support for the injured left leg.

60. Correct Answer: 3

Rationale: A nursing goal in the care of a patient experiencing severe alcohol withdrawal symptoms is the promotion of safety and comfort. Anxiety, agitation, insomnia, diaphoresis, tremors, delirium, and seizures are possible symptoms of alcohol withdrawal. To promote safety during severe withdrawal, a patient should not be allowed to ambulate alone.

61. Correct Answer: 1

Rationale: The installation of handrails or grab bars in the bathroom, a high-traffic area of the home, can help to prevent falls.

62. Correct Answers: 1, 2, 3, 4

Rationale: The acronym RACE is often used to assist the nurse with remembering the priority actions associated with a fire. The first priority is rescue or removal of the patient from immediate danger. The second action is activation of the fire alarm system. The third action should be the confinement of the fire by closing doors and windows. The final action is to extinguish the fire, if possible, using an available fire extinguisher. The first priority is *always* the safety of patients and personnel; if attempts to extinguish a fire would compromise the safety of either group, the nurse should await the arrival of trained fire personnel.

63. Correct Answer: 1

Rationale: Establishment and maintenance of a patent airway is a primary goal after a facial injury. Bedside equipment that should be available would include suction equipment.

64. Correct Answer: 1

Rationale: The patient who is at greatest risk for falls is the one who is elderly and confused, is incontinent, and whose bed is left in high position. Interventions to prevent falls in this patient scenario would include leaving the bed in the lowest position, frequent regular toileting, and reorientation of the patient to the environment.

65. Correct Answer: 1

Rationale: Neuromuscular blocking agents prevent acetylcholine from activating receptors on the skeletal muscles and result in muscle relaxation. These agents can cause respiratory arrest owing to the relaxation of the respiratory muscles. A bag-valve-mask device and oxygen should be immediately available at the bedside of any patient who is receiving such a medication to ensure the safe delivery of care.

66. Correct Answer: 2

Rationale: An occupational infection or disease transmission can occur by inoculation of tissues with a needle contaminated with blood-borne pathogens. The immediate care of the contaminated area would include flushing and washing the area with soap and water.

SECTION I
SECTION II
SECTION III
SECTION IV
SECTION V
SECTION VI
SECTION VII
SECTION VIII
SECTION IX
SECTION X

HEALTH PROMOTION AND MAINTENANCE

67. Correct Answers: 1–7

Rationale: A neurovascular assessment is done to determine any associated damage to the vasculature and peripheral nervous system that might occur with an extremity fracture. The essential components of the assessment include pain, pulses, sensation, movement, color, temperature, and capillary refill.

68. Correct Answer: 1

Rationale: A pregnant patient will see a gradual, forward curving of the spine as the growth of the fetus pulls the pelvis forward. The lordosis will resolve after delivery.

69. Correct Answer: 4

Rationale: An excess of body weight can place increased stress on the structures of the lower back. Goals should be established if weight reduction is needed and interventions individualized that will promote a patient's success in weight reduction.

70. Correct Answer: 2

Rationale: When teaching an illiterate patient, the nurse should use short, simple words, teach essential information first, repeating as necessary, and use understandable analogies. The nurse can ask the patient to restate, review, or demonstrate skills to ensure an understanding of the content.

71. Correct Answer: True

Rationale: Warm-up exercises prelengthen tissues, increase the temperature of a muscle, and contribute to increased metabolism and better oxygenation of the muscles during activity. Stretching is thought to increase kinesthetic awareness and lessen the chance for uncoordinated movement.

72. Correct Answer: 1

Rationale: There are two sources of vitamin D: sunlight and diet. Increasing a patient's daily exposure to sunlight will increase the amount of cholecalciferol (vitamin D_3) that is naturally produced when the skin is exposed to sunlight.

73. Correct Answer: 4

Rationale: Measures that promote bone strength can help to reduce the risk of osteoporosis. One measure includes an adequate intake of calcium. Calcium is needed to maintain bone integrity in an aging patient. The recommended calcium intake for a patient aged 51 or older is 1,200 mg/day.

74. Correct Answer: 2

Rationale: A ballottement test is a physical assessment technique used to check for the presence of fluid or effusions on the patella. Downward pressure on the suprapatellar pouch is applied to an extended knee. The patella is pushed down against the femur and released. If fluid is present, the patella will float outward.

75. Correct Answer: 3

Rationale: The childhood immunization schedule for DTaP includes a four-shot series at ages 2 months, 4 months, 6 months, and 15–18 months. The DTaP is recommended to be given at ages 11 or 12 for patients who received the full childhood vaccination series. A 22-year-old patient should receive one dose of the tetanus toxoid if the individual was fully immunized during childhood and received a DTaP around the age of 11 or 12.

76. Correct Answer: 2

Rationale: An elderly patient should use ramps provided in buildings and street corners to prevent falls and avoid added stress on the musculoskeletal system.

77. Correct Answer: 3

Rationale: Obesity is a risk factor for the development of osteoarthritis. Maintenance of an ideal weight is one means by which a patient can prevent added wear and tear on a joint and promote joint health.

78. Correct Answer: 2

Rationale: Assessment of visual impairment provides data that the nurse can use when planning for appropriate teaching strategies. The use of auditory or tactile materials would be an appropriate intervention to ensure individualization of the teaching plan and achieve desired educational goals.

79. Correct Answers: 1, 3, 4

Rationale: Occupations that require continuous wrist movement place a person at risk for the development of carpal tunnel syndrome. A hair stylist, computer operator, and seamstress are all examples of occupations that require continuous wrist movement.

80. Correct Answer: **2**

Rationale: Weight-bearing exercises are essential for the maintenance of bone mass. Walking would be the best type of activity for an elderly patient to promote weight bearing and the maintenance of bone mass.

81. Correct Answer: **1**

Rationale: Musculoskeletal changes associated with aging would include a decrease in muscle elasticity and tone.

82. Correct Answers: **1, 2, 6**

Rationale: Factors that have been linked to the development of osteoarthritis include obesity, family history of the disease, and regular strenuous exercise that places wear and tear on joints.

83. Correct Answer: **4**

Rationale: The knee is the largest joint in the body and the one most susceptible to a sports-related injury.

84. Correct Answer: **1**

Rationale: Scoliosis screening is performed in the pre-adolescence/adolescence period. Screening is recommended for girls in grades 5 through 7, and for boys in grade 8 or 9.

85. Correct Answer: **1**

Rationale: Gout is a disease characterized by the presence of urate crystals in the joint cavity. Potential causes include hyperuricemia from an overproduction of uric acid and a decreased ability of the kidney to excrete excess uric acid. Uric acid is a product of purine metabolism. The patient should be instructed to reduce the amount of liver, sardines, and shrimp in the diet, as these substances are high in purines.

86. Correct Answer: **3**

Rationale: Regular weight-bearing exercise is needed to promote bone health. Bone formation is enhanced by weight-bearing activities such as walking.

PSYCHOSOCIAL INTEGRITY

87. Correct Answer: **2**

Rationale: The fear of anesthesia is not uncommon for a patient. Concerns can be caused by past experience or the past experience of others and by fear of loss of control. Given that the nurse is unaware of the basis of the patient's fears, an open-ended response that will elicit more information will assist the nurse in planning for the most appropriate intervention.

88. Correct Answer: **1**

Rationale: The patient has expressed a wish to go home. The nurse should discuss the availability of resources that can assist with the care of the patient and determine the appropriateness of the use of the resources for the family. Home health and hospice care are both resources that could provide support for the care of the patient.

89. Correct Answer: **1**

Rationale: Assertive communication is the ability to express thoughts in an open, honest, and direct manner that demonstrates respect both for oneself and for others. The use of "I" statements, maintaining eye contact, and congruent verbal and facial expressions are all components of assertiveness skills. The statement, "I feel as though I met the standard of care," is direct and specific to the expectations of patient care in the situation. The nurse also demonstrates respect for the opinion of the other nurse by asking for feedback and the reason for the concerns.

90. Correct Answer: **3**

Rationale: Hospitalization of the mother will most likely affect the family members' roles and tasks. Responsibilities will need to be reallocated within the family while the mother recovers from her injuries.

91. Correct Answer: **3**

Rationale: The patient has experienced the actual loss of an extremity. Grief is the emotional reaction to loss. Kübler-Ross (1969) defines five stages of grief: (1) denial and isolation, (2) anger, (3) bargaining, (4) depression, and (5) acceptance. Although each individual experiences grief differently, the first stage is often denial.

92. Correct Answer: **3**

Rationale: The open-ended statement is a means of focusing in on the problem and obtaining more information about the patient's concerns. Focusing helps the nurse to zero in on a topic until the issues and concerns are clearly identified.

SECTION I
SECTION II
SECTION III
SECTION IV
SECTION V
SECTION VI
SECTION VII
SECTION VIII
SECTION IX
SECTION X

93. Correct Answer: 4

Rationale: Systemic lupus erythematosus is a chronic, inflammatory, systemic disease. There is female predominance in the disease's incidence. The incidence of the disease is also higher in African American, Latin American, and Asian populations.

94. Correct Answer: 1

Rationale: Defense mechanisms are reactions to stressors. The 28-year-old patient used denial to refuse to acknowledge a chronic disease.

95. Correct Answer: 2

Rationale: The football player used the defense mechanism of displacement. The patient transferred an emotional reaction related to the injury and inability to play to the provider and the chair.

96. Correct Answer: 3

Rationale: The patient used rationalization as a defense mechanism for the adverse medication event. Even though the patient had been told not to drink, a rationalization that "One drink won't hurt" was made.

97. Correct Answer: 1

Rationale: NANDA defines the nursing diagnosis of disturbed body image as confusion about and/or dissatisfaction with the mental picture of one's physical self. The patient who looks into the mirror and sees only a person without a leg has a disturbed body image.

98. Correct Answer: 3

Rationale: Many Asian Americans believe that there are points on the body that are located on energy pathways. When energy flow is out of balance, treatment modalities for the pathways include acumassage, acupressure, and acupuncture. These treatments are thought to restore equilibrium.

99. Correct Answer: 1

Rationale: Food preferences for Hispanic patients often include beans and tortillas. These foods are a staple in the Hispanic diet.

100. Correct Answer: 3

Rationale: This patient has described a situational crisis that resulted in an inability to sleep, fatigue, and problems with concentration. One response by patient to this situation has been to increase alcohol consumption. According to NANDA, ineffective coping is the inability to form a valid appraisal of the stressors, inadequate choices of practiced responses, and/or inability to use available resources. This scenario describes a patient who is ineffective in coping with the situational crisis that was experienced.

101. Correct Answer: 1

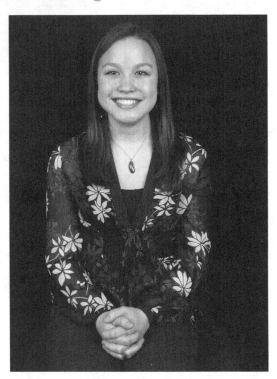

Rationale: An osteosarcoma is an aggressive, malignant tumor of the bone. A patient who demonstrates positive, nonverbal behaviors after receiving news of a malignant diagnosis would require further assessment for understanding of the diagnosis.

102. Correct Answer: 4

Rationale: Religious beliefs prevent Seventh Day Adventists from eating pork. Pork is believed to be an unclean meat.

103. Correct Answer: 3

Rationale: In the denial stage of grief and loss, the nurse should be supportive of the patient, and then act as the opportunity arises to increase the patient's awareness of the situation.

104. Correct Answer: 2

Rationale: Patients with spinal cord injury can experience an overwhelming sense of loss, and major depression may be one response. Depression is a depressed mood state. Symptoms affect the emotional (feeling of sadness), cognitive (difficulty concentrating), and behavioral and social (social withdrawal) realms.

105. Correct Answer: <u>1</u>

Rationale: Relaxation is an intervention used to control stress. Physiologic outcomes associated with the use of relaxation techniques include rhythmic breathing, decreased heart rate, and reduced muscle tension.

106. Correct Answer: <u>3</u>

Rationale: Self-esteem is the need to feel good about oneself and to believe that others hold one in high regard. A change in body image that occurs unexpectedly can influence a patient's self-esteem.

BASIC CARE AND COMFORT

107. Correct Answers: <u>3, 4, 5, 6</u>

Rationale: Immobility can have an effect on every body system. Venous pooling occurs due to decreased resistance in the vasculature. Muscles atrophy from non-use. There is a slowed gastrointestinal muscular activity that can result in constipation. Urinary stasis occurs when urine remains in the renal pelvis longer because gravity is not facilitating the movement to the ureters and bladder.

108. Correct Answer: <u>4</u>

Rationale: Preoccupation with stimuli other than pain has been found to reduce pain. Listening to music is a type of auditory distraction. Distraction has been found to be effective for brief episodes of severe pain, as a non-pharmacologic adjunct to analgesics, and for the relief of mild pain.

109. Correct Answer: <u>3</u>

Rationale: A liquid diet includes only foods that are clear at room or body temperature. Pudding contains milk and would not be a selection on a clear liquid diet.

110. Correct Answer: <u>2</u>

Rationale: A fracture bedpan is smaller and flatter than a regular bedpan. It is easier to place under a patient than a regular bedpan. A patient who has difficulty with easily raising himself or herself onto a regular bedpan, has femur or lower spine fractures, is immobile, or has limited movement should use a fracture pan.

111. Correct Answer: <u>4</u>

Rationale: The three-point gait is used for patients who may bear weight on only one foot. Weight bearing is permitted on only one foot, while the other foot acts as a balance and does not support the individual's weight.

112. Correct Answer: <u>1</u>

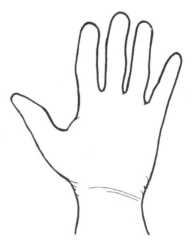

Rationale: Abduction of the fingers is seen in the figure where the fingers are spread apart.

113. Correct Answer: <u>2</u>

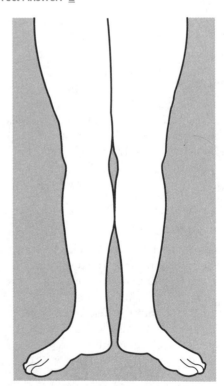

Rationale: External rotation of the hip is seen in the figure where the foot and leg are moved outward and away from the other leg.

SECTION
I

SECTION
II

SECTION
III

SECTION
IV

SECTION
V

SECTION
VI

SECTION
VII

SECTION
VIII

SECTION
IX

SECTION
X

114. Correct Answer: **3**

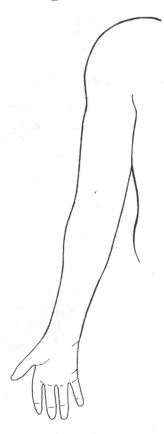

Rationale: Supination is seen in the figure that shows the lower arm rotated so that the palm of the hand is up.

115. Correct Answer: **3**

Rationale: The use of massage therapy may promote increased circulation and reduce the stiffness associated with osteoarthritis. The cutaneous stimulation of massage may also prevent pain by controlling the gating mechanism for pain impulses in the central nervous system.

116. Correct Answer: **1**

Rationale: Isometric exercises involve muscle contraction without a shortening of the muscle fibers. An example of an isometric exercise is contraction and relaxation of the quadriceps muscle. The benefits of isometric exercise include increased muscle mass, tone, and strength. The circulation to the muscle is also improved.

117. Correct Answer: **4**

Rationale: A medium stalk of cooked broccoli would contain the largest amount of calcium,

approximately 158 mg. The apple, beef, and cream cheese contain less than 50 mg of calcium and are relatively poor sources of calcium.

118. Correct Answer: **2**

Rationale: Low back pain is a common clinical manifestation of a herniated lumbar disc. A side-lying position with knee flexion will often relax the lumbar muscles and promote comfort for the patient.

119. Correct Answer: **1**

Rationale: Rest is an intervention for patients with rheumatoid arthritis. This intervention reduces the stress on the joint, thereby relieving pain.

120. Correct Answer: **4**

Rationale: In the assessment, the nurse has diagnosed the problem of sleep pattern disturbance. This problem is related to the patient's fear of impending surgery. Based on the diagnosis, the most appropriate intervention by the nurse would be allowing the patient an opportunity to discuss any concerns about the surgery.

121. Correct Answer: **4**

Rationale: Cayenne (capsicum) is an herbal product that is derived from red peppers. It is used as an ingredient in topical preparations used for osteo and rheumatoid arthritic conditions. Capsicum is thought to reduce the pain associated with inflammation by interfering with substance P, which is responsible for the transmission of pain impulses.

122. Correct Answer: **1**

Rationale: Paraplegia is the loss of motor and/or sensory functions of the lower trunk and limbs. A patient with a lumbar fracture and complete spinal cord transection would exhibit paraplegia.

123. Correct Answer: **2**

Rationale: The amount of sleep needed for young adults depends on individual needs. The recommendation for the average amount of sleep a young adult should get is 8 hours per night.

124. Correct Answer: **3**

Rationale: Halitosis is defined as a strong mouth odor or a persistent bad taste in the mouth.

125. Correct Answer: <u>1</u>

Rationale: Decreased bowel motility is an effect of anesthesia. A postoperative surgical patient should be encouraged to ambulate and increase fluid and fiber intake as tolerated to promote a return to normal bowel habits.

126. Correct Answer: <u>2</u>

Rationale: The normal intake and output of a patient should be approximately 2,500 cc. Intake should approximate output or the ingestion of liquids should be close to the urine output.

PHARMACOLOGICAL AND PARENTERAL THERAPIES

127. Correct Answer: <u>2</u>

Rationale: There are structural similarities between the cephalosporins and the penicillins. As a consequence, there is a chance for a cross-sensitivity reaction in a patient who receives a cephalosporin and is allergic to penicillin. Patients with a history of severe penicillin allergies should not receive a cephalosporin. The safest action by the nurse is to confirm the orders with the prescriber.

128. Correct Answer: <u>1</u>

Rationale: Salicylism develops when aspirin levels exceed therapeutic levels. Clinical manifestations associated with the problem include tinnitus, sweating, headache, dizziness, and hyperventilation. If left untreated, acute salicylate poisoning can develop.

129. Correct Answer: <u>2</u>

Rationale: Prior to initiating treatment with Plaquenil, a vision exam should be completed. Retinal damage is a toxicity that has been associated with the administration of this drug. It is recommended that the patient undergo an initial vision examination and follow-up exams every 6 months.

130. Correct Answer: <u>4 tablets</u>

Rationale: The first step is the conversion of the 1.3 g dose to milligrams: 1,000 mg = 1 g; 1.3 g × 1,000 mg = 1,300 mg. Once converted to milligrams, the dose is divided by the amount of drug supplied (325 mg): 1,300 mg/325 mg = 4 tablets.

131. Correct Answer: <u>4</u>

Rationale: Patient-controlled analgesia is a method of delivering pain medication through an electronic infusion device that allows the patient to administer pain medication on an as-needed basis. The ability of the patient to maintain an effective level of pain medication to control pain and minimize side effects is the goal of the therapy. A patient who is not achieving adequate pain control should notify the nurse so that the plan of care and the use of the PCA device can be evaluated.

132. Correct Answer: <u>3</u>

Rationale: Intra-articular injection is the injection of medication into a joint space.

Hydrocortisone is given as an intra-articular injection to suppress inflammation. The primary actions of the glucocorticoid administered via this route are local and not systemic.

133. Correct Answer: <u>1</u>

Rationale: Esophagitis and resultant ulceration are adverse effects of the administration of Fosamax. Prolonged contact with the esophageal mucosa resulting from incomplete passage of the drug is the cause of the esophagitis. One intervention to promote drug passage includes avoidance of the supine position for at least 30 minutes after the drug is administered.

134. Correct Answer: <u>4</u>

Rationale: High-dose, long-term use of glucocorticoids causes bone loss through three mechanisms. First, osteoblasts are suppressed, decreasing bone formation. Second, there is an increase in bone resorption by osteoclasts. Third, a reduction in the intestinal absorption of calcium results in hypocalcemia and an increase in parathyroid hormone, which causes calcium to be mobilized from the bone. The long-term use of glucocorticoids can result in a decrease in bone mineral density, with fractures as a resultant complication.

135. Correct Answer: <u>2</u>

Rationale: The primary organ responsible for the metabolism of many drugs is the liver. A patient with a chronic history of alcoholism and resultant liver damage would be at the greatest risk for a drug metabolism problem.

SECTION I

SECTION II

SECTION III

SECTION IV

SECTION V

SECTION VI

SECTION VII

SECTION VIII

SECTION IX

SECTION X

136. Correct Answer: **5 hours**

Rationale: 1,000 mL/x h = 200 mL/1 h; 1,000 mL = 200 mL(x h); x = 1,000 mL/200 mL/h; = 5 h.

137. Correct Answer: **2**

Rationale: Cogentin is an anticholinergic medication that is prescribed to decrease the rigidity and tremors associated with Parkinson's disease. Dry mouth, blurred vision, urinary retention, and constipation are all adverse effects associated with this drug.

138. Correct Answer: **3**

Rationale: Absorption is the movement of a drug from the site of administration into the bloodstream. An intramuscular injection is absorbed through the walls of the capillary beds. The most rapid route for absorption would be the intramuscular injection, as the drug would not need to cross cell membranes to enter the bloodstream.

139. Correct Answer: **1.3 mL**

Rationale: The problem is set up as a ratio proportion where 125 mg/2 mL = 80 mg/x mL. The nurse solves for x by cross-multiplying: 125 mg(x) = 160 mg/mL(x) = 160 mg/mL/125 mg; x = 1.28 mL, when rounded to the nearest tenth would be 1.3 mL.

140. Correct Answer: **3**

Rationale: Dalteparin is a low-molecular-weight heparin that is given to promote anticoagulation. Low-molecular-weight heparins are administered via the subcutaneous route.

141. Correct Answer: **3**

Rationale: The major reason why the carbidopa–levodopa combination is preferred over levodopa monotherapy is because more dopamine is made available in the basal ganglia. Carbidopa inhibits the enzyme decarboxylase within the peripheral nervous system, which allows more of the levodopa to cross the blood–brain barrier and be converted to dopamine in the brain. If levodopa is given alone, the drug is converted to dopamine in the peripheral nervous system, leaving only about 1% of the levodopa to cross the blood–brain barrier and reach the site of action. Levodopa, once converted to dopamine in the peripheral nervous system, will not cross the blood–brain barrier.

142. Correct Answer: **2**

Rationale: Flexeril is a central-acting muscle relaxant that is used to relieve muscle spasms. Its mechanism of action for spasm relief is unclear.

143. Correct Answer: **2**

Rationale: Zofran is an antiemetic drug that is used for the prevention of acute emesis. The drug blocks the type 3 serotonin receptors in the chemoreceptor trigger zone of the brain and afferent vagal neurons of the upper gastrointestinal system.

144. Correct Answer: **3**

Rationale: 30 mL = 1 oz; 0.5 oz = 15 mL.

145. Correct Answer: **2**

Rationale: Neupogen is given to stimulate the production of leukocytes in patients with cancer who are receiving chemotherapy and in patients with severe chronic neutropenia. The drug acts on the bone marrow to increase the production of neutrophils.

146. Correct Answer: **1**

Rationale: Aspirin inhibits cyclooxygenase (COX). Cyclooxygenase is an enzyme that converts arachidonic acid into prostaglandins. With tissue injury, COX synthesizes prostaglandins, which in turn sensitize receptors to painful stimuli. Blocking the action of COX with the administration of aspirin will, therefore, reduce pain at the site of tissue injury.

147. Correct Answer: **1**

Rationale: The U.S. Food and Drug Administration classifies medications according to their possible risks to the fetus. This system includes five categories: A, B, C, D, and X. Drugs in category A are least dangerous to the fetus, whereas those in category X are most dangerous to the fetus. The nurse should interpret a category X drug as one where the potential harm to the fetus outweighs the benefits of its administration. The risks and benefits of drug administration to a pregnant patient should always be discussed with the prescriber.

148. Correct Answer: **2**

Rationale: Heparin is an anticoagulant that is used to prevent the enlargement of an existing clot and to prevent new clots from forming. This medication does not dissolve existing clots.

149. Correct Answer: 3

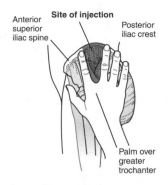

Rationale: The landmarks for intramuscular injection into the ventrogluteal site include the greater trochanter of the femur, the iliac spine, and the iliac crest. The site is identified by placing the palm of the hand on the trochanter with the index finger pointed toward the iliac crest and the middle finger pointed toward the iliac spine. A "V" is formed, and the IM injection is given in the "V" area.

150. Correct Answer: 2

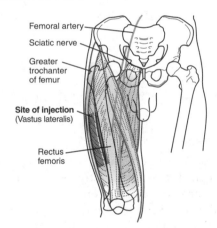

Rationale: The landmarks for IM injection into the anterolateral thigh are the greater trochanter and the knee. The site is one-third the distance from the trochanter to the knee, between the anterior and outer lateral thigh.

151. Correct Answer: 1

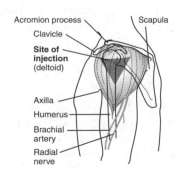

Rationale: The landmarks for the IM injection into the deltoid are the acromion process and the insertion point of the deltoid muscle. The site is two fingerbreadths above the insertion of the deltoid in the lateral aspect of the arm.

152. Correct Answer: 1

Rationale: The 0.9% normal saline is an isotonic solution. Red blood cells should be administered with an isotonic solution to prevent cell damage.

153. Correct Answer: 4

Rationale: Aspirin suppresses the action of cyclooxygenase (COX). One action of cycloxygenase-1 is the promotion of platelet aggregation through the synthesis of prostaglandins and the compound thromboxane A_2. The administration of aspirin blocks the action of COX-1 and acts to decrease platelet aggregation. Bleeding can be an adverse effect of a decrease in platelet aggregation. A patient who is taking regular doses of aspirin should be cautioned to observe for and report any unusual bruising or bleeding.

154. Correct Answer: 1

Rationale: Lioresal reduces the hyperactive reflexes involved in muscle movement and relieves or decreases spasticity.

155. Correct Answer: 3

Rationale: To maximize its absorption, the drug should be taken in the morning prior to eating meals. A full glass of water should be taken with the medication. The patient should not ingest anything for approximately 30 minutes after taking the medication.

156. Correct Answer: 2

Rationale: Serum drug levels are used for determining the appropriate dosing of aminoglycosides. A trough level should be low enough to minimize drug toxicity. A peak level should be high enough to inhibit bacterial growth. A trough level should be drawn just prior to the administration of a dose of the drug.

157. Correct Answer: C

Rationale: Colchicine is prescribed to decrease the inflammatory symptoms associated with an acute attack of gout. This drug inhibits the migration of leukocytes to the inflamed site.

158. Correct Answer: 4

Rationale: For an emergent situation, type O blood would be the most rapidly available product and can be given until type-specific or fully type and cross-matched blood is available. A full type and cross match takes approximately 30 to 45 minutes to complete. Type-specific matching will take approximately 10 to 15 minutes.

159. Correct Answer: **4**

Rationale: Heparin is an anticoagulant medication that is used to prevent the extension of the existing clot. Heparin promotes anticoagulation by inactivating thrombin and factor Xa through the action of antithrombin. Heparin is a rapid-acting anticoagulation and takes effect within minutes when administered intravenously.

REDUCTION OF RISK POTENTIAL

160. Correct Answer: **3**

Rationale: Surgical drains allow for fluids and blood to be removed from a wound. The bulb on a Jackson-Pratt drain should be compressed and the bulb plugged to establish a constant, low suction of the wound site.

161. Correct Answer: **1**

Rationale: A pathological fracture is a discontinuity in the bone that is weakened by disease or tumors. The 84-year-old-female with osteoporosis—a condition characterized by loss of bone mass and deterioration in cancellous bone—would be at the greatest risk for a pathological fracture.

162. Correct Answer: **2**

Rationale: The use of heat to promote blood flow and reduce swelling is recommended approximately 24 to 48 hours after the acute injury phase.

163. Correct Answer: **1**

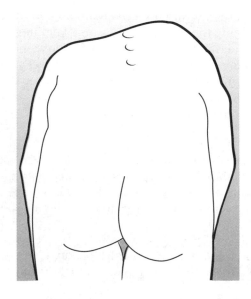

Rationale: Scoliosis is an abnormal lateral deviation of the spine that may or may not include rotation or deformity of the vertebrae. Characteristics of scoliosis include uneven shoulders or iliac crests, prominent scapula on the convex side of the curve, malalignment of the spinous processes, asymmetry of the flanks, and paraspinal muscle prominence when bending forward.

164. Correct Answer: **2**

Rationale: Hemorrhage and shock are the most serious complications associated with a femur fracture. Blood loss between 1,000 and 3,000 mL into the thigh and resultant hypovolemic shock has occurred in association with femur fractures.

165. Correct Answer: **2**

Rationale: A splintered or displaced rib fracture can be associated with damage to the lungs and pleura. A hemothorax is an accumulation of blood in the pleural space. A chest tube is placed to remove the blood, fluid, and air from this space and allow the lung to re-expand.

166. Correct Answer: **3**

Rationale: The inability of a patient to smile or elevate the eyebrows is suggestive of a motor problem with cranial nerve VII, the facial nerve.

167. Correct Answer: **2**

Rationale: The XI cranial nerve innervates the sternocleidomastoid and trapezius muscles, which promote the movement of the head and shoulders. Assessment of these muscles is accomplished by asking the patient to shrug the shoulders against resistance and to turn the head to either side against resistance.

168. Correct Answer: **2**

Rationale: An electromyelogram (EMG) is a recording of electrical activity associated with nervous innervation of skeletal muscle. This diagnostic tool is used to identify problems with muscle or nervous innervation of the muscle, such as lower motor neuron disease or peripheral neuropathy.

169. Correct Answer: **2**

Rationale: Several theories have been proposed for the postoperative sensation of phantom limb pain. This neurological pain is commonly experienced by patients after an amputation.

170. Correct Answer: 1

Rationale: Neuropathy is a risk factor for the development of diabetic foot ulcers. Neuropathy is damage to the nerve caused by a thickening of vessel walls that supply the nerve and demyelinization. Sensory neuropathy is common in diabetics. The loss of the protective sensation of pain and discomfort, found with a sensory neuropathy, can lead to soft-tissue damage and foot ulcerations.

171. Correct Answer: 1

Rationale: Assessment of the pin site should be made prior to the implementation of pin care. Assessment would include inspection and palpation of the pin insertion sites.

172. Correct Answers: 3, 6

Rationale: Age-related bone loss occurs after 50 years. Postmenopausal females are at increased risk for osteoporosis due to a decrease in estrogen levels following menopause. Decreased estrogen levels are associated with decreased bone mineral density and increased risk of fractures.

173. Correct Answer: 2

Rationale: A dislocation is an injury to ligamentous structures surrounding a joint that results in the displacement of the articular surfaces of the joint. A dislocation is considered an orthopedic emergency. The hip is particularly susceptible to avascular necrosis, a complication that can occur the longer a joint remains without reduction. Avascular necrosis is the death of bone cells as a result of inadequate blood supply.

174. Correct Answer: 4

Rationale: Compartment syndrome is a condition where intracompartmental pressures are increased in the myofascial compartment and neurovascular function of the tissues is compromised. Prompt diagnosis is critical to preserve function. A fasciotomy is a procedure that would decrease the intracompartmental pressure. A fasciotomy creates a surgical opening in the fascia that surrounds the muscle and results in decompression of the compartment and surrounding structures.

175. Correct Answer: 1

Rationale: Foot drop is a complication that occurs when the feet are not supported in the dorsiflexion position and damage occurs to the peroneal nerve; that is, the feet are unable to maintain a perpendicular position. The use of a footboard can help to prevent this problem in patients who are at risk for its development.

176. Correct Answer: 2

Rationale: Tetanus results from a neurotoxin that is released by anaerobic bacillus bacteria, *Clostridium tetani*. This bacterium is found in soil, garden mold, and manure. It enters the body through a wound, which has a low-oxygen environment that allows the organism to mature and produce toxin. The farmer with the open wound in a newly plowed field would be at the greatest risk for the development of tetanus, as the organism is often found in soil.

177. Correct Answers: 1–6

Rationale: Pain is often elicited when a patient with a rib fracture attempts to breathe deeply. Such patients are predisposed to shallow respirations because of the associated pain. Goals of care for a patient with a rib fracture include the promotion of adequate chest expansion and the prevention of atelectasis. All of the listed interventions are used to achieve these goals.

178. Correct Answer: 1

Rationale: A pulmonary embolism is a blood clot that originated in the venous system on the right side of the heart. A thrombus forms in the venous system, dislodges, and becomes an embolus that ultimately lodges in the pulmonary vasculature and obstructs blood flow there. Dyspnea and anxiety are clinical manifestations that result when the lungs are not adequately perfused. That is, the lungs are ventilated in pulmonary embolism, but the inability to perfuse the lung prevents adequate gas exchange. The body compensates by trying to increase ventilation. As hypoxia from inadequate perfusion increases, the patient's anxiety level increases. The symptoms of pulmonary embolism depend on the size of the embolus and its location in the pulmonary vasculature.

179. Correct Answer: 4

Rationale: Crutchfield tongs are a type of skeletal traction. The tongs are attached to the skull for the purposes of immobilization and alignment of the cervical vertebrae after an injury. The nurse would assess both motor and sensory functions to detect any neurological deterioration. Hand strength is one means of identifying spinal compression of the motor nerves.

180. Correct Answer: **2**

Rationale: A dual-energy x-ray absorptiometry measures bone mineral density. Bone mass of the spine, femur, forearm, and total body can be measured by this means. The test is used to diagnose metabolic bone disease and to monitor the effectiveness of treatment.

181. Correct Answer: **2**

Rationale: A patient may be predisposed to hip dislocation after surgical placement of a prosthesis when assuming positions of greater than 90° flexion, adduction, or internal rotation. A patient who crosses his or her legs when seated would also be at risk for dislocation.

182. Correct Answer: **2**

Rationale: A stress fracture is an overuse injury that results from repeated wear on a bone. The individual at greatest risk for the development of a stress fracture would be the 24-year-old marathon runner.

183. Correct Answer: **3**

Rationale: Bone healing is influenced by individual and local factors and the type of injury experienced. Non-union is the failure of the fracture to heal before the bone repair process stops.

184. Correct Answer: **2**

Rationale: Bone healing is influenced by individual and local factors and the type of injury experienced. Delayed union is a slower-than-normal fracture healing process.

185. Correct Answer: **1**

Rationale: Bone healing is influenced by individual and local factors and the type of injury experienced. Malunion is a fracture that heals with some type of deformity, angulation, or rotation.

186. Correct Answer: **1**

Rationale: Because the normal protective structures of the brain are compromised with a skull fracture and there is the potential for invasion of the open area with microorganisms, the nurse should be alert for clinical manifestations of infection in a patient who has an open, depressed skull fracture.

187. Correct Answer: **4**

Rationale: The greatest blood loss and potential for hypovolemic shock are associated with fractures of the pelvis and femur.

188. Correct Answer: **4**

Rationale: Compartment syndrome is an elevation of the pressure within a confined myofascial compartment. This elevated pressure can result in neurovascular compromise of the tissue. Pain caused by ischemia, that is not relieved by the use of narcotics is one clinical finding associated with compartment syndrome.

189. Correct Answer: **1**

Rationale: Rhabdomyolysis is a disease characterized by the breakdown of skeletal muscle, such as with a severe crushing injury. With this type of injury, myoglobin is released from the damaged muscles and excreted in the urine. The nurse should monitor urine lab values for the presence of myoglobin to determine the effectiveness of treatment.

190. Correct Answer: **3**

Rationale: Guillain-Barré syndrome is an acute, progressive form of polyneuritis. It affects the peripheral nervous system and is characterized by a loss of myelin, which results in edema and inflammation of the nerves. The most serious complication associated with Guillain-Barré syndrome is respiratory failure. This complication is caused by damage to the nerves that innervate the respiratory muscles and leads to hypotonia or paralysis and the inability to breathe.

191. Correct Answer: **2**

Rationale: The fracture described in the scenario communicates with the external environment through the skin and has multiple fragments. It would be classified as an open, comminuted fracture.

192. Correct Answer: **3**

Rationale: Fat embolism can occur after a long bone fracture. It results from the release of fat droplets from the bone marrow into the circulation and embolization in end organs such as the lungs. Clinical manifestations of this complication include chest pain, tachypnea, ap-

Answers and Rationales   327

SECTION
I

SECTION
II

SECTION
III

SECTION
IV

SECTION
V

SECTION
VI

SECTION
VII

SECTION
VIII

SECTION
IX

SECTION
X

prehension, confusion, and the presence of petechiae on the chest, neck, axillae, and shoulders. The petechiae are thought to be caused by skin capillary embolization.

PHYSIOLOGICAL ADAPTATION

193. Correct Answer: 1

Rationale: The application of cold to a sprained ankle will promote vasoconstriction and prevent swelling and decrease the transmission of nerve impulses to reduce pain.

194. Correct Answer: 4

Rationale: Internal hip rotation is the turning of the foot and leg inward toward the other leg.

195. Correct Answer: 2

Rationale: A first-day postoperative patient would be expected to be out of bed with weight bearing on the non-operative side.

196. Correct Answer: 1

Rationale: A comminuted fracture is a fracture that has more than two fragments.

197. Correct Answer: 2

Rationale: An oblique fracture is a slanted fracture that occurs along a bone's long axis.

198. Correct Answer: 3

Rationale: A transverse fracture is a fracture at a right angle to the long axis of the bone.

199. Correct Answer: 2

Rationale: Somatic pain is a type of nociceptive pain. An injury to bone, joint, muscle, skin, or connective tissue is often the source of the pain. Characteristics of somatic pain include aching, throbbing, and well-localized pain.

200. Correct Answer: 3

Rationale: Multiple sclerosis is an autoimmune disorder that attacks the myelin sheaths of nerve fibers in the central nervous system and produces lesions known as plaques.

201. Correct Answer: 4

Rationale: Foreign objects should not be inserted inside the cast. Injury to the tissues could occur and not be detected until removal of the cast.

202. Correct Answer: 1

Rationale: Parkinson's disease is a degenerative disorder of the basal ganglia. Clinical manifestations include bradykinesia, rigidity, and tremors. Bradykinesia is characterized by slowness in the initiation and performance of movements and difficulty in stopping sudden, unexpected voluntary movements. Rigidity is resistance to flexion and extension in the range of motion. Tremors are seen in the distal portions of the extremities.

203. Correct Answer: 1

Rationale: A basilar skull fracture occurs from force exerted at the base of the skull. Clinical manifestations of the injury to the middle fossa include Battle's sign (ecchymosis noted over the mastoid process), otorrhea caused by CSF leaking from the ear, and facial paralysis associated with injury to the cranial nerve.

204. Correct Answers: 1, 2, 3, 4

Rationale: There are four stages of bone healing. The initial stage of healing, which occurs within the first several days after a fracture, is hematoma formation. The hematoma is formed by the disruption of blood vessels in the area of the fracture. Next, a callus forms. Fibroblasts and osteoblasts migrate to the fracture and begin to reconstruct the damaged bone. The third stage of bone healing is ossification, which is characterized by the deposition of mineral salts into the callus as bone begins to replace the callus. The final stage of bone healing is remodeling, which involves resorption of excess bony callus; the shape and outline of the bone also become reestablished when weight bearing resumes.

205. Correct Answer: 1

Rationale: Immobilization of a fractured extremity as an initial intervention prevents unnecessary movement and further damage or neurovascular complications that could result from bone fragments.

206. Correct Answer: 1

Rationale: Osteodystrophy comprises skeletal complications associated with end-stage renal disease. It results from an inadequate vitamin D level, a decreased serum calcium level, an increased phosphate level, and hyperparathyroidism. Patients with renal failure cannot activate vitamin D to promote calcium absorption in the intestine, resulting in hypocalcemia. As a consequence, they are unable to eliminate phosphate and so develop hyperphosphatemia. The parathyroid gland responds to the hypocalcemia and hyperphosphatemia by secreting parathyroid hormone which stimulates increased bone resorption. The result is abnormal bone resorption and defective bone remodeling.

207. Correct Answer: 3

Rationale: An osteosarcoma is a malignant, rapid-growing tumor that often moves from the metaphysic of the bone into the periosteal surface. It can occur in any bone but most commonly arises in the area of the knee or the proximal humerus.

208. Correct Answer: 1

Rationale: Bursae are small sacs of connective tissue that are lined with synovial membrane and contain synovial fluid. These structures provide cushioning in areas of the body where friction occurs between moving parts, such as the movement of a tendon over a bone. Bursae are not a part of the joint.

209. Correct Answers: 1, 3

Rationale: Osteoarthritis is characterized by changes in the articular cartilage associated with the "wear and tear" of the joint. The loss of cartilage results in changes to the subchondral bone. Osteophytes—bony outgrowths at the joint margins—also form as the disease progresses.

210. Correct Answer: 2

Rationale: A patient with a herniated lower lumbar disc may experience clinical manifestations of altered sensory and motor functions to the area of the body innervated by the nerve roots. Common symptoms include pain, depressed reflexes, paresthesias, or muscle weakness.

211. Correct Answer: 3

Rationale: Paget's disease is characterized by excessive bone destruction and unorganized bone repair. Treatments for this bone disease may include nonsteroidal anti-inflammatory drugs (NSAIDs) to control pain, and biphosphonates or calcitonin to decrease bone resorption. The patient should also take the recommended doses of calcium and vitamin D.

212. Correct Answer: 3

Rationale: Vitamin D is obtained through ingestion of food containing the substance or exposure to sunlight. Once absorbed, the substance is metabolized by the kidneys and liver into an activated form. Activated vitamin D is needed for the absorption of calcium from the intestine.

213. Correct Answer: 4

Rationale: The cerebellum coordinates voluntary movement and maintains trunk stability and equilibrium.

214. Correct Answer: 1, Buck's traction

Rationale: Buck's traction is a type of skin traction used to immobilize, position, or align a lower extremity. It is used for the treatment of contracture and hip and knee problems. Pull is exerted on the lower extremity with a system of ropes, pulleys, and weights.

215. Correct Answer: 2

Rationale: Osteoblasts are bone-building cells that are responsible for the formation of bone matrix.

216. Correct Answer: 2

Rationale: Hyperextension injuries result from an upward or excessive force that throws the spine backward. The spinal cord becomes injured with the hyperflexive movements of the spine.

217. Correct Answer: 3

Rationale: Carpal tunnel syndrome is caused by compression of the median nerve. This nerve is a branch of the brachial plexus that extends along the radial parts of the forearm and hand.

218. Correct Answer: 4

Rationale: Hallux valgus is a painful deformity of the great toe. The toe angles toward the second toe, and there is bony enlargement of the medial side of the first metatarsal head accompanied by the formation of a bursa or a callus. This condition is commonly called a bunion.

219. Correct Answer: 1

Rationale: A patient who experienced a complete spinal cord transection at the level of the fourth cervical vertebrae would be expected to have head and neck control and some shoulder elevation.

220. Correct Answer: 2

Rationale: Signs and symptoms of choking include inability to speak; clutching of the neck with the hands; poor, ineffective cough; cyanosis; stridor; and difficulty breathing. The Heimlich maneuver is an emergency procedure used for a conscious, choking patient.

221. Correct Answer: <u>1</u>

Rationale: A laminectomy is a surgical treatment for a patient with a herniated disc. This procedure is performed to relieve compression of the spinal cord that results from a degenerated, damaged, or displaced disc. It involves the removal of the vertebral arch of one or more vertebrae.

222. Correct Answer: <u>4</u>

Rationale: Rheumatoid arthritis is a systemic, inflammatory disease that results from an immune response. Boutonniere deformity of the joints is characteristic of rheumatoid arthritis.

Care of Patients with Hypertension and Cardiac Problems

MANAGEMENT OF CARE

Multiple Choice

1. The night shift nurse notices the odor of alcohol on the oncoming nurse's breath while giving report. What is the priority action by the night nurse?

1. Confront the nurse with the assessment.
2. Observe the nurse throughout the shift for any other symptoms of alcohol abuse.
3. Notify the nurse manager.
4. Contact a member of an impaired nurse program.

2. A competent, alert patient, after discussion with the physician, requests no resuscitation efforts. The family wants all resuscitation measures utilized. The physician writes a "do not resuscitate" order on the patient's chart. What is the predominant ethical principle in the scenario?

1. Beneficence.
2. Justice.
3. Autonomy.
4. Veracity.

3. The nurse is preparing to counsel a patient on tobacco cessation as an intervention to reduce cardiovascular risk factors. Which question would be most important for the nurse to ask?

1. "Will your family be supportive of your decision to stop smoking?"
2. "Are you ready to quit smoking?"
3. "Do you know what community resources are available to assist you?"
4. "What is your understanding about smoking and cardiovascular disease?"

4. A postoperative heart transplant patient is receiving immunosuppressive therapy. What is the best action by the nurse to prevent infection?

1. Implementation of neutropenic precautions.
2. Hand washing before and after care.
3. Moving the patient to a positive air flow room.
4. Ensuring that all visitors wear masks, gloves, and gowns.

5. The nurse is using a clinical pathway or care map. With which type of nursing care delivery system are pathways or care maps most commonly associated?

1. Partnership models.
2. Primary care nursing.
3. Case management.
4. Total patient care.

6. While out to dinner, a nurse overhears another healthcare provider discussing the details of a patient's care with a friend. The healthcare provider mentions the name of the patient during the discussion. The nurse understands that this conversation is in violation of which ethical principle?

1. Fidelity.
2. Veracity.
3. Malfeasance.
4. Confidentiality.

7. The demand for heart transplants currently exceeds the available supply of donor hearts. A computerized database was established to ensure equitable distribution of organs. Which ethical principle applies to this situation?

1. Autonomy.
2. Distributive justice.
3. Veracity.
4. Beneficence.

8. A nurse goes in to a patient's room and, upon assessment, finds the patient unresponsive and without respiratory effort. What is the priority for the care of this patient?

1. Open the airway and ventilate the patient.
2. Obtain the emergency resuscitation cart.
3. Call a code and wait for the code team to arrive.
4. Insert an oropharyngeal airway and perform pharyngeal suction.

9. Which situation would not require written informed consent for giving care?

1. An incompetent patient who has family present.
2. A provider who gives free healthcare services.
3. A patient who is unable to read or write.
4. An emergency situation.

Matching

Using the terms below, match the description with the appropriate organization or program.

10. Prospective inpatient reimbursement system for Medicare and Medicaid patients that establishes a predetermined payment schedule for a given surgery or episode of illness.

11. A federally run program that provides health insurance coverage for cardiovascular, as well as other, patient populations who are ages 65 and older.

12. The accrediting body that establishes national patient safety goals and reviews organizations for their demonstrated effectiveness in meeting these goals.

13. An unstable patient experiencing acute coronary syndrome needed to be transferred from one facility to another for emergency medical care; this federal legislation sets forth the requirements for the patient's care and transfer.

14. A national voluntary health agency whose mission is to reduce disability and death from cardiovascular diseases and stroke.

1. Medicare.
2. Medicaid.
3. Joint Commission on Accreditation of Healthcare Organizations.
4. Emergency Treatment and Active Labor Act (EMTALA).
5. Social Security Act.
6. American Nurses Association.
7. American Heart Association.
8. Diagnosis-related groups.

Multiple Choice

15. A charge nurse completed shift assignments for the unlicensed personnel in the department. In which situation would the charge nurse be most likely to have liability for the actions of the unlicensed personnel?

1. An alert patient who falls when getting out of bed, with the call light in place and all bed rails in the proper position.
2. Unlicensed personnel are socializing with other staff after assignments have been completed.
3. Performance of a procedure for which a competency-based skills check off has not been completed.
4. Notification of the charge nurse that a patient is requesting to leave against medical advice.

16. A patient is referred to a cardiac rehabilitation facility in the community after discharge from an acute care facility. Which level of community-based preventive, care practice would the referral be considered?

1. Primary prevention.
2. Secondary prevention.
3. Tertiary prevention.
4. Quarternary prevention.

17. The discharge care plan for a patient admitted with a sternal wound infection includes the administration of intravenous antibiotics through a peripherally inserted central venous catheter. Which type of referral would the nurse anticipate needing for the patient to ensure continuity of care with the antibiotic therapy?

1. Home healthcare nursing services.
2. Assisted living facility.
3. Public health services.
4. Outpatient physical therapy services.

18. A nurse achieves certification in cardiovascular nursing practice. Which statement about certification is true?

1. Certification is available only through the American Nurses Association.
2. Certification demonstrates an individual's basic competency for entry into practice.
3. Certification is a type of credentialing that has professional status within the defined area of practice.
4. Certification provides written proof of the individual's nursing qualifications.

19. A patient expresses a desire to designate someone to make healthcare decisions should she become unable to make those decisions for herself. Which document is needed for this purpose?

1. Estate planning tool.
2. Living will.
3. Deposition.
4. Durable power of attorney for health care.

20. The nurse is assessing a patient with the rhythm shown below. The patient is not breathing and is pulseless. What is the priority treatment for the rhythm?

1. Pacemaker insertion.
2. Administer lidocaine (Xylocaine).
3. Defibrillation.
4. Administer verapamil (Calan).

21. While the nurse is obtaining a health history on a patient, the patient indicates that he does not have money to pay for medications. The nurse responds by saying, "I understand that you do not have the money to pay for your medicines." Which type of therapeutic communication technique did the nurse utilize?

1. Reflection.
2. Restating.
3. Clarification.
4. Focusing.

22. The nurse obtains a blood pressure reading of 50/30. The patient is awake, alert, and talking calmly with his family. Which action should the nurse take?

1. Ask the family to immediately leave the room.
2. Recheck the blood pressure.
3. Place the patient in the Trendelenburg position.
4. Prepare for resuscitation procedures.

23. Assessment findings reveal that a patient is concerned about her ability to pay for medications once discharged. Which healthcare team member would be most helpful in planning the patient's care?

1. Respiratory therapist.
2. Social worker.
3. Community pharmacist.
4. Utilization reviewer.

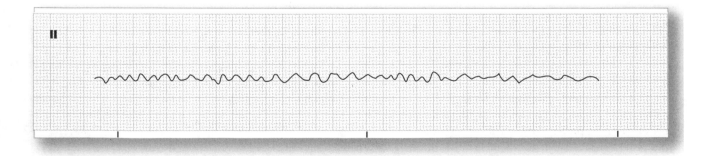

24. A patient is diagnosed with severe cardiomyopathy and is unable to perform activities of daily living. The patient is expected to be discharged home sometime in the next 2 days. To ensure continuity of care, which priority factor should the nurse assess the patient for?

1. A plan for who will provide for the patient's activities of daily living.
2. Availability of a community meal delivery program.
3. Type of adaptive equipment the patient currently has to support his care.
4. The patient's ability to pay for home healthcare services.

25. Which patient should receive the priority referral to a dietician?

1. A patient with nausea and vomiting relieved by medication.
2. A patient whose only intake has been D_5W at a "keep open rate" for 48 hours.
3. A patient who ate only 25% of one meal.
4. A patient who indicated that the meal was not hot enough when received.

26. Which statement describes a discharge teaching need for a patient with congestive heart failure?

1. Vigorous exercise should occur daily.
2. Weight should be measured at the same time each day.
3. A monthly troponin level will need to be drawn.
4. Fluid intake should be at least 3 liters per 24 hours.

27. Two nurses want the same weekend off. Nurse Jones approaches Nurse Smith and states, "If you would work the upcoming weekend for me, I will work any other day for you that you choose." Identify Nurse Jones's personal style for dealing with conflict.

1. Avoiding (withdrawing).
2. Accommodating (smoothing).
3. Forcing the issue (competing).
4. Compromising (negotiating).

28. A nurse manager is concerned about an increase in the number of pressure ulcers in patients over the past month. Which hospital resource could the nurse ask for assistance in investigating the problem?

1. Utilization management.
2. Quality management.
3. Products committee.
4. Epidemiology/infection control.

29. An embolectomy is performed for an arterial thrombus in a patient's lower extremity. What is the priority nursing action in the immediate postoperative period?

1. Pain management.
2. Active and passive range of motion.
3. Neurovascular assessment.
4. Monitoring for fluid excess.

30. A patient is alert and oriented, but unable to read or write. Which steps should be included to obtain informed consent for surgery? (Select all that apply.)

1. The surgeon explains the procedure and complications.
2. The patient's questions about the procedure are addressed.
3. A healthcare provider reads the consent to the patient.
4. The patient's next of kin signs the consent.
5. The patient signs the consent with a mark or X.
6. A guardian must be appointed by the court for the patient.

31. A patient is having premature ventricular bigeminy. What is the priority nursing action?

1. Assess the patient.
2. Notify the physician.
3. Prepare to administer amniodarone.
4. Call a code.

32. A nurse has contacted a respiratory services company to make arrangements for a patient's home oxygen therapy upon discharge. Which information would be most appropriate for the nurse to have available upon initial referral to the company?

1. Oxygen saturation (SaO_2) measurements for the past 72 hours.
2. The delivery device and amount of oxygen used.
3. The knowledge base of the patient related to oxygen therapy.
4. The patient's vital signs for the past 24 hours.

33. Which factor has contributed to the increasing cost of cardiovascular care?

1. New technology.
2. Decrease in litigation.
3. Development of critical pathways.
4. Managed care organizations.

Identification

34. Nurse Smith (initials "NS") documented a blood pressure measurement of 120/60 on a patient's medical record. The blood pressure should have read 120/80. Identify the most appropriate way to correct the error.

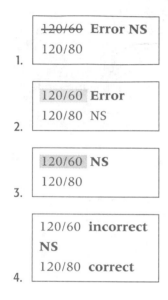

1.
~~120/60~~ **Error NS**
120/80

2.
120/60 **Error**
120/80 **NS**

3.
120/60 **NS**
120/80

4.
120/60 **incorrect**
NS
120/80 **correct**

Multiple Choice

35. When the nurse is turning a patient in bed, a chest tube is accidentally discontinued. What should the nurse do first?

1. Notify the physician.
2. Assess lung sounds.
3. Apply a dressing with three sides taped.
4. Gather supplies for tube reinsertion.

36. The nurse is preparing a patient for a diagnostic cardiac catheterization. Which task would be appropriate for the nurse to delegate to a certified nursing assistant?

1. Assessment of the patient's peripheral pulses.
2. Obtaining vital signs.

3. Documentation of a pre-procedure note on the medical record.
4. Teaching the patient's family about patient discharge needs.

37. The night-shift charge nurse asks the nurse manager for assistance in dealing with an employee whose skills are marginal when caring for a patient with a pulmonary artery catheter who requires cardiac output measurements. Which intervention should the nurse manager take first?

1. Terminate the employee.
2. Assess the reason for the marginal performance.
3. Send the employee to a course on cardiac output measurements.
4. Establish goals and a timeline for improvement.

38. As part of orientation, a new nurse completed a skills check-off on the use of chest drainage systems. Which type of competency was assessed?

1. Cultural.
2. Interpersonal.
3. Psychomotor.
4. Decision making.

Identification

39. Review the three ECG rhythms and, based on the rhythm, identify which patient the nurse should assess first.

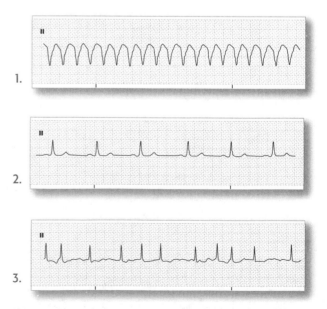

Multiple Choice

40. A nurse applies for a position in a cardiovascular intensive care unit and indicates on her résumé that she has obtained certification in critical care nursing. The nurse does not actually have this certification. This situation is an example of which legal issue?

1. Libel.
2. Slander.
3. Fraud.
4. Negligence.

41. A Hispanic patient who does not speak English requires open heart surgery. Informed consent for the surgery is required. What is the most appropriate action by the nurse when obtaining the patient's informed consent?

1. Contact a member of the patient's family who can speak English.
2. Obtain a trained medical interpreter.
3. Notify the operating room that the patient is unable to give informed consent.
4. Use gestures and nonverbal techniques to communicate with the patient.

42. Priority management of a patient with pheochromocytoma would include which intervention?

1. Blood pressure measurement.
2. Monitoring urine output.
3. Neurological checks.
4. Obtaining serum glucose levels.

43. Four patients have been evaluated in the emergency room and are awaiting bed assignments on a cardiovascular telemetry unit. One bed is currently available. Which patient should be assigned to the available telemetry bed?

1. A 70-year-old patient currently in normal sinus rhythm who experienced syncope.
2. A 45-year-old patient with a myocardial infarction who was administered thrombolytic therapy in the emergency room.
3. A 57-year-old patient with a possible deep vein thrombosis who was started on heparin therapy.
4. A 62-year-old patient with renal insufficiency who is scheduled to undergo a diagnostic cardiac catheterization.

44. A patient diagnosed with an acute coronary syndrome has expressed a willingness to stop smoking. From which discharge plan would the patient benefit most?

1. Provision of a 1-week supply of nicotine patches.
2. Referral to a community agency with smoking cessation resources.
3. Prescription for an antidepressant medication.
4. Smoking cessation educational materials.

SAFETY AND INFECTION CONTROL

Identification

45. Admission orders are written for a patient with congestive heart failure (below). Review the orders and identify the one that requires further clarification.

Admission Orders					
Patient Name: Jones, Teri					
Patient Number: #3-11316-7					
Date	Time Written	Orders	Order Checked	Time Noted	Nurse's Signature
1/31/07	0930	① Digoxin 0.125 mg p.o. daily	✓		
		② Lasix 40 mg b.i.d.	✓		
		③ K-lyte 25 mEq p.o. now	✓		
		④ Aspirin 81 mg p.o. daily	✓	1000	*N. Nurse RN*

Multiple Choice

46. Which statement demonstrates an understanding of the precautions that should be taken for a patient to promote the safe operation of an implanted permanent pacemaker?

1. Microwave ovens should be avoided.
2. Large magnetic fields should be avoided.
3. Cellular phone use should be avoided.
4. X-rays should be avoided.

47. A postoperative order reads, "Chest drainage system to 20 cm of suction." Upon assessment, the nurse finds the suction to be 15 cm. Which action would the nurse take to change the suction amount to the prescribed level?

1. Add sterile water to the suction chamber up to the 20-cm mark.
2. Increase wall suction to 20 mm Hg.
3. Instill tap water into the water seal chamber to the 20-cm mark.
4. Remove 5 cc of water from the suction chamber to achieve 20 cm of suction.

48. Safe administration of transdermal nitroglycerin would include which nursing action?

1. Instruct the patient to inhale the nitroglycerin spray.
2. Administer nitroglycerin in a plastic IV bottle with polyvinyl chloride tubing.
3. Write the opening date on a tablet bottle and discard it after 2 years.
4. Apply the patch to a hairless area on the skin.

49. A preceptor observes a new nurse perform a sterile dressing change. Just prior to applying the dressing to the wound, the new nurse contaminates the dressing. What is the most appropriate action by the preceptor?

1. Offer to obtain another sterile dressing to use to complete the procedure.
2. Discuss the break in procedure after the dressing change is completed.
3. Ignore the incident, as there is minimal chance of an infection occurring.
4. Excuse the new nurse and complete the procedure yourself.

50. The nurse observes the following rhythm on the continuous cardiac monitor. The nurse rushes to the patient's bedside and finds the patient awake, alert, and without complaints. Which action should the nurse take?

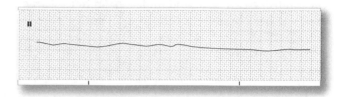

1. Check the EKG leads to see if they have become disconnected.
2. Call for the rapid response team.
3. Observe the patient for a delayed response to the rhythm.
4. Initiate cardiopulmonary resuscitation.

51. Which statement would indicate a need for further teaching for a patient who is to be discharged on warfarin (Coumadin)?

1. "I need to observe my bowel movements for blood."
2. "I will need to return to the clinic so that a prothrombin time (PT) can be performed."
3. "I should use an electric razor when shaving."
4. "I will need to decrease my sodium intake."

52. Which action should be questioned in a patient who is receiving a thrombolytic medication?

1. Intravenous injection into an existing site.
2. Performing an arterial puncture to obtain a blood gas.
3. Shaving a patient with an electric razor.
4. Application of cold packs to a swollen area.

53. The nurse administers morphine 4 mg IV at 1400 hours. An incorrect dose was administered—morphine 2 mg IV should have been administered instead. Select the best way to document the incorrect dosage in the medical record.

1. An incorrect dose of medication given to the patient. Morphine 4 mg IV was administered at 1400 instead of the 2 mg IV that was ordered.
2. Morphine 4 mg IV given at 1400.
3. Morphine 4 mg IV was accidentally given instead of 2 mg IV.
4. Morphine 4 mg IV given at 1400 in error.

54. At 2:00 P.M. a patient is administered a dose of medication. A 24-hour clock (i.e., military time) is used at the hospital. What would be the appropriate time to document medication administration?

1. 0200.
2. 1400.
3. 1600.
4. 1800.

55. A patient is undergoing synchronized cardioversion and will receive sedation prior to the procedure. Which equipment must the nurse have at the bedside to ensure the safe delivery of care?

1. Bag-valve-mask device.
2. Infusion pump.
3. Nasogastric tube.
4. Mechanical ventilator.

56. Which medication order should the nurse verify with the prescriber?

1. Digoxin 25 mg PO daily.
2. Metoprolol 50 mg PO bid.
3. Epinephrine 1 mg IV now.
4. Enoxaparin 80 units SQ daily.

Identification

57. A patient collapses in a department store and is pulseless. An automatic external defibrillator (AED) is immediately available at the scene. Prioritize the steps that a nurse would take to ensure the safe use of the equipment.

1. Attach the AED pads to the victim's chest.
2. Turn on the power.
3. Announce, "Stand clear."
4. Wait for the shock to be delivered.
5. Push the "Analyze" button.
6. Deliver up to three shocks if indicated.

Multiple Choice

58. Which measure should the nurse take to prevent a sternal wound infection in a patient who has had postoperative coronary artery bypass grafts?

1. Implement standard precautions.
2. Wear a mask, gloves, and gown with every direct patient contact.
3. Restrict the number of visitors.
4. Utilize clean technique with each dressing change.

59. A nursing assistant reports a blood pressure on an adult patient. The nurse notes that the cuff used to obtain the blood pressure was too small. What effect will the size of the cuff have on the blood pressure reading?

1. No effect.
2. The measurement will be one-half of the normal reading.
3. The measurement will be too high.
4. The measurement will be too low.

60. Which measure, if used by the nurse, would be most effective in prevention of the transfer of methicillin-resistant *Staphylococcus aureus* (MRSA) between postoperative patients on a cardiothoracic unit?

1. Use of gloves for handling all body fluids.
2. Placing the patient in a private room.
3. Use of a mask, gloves, and gown.
4. Hand hygiene.

61. A patient with angina is prescribed isosorbide dinitrate (Isordil). Which activity could pose a safety risk for this patient?

1. Relaxing in a hot tub.
2. Swimming in a pool.
3. Daily brisk walks.
4. Drinking a hot liquid.

62. The nurse is assisting with the insertion of a triple-lumen central venous catheter in a patient with congestive heart failure. When placing the catheter on the sterile field, the catheter tip touches the nurse's scrubs. What is the best action by the nurse?

1. Obtain a new triple-lumen catheter.
2. Wipe off the catheter with an alcohol swab.
3. Cleanse the insertion site with additional antiseptic solution.
4. Flush the catheter with normal saline multiple times.

63. The nurse is preparing to defibrillate a pulseless, adult patient. Which action demonstrates safe, appropriate use of the defibrillator?

1. Apply the paddles to the right anterior and right posterior chest.
2. Do not take the time to remove nitroglycerin ointment.

3. Ensure that the device is placed on cardiovert.

4. Notify all beside personnel to stand clear immediately prior to defibrillation.

Short Answer

64. An intravenous fluid order reads as follows: D_5 $\frac{1}{2}$ NS with 20 mEq KCl to infuse at 125 mL/h. The intravenous fluid bag label is shown below. Is it safe for the nurse to administer the fluid?

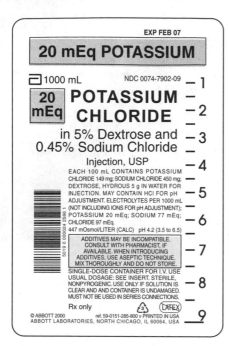

Multiple Choice

65. The nurse discovers a patient lying on the floor after a fall. Which actions should the nurse take first?

1. Assess the patient and provide needed care.

2. Document all observations immediately in the medical record.

3. Contact the physician and the nursing supervisor.

4. Go to the nurses' station and get help to move the patient.

66. When the nurse is taking a medication history, the patient identifies the use of herbal supplements. The patient asks the nurse about the safety of taking over-the-counter supplements. What is the nurse's best response?

1. "Information on the safety and efficacy of medicinal herbs is provided on the product label."

2. "Manufacturing of medicinal herbs is regulated by the Food and Drug Administration."

3. "Dietary supplements can be marketed without proof of safety or efficacy."

4. "All medicinal herbs are tested in clinical trials to ensure their safety."

HEALTH PROMOTION AND MAINTENANCE

Multiple Choice

67. Reduction of sodium intake is one type of non-pharmacological treatment for hypertension. What is the expected effect of this treatment?

1. Promotes weight loss through diuresis.

2. Decreases vascular fluid volume.

3. Stimulates parasympathetic nervous system activity.

4. Increases serum osmolality and vascular volume.

68. A patient who has been diagnosed with severe congestive heart failure states, "I can't seem to lie flat to sleep. I have to sleep with my head on three pillows at night in order to breathe. Why do I have to do that?" What is the nurse's best response?

1. "Sleeping with the head elevated will decrease the amount of venous blood returning to the heart."

2. "Elevation of the head of the bed promotes improved air exchange by allowing maximum diaphragm expansion."

3. "Tracheal alignment and gas exchange are promoted by elevation of the head."

4. "There is no reason your husband should need to sleep on three pillows at night."

69. Which method would be most effective for evaluating an adult patient's ability to obtain an accurate pulse rate?

1. Have the patient describe how to take a pulse.

2. Observe the patient demonstrate and practice how to take his or her own pulse.

3. Give the patient written instructions to read when needed.

4. Ask the patient to write down the steps for how to take a pulse.

Identification

70. A patient who has been diagnosed with cardiovascular disease is 65 inches tall and weighs 160 pounds. Using the body mass index chart, identify whether this patient should consider weight reduction strategies to promote cardiovascular health.

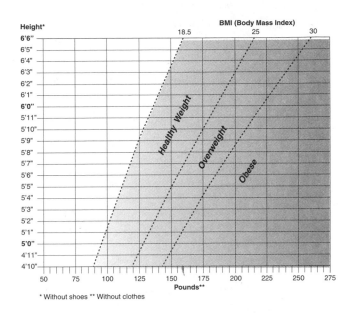

* Without shoes ** Without clothes

Multiple Choice

71. To assess for jugular vein distention, a patient should be placed in what position?

1. Semi-Fowler's.
2. Prone.
3. Trendelenburg.
4. Supine.

72. The nurse is preparing a continuing education class on health disparities associated with cardiovascular disease. Which group of patients should the nurse include because they often have atypical presentations of acute myocardial infarction?

1. Caucasians.
2. Women.
3. Middle-aged males.
4. Native Americans.

73. Which group is at the greatest risk for the development of hypertension?

1. Native Americans.
2. African Americans.
3. Pacific Islanders.
4. Asians.

74. A patient with Raynaud's disease should be taught to avoid which environmental factor?

1. Cold temperatures.
2. Exposure to secondhand smoke.
3. Contact with pesticides.
4. High levels of smog.

75. Which factor could increase an individual's risk for developing varicose veins? (Select all that apply.)

1. Obesity.
2. Pregnancy.
3. Male gender.
4. African American ethnicity.
5. Congenital weakness of the artery.
6. Sedentary lifestyle.

76. Which health behavior will be essential for the patient with thromboangiitis obliterans (Buerger's disease) to modify?

1. Ingestion of alcohol.
2. Smoking.
3. Caffeine ingestion.
4. Sedentary lifestyle.

77. Which risk factor for coronary artery disease is modifiable?

1. Sedentary lifestyle.
2. Family history.
3. Gender.
4. Age.

78. The nurse is providing discharge teaching for a patient's family member on the administration of enoxaparin (Lovenox). Which action by the family member would indicate an understanding of the administration procedure for the drug?

1. An 18-gauge, 1½-inch needle is selected for injection.
2. The family member administers the medication subcutaneously.
3. The family member aspirates for blood return after the needle is inserted in the muscle.
4. The same administration site is used for every injection.

79. The nurse is assessing a patient in an outpatient clinic. The patient was started on furosemide (Lasix) 40 mg PO daily, 1 week ago. Which statement by the patient indicates the need for further education?

   1. "Since my hands aren't as swollen, I can wear my rings again."

   2. "I have lost 3 pounds since last week. I weigh myself every day."

   3. "I'm not getting enough sleep because I have to get up and go to the bathroom so much at night."

   4. "I'm taking the potassium supplements with breakfast each morning."

80. Which cardiovascular changes are normally found in a geriatric patient? (Select all that apply.)

   1. Decreased elasticity of the heart.

   2. Thickening and stiffening of heart valves.

   3. Increased response to sympathetic nervous system stimulation.

   4. Shortened conduction time through the atria.

   5. More pronounced auscultation of S_1 and S_2.

   6. Increased elasticity of the arteries.

81. A low-fat, low-cholesterol diet is prescribed for a patient with a history of coronary artery disease. The nurse knows that the patient understands the diet plan if which entree is selected?

   1. Fried cod.

   2. Grilled chicken breast.

   3. Pasta with cream sauce.

   4. Broiled T-bone steak.

82. How does exercise affect elevated cholesterol levels?

   1. Decreases high-density lipoproteins (HDL).

   2. Increases very-low-density lipoproteins (VLDL).

   3. Decreases low-density lipoproteins (LDL).

   4. Increases apolipoproteins.

83. Which risk factor for atherosclerosis is nonmodifiable?

   1. Hyperlipidemia.

   2. Uncontrolled hypertension.

   3. Obesity.

   4. Increasing age.

84. A patient with a history of deep vein thrombosis asks the nurse, "What can I do to prevent this from happening again?" Which activity would reduce the risk of the development of deep vein thrombosis?

   1. Keep your legs crossed when sitting to decrease blood flow.

   2. Avoid sitting for prolonged periods of time.

   3. Elevate your feet when sitting for extended periods.

   4. Tight, constrictive hosiery should be worn.

Identification

85. Identify the location on the chest where the nurse would take an apical pulse.

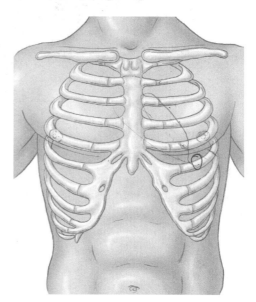

Multiple Choice

86. Upon completing a patient history, the nurse finds that the patient leads a sedentary lifestyle, has a body mass index of 36, and has a good appetite. What is the most appropriate nursing diagnosis for this patient?

   1. Risk for metabolic syndrome X related to sedentary lifestyle.

   2. Obesity related to lack of exercise.

   3. Altered nutrition; more than body requirements related to caloric intake greater than calories expended.

   4. Altered nutrition; less than body requirements related to an abnormal body mass index.

PSYCHOSOCIAL INTEGRITY

Multiple Choice

87. A patient states, "My parents were Baptist. When I left for college, I stopped going to church; there was always something else to do. Now that I have been diagnosed with cardiomyopathy, I think it is time to return to my church and begin to explore my purpose in life." Which nursing diagnosis is appropriate for this patient?

1. Spiritual well-being, readiness for enhanced.
2. Spiritual distress, risk for.
3. Sorrow, chronic.
4. Spiritual deficit, alienation.

88. Which religious affiliation does the nurse understand includes religious beliefs that would affect the administration of blood and/or blood products?

1. Roman Catholic.
2. Presbyterian.
3. Jehovah's Witness.
4. Hinduism.

89. Risk factor modification is discussed with a patient during recovery from a myocardial infarction. The patient states, "I don't understand why it is so important to change my lifestyle when I am going to die anyway." What is the nurse's best response?

1. "A reduction in risk factors can slow the progression of the disease and lessen the chance for further myocardial damage."
2. "Aggressive risk factor reduction can add at least 15 years to your life, if you begin those interventions now."
3. "It will be difficult to change your lifestyle, but you should not let that stop you."
4. "You should want to live the healthiest lifestyle possible for your family's sake."

90. A chronic smoker has developed a physical dependence on nicotine. The patient is hospitalized and has been unable to smoke for the past 48 hours. Which symptoms of tobacco withdrawal would the nurse observe for?

1. Decreased appetite, weight loss.
2. Irritability, restlessness.
3. Improved cognition, reduced aggression.
4. Hallucinations, visual impairment.

91. A new graduate nurse on orientation witnessed a sudden, unexpected cardiac arrest in a patient she was caring for. The graduate nurse is visibly disturbed by the situation. What is the best way for the preceptor to reduce the new nurse's stress?

1. Recommend that the graduate nurse schedule an appointment with a psychiatrist.
2. Ask the graduate nurse to share her thoughts and feelings about the situation.
3. Request that the nurse manager schedule an extra day off for the graduate nurse.
4. Encourage the nurse to keep busy and to not think about the situation.

Matching

Using the terms below, match the patient response with the appropriate issue it demonstrates.

92. After experiencing a myocardial infarction, a patient states, "What is everyone so concerned about? I just had really bad indigestion. I'm fine."

93. A patient tells the nurse after being diagnosed with coronary artery disease, "There is nothing I can do that will ever help to make me better."

94. A patient admitted with chest pain tells the nurse, "My father died of a heart attack, and my uncle died on the operating room table while having open heart surgery. I am afraid I am going to die, too."

95. During a visit to the outpatient clinic for a blood pressure check, a patient diagnosed with essential hypertension states, "I know I have high blood pressure, but I don't feel bad and I don't see the need to make any changes in the way I live. I'm going to die some day anyway."

1. Denial, ineffective.
2. Hopelessness.
3. Fear.
4. Adjustment, impaired.

Multiple Choice

96. Which statement by the nurse would promote therapeutic communication with the patient?

1. "Did you have a restful morning?"
2. "Are you ready to get up and try walking down the hall?"
3. "Don't worry at all about the procedure. It's been done a million times."
4. "Tell me about the night you had."

97. The nurse is preparing a patient who experienced a myocardial infarction for discharge. The patient expresses concern about having sex with his wife when he returns home. Which response by the nurse would be most helpful in lessening the patient's fears?

1. "It is common for patients to worry about resuming sexual activities. Tell me about your concerns."

2. "There is nothing to worry about. You can continue at the same sexual activity level you had prior to the illness."

3. "You should refrain from all sexual activity for at least the next 6 weeks. Would you like me to discuss this with your wife?"

4. "Impotence can be a side effect of your medications. You and your wife should refrain from sexual activity while you are being treated for the illness."

98. A patient diagnosed with a myocardial infarction tells the nurse, "I am afraid I won't be able to deal with all the issues my illness has created." Which nursing action would be most supportive of the patient's coping behaviors?

1. Encourage the patient to comply with the plan of care.

2. Assist the patient to identify available supportive resources.

3. Tell family members to assume more responsibilities.

4. Work with the patient to identify all the adverse effects of the illness.

99. A patient is transported to the emergency room via ambulance for treatment of crushing chest pain. Before the family members arrive, the patient dies. What is the best response by the nurse upon arrival of the family to the emergency room?

1. Ask the ER physician to have sedation available for the family members.

2. Escort the family members to a private location and notify them of the patient's death.

3. Notify the family of the death immediately upon their arrival in the waiting room.

4. Assess the family members for the one who is the most emotionally stable and notify that person of the death.

100. An elderly patient's wife begins to cry and indicates that she is worried about her husband's impending open heart surgery. What is the most appropriate nursing action?

1. Contact the physician and ask him to review the surgical procedure with the wife and husband.

2. Encourage the wife to discuss her feelings and concerns.

3. Talk with the wife about the patient's care needs upon discharge.

4. Reinforce to the wife the physician's surgical outcome data.

101. A patient states, "I am afraid I will become addicted to morphine if I take the medication to help control my post-operative pain." What is an appropriate nursing diagnosis for the patient?

1. Impaired adjustment related to need to control pain.

2. Disturbed thought processes due to post-operative anesthetic effects.

3. Knowledge deficit related to the effects and use of morphine.

4. Powerlessness related to lack of pain control.

102. A patient who is awaiting a heart transplant for severe cardiomyopathy asks if she will die before a transplant becomes available. What is the nurse's best response?

1. "Because you are so ill, you will be high on the transplant list."

2. "Let's talk about what makes you think you are going to die."

3. "You should discuss your concerns with the physician."

4. "Would you like to speak with a chaplain?"

103. A patient reports chronic use of "crack" cocaine. The patient was admitted with chest pain and asks the nurse, "What does my cocaine use have to do with my heart?" Which statement best describes the cardiovascular effects of cocaine?

1. Cocaine acts as a stimulant and can cause angina due to vasoconstriction and increased myocardial workload.

2. Cocaine stimulates the parasympathetic nervous system and slows electrical conduction in the ventricles.

3. Cocaine decreases respiratory effort and oxygen delivery to myocardium due to its depressant actions.

4. Cocaine competes for $beta_2$ receptor sites and decreases myocardial contractility.

104. To prevent increased anxiety in a patient who is awaiting a percutaneous angioplasty procedure,

which action would be most appropriate for the nurse to take?

1. Tell the patient not to worry—the complication rate for this procedure is very low.
2. Talk with the patient about any questions or concerns he or she has regarding the procedure.
3. Prepare to administer haloperidol (Haldol) to control the patient's anxiety.
4. Notify the cardiac catheterization lab staff to have additional anti-anxiety medication available.

105. While the nurse is caring for a patient with cardiovascular disease, he becomes physically abusive to the nurse. What is the priority of care for the patient?

1. Put the patient in an isolated area.
2. Assign a nursing assistant to sit with the patient.
3. Assist the patient to restore self-control.
4. Place the patient in restraints.

106. A patient has a history of alcohol dependence. Which symptoms should the nurse monitor for that would indicate the patient is experiencing early alcohol withdrawal?

1. Bradycardia and hypotension.
2. Hallucinations and tremors.
3. Decreased temperature and leg cramps.
4. Depression and an increased need for sleep.

BASIC CARE AND COMFORT

Multiple Choice

107. According to Abraham Maslow, the need for sleep, rest, activity and nutrition would be classified under which patient need?

1. Self-actualization.
2. Safety and security.
3. Physiologic needs.
4. Human needs.

108. A 12-lead electrocardiogram (ECG) is being done on a patient with a complaint of chest pain. Which action by the patient would be most likely to create artifact on the recording?

1. Supine, lying in bed.
2. Arm movement.
3. Talking softly.
4. Lying quietly with slight head elevation.

109. A patient asks the nurse the reason for use of incentive spirometry. What is the nurse's best response?

1. "Incentive spirometry helps to maximize lung inflation and prevent atelectasis."
2. "Incentive spirometry uses gravity to assist in the removal of bronchial secretions."
3. "Incentive spirometry loosens thick secretions."
4. "Incentive spirometry ensures a patent airway and prevents obstruction."

110. Which nursing intervention would promote comfort in a patient with a nasogastric tube?

1. Use moistened, cotton-tip swabs to clean the nose.
2. Encourage intake of oral fluids to increase hydration.
3. Provide mouth care every other day to prevent dehydration.
4. Apply tension to the tube to prevent movement.

Short Answer

111. A patient with congestive heart failure has been monitoring her daily weight at home. The patient presents for a clinic visit and reports a 10-pound weight gain over the past week. Calculate how many kilograms the patient gained.

Multiple Choice

112. A patient with peripheral vascular disease has venous congestion in the lower extremities. Which intervention would decrease congestion and improve venous return?

1. Increase the amount of time the patient stands.
2. Elevate the extremities above the level of the heart.
3. Use constrictive clothing to decrease the swelling.
4. Encourage decreased ambulation until the swelling decreases.

113. A patient with a large sternal wound complains of incisional pain with coughing. The patient has just been medicated for pain. Which non-pharmacological action might the nurse take to decrease the patient's incisional pain?

1. Provide a pillow to splint the incision.
2. Place the patient in a prone position.

3. Change the patient's position more frequently.

4. Increase the patient's physical activity.

114. Which statement about the use of garlic as a complementary therapy for cardiovascular disease is true?

1. Garlic promotes blood pressure reduction through vasodilation of blood vessels.

2. Garlic lowers cholesterol by interfering with absorption of the substance in the gastrointestinal tract.

3. Garlic increases platelet aggregation and promotes clotting.

4. Garlic inhibits the synthesis of prostaglandins and promotes an anti-inflammatory effect.

115. Which intervention would be appropriate for a nurse to include when discussing foot care with a patient with peripheral vascular disease? (Select all that apply.)

1. Dry the feet thoroughly after bathing.

2. Cut off all corns and calluses.

3. Educate the patient to break in new footwear to prevent tissue injury.

4. Sit with the legs crossed to decrease swelling.

5. Use constrictive clothing on the feet and ankles.

6. Wash the feet with mild soap and warm water.

7. Use heating pads to improve circulation to the feet.

116. A patient is receiving oxygen at a rate of 2 L/min. The patient's oxygen saturation levels decrease, so the nurse increases the oxygen delivery rate to 3 L/min. What is the approximate concentration of oxygen that is being delivered by the nasal cannula?

1. 21%.

2. 24%.

3. 28%.

4. 32%.

117. What is the expected outcome from teaching a patient biofeedback techniques?

1. Promotion of muscle contraction.

2. Greater control over physiologic processes.

3. Greater contentment with life.

4. Increased self-esteem.

118. After the patient starts on a low-fat, low-sodium diet, the nurse notices that the patient consumes less than 10% of meals. The patient had previously eaten 75% to 100% of meals. Based on the assessment, what is the nurse's best action?

1. Contact the dietician to speak with the patient about menu selections.

2. Report the findings to the physician.

3. Ask the family to bring in meals that include all of the patient's favorite foods.

4. Add in a few high-fat and high-sodium selections to encourage the patient to eat.

Short Answer

119. Based on the following items, calculate the fluid intake, in milliliters, for the patient.

Apple juice: 8 ounces

Carbonated beverage: 12 ounces

Broth: 6 ounces

Water with medications: 4 ounces

Multiple Choice

120. A patient diagnosed with angina is instructed to rest when having an episode of chest pain. What is the best explanation for how rest relieves the pain associated with angina?

1. Coronary blood vessels dilate and increase myocardial cell perfusion.

2. Increased venous return to the heart decreases myocardial oxygen needs.

3. Coronary arteries constrict and shunt blood to vital areas of the myocardium.

4. A balance between myocardial cellular needs and demand is achieved.

121. A patient is prescribed total parenteral nutrition. Which finding indicates that a desired nutritional goal has been achieved?

1. Total serum protein, 6.5 g/dL.

2. Blood urea nitrogen, 45 mg/dL.

3. Serum albumin, 2.0 g/dL.

4. Serum transferrin, 150 mg/dL.

122. A nursing diagnosis of "activity intolerance related to dyspnea" is formulated for a patient. Which finding would support this diagnosis?

1. Three-pillow orthopnea when sleeping at night.

2. Inability to walk to the bathroom without shortness of breath.

3. Rales, rhonchi, and tachypnea upon assessment.

4. Complaints of lightheadedness when sitting up in bed.

Identification

123. Review the nutrition label from the food product and determine what advice the nurse should give to a patient with arteriosclerosis regarding this food choice.

Nutrition Facts

Serving Size 1 cup (228 g)
Servings Per Container 2

Amount per Serving

Calories 250	Calories from Fat 110

% Daily Value*

Total Fat 12g	**18%**
Saturated Fat 3g	**15%**
Trans Fat 1.5g	
Cholesterol 30mg	**10%**
Sodium 470g	**20%**
Total Carbohydrate 31g	**10%**
Dietary Fiber 0g	**0%**
Sugars 5g	
Protein 5g	

Vitamin A	4%	•	Vitamin C	2%
Calcium	20%	•	Iron	4%

* Percent Daily Values are based on a 2,000 calorie diet. Your daily values may be higher or lower depending on your calorie needs:

		Calories	2,000	2,500
Total Fat	Less than		65g	80g
Sat Fat	Less than		20g	25g
Cholesterol	Less than		300mg	300mg
Sodium	Less than		2,400mg	2,400mg
Total Carbohydrate			300g	375g
Dietary Fiber			25g	30g

Multiple Choice

124. You are caring for a patient with a urine output of 350 cc in a 24-hour period. Which term would you use to describe this finding?

1. Polyuria.
2. Anuria.
3. Dysuria.
4. Oliguria.

125. A post-operative patient who underwent an abdominal aortic aneurysm repair has a nasogastric tube set to low intermittent suction. The patient complains of nausea, is vomiting, and has abdominal discomfort. Which action should the nurse take first?

1. Administer pain medication.
2. Check the abdominal dressing.

3. Assess the nasogastric tube for proper operation.
4. Contact the physician to discuss the need for an antiemetic.

126. A post-operative cardiac surgery patient is started on enteral nutrition. Which statement regarding enteral nutrition is true?

1. Enteral nutrition does not require a functional gastrointestinal tract.
2. Enteral nutrition is more costly than parenteral nutrition.
3. The subclavian vein is the most common site for enteral catheter insertion.
4. Aspiration pneumonitis is a complication of enteral therapy.

PHARMACOLOGICAL AND PARENTERAL THERAPIES

Multiple Choice

127. The nurse is preparing to administer a loading dose of lidocaine for a patient in ventricular tachycardia. The patient weighs 154 pounds. The order reads as follows: "Administer lidocaine 1 mg/kg IV bolus for ventricular tachycardia." The medication is supplied in a 100-mg syringe (10 mg/mL). How many milliliters of the medication would the nurse need to administer?

1. 0.7 mL.
2. 3.8 mL.
3. 7 mL.
4. 38 mL.

128. A blood pressure of 230/150 mm Hg is found when a patient presents to the emergency room. The patient is given nitroprusside (Nipride). What is the desired action of this drug?

1. It relaxes the smooth muscles of the arterioles and veins.
2. It reduces blood volume.
3. It blocks the action of angiotensin II.
4. It blocks the action of aldosterone on the kidneys.

129. A patient was recently started on an angiotensin-converting enzyme (ACE) inhibitor. The patient presents to the outpatient clinic with a complaint of a dry, irritating, nonproductive cough. Which action should the nurse take?

1. Assess the patient further for symptoms of a respiratory problem.

2. Notify the prescriber; these findings indicate an adverse effect of the medication.

3. These findings are a desired action of the medication.

4. Discontinue the medication; ACE inhibitors are contraindicated in patients with respiratory problems.

130. A patient is prescribed hydrochlorothiazide (HydroDiuril) for the initial treatment of hypertension. What is the action of this drug?

1. It blocks stimulation of beta$_1$ receptors in the sympathetic nervous system.

2. It decreases the reabsorption of sodium and water in the distal renal tubule.

3. It promotes the movement of extravascular fluids into the vascular compartment by osmotic pressure.

4. It prevents angiotensin II from binding with receptor sites.

131. An adult patient's prescription reads as follows: "Infuse 80 mEq of potassium chloride in 100 cc D$_5$W over 30 minutes." Based on the nurse's understanding of potassium administration, what is the most appropriate action?

1. Administer the medication.

2. Contact the prescriber about the order.

3. Monitor the EKG during the medication's administration.

4. Switch the administration route to oral.

132. The nurse is administering furosemide (Lasix) to a patient who has edema associated with congestive heart failure. What is the most appropriate parameter for the nurse to monitor regarding the effectiveness of this drug?

1. Serum potassium level.

2. Daily weight.

3. Abdominal girth measurement.

4. Urine specific gravity.

133. The nurse is monitoring a patient who is routinely taking newly prescribed nitroglycerin. The patient tells the nurse that he has been experiencing a pounding headache. What is the most likely reason for this finding?

1. It is a symptom of drug toxicity.

2. It is an adverse effect of the drug.

3. The finding has no association with the drug therapy.

4. The patient has developed a nitrate tolerance.

Matching

Match the medication with the correct statement about the drug's indication, action, and side effect.

134. Gemfibrozil (Lopid).

135. Nicotinic acid (Niacin).

136. Simvistatin (Zocor).

137. Ezetimibe (Zetia).

1. Reduces VLDL and increases HDL levels. Gastrointestinal disturbances and an increased risk of gallstones may occur.

2. Lowers LDL cholesterol and VLDL triglyceride levels; raises HDL. May cause severe flushing.

3. Lowers LDL level, increases HDL level, and slows progression of coronary artery disease. Adverse effects may include myopathy and hepatotoxicity.

4. Lowers LDL, triglycerides, and apolipoprotein B levels by blocking absorption in the gastrointestinal tract. Minimal adverse effects have been identified.

Multiple Choice

138. A patient with acute coronary syndrome is administered thrombolytic therapy. Which portion of the EKG tracing would the nurse observe to determine the effectiveness of the medication?

1. PR interval.

2. Width of QRS complex.

3. ST-segment.

4. QT interval.

139. A postoperative cardiac surgery patient is being discharged with a prescription for acetaminophen/oxycodone (Percocet) for pain control. Which statement by the patient indicates a need for further education about the medication by the nurse?

1. "If I experience constipation, I should maintain my level of physical activity, increase my fluid intake, and take a stool softener."

2. "I should not drive when taking the medication because it can make me drowsy."

3. "I should take an extra dose of the medication if the pain is not controlled."

4. "If I get dizzy and lightheaded, I should sit or lie down and then move slowly when getting back up."

140. When completing discharge teaching for a patient who has experienced a myocardial infarction, the patient asks the nurse why aspirin has been prescribed daily. What is the nurse's best response?

1. "Aspirin is used as a prophylactic analgesic to reduce pain."

2. "The medication helps to maintain coronary blood flow by decreasing platelet aggregation in the coronary arteries."

3. "Aspirin is used to prevent fever associated with the inflammatory response in myocardial infarction."

4. "The medication increases the amount of blood in the coronary arteries."

141. The nurse is preparing to administer digoxin (Lanoxin) to an adult patient. Given the nurse's knowledge of the medication, which assessment should the nurse complete prior to administering the digoxin?

1. Assess the apical pulse rate.
2. Obtain a blood pressure.
3. Check a radial pulse.
4. Ask the patient if he has experienced any chest pain.

142. Verapamil (Calan) is administered to a patient with supraventricular tachycardia (SVT). What is the expected outcome of this medication's administration?

1. Reduced heart rate.
2. Increased heart rate.
3. Improved strength of myocardial contractility.
4. Decreased blood pressure.

143. An infusion device malfunctions, causing a patient to receive the entire contents of a 250 cc IV bag of heparin solution in less than 15 minutes. The bag contained 25,000 units of heparin in 250 cc of D_5W. What is the first-line pharmacologic treatment for a heparin overdose?

1. Vitamin K.
2. Coumadin.
3. Protamine sulfate.
4. Calcium gluconate.

144. What education will be required for a patient who is prescribed transdermal nitroglycerin?

1. Wipe off the previous dose before applying a new dose.
2. Apply the medication over a hairy area of the body.
3. Use the same site of application with each dose.
4. Vary the time of application for each daily dose.

Short Answer

145. The nurse is preparing to administer digoxin (Lanoxin) 0.125 mg by mouth. Tablets are available that contain 0.25 mg of medication. How many tablets would the nurse administer?

Multiple Choice

146. Aminoglycosides are administered to a patient for a postoperative infection. Which finding would be an indicator of an adverse effect of the therapy?

1. BUN, 11 mg/dL; creatinine, 1.2 mg/dL.
2. Complaints of changes in hearing.
3. WBC, 5.5 mm^3.
4. Jaundice and pruritus.

147. A patient is receiving intravenous fluids for the management of hypovolemic shock. What is the primary effect of this kind of fluid therapy?

1. Increases preload.
2. Decreases preload.
3. Increases afterload.
4. Decreases afterload.

148. Which factor, if present in a patient's history, should the nurse recognize as likely to interfere with the action of a prescribed antihypertensive medication?

1. Participation in a weekly exercise program.
2. Loss of 6 pounds in 1 month.
3. Use of an over-the-counter nasal decongestant.
4. Daily fluid intake of 2 L.

149. The nurse is caring for a patient with acute coronary syndrome who is receiving alteplase (tPA). Which adverse effect should the nurse monitor the patient for?

1. Fluid retention.
2. Bleeding.
3. Muscle pain.
4. Hepatomegaly.

150. What is the desired effect of metoprolol (Lopressor) when it is used to treat angina pectoris?

1. Decrease the workload of the myocardium.
2. Reduce coronary perfusion by constriction of the coronary veins.
3. Promote impulse conduction through the sino-atrial node.
4. Increase preload and venous return to the heart.

151. Which statement is true regarding the administration of reteplase (Retavase) in the treatment of acute coronary syndrome?

1. A patient will continue to take thrombolytics by mouth for several months following an acute myocardial infarction to prevent re-occlusion of the coronary artery.
2. The most appropriate way to monitor the effectiveness of thrombolytic therapy is to observe the patient for signs of decreased edema.
3. A generalized rash is the adverse effect most commonly associated with the administration of thrombolytics.
4. Thrombolytic therapy should be initiated within the first 4 to 6 hours from the onset of chest pain.

152. Which antihypertensive medication prevents the conversion of angiotensin I to angiotensin II?

1. Alpha-receptor antagonist.
2. Angiotensin-receptor blocker.
3. Beta-adrenergic blocker.
4. Angiotensin-converting enzyme (ACE) inhibitor.

153. The cardiac monitor indicates the patient has a bradycardia with a rate of 40. Upon assessment, the patient is diaphoretic and complains of chest pain. Which pharmacologic intervention would the nurse anticipate administering in this scenario?

1. Lidocaine.
2. Adenosine.
3. Epinephrine.
4. Atropine.

154. For which patient is administration of alteplase (Activase) for treatment of a myocardial infarction contraindicated?

1. A 26-year-old man who smokes cigarettes.
2. A 30-year-old woman who was in a motor vehicle accident 6 months ago.
3. A 42-year-old man who has a bleeding gastric ulcer.
4. A 48-year-old woman who is postmenopausal.

155. A patient's medicinal history includes the use of the herbal medication garlic and the prescribed medication warfarin (Coumadin). Based on the nurse's knowledge of drug–drug interactions, which problem could occur when a patient takes both of these products concurrently?

1. Increased bleeding potential.
2. Elevated blood pressure.
3. Decreased immune function.
4. Altered renal perfusion.

156. How does a calcium-channel blocker affect vascular smooth muscle?

1. It blocks the influx of calcium into the smooth muscle cells and prevents vasoconstriction.
2. It prevents parasympathetic stimulation of the smooth muscle and promotes vasodilation.
3. It promotes myocardial venous circulation by blocking calcium entry into myocardial cells.
4. It improves the automaticity of myocardial cells by blocking the influx of calcium and increases the heart rate.

157. The nurse is preparing to administer carvedilol (Coreg) to a patient. Which action should the nurse take first?

1. Assess the patient's current pulse and blood pressure.
2. Review the patient's urine output as recorded by nurses on the previous shift.
3. Check the patency of the patient's IV line.
4. Find the results of the patient's last blood pressure measurement.

158. A patient with congestive heart failure was prescribed digoxin. The lab reports a digoxin level of 2.9 ng/mL. The next dose of digoxin is due to be administered now. Which action should the nurse take?

1. Assess the patient for cardiac symptoms of toxicity; if none are identified, administer the drug.

2. Administer the medication; the patient's digoxin level is within the therapeutic range.

3. Assess the apical pulse rate. If the pulse is normal, administer the medication.

4. Hold the medication and contact the prescriber.

Short Answer

159. A patient has been diagnosed with a myocardial infarction, and heparin therapy is initiated. The order is for heparin 25,000 units/250 cc D₅W to infuse at 1,100 units/hour. Which rate would the nurse set on the infusion device?

REDUCTION OF RISK POTENTIAL

Short Answer

160. The nurse is asked to calculate a risk prediction score for a patient with no currently known heart disease. Use the tables for calculating a Framingham risk prediction score for a male, Caucasian patient with the following risk factors for coronary heart disease:

> Age: 62
> Total cholesterol: 230 mg/dL
> Smoker
> History of diabetes
> HDL: 42 mg/dL
> Blood pressure with treatment: 148/92

Coronary Disease Risk Production Score Sheet for Men Based on Total Cholesterol Level

Step 1

Age

Years	Points
30-34	-1
35-39	0
40-44	1
45-49	2
50-54	3
55-59	4
60-64	5
65-69	6
70-74	7

Step 2

Total Cholesterol

(mg/dl)	(mmol/L)	Points
<160	<4.14	-3
160-199	4.15-5.17	0
200-239	5.18-6.21	1
240-279	6.22-7.24	2
>280	>7.25	3

Step 3

HDL - Cholesterol

(mg/dl)	(mmol/L)	Points
<35	<0.90	2
35-44	0.91-1.16	1
45-49	1.17-1.29	0
50-59	1.30-1.55	0
>60	>1.56	-2

Step 4

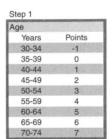

Blood Pressure

Systolic	Diastolic (mmHg)				
	<80	80-84	85-89	90-99	?100
<120	0				
120-129		0 pts			
130-139			1		
140-159				2	
?160					3 pts

Note: When systolic and diastolic pressures provide different estimates for point scores, use the higher number.

Step 5

Diabetes	Points
No	0
Yes	2

Step 6

Smoker	Points
No	0
Yes	2

Step 7 (sum from steps 1 - 6)

Adding up the points

Age	_____
Total Cholesterol	_____
HDL Cholesterol	_____
Blood Pressure	_____
Diabetes	_____
Smoker	_____
Points Total	_____

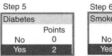

Key

Color	Risk
green	Very low
white	Low
yellow	Moderate
rose	High
red	Very high

Step 8 (determine CHD risk from point total)

CHD Risk

Point Total	10 Yr CHD Risk
?1	2%
0	3%
1	4%
2	4%
3	5%
4	7%
5	8%
6	10%
7	13%
8	16%
9	20%
10	25%
11	31%
12	37%
13	45%
?14	?53%

Step 9 (compare to man of same age)

Comparative Risk

Age (years)	Average 10 Yr CHD Risk	Low* 10 Yr CHD Risk
30–34	3%	2%
35–39	5%	3%
40–44	7%	4%
45–49	11%	4%
50–54	14%	6%
55–59	16%	7%
60–64	21%	9%
65–69	25%	11%
70–74	30%	14%

*Low risk was calculated for a man the same age, normal blood pressure, total cholesterol 160–169 mg/dL, HDL cholesterol 45 mg/dL, non-smoker, no diabetes

Risk estimates were derived from the experience of the NHLBI's Framingham Heart Study, a predominantly Caucasian population in Massachusetts, USA

Multiple Choice

161. Which predisposing factors are associated with the development of infective endocarditis?

1. Antibiotic treatment and coronary artery disease.
2. Damaged endocardial surface and a portal for organism entry.
3. Increased release of myoglobin, which interacts with viral organisms.
4. Existing infection and a damaged pericardium.

162. Which clinical presentation is consistent with chronic anemia?

1. Fatigue, dyspnea at rest, pallor, tachycardia.
2. Hemarthrosis, bruising, prolonged nose bleeds, hematuria.
3. Enlarged lymph nodes, night sweats, fatigue, infections.
4. Fever, lymphadenopathy, sore throat, decreased appetite.

163. Which complication can develop within the heart as a result of prolonged, uncontrolled hypertension in an adult patient?

1. Stroke.
2. Left ventricular hypertrophy.
3. Retinopathy.
4. Carotid stenosis.

164. Which measurement is the best indicator of tissue perfusion?

1. Systolic blood pressure.
2. Diastolic blood pressure.
3. Mean arterial blood pressure.
4. Pulse pressure.

165. A postoperative cardiac surgery patient is administered morphine sulfate 4 mg IV for pain at 0900. The following vital signs, obtained before pain medication administration and 30 minutes after the administration, are noted on the flow sheet:

Time	Nurse Initials	Blood Pressure	Pulse	Respirations	Temperature
0855	NS	142/86	92 bpm	14/min	98.0°F
0930	NS	130/60	80 bpm	6/min	98.2°F

Based on these findings, which action would the nurse anticipate taking?

1. Let the patient continue to sleep.
2. Prepare to administer naloxone (Narcan).
3. Increase the intravenous fluid rate.
4. Place the patient on a cardiac monitor.

166. A patient with congestive heart failure has gained 4 pounds in the past week and states, "I get short of breath when I walk even a few steps." What is the nurse's best response?

1. "Your appetite seems to have improved since your last visit."
2. "Describe how you have been following your treatment plan."
3. "Have you overexerted yourself with your exercise regimen?"
4. "Does your shortness of breath improve with rest?"

167. Sequential pneumatic compression devices are used to prevent which postoperative complication?

1. Atelectasis.
2. Edema.
3. Venous thrombosis.
4. Bleeding.

168. A fluid challenge of 250 mL of normal saline is given to a patient who has pre-renal failure. What is the purpose of this fluid challenge?

1. To dilute the waste products in the intravascular fluid.
2. To cause interstitial fluids to move into the intravascular space.
3. To decrease the pressure in Bowman's capsule so as to promote renal perfusion.
4. To increase cardiac output and promote renal perfusion.

169. Upon assessment, the nurse finds an intravenous access site to be swollen, reddened, cool, and painful to palpation. Which action should the nurse take first?

1. Discontinue the intravenous infusion.
2. Flush the device with saline.
3. Apply a warm compress.
4. Elevate the area.

170. A nurse is assessing a surgical incision for signs of infection. Which signs would the nurse look for?

1. Large amounts of serosanguinous drainage.
2. Eschar formations over the incision line.
3. Granulosis around the edges of the wound.
4. Redness, swelling, and cloudy drainage.

171. A patient with blood loss anemia is receiving a unit of packed red blood cells. The patient's vital signs were taken immediately prior to transfusion at 0725 and again at 0740, 15 minutes after the transfusion had been started. The vital signs were documented on the flow sheet as follows:

Time	Nurse Initials	Blood Pressure	Pulse	Respi- rations	Temper- ature
0725	NS	120/50	88 bpm	14/min	98.4°F
0740	NS	100/60	106 bpm	26/min	101.5°F

Which action should the nurse take first?

1. Increase the rate of infusion.
2. Assess the incision site for signs of infection.
3. Elevate the head of the bed.
4. Stop the transfusion.

172. An expected outcome for a patient who has experienced a myocardial infarction is a gradual increase in activity. The patient states, "How will I know if I am overdoing it?" What is the nurse's best response?

1. "A 50% increase in heart rate from baseline would indicate your readiness to increase activity."
2. "Any sign or symptom of muscle strain would indicate the need to cut back on activity and notify your physician."
3. "At the first sign of chest pain or shortness of breath, you should stop and rest."
4. "The presence of edema in the extremities would indicate a need to cut back on activity."

173. A patient with a history of rheumatic fever is at risk for damage to which part of the cardiovascular system?

1. Aorta.
2. Heart valves.
3. Thoracic baroreceptors.
4. Electrical conduction pathways.

174. A patient is placed on complete bed rest. The nurse understands that this patient is at risk for the development of which venous complication?

1. Thrombophlebitis.
2. Aneurysm.
3. Varicose veins.
4. Thromboangiitis obliterans.

175. Which individual has the highest risk for developing thrombophlebitis?

1. A 35-year-old farmer.
2. A 45-year-old automobile mechanic.
3. A 55-year-old computer programmer.
4. A 62-year-old college football coach.

Identification

176. Which EKG finding should the nurse recognize as an early indicator of hyperkalemia?

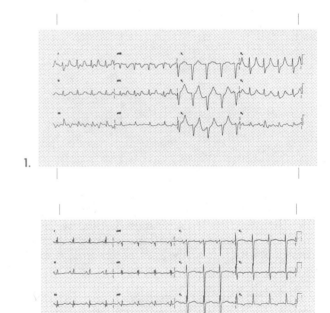

1.

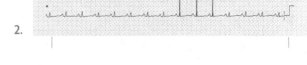

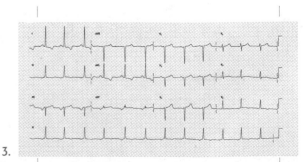

2.

3.

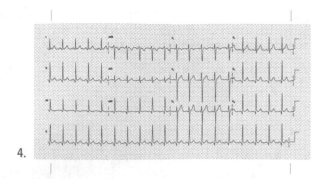

4.

Multiple Choice

177. A normally healthy patient presents to the outpatient clinic with complaints of episodes where the fingers become numb and pale, followed by a period where the fingers are red, throbbing, and painful. These episodes seem to be triggered by cold weather. Based on this information, which problem does the nurse suspect?

1. Venous thrombosis.
2. Raynaud's disease.
3. Buerger's disease.
4. Aneurysm dissection.

178. Which lab test provides the most specific marker for myocardial cell damage?

1. Troponin.
2. Creatinine kinase.
3. D-dimer.
4. LDH.

179. The nurse is caring for a patient in the immediate postoperative period following coronary artery bypass graft surgery. Which finding should the nurse discuss with the physician?

1. Serum sodium of 140 mEq/L.
2. Total urine output of 20 cc for 2 hours.
3. Mediastinal tube drainage of 50 cc in the last 30 minutes.
4. Pulse rate of 90 beats/min.

180. An EKG tracing in lead II is completed. Which finding is normal? (Select all that apply.)

1. Inverted P wave.
2. PR interval is 0.12 to 0.20 second.
3. ST segment is elevated.

4. R-to-R interval is regular.
5. QRS interval is 0.21 second or greater.
6. R wave has a negative deflection.

181. A patient suspected of having cardiac valvular disease undergoes a transesophageal echocardiogram. Nursing care of the patient following this procedure would include observation for which problem?

1. Chest pain.
2. Renal insufficiency.
3. Anxiety.
4. Difficulty swallowing.

182. What is the most serious complication associated with the development of deep vein thrombosis?

1. Edema.
2. Pulmonary embolus.
3. Decubiti.
4. Air embolus.

183. Which factor is associated with the development of secondary hypertension?

1. Family history of hypertension.
2. High dietary sodium intake.
3. Cigarette smoking.
4. A tumor of the adrenal gland.

184. A patient's labwork shows a total cholesterol level of 298 mg/dL and an LDL level of 180 mg/dL. Which statement about the lab values is correct?

1. The LDL level is high, and the total cholesterol level is low.
2. Both values are high.
3. The LDL level is low and the total cholesterol level is high.
4. Both values are normal.

185. Which complication is often associated with the rhythm shown below?

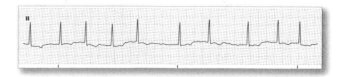

1. Cardiac tamponade.
2. Pericarditis.
3. Emboli.
4. Ventricular hypertrophy.

186. The nurse is assessing several patients in an outpatient clinic. Which patient would it be most important for the nurse to monitor for orthostatic hypotension?

1. A 35-year-old patient with pre-hypertension that is adequately controlled by diet.
2. A 43-year-old patient who complains of dizziness from an inner ear infection.
3. A 68-year-old patient who is taking a loop diuretic.
4. A 72-year-old patient with fluid volume excess.

187. When performing a physical assessment on a patient with left-sided congestive heart failure, which finding would the nurse expect to find?

1. Dependent edema.
2. Hepatomegaly.
3. Distended jugular veins.
4. Bibasilar rales.

188. Which problem would result in an increased hematocrit?

1. Dehydration.
2. Fluid excess.
3. Hypertension.
4. Hypokalemia.

189. The nurse is caring for a patient with an acute coronary syndrome who has been admitted to the intensive care unit. The patient has begun to have cardiac dysrhythmias. What is the most probable cause of these dysrhythmias?

1. Respiratory alkalosis.
2. Tissue ischemia.
3. Hyperglycemia.
4. Digitalis toxicity.

190. A patient with severe cardiomyopathy has been on bed rest and has now developed a pressure ulcer. Identify the stage of pressure ulcer that is seen in the picture.

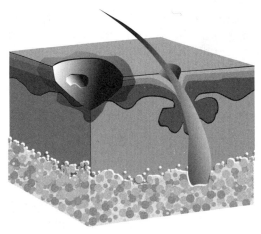

1. Stage I.
2. Stage II.
3. Stage III.
4. Stage IV.

191. A patient is admitted with blunt chest trauma following a motor vehicle accident. A myocardial contusion is suspected. Which diagnostic procedures should the nurse anticipate performing?

1. Chest x-ray and CBC with differential.
2. 12-lead EKG and cardiac enzymes.
3. Cardiac catheterization and coagulation studies.
4. CT scan and basic metabolic profile.

192. Which patient is the most likely candidate to undergo a minimally invasive direct coronary artery bypass grafting (MIDCABG) procedure?

1. A 55-year-old patient with single-vessel coronary artery disease for whom medical management is not effective.
2. A 39-year-old patient with multiple-vessel coronary artery disease with ECG findings of ST depression.
3. A 70-year-old patient with right coronary and circumflex artery occlusions who cannot tolerate myocardial revascularization.
4. A 47-year-old patient with EKG findings indicative of an ST-elevation myocardial infarction.

PHYSIOLOGICAL ADAPTATION

Multiple Choice

193. A patient reports being abruptly awakened from sleep at night with shortness of breath. Which finding would the nurse document?

1. Paroxysmal nocturnal dyspnea.
2. Orthopnea.
3. Cheyne-Stokes respirations.
4. Kussmaul respirations.

194. Which treatments would the nurse anticipate for a patient who is experiencing cardiogenic shock?

1. Corticosteroids, epinephrine, and oxygen.
2. Oxygen, fluids, and O-negative blood.
3. IV nitroglycerin, diuretics, and an intra-aortic balloon pump.
4. Oxygen, dopamine, and lidocaine.

195. Immediately after the initiation of a blood transfusion, the patient complains of tightness in the throat, shortness of breath, and chest pain. What is the priority nursing intervention?

1. Notify the physician.
2. Complete a head-to-toe physical assessment of the patient.
3. Stop the transfusion.
4. Administer sublingual nitroglycerin.

196. Which patient symptoms are associated with right-sided heart failure? (Select all that apply.)

1. Bibasilar rales.
2. Abdominal discomfort.
3. Orthopnea.
4. Hepatomegaly/splenomegaly.
5. Swollen ankles.
6. Ascites.

197. Which procedure would a nurse anticipate preparing for when caring for a patient with cardiac tamponade?

1. Thoracentesis.
2. Mediastinal tube insertion.
3. Pulmonary artery catheter insertion.
4. Pericardiocentesis.

198. What is the cause of cardiogenic shock?

1. Loss of fluid from the vascular space.
2. Increased size of the vascular compartment.
3. Inability of the heart to pump adequately.
4. Obstruction of flow in the vasculature.

199. An emergency medical technician reports that a patient was involved in a frontal impact collision in which the steering wheel was noted to be depressed. Based on the EMT report and the clinical findings of hypotension, muffled heart tones, and distended neck veins, which problem would the nurse suspect?

1. Laceration of the pulmonary vein.
2. Pneumothorax.
3. Cardiac tamponade.
4. Acute coronary syndrome.

200. Which statement provides an explanation for the hypertension associated with polycystic kidney disease?

1. Afterload is increased due to pressure on the abdominal aorta.
2. Bleeding into the cysts results in an increased intravascular volume.
3. Compression of intrarenal blood vessels results in activation of the renin–angiotensin–aldosterone mechanism.
4. Erythropoietin is released and promotes an increase in circulating blood volume.

201. Which statement is true about the renin–angiotensin–aldosterone mechanism?

1. Aldosterone acts on the renal tubules and promotes the elimination of sodium and water through the urine.
2. Angiotensinogen is the catalyst for the conversion of angiotensin I to angiotensin II.
3. Renin is released from the juxtaglomerular cells and is the substance responsible for the conversion of angiotensinogen to angiotensin I.
4. The stimulus for the release of renin from the renal tubule is an elevation in the blood pressure.

202. What is the cardiac output of a patient who weighs 78 kg, has a stroke volume of 70 mL, and has a pulse of 85 beats/min?

1. Not enough data is provided to calculate the answer.
2. 5,460 mL.
3. 5,950 mL.
4. 6,630 mL.

203. Upon assessment, the nurse notes that the patient has a thready pulse. Which term best describes the pathophysiology of this finding?

1. Hypertension.
2. Circulatory overload.
3. Inflammation of the vessel.
4. Decreased cardiac output.

204. Which term best describes angina that is caused by spasm of a coronary blood vessel?

1. Classic angina.
2. Variant (Prinzmetal) angina.
3. Unstable angina.
4. Crescendo angina.

205. Which is the best description of the pathophysiology of an increased systolic blood pressure in atherosclerosis?

1. Increased arterial elasticity and lumen diameter.
2. Increased arterial elasticity and decreased lumen diameter.
3. Decreased arterial elasticity and increased lumen diameter.
4. Decreased arterial elasticity and lumen diameter.

206. In which type of vessel are gases, nutrients, and wastes exchanged?

1. Lymphatic vessels.
2. Arterioles.
3. Capillaries.
4. Venules.

207. A patient experiences stimulation of the vagus nerve. What is the major effect that this nerve stimulation would have on the cardiovascular system?

1. Decreased heart rate.
2. Strengthened contractility.
3. Increased stroke volume.
4. Vasodilation of blood vessels in the skin.

208. Which statement best describes the physiologic factors that influence blood pressure?

1. Chemoreceptors respond to a decreased oxygen level in the blood by stimulating the renin–angiotensin–aldosterone system to dilate the blood vessels.
2. Baroreceptors respond to sudden changes in blood pressure by stimulating the autonomic nervous system.
3. Decreased stroke volume stimulates the parasympathetic nervous system.
4. Antidiuretic hormone is released in response to stimulation of the renin–angiotensin–aldosterone system.

209. Which phase of the electrocardiogram represents atrial depolarization?

1. P wave.
2. QRS complex.
3. T wave.
4. ST segment.

Matching

Match the symptom of hypovolemic shock with its physiologic cause.

210. Cool, pale skin.

211. Increased rate and depth of respirations.

212. Increased urine specific gravity.

213. Increased pulse rate.

1. Increased release of antidiuretic hormone.
2. Vasoconstriction of peripheral vessels.
3. Compensatory mechanism related to metabolic acidosis.
4. Stimulation of beta$_1$ receptors of the sympathetic nervous system.

214. A patient with a ruptured aortic aneurysm is in hypovolemic shock. The patient has a pulmonary artery catheter in place. Which hemodynamic information would the nurse anticipate finding?

1. Mean arterial pressure: 80 mmHg.
2. Central venous pressure: 0 mmHg.
3. Pulmonary capillary wedge pressure: 10 mmHg.
4. Cardiac output: 4 L/min.

Multiple Choice

215. A carotid bruit is identified upon completion of a patient's physical assessment. Which underlying pathophysiology is associated with the development of a bruit?

1. Arterial occlusive disease.
2. Pericarditis.
3. Congestive heart failure.
4. Valvular defect.

216. Which valvular disorder results in an impedance of forward blood flow into the left ventricle and increased workload of the left atrium?

   1. Aortic insufficiency.
   2. Mitral stenosis.
   3. Tricuspid regurgitation.
   4. Pulmonic incompetence.

217. What is the pathophysiologic basis for the pain associated with angina?

   1. Pressure on the phrenic nerve during diastole.
   2. Inability of the left ventricle to contract fully.
   3. Myocardial oxygen demand that exceeds supply.
   4. Incompetent cardiac valves during systole.

218. Upon physical assessment of a patient's lower extremities, the nurse observes warm skin, with brown pigmentation noted around the ankles. Which condition should the nurse suspect?

   1. Venous insufficiency.
   2. Arterial occlusive disease.
   3. Venous stasis ulcers.
   4. Arterial aneurysm.

219. To achieve effective chest compressions in an adult who requires cardiopulmonary resuscitation, what depth of compression should be achieved?

   1. $\frac{1}{2}$ to 1 inch.
   2. 1 to 1$\frac{1}{2}$ inches.
   3. 1$\frac{1}{2}$ to 2 inches.
   4. 2 to 2$\frac{1}{2}$ inches.

220. Prior to pushing intravenous medications during cardiopulmonary resuscitation, which action would be a priority for safe care?

   1. Assess the site for signs of infection.
   2. Flush the IV line with normal saline.
   3. Insert a second IV.
   4. Ensure the patency of the IV line.

221. What is the most common clinical manifestation of cardiac ischemia?

   1. Nausea.
   2. Pain.
   3. Jugular vein distention.
   4. Hypothermia.

222. The nurse is unable to palpate a carotid pulse on an adult patient with chest compressions in progress. Which priority action should the nurse take?

   1. Stop the compressions and assess for a femoral pulse.
   2. Continue the compressions and assess for a brachial pulse.
   3. Notify the compressor to reposition the hands and increase the depth of the compressions.
   4. Implement the cricoid pressure maneuver.

MANAGEMENT OF CARE

1. Correct Answer: **3**

Rationale: To ensure the safety of patients, the night-shift nurse should immediately notify the nurse manager of the problem. In the absence of the nurse manager, the charge nurse or nursing supervisor should be notified. The manager/charge nurse/nursing supervisor can then pursue the appropriate administrative actions for the situation.

2. Correct Answer: **3**

Rationale: The ethical principle of autonomy applies to this situation, in that a competent patient has the right to make decisions for himself or herself. Autonomy is the right of a person to make his or her own decisions.

3. Correct Answer: **2**

Rationale: The patient's readiness to quit smoking is the key factor in beginning a smoking cessation program. Tobacco cessation strategies will be most effective in a patient who demonstrates a readiness to stop smoking.

4. Correct Answer: **2**

Rationale: The most frequent cause of nosocomial infection is contamination caused by the transmission of organisms on the hands of healthcare workers. In an acute care setting, healthcare workers can carry organisms that have a strong pathogenic potential. A patient who received a heart transplant is at an increased risk for infection owing to suppression of the immune system by medications to prevent transplant rejection. Hand washing will reduce the amount of bacteria to which patients are exposed and decrease the risk of transmission of organisms to patients.

5. Correct Answer: **3**

Rationale: Case management is a type of patient care delivery system that is designed to achieve maximum patient outcomes and control costs. A clinical pathway or care map is an interdisciplinary tool for care planning within a case management delivery model. The tools are used as a plan for care and to track patient progress toward identified outcomes within specific time frames.

6. Correct Answer: **2**

Rationale: Confidentiality is related to the concept of privacy. Information obtained from or related to the care of an individual should not be discussed without the permission of that individual unless there is a direct threat to the social good. The nurse violated the patient's confidentiality when discussing his or her specific case with another individual who was not directly involved in the management of the patient's care.

7. Correct Answer: **2**

Rationale: The allocation of a resource that is in short supply is the basis for this scenario. The ethical principle of justice (i.e., "like cases being treated alike") applies here. Specifically, distributive justice refers to the allocation of social benefits and burdens based on equality, individual need, effort, societal contribution, individual merit, and legal entitlement. The establishment of the computerized database and a fair means of distributing organs to those patients most in need would be an example of distributive justice.

8. Correct Answer: **1**

Rationale: The appropriate prioritization to be considered for the scenario is airway, breathing, and circulation. Opening the airway and ventilating the patient focuses on the priorities of airway and breathing.

9. Correct Answer: **4**

Rationale: Voluntary consent given in writing by the patient is required before a non-emergent surgery or other invasive procedure can be performed. Informed consent occurs when a patient has the full understanding of the procedure, its risks, its potential complications, and alternatives to care. The giving of consent protects both the patient and the physician. Although every effort should be made to obtain informed consent, in a life-saving situation or emergency, the physician may proceed without consent. The doctrine of implied consent is applied to emergent/life-saving situations.

10. Correct Answer: **8**

Rationale: Diagnosis-related groups were created in 1983. They are a prospective inpatient reimbursement system for Medicare and Medicaid patients for a given surgery or episode of illness. This system was established as a means to control healthcare costs.

11. Correct Answer: **1**

Rationale: Medicare is a federally run program that was established in 1965 under the Social Security Act and provides health insurance to people age 65 and older.

12. Correct Answer: **3**

Rationale: National Patient Safety goals target critical areas where patient safety can be improved through specific actions by healthcare organizations. The Joint Commission on Accreditation of Healthcare Organizations is the agency responsible for establishing these goals. The organization also surveys hospitals to determine their compliance in meeting the goals.

13. Correct Answer: **4**

Rationale: The Emergency Transfer and Active Labor Act passed in 1986 as a part of the Consolidated Omnibus Budget Reconciliation Act. With regard to emergency care and treatment, the act indicates that any patient who comes to an Emergency Department and requests examination or treatment for a medical condition must be provided with an appropriate medical screening examination to determine whether he or she is suffering from an emergency medical condition. If the patient has such a condition, then the hospital is obligated to either provide him or her with treatment until the individual is stable or to transfer the patient to another hospital as outlined by the statute's directives.

14. Correct Answer: **7**

Rationale: The American Heart Association is a national voluntary health agency whose mission is to reduce disability and death from cardiovascular diseases and stroke. The organization provides numerous resources to achieve its established mission.

15. Correct Answer: **3**

Rationale: A liability is an obligation that can be enforced by law and determined by a court. A nurse is legally liable for his or her actions. The charge nurse is responsible for delegating the right task, in the right circumstance, to the right person, with the right direction/communication and the right supervision/evaluation. In this scenario, the charge nurse has delegated an assignment (wrong task) to an unlicensed person (wrong person) who does not have documented skill or competency in the procedure. The charge nurse could be liable for inappropriate delegation of an assignment to unlicensed personnel.

16. Correct Answer: **3**

Rationale: Nurses in a community-based practice setting utilize three levels of preventive care: primary, secondary, and tertiary. Tertiary prevention focuses on improving quality of life and preventing deterioration once illness or a disease has occurred. A cardiac rehabilitation program begins during hospitalization and progresses to the community upon patient discharge. The purpose of such a rehabilitation program is to promote progressive activity and reduce risk factors associated with an existing disease.

17. Correct Answer: **1**

Rationale: The purpose of the referral is the administration of antibiotics to treat a sternal wound infection. The most appropriate referral choice based on the patient's need would be a home healthcare service. Nursing services required based on this scenario would include intravenous therapy, wound management, and patient/family teaching.

18. Correct Answer: **3**

Rationale: Certification is one type of credentialing. It is defined as the documented validation of specific qualifications demonstrated by the individual registered nurse in the provision of professional nursing care within a defined area of practice. It is one means by which competency can be assessed. Certification is usually awarded by a professional organization and is not a legal credential. The American Nurses' Credentialing Center is one example of a professional organization that is responsible for the certification of nurses in a variety of practice areas.

19. Correct Answer: **4**

Rationale: The 1991 Patient Self-Determination Act encourages people to prepare advance directives, such as the durable power of attorney for health care. With a durable power of attorney for health care, the patient designates another individual to make healthcare decisions on his or her behalf if the patient should become incapacitated.

20. Correct Answer: **3**

    Rationale: Ventricular fibrillation is a life-threatening dysrhythmia that is treated by defibrillation. In defibrillation, an electrical current causes simultaneous depolarization of myocardial cells. When the cells repolarize, the goal is to have the sinus node regain pacemaker status.

21. Correct Answer: **2**

    Rationale: In this scenario, the nurse is using the therapeutic communication technique of restating. Restating is used to demonstrate to the patient that the nurse is listening to what has been said and to reinforce important components of a conversation.

22. Correct Answer: **2**

    Rationale: Through the use of critical thinking skills, the nurse should recognize that the patient observations are not congruent with the vital signs. For this reason, the nurse should validate the blood pressure measurement to ensure its accuracy and avoid a potential measurement error.

23. Correct Answer: **2**

    Rationale: Social workers assist patients and families in arranging the necessary support to facilitate discharge to the community. As an intervention, the nurse could refer the patient's case to a social worker for identification of available resources for medication payment assistance.

24. Correct Answer: **1**

    Rationale: In the scenario, the patient is unable to perform activities of daily living (ADLs) on his own and will need assistance and support to perform these ADLs. The priority factor for the nurse to assess is identification of who will provide the patient care upon discharge. Identification of the person who will assume the responsibility for care is a critical factor in the establishment of the discharge plan.

25. Correct Answer: **2**

    Rationale: The priority referral to dietary services should be for the patient who has not had an adequate caloric intake for 2 days. The infusion of 1,000 cc of D_5W will provide only approximately 180 calories.

26. Correct Answer: **2**

    Rationale: Daily weights are an important intervention and a focus of a discharge teaching plan to ensure effective management of fluid volume. At the same time each day, the patient should perform and record a daily weight. Weight gains greater than 0.9 to 1.4 kg or per parameters as identified by the healthcare provider, should be reported, as they can be indicative of fluid volume excess.

27. Correct Answer: **4**

    Rationale: This scenario represents a compromising or negotiating style for dealing with conflict. Such a conflict management style allows for the nurses to come to a compromise that is acceptable to both of them.

28. Correct Answer: **2**

    Rationale: Hospitals need to continually improve the care that they deliver to patients. Such quality-related activities are often mandated by accrediting agencies. To ensure ongoing improvement, organizations should work with their employees to identify quality issues. Resources, such as quality management staff, are available to assist with analysis of problems such as an increase in pressure ulcers.

29. Correct Answer: **3**

    Rationale: An embolectomy is a procedure used on a viable extremity to remove an arterial thrombus and restore blood flow to the involved lower extremity. Neurovascular assessment of the extremity is a priority action in the first 24 hours after the procedure to assess for any signs that may be indicative of reocclusion. The goal of treatment is to promote tissue perfusion, prevent cellular ischemia, and avoid any additional complications.

30. Correct Answers: **1, 2, 3, 5**

    Rationale: Informed consent is knowledgeable, voluntary permission obtained from a patient to perform a test or procedure. The consent is written, identifies the procedure to be performed, and is signed by the patient or the person who is legally responsible for the patient. It is the responsibility of the surgeon to explain the procedure, alternative treatments, and any risks to the patient. The patient must have the opportunity to ask questions. Given that this patient is illiterate, the consent form must be read to the patient. Once this is completed, the patient is competent to sign the consent with an X or other mark.

SECTION I

SECTION II

SECTION III

SECTION IV

SECTION V

SECTION VI

SECTION VII

SECTION VIII

SECTION IX

SECTION X

31. Correct Answer: **1**

Rationale: The priority action is a patient assessment. Ventricular bigeminy will affect cardiac output, so the patient must first be assessed to determine the individual effect of the rhythm on cardiac output and his or her response to the dysrhythmia.

32. Correct Answer: **2**

Rationale: Initially, the company will need to know the type of oxygen delivery device and the amount of oxygen ordered for home therapy. This information will provide the company with baseline information to set up the service.

33. Correct Answer: **1**

Rationale: New technology has contributed to the increasing cost of cardiovascular care and health care overall. Intracoronary stents, automated internal cardioverter defibrillators, positron emission tomography (PET) scans, and ventricular assist devices are all examples of costly technologies that can be used in the provision of cardiovascular care.

34. Correct Answer: **1**

> ~~120/60~~ **Error NS**
> 120/80

Rationale: The medical record is a legal document. To correct an error, the nurse should draw a single line through the error, write "error," initial the error, and then write in the correct information.

35. Correct Answer: **3**

Rationale: The first action a nurse should take upon accidental removal of a chest tube is to cover the chest tube insertion site with a dressing that is taped on three sides. The three-sided dressing allows air to escape from the site, but promotes coverage of the wound and occlusion to prevent air from reentering the pleural space.

36. Correct Answer: **2**

Rationale: A task or procedure can be delegated if it does not require any independent nursing judgment, assessment, complex observation, or critical thinking. The licensed nurse should consider the "five rights" of delegation when determining whether a task should be delegated: right task, right circumstances, right person, right communication or direction, and right evaluation or feedback. Obtaining vital signs is a standard task that can be delegated to a nursing assistant. This skill must be performed within the scope of the unlicensed staff member's job description. In addition, the assistant must have been trained in the skill of vital sign measurement and have experience with the task.

37. Correct Answer: **2**

Rationale: Before establishing a performance improvement plan for the nurse, the manager needs to have an understanding of which performance domain the issue is associated with. Domains of performance include cognitive, interpersonal, psychomotor/technical, decision-making and cultural. The manager will need to make an assessment of the reason for the marginal performance by discussing the problem with the employee.

38. Correct Answer: **3**

Rationale: A competency is a demonstrated skill or ability that a nurse needs to function in health care. Nursing competency can be assessed in the cognitive, interpersonal, decision-making, and psychomotor/technical domains through a variety of methods such as exams, tests, interviews, and observations. A skills check-off would assess the nurse's ability to perform a skill safely, effectively, and efficiently. Performance of a skill assesses the psychomotor/technical domain of competence.

39. Correct Answer: **Ventricular tachycardia**

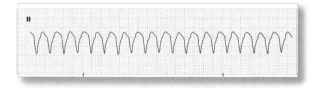

Rationale: The patient with ventricular tachycardia should be assessed first. Ventricular tachycardia is an electrical rhythm that originates in the ventricles of the heart. The rhythm is characterized by at least three consecutive ventricular complexes with a rate greater than 100 beats/min. Two types of ventricular tachycardia are distinguished: stable and unstable. Further assessment of the patient will determine the type of ventricular tachycardia and the necessary treatment priorities.

40. Correct Answer: 3

Rationale: Fraud is a deliberate deception for personal gain. In this scenario, the nurse has attempted to gain a position by providing incorrect information (certification status) to the employer. The false declaration of certification is an attempt by the nurse to defraud the employer. Fraud can be prosecuted as a crime.

41. Correct Answer: 2

Rationale: Informed consent is a patient's permission to proceed with a procedure or test. This permission must be given without coercion and with a complete understanding of the procedure or test to be performed and the alternative treatment options available. The document must be written or translated into a language understood by the patient and consent obtained by the person performing the procedure or test. The availability of a trained medical interpreter for the Spanish-speaking patient is necessary for the informed consent process. The ideal situation would be a combination of a trained medical interpreter for the explanation of the procedure or test coupled with a written consent form in the patient's language. The U.S. Department of Health and Human Services provides National Standards on Culturally and Linguistically Appropriate Services for healthcare organizations.

42. Correct Answer: 1

Rationale: A pheochromocytoma is a benign tumor of the adrenal glands. Such a tumor often arises from the adrenal medulla. One function of the adrenal medulla is the release of catecholamines in response to sympathetic nervous system stimulation. Monitoring a patient's blood pressure is an important aspect of nursing management, because catecholamines promote vasoconstriction. The result of vasoconstriction is increased blood pressure. As a consequence, a pheochromocytoma can be a secondary cause of new-onset hypertension.

43. Correct Answer: 2

Rationale: When establishing priorities, the nurse should consider which patient requires immediate attention and which can be put off. The priority assignment of the telemetry bed would be the patient with chest pain who was administered a thrombolytic medication. The patient with a known myocardial infarction who received treatment in the form of thrombolytic therapy would require continuous monitoring for signs of adequate tissue perfusion and prevention of complications such as dysrhythmias.

44. Correct Answer: 2

Rationale: A referral to a community agency will allow the patient to have a contact regarding available smoking cessation resources and promote continuity of care after the acute care hospitalization ends. To achieve the desired smoking cessation outcome, the agency can then match the patient's needs with the appropriate services.

SAFETY AND INFECTION CONTROL

45. Correct Answer: 2

Rationale: The Lasix order is incomplete, because no route of administration is identified. The nurse should clarify the route of administration with the prescriber to avoid a medication error.

Admission Orders					
Patient Name: Jones, Teri					
Patient Number: #3-11316-7					
Date	**Time Written**	**Orders**	**Order Checked**	**Time Noted**	**Nurse's Signature**
1/31/07	0930	① Digoxin 0.125 mg p.o. daily	✓		
		② Lasix 40 mg b.i.d.	✓		
		③ K-lyte 25 mEq p.o. now	✓		
		④ Aspirin 81 mg p.o. daily	✓	1000	*N. Nurse RN*

46. Correct Answer: <u>2</u>

Rationale: Areas of large magnetic fields, such as those found with magnetic resonance imaging (MRI) devices or arc welding equipment and electrical substations, should be avoided. The magnetic field may potentially result in deactivation of certain pacemakers.

47. Correct Answer: <u>1</u>

Rationale: In a traditional chest drainage unit, suction is determined by the water level in the suction control chamber. Sterile water should be added to the system to achieve the prescribed level of suction.

48. Correct Answer: <u>4</u>

Rationale: Transdermal nitroglycerin is absorbed through the skin. Application to a hairless area will promote delivery of the medication via absorption.

49. Correct Answer: <u>1</u>

Rationale: Prevention of infection is a key role of the nurse. The preceptor, upon observing the break in procedure, should offer to obtain another dressing for the nurse. That is, the preceptor should bring the contamination problem to the attention of the new nurse and prevent completion of the procedure with a contaminated dressing.

50. Correct Answer: <u>1</u>

Rationale: The rhythm is a flat-line rhythm. Interpretation of the rhythm will vary based on the patient assessment. This patient shows no signs of distress. Critical thinking would, therefore, lead the nurse to assess for an alternative reason for the flat-line ECG appearance. One alternative would be to check the equipment for any malfunction such as a loose or disconnected ECG lead.

51. Correct Answer: <u>4</u>

Rationale: Warfarin (Coumadin) is an anticoagulant. Care of a patient who is discharged on warfarin should include lab monitoring of the treatment (PT) and minimization of adverse drug effects (bleeding). A patient who believes it is necessary to decrease sodium intake due to the prescription would require further education.

52. Correct Answer: <u>2</u>

Rationale: Thrombolytic drugs degrade existing clots and disrupt the clotting cascade so as to prevent new clots from forming. Bleeding is a complication associated with the use of thrombolytics. Interventions that could result in bleeding, such as arterial puncture, should be avoided during the administration of these drugs.

53. Correct Answer: <u>2</u>

Rationale: The nurse should include the facts of the medication error in the medical record documentation. The factual information for the scenario includes the type, amount, route, and time the medication was administered.

54. Correct Answer: <u>2</u>

Rationale: On a 24-hour clock, the time after 12:00 noon is calculated as 12 + the number of hours past noon (meridian). On a traditional clock, 2:00 P.M. is 2 hours post-meridian (12 + 2) and would be documented as 1400 hours.

55. Correct Answer: <u>1</u>

Rationale: The priorities of emergency care are airway, breathing, and circulation. A bag-valve-mask device is needed to ventilate the patient in the event the patient suffers complications from the cardioversion that result in respiratory or cardiac arrest.

56. Correct Answer: <u>1</u>

Rationale: The normal daily dose of digoxin is 0.125 to 0.25 mg. A dose of 25 mg of digoxin is an overdose of the medication.

57. Correct Answers: <u>2, 1, 5, 3, 4, 6</u>

Rationale: According to basic life support protocols, the first step in the application of an AED is to turn the power on. The second step is to attach the pads to the victim's chest, followed by pushing the "Analyze" button. The device will often announce "Stand clear," and the equipment operator should also ensure that all bystanders are clear of the patient. If indicated, a shock will be delivered. If indicated, a total of three shocks are delivered before the patient is assessed for the presence of a pulse.

58. Correct Answer: <u>1</u>

Rationale: Standard precautions are used in the care of all patients regardless of their diagnosis. The correct implementation of the precautions and associated barrier techniques minimizes the risk that the patient will develop a hospital-acquired infection.

59. Correct Answer: **3**

Rationale: One aspect of accurate blood pressure measurement requires the appropriate use of equipment. The use of a blood pressure cuff that is too small will result in a falsely high blood pressure reading.

60. Correct Answer: **4**

Rationale: Hand hygiene is the most effective way to prevent the spread of infectious organisms. Hand hygiene incorporates hand washing with soap and water, surgical hand washing, and the use of hand rubs such as an alcohol-based product.

61. Correct Answer: **1**

Rationale: Isosorbide dinitrate acts on vascular smooth muscle to promote vasodilation. The vasodilator action primarily affects veins and reduces preload. The high temperatures in a hot tub also promote vasodilation. The combined effects of medication and the hot-tub temperature could potentially result in a hypotensive episode. Patients with angina should be cautioned about this risk to their safety.

62. Correct Answer: **1**

Rationale: The catheter tip was contaminated when it came in contact with the scrubs. A new sterile catheter should be obtained for the procedure.

63. Correct Answer: **4**

Rationale: Defibrillation is the delivery of an electrical current to depolarize a critical mass of myocardial cells. Prior to defibrillation of a patient, a verbal announcement of an impending shock must be made, to ensure that everyone is clear of contact with the patient, bed, and equipment touching the patient. Contact with the patient, bed, or equipment during the delivery of the shock could result in electrical injury to the person involved.

64. Correct Answer: **No**

Rationale: The type of fluid and additives are correct, but the fluids should not be hung as the expiration date was February 2007. To ensure safe care, expired IV fluids should be discarded or returned to the pharmacy; they should not be infused into patients.

65. Correct Answer: **1**

Rationale: The first responsibility the nurse has upon finding a patient on the floor is to assess the patient. The priority is assessment and treatment of any immediate needs.

66. Correct Answer: **3**

Rationale: Approximately 33% of Americans take some form of herbal supplement. Supplements can be marketed without proof of their safety or efficacy, and the quality of the manufacturing of the products is not regulated by governmental agencies.

HEALTH PROMOTION AND MAINTENANCE

67. Correct Answer: **2**

Rationale: A decrease in dietary intake of sodium is one type of initial lifestyle modification that a patient with hypertension should consider. The presence of increased amounts of sodium in the vasculature, can cause the movement of interstitial fluids into the vessels, thus increasing blood volume and resulting in increased pressure. By decreasing sodium consumption to a recommended level of 2.4 g/day, the patient could experience an associated decrease in the amount of vascular fluid volume.

68. Correct Answer: **1**

Rationale: The patient is experiencing orthopnea. Orthopnea is an abnormal condition in which a person must sit or stand to promote comfortable respiratory effort. Elevation of the head with pillows to promote comfortable respiratory effort results in vascular volume reduction. Gravity pulls fluids into the lower extremities, leading to a decreased preload and a lessened cardiac volume workload.

69. Correct Answer: **2**

Rationale: Demonstration and practice are essential aspects of teaching skills. The demonstration and practice allow the nurse to evaluate the patient's implementation of a skill and to determine whether any reinforcement or additional teaching is needed.

70. Correct Answer: **Yes, for cardiovascular health the patient should consider weight reduction strategies.**

Rationale: First, a conversion of inches to feet needs to be done. A patient who is 65 inches tall is 5 feet, 5 inches tall (1 ft = 12 in.). A

SECTION I
SECTION II
SECTION III
SECTION IV
SECTION V
SECTION VI
SECTION VII
SECTION VIII
SECTION IX
SECTION X

patient who is 5 feet, 5 inches tall and weighs 160 pounds has a body mass index of 27 and is overweight. Weight reduction strategies should be considered for this patient.

71. Correct Answer: **1**

Rationale: To assess for jugular vein distention, the patient should be placed in a semi-Fowler's position. The presence of distended, protruding, or bulging veins in the semi-Fowler's position would be an abnormal finding.

72. Correct Answer: **2**

Rationale: Not all patients have classic presentations of myocardial infarction. Women have been found to have atypical presentations of chest pain and often complain of shortness of breath and fatigue when experiencing a myocardial infarction.

73. Correct Answer: **2**

Rationale: Epidemiological studies indicate that African Americans have the highest risk for the development of hypertension.

74. Correct Answer: **1**

Rationale: Raynaud's disease is characterized by attacks of vasospasm in the small arteries and arterioles of the fingers and sometimes the toes. The disease primarily affects young women and can be triggered by exposure to cold.

75. Correct Answers: **1, 2, 6**

Rationale: Varicose veins are tortuous, dilated veins with incompetent valves. Risk factors for the development of varicose veins include gender, genetic predisposition, sedentary lifestyle, age, and ethnicity. Women are four times more likely to develop varicose veins than men. In pregnancy, hormonal levels weaken vein walls, which in turn leads to incompetent valves. A sedentary lifestyle results in venous pooling and compromised valves. With age, there is decreased vascular elasticity and a risk for varicosity. African Americans have more venous valves and are less susceptible to varicose veins than Caucasians.

76. Correct Answer: **2**

Rationale: Thromboangiitis obliterans is a non-atherosclerotic, inflammatory disorder of the medium-sized arteries, veins, and nerves of the upper and lower extremities. Patients with this disease must stop smoking or other use of tobacco. The pathophysiology of the disease is uncertain, but smoking is known to be linked with the problem.

77. Correct Answer: **1**

Rationale: A modifiable risk factor for coronary artery disease is a circumstance over which a person has control. A sedentary lifestyle is a modifiable risk factor that a patient can control by increasing activity and establishing a program for regular exercise.

78. Correct Answer: **2**

Rationale: Lovenox is an anticoagulant medication that is administered via the subcutaneous route.

79. Correct Answer: **3**

Rationale: Furosemide is a diuretic. When administered orally, it has an onset of action within 60 minutes and its duration of action lasts for 6 to 8 hours. The patient should be taught to take the medication in the morning to avoid disruption of normal sleep patterns associated with the diuretic action of the drug.

80. Correct Answers: **1, 2**

Rationale: Gerontological changes in the cardiovascular system include decreased elasticity of the heart associated with increased collagen and decreased elastin, as well as thickening and stiffening of heart valves from lipid accumulation.

81. Correct Answer: **2**

Rationale: A reduction in intake of fat and cholesterol can reduce a person's risk of cardiovascular disease. The patient should consider both the type of food consumed and the method of preparation. Grilled chicken would be the best selection for a patient on a low-fat, low-cholesterol diet.

82. Correct Answer: **3**

Rationale: Regular exercise can reduce LDL cholesterol levels, increase HDL cholesterol levels, and decrease the risk of coronary heart disease.

83. Correct Answer: **4**

Rationale: A non-modifiable risk factor for coronary artery disease is a circumstance over which a person has no control. Age is a non-modifiable risk factor.

84. Correct Answer: **2**

Rationale: A patient with a history of deep vein thrombosis should avoid sitting for prolonged periods of time. Prolonged sitting and immobility can result in venous stasis, which is thought to be a risk factor for the development of deep vein thrombosis.

85. Correct Answer: <u>**Midclavicular line, fifth intercostal space, left chest.**</u>

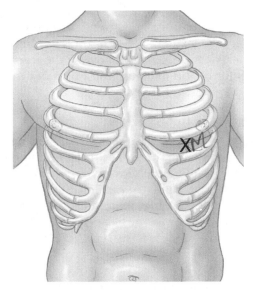

Rationale: The apical pulse should be auscultated on the left side of the chest at the fifth intercostal space, at the midclavicular line.

86. Correct Answer: **3**

Rationale: A patient with a body mass index of 36 is obese. Obesity coupled with a sedentary lifestyle would be indicative of a nutritional problem in which caloric intake exceeded caloric expenditures. The result is continued weight gain without intervention.

PSYCHOSOCIAL INTEGRITY

87. Correct Answer: **1**

Rationale: The patient has expressed a desire and readiness to return to his church to explore his spirituality and purpose in life. The NANDA definition of the nursing diagnosis is the ability to experience and integrate meaning and purpose in life through a person's connectedness with self, others, art, music, literature, nature, or a power greater than oneself.

88. Correct Answer: **3**

Rationale: Jehovah's Witnesses believe that blood transfusions violate God's law. Alternative treatments such as autotransfusions and surgical techniques that decrease blood loss may need to be considered for patients who refuse transfusions owing to their religious beliefs.

89. Correct Answer: **1**

Rationale: The nurse should assist the patient in recognizing the choices he or she has regarding disease progression through risk factor modification. A reduction in risk can slow disease progression and lessen the chance of further myocardial damage. It is up to the patient to make an informed choice about whether he or she will implement any risk reduction strategies. It is the responsibility of the nurse to assist the patient in understanding his or her choices.

90. Correct Answer: **2**

Rationale: Chronic cigarette smoking can result in physical dependence on nicotine. Symptoms of tobacco withdrawal may include craving, nervousness, restlessness, irritability, impatience, increased hostility, impaired concentration, and increased appetite and weight gain.

91. Correct Answer: **2**

Rationale: An unexpected arrest is a stressful situation for a nurse. The nurse should be encouraged to share his or her thoughts and feelings about the situation. One of the most successful ways to reduce stress after emergency situations is to talk about the situation.

92. Correct Answer: **1**

Rationale: The patient is denying that a myocardial infarction was experienced. The nursing diagnosis of "denial, ineffective" is defined by NANDA as a conscious or unconscious attempt to disavow the knowledge or meaning of an event so as to reduce anxiety and fear, but leading to the detriment of health.

93. Correct Answer: **2**

Rationale: The nursing diagnosis of "hopelessness" is defined by NANDA as the subjective state in which an individual sees limited or no

SECTION I
SECTION II
SECTION III
SECTION IV
SECTION V
SECTION VI
SECTION VII
SECTION VIII
SECTION IX
SECTION X

alternatives or personal choices available and is unable to mobilize energy on his or her own behalf.

94. Correct Answer: **3**

Rationale: The nursing diagnosis of "fear" is defined by NANDA as the response to a real or imaginary perceived threat that is continuously recognized as a danger.

95. Correct Answer: **4**

Rationale: The definition of the nursing diagnosis "adjustment, impaired" is defined by NANDA as the inability to modify one's lifestyle or behavior in a manner consistent with a change in one's health status.

96. Correct Answer: **4**

Rationale: An open-ended question should be used to allow the patient a wide range of responses. A closed question that elicits a yes-or-no answer and comments that use clichés are both barriers to therapeutic communication.

97. Correct Answer: **1**

Rationale: The patient's concern about sexual activity after cardiac illness should be addressed as a part of the plan of care. Using an open-ended statement such as "Tell me about your concerns" allows the nurse to focus on the information most needed by the patient and his or her partner.

98. Correct Answer: **2**

Rationale: The nurse can facilitate a patient's ability to cope with illness by maximizing strengths, teaching, and referring the patient to available supportive resources.

99. Correct Answer: **2**

Rationale: Family members should be provided with a private place to begin their grieving process once notified of the sudden death of a family member. The nurse should be an attentive listener and provide support to a family in the grieving process.

100. Correct Answer: **2**

Rationale: The nurse should allow time and encourage the wife to discuss her feelings and concerns about the impending surgery so as to facilitate a helping relationship for both the patient and the family.

101. Correct Answer: **3**

Rationale: The development of an addiction to opioids as a result of clinical exposure is extremely rare when opioids are given to acutely control pain, as is the case in a postoperative situation. A knowledge deficit exists for the patient about the use and effects of morphine and the addiction potential of the drug.

102. Correct Answer: **2**

Rationale: The use of an open-ended question will allow the patient an opportunity to freely verbalize her concerns and provide the nurse with information to determine a plan of care related to those concerns.

103. Correct Answer: **1**

Rationale: "Crack" cocaine is a central nervous system stimulant. This drug stimulates the sympathetic nervous system, which can result in increased heart rate, contractility, and vasoconstriction. Chest pain can result from the increased work of the heart and vasoconstriction.

104. Correct Answer: **2**

Rationale: Varying degrees of anxiety can be expected when a patient experiences a new situation. Enhancing the patient's knowledge about what to expect and facilitating his or her ability to ask questions is one strategy to assist in reducing anxiety.

105. Correct Answer: **3**

Rationale: The nurse should utilize the nursing process to assess the reason for the behavior, implement interventions that could help the patient restore self-control, and evaluate the effectiveness of the interventions.

106. Correct Answer: **2**

Rationale: Abrupt withdrawal of alcohol from a patient with a high degree of alcohol dependence can result in withdrawal syndrome. The clinical manifestations of this syndrome may include hallucinations; tremors; increased heart rate, blood pressure, and temperature; vomiting; cramping; and possibly seizures.

BASIC CARE AND COMFORT

107. Correct Answer: 3

Rationale: Abraham Maslow ranked human needs according to a hierarchy. At the base of the needs hierarchy are physiologic needs, followed by safety and security needs, belongingness and affection needs, esteem and self-respect needs, and self-actualization needs. Rest, sleep, activity, and nutrition are examples of physiologic needs. According to Maslow, the physiologic needs are always present and must be met before an individual can move to address needs at a higher level in the hierarchy.

108. Correct Answer: 2

Rationale: An electrocardiogram is a recording of the electrical activity of the heart. Movement of the limbs or parts of the body where leads to record impulse transmission are attached can result in artifact, or an artificial disturbance on the ECG tracing.

109. Correct Answer: 1

Rationale: An incentive spirometer helps to maximize lung inflation and prevent atelectasis. A volume incentive spirometer uses visual feedback to assist the patient in achieving preset goals for inspiratory volumes.

110. Correct Answer: 1

Rationale: A nasogastric tube can cause irritation to the nasal mucosa. Regular nasal hygiene should be provided as a part of the care of a patient with a nasogastric tube.

111. Correct Answer: 4.5 kg

Rationale: 1 lb = 2.2 kg. To convert pounds to kilograms, divide the number of pounds by 2.2 kg: 10/2.2 = 4.5.

112. Correct Answer: 2

Rationale: Elevation of the extremities above the level of the heart in a patient with venous congestion can promote venous return to the heart by gravity and decrease venous congestion.

113. Correct Answer: 1

Rationale: Deep breathing and coughing are important post-operative interventions to prevent respiratory complications such as atelectasis. Splinting the sternal area with a pillow or blanket to provide incisional support will aid the patient in deep breathing and coughing and help to reduce discomfort.

114. Correct Answer: 1

Rationale: Ingestion of garlic is thought to increase the activity of an enzyme called nitric oxide synthetase. This enzyme acts to promote relaxation of vascular smooth muscle. The result is vasodilation of the blood vessels and a lowering of blood pressure.

115. Correct Answers: 1, 3, 6

Rationale: The goal of foot care in a patient with peripheral vascular disease is to maintain and promote tissue integrity. Prevention of tissue damage acts to prevent potential complications such as ulceration, infection, and gangrene. Interventions that will facilitate maintenance of tissue integrity include washing the feet with a mild soap and warm water, drying the feet thoroughly after bathing, and breaking in new footwear.

116. Correct Answer: 4

Rationale: The oxygen concentration of room air is approximately 21%. When using a nasal cannula, each 1 L of oxygen increases the oxygen concentration by approximately 4% from room air. Therefore a patient on 2 L/min nasal cannula would be receiving approximately 28% oxygen. An increase to 3 L/min would increase the oxygen concentration to approximately 32%.

117. Correct Answer: 2

Rationale: Biofeedback is an alternative mind–body therapy that assists individuals in gaining conscious control over body processes. The individual is provided with visual or auditory information about physiologic processes such as blood pressure, heart rate, and muscle tension through the use of instruments, and is then taught interventions that will help him or her to control these processes.

118. Correct Answer: 1

Rationale: Based on the scenario, the change in diet is the reason for the reduction in nutritional intake. Contacting the dietician to discuss menu selections that the patient enjoys could promote better compliance with the dietary plan and improve the patient's nutritional intake.

SECTION I

SECTION II

SECTION III

SECTION IV

SECTION V

SECTION VI

SECTION VII

SECTION VIII

SECTION IX

SECTION X

119. Correct Answer: **900 mL**

    Rationale: The patient's total intake was 30 oz. The ounces then need to be converted to milliliters. 1 oz = 30 mL; 30 oz × 30 mL/oz = 900 mL.

120. Correct Answer: **4**

    Rationale: Rest is a condition where the body is in a decreased state of activity. In a patient with angina, rest—by decreasing the body's and cardiac cells' metabolic needs—allows the existing coronary circulation to better meet the individual's myocardial cellular needs. Rest facilitates obtaining a balance between myocardial cellular needs and demand through the reduction of activity.

121. Correct Answer: **1**

    Rationale: Components of parenteral nutritional therapy needed to maintain nutrition are proteins, carbohydrates, and fats. Additional elements may include vitamins, electrolytes, and minerals. An increase in the total serum protein to a normal level (6.0–8.0 mg/dL) would indicate that the patient is receiving adequate amino acids to support his or her protein requirements.

122. Correct Answer: **2**

    Rationale: The nursing diagnosis is activity intolerance related to dyspnea. The only patient finding that addresses activity is the inability to walk to the bathroom without shortness of breath.

123. Correct Answer: **The nurse should counsel the patient to select food items that are lower in cholesterol and to reduce his or her intake of saturated fats. Minimal trans fats should be ingested.**

    Rationale: A high-fat diet contributes to the development of atherosclerosis. A patient who has been diagnosed with atherosclerosis should incorporate therapeutic lifestyle changes into his or her management plan for the disease. Dietary modifications should include a reduction in the amount of fat ingested. The amount of saturated fat ingested should not exceed 7% of the total daily calories, and the daily cholesterol intake should be no more than 200 mg. The total daily dietary fat intake should be approximately 25% to 35% of the total calories ingested.

124. Correct Answer: **4**

    Rationale: Oliguria is defined as urine output less than 500 mL but more than 100 mL in a 24-hour period. A urine output of 350 mL in a 24-hour period would fall within the parameters that define oliguria.

125. Correct Answer: **3**

    Rationale: A nasogastric tube is used in a postoperative patient to decompress the stomach and drain the gastric contents until gastric motility returns. Symptoms of nausea and abdominal discomfort could be indicative of a tube that is not draining properly. The nurse should assess the tube for proper position and operation.

126. Correct Answer: **4**

    Rationale: A complication of enteral nutritional therapy is aspiration pneumonitis. The condition may prove fatal in some patients. Interventions to prevent aspiration would include ensuring proper tube placement, elevating the head of the bed during feeding, and assessing the patient for residuals, among other things.

PHARMACOLOGICAL AND PARENTERAL THERAPIES

127. Correct Answer: **3**

    Rationale: There are several steps to answering this problem:

    1. Pounds must be converted to kilograms: 1 lb = 2.2 kg; 154 lb/2.2 kg/lb = 70 kg.

    2. To give a 1 mg/kg bolus, the nurse will need to administer a 70 mg bolus of the drug.

    3. The drug is supplied as 10 mg/mL. The problem should be set up as a ratio proportion where 70 mg/x mL = 10 mg/1 mL; 70 mg (1 mL) = 10 mg(x mL); x mL = 70 mg (1 cc); 10 mg(x) = 7 mL.

128. Correct Answer: **1**

    Rationale: Nitroprusside is often the first-line medication used to manage hypertensive emergencies. This drug is administered by continuous intravenous infusion and is rapid acting. By relaxing the smooth muscles of the arterioles and veins, nitroprusside promotes vasodilation and reduces blood pressure.

129. Correct Answer: 2

Rationale: Cough is an adverse effect of therapy with ACE inhibitors and occurs in 5% to 10% of patients. The cough is thought to be caused by the accumulation of bradykinin.

130. Correct Answer: 2

Rationale: Hydrochlorothiazide is a thiazide diuretic. This drug promotes diuresis by decreasing the reabsorption of sodium, water, and chloride in the distal convoluted renal tubules. With the reduction of blood volume by diuresis, blood pressure is reduced.

131. Correct Answer: 2

Rationale: Intravenous potassium is generally administered at a rate no faster than 10 mEq/h. The order should be questioned because it calls for the administration of 80 mEq of potassium in 30 minutes, which is much more than the recommended dose of 10 mEq/h and could result in cardiac complications and hyperkalemia.

132. Correct Answer: 2

Rationale: Loop diuretics such as Lasix lower blood pressure by reducing the blood volume through diuresis and decreasing arterial resistance. Weight is an excellent indicator of fluid status, whereas a loss or gain of approximately 1 L of fluid = 1 kg. For patients receiving Lasix therapy, the loss of fluid volume can be assessed by measuring daily trends in weight gain or loss.

133. Correct Answer: 2

Rationale: Nitroglycerin results in vasodilation. Headache is often an initial adverse side effect of nitrate therapy. This effect will often diminish with continued use.

134. Correct Answer: 1

Rationale: Gemfibrozil acts on receptors in the liver to increase the clearance of VLDL levels (triglycerides) and increase HDL production. The drug is generally well tolerated, but side effects can include gastrointestinal disturbances such as nausea, abdominal pain, and diarrhea. In addition, there is an increased risk for gallstones with use of this drug because of the increased biliary saturation level of cholesterol.

135. Correct Answer: 2

Rationale: One action of nicotinic acid is the reduction of lipolysis in adipose tissue. As a consequence, this drug reduces both VLDL and LDL levels. Adverse effects include an intense flushing of the face, neck, and ears of almost all patients who take this drug.

136. Correct Answer: 3

Rationale: Through its action on hepatocytes and inhibition of HMG-CoA reductase, simvistatin acts to lower LDL levels and increase HDL levels. The statins are also thought to have a non-lipid cardiovascular action that acts to stabilize plaque and reduce inflammation at the plaque site—both actions can reduce the risk of a cardiovascular event. Two of the most serious adverse effects associated with simvistatin are myopathy and hepatotoxicity.

137. Correct Answer: 4

Rationale: Ezetimibe reduces total cholesterol, LDL, triglycerides, and apolipoprotein B levels by blocking the absorption of cholesterol in the small intestine. This drug has minimal adverse effects and is generally well tolerated.

138. Correct Answer: 3

Rationale: A thrombolytic agent is used to dissolve an existing thrombus and restore blood flow through the coronary artery in a patient with acute coronary syndrome (ACS). An ST segment represents ventricular repolarization and should be seen as an isoelectric line on ECG. An elevation of greater than 1 mm on the ECG can indicate acute myocardial injury from blockage of blood flow (such as would be caused by a thrombus in ACS) to the myocardium. Timely administration of a thrombolytic agent can result in dissolution of the thrombus and restoration of blood flow to the myocardium, resulting in a decrease in the ST-segment elevation. The ECG is used in conjunction with lab values and patient assessment to determine the extent of injury and confirm a diagnosis.

139. Correct Answer: 3

Rationale: Percocet is a combination drug composed of acetaminophen and oxycodone (an opioid). The action of the drug is to produce analgesia and sedation. The patient should take the medication only as prescribed. Taking an extra dose of the medication could result in adverse effects.

SECTION I

SECTION II

SECTION III

SECTION IV

SECTION V

SECTION VI

SECTION VII

SECTION VIII

SECTION IX

SECTION X

140. Correct Answer: **2**

Rationale: Normally, cyclooxygenase-1 (COX-1) acts on thromboxane A (TXA_2) to promote platelet aggregation and on vascular smooth muscle to cause vasoconstriction. Aspirin acts as a cyclooxygenase inhibitor, preventing both platelet aggregation and vasoconstriction. The antiplatelet and anti-vasoconstrictive effects decrease the chance of a thrombus forming in the coronary arteries. Aspirin is prescribed to patients with a history of myocardial infarction as a secondary means to prevent reinfarction.

141. Correct Answer: **1**

Rationale: Digoxin is a cardiac glycoside that affects both the mechanical and electrical aspects of the heart. The drug increases the force of ventricular contraction and reduces heart rate. Because of its effects on heart rate, the nurse should assess the patient's apical pulse before administering the drug, as this pulse would be the most reliable indicator of heart rate. If the pulse is less than 60 beats/min, the nurse should notify the prescriber before administering the medication. A further decrease in heart rate could result in decreased cardiac output and adverse effects for the patient.

142. Correct Answer: **1**

Rationale: Verapamil (Calan) acts by blocking calcium channels in blood vessels and the heart. In this scenario, the patient is experiencing a supraventricular tachycardia. Verapamil decreases the ventricular rate by blocking electrical impulses at the sino-atrial node, thereby decreasing the heart rate.

143. Correct Answer: **3**

Rationale: Heparin is an anticoagulant. The infusion of 25,000 units of this medication over a short period can result in an overdose of the drug. Protamine sulfate is used for the treatment of a heparin overdose. It bonds with heparin to produce a heparin–protamine complex that does not have anticoagulant activity. One milligram of protamine inactivates approximately 100 units of heparin.

144. Correct Answer: **1**

Rationale: Nitroglycerin is an antianginal drug that acts as a vasodilator. When using a transdermal patch, the route of drug absorption is through the skin. Any remaining residual medication should be removed prior to the application of a new dose to avoid excessive dosing of the drug.

145. Correct Answer: **½ tablet**

Rationale: The problem is set up as a ratio proportion where 0.25 mg/1 tablet = 0.125 mg/x tablet. The nurse solves for x by cross-multiplying: 0.25 mg(x) = 0.125 mg (1 tablet); x = 0.125 mg/1 tablet/0.25 mg; x = 0.5 = ½ tablet. One-half of a 0.25 mg digoxin tablet is equal to a 0.125 mg dose of digoxin.

146. Correct Answer: **2**

Rationale: Aminoglycosides can accumulate in the inner ear and result in injury that impairs hearing and/or balance. The toxic levels accumulate when the drug is unable to move out of the inner ear cells. With prolonged exposure to the drug, cells in the inner ear can be damaged. Thus an adverse effect of these drugs is ototoxicity.

147. Correct Answer: **1**

Rationale: In hypovolemic shock, the patient loses vascular volume. The administration of intravenous fluids is one means by which vascular volume may be replaced. Increasing the vascular volume results in an increased preload—that is, an increase in the amount of volume that is returned via the venous circulation to the heart.

148. Correct Answer: **3**

Rationale: Nasal decongestants that are administered orally act by stimulating alpha$_1$-adrenergic receptors on blood vessels. The result is vasoconstriction of the vessels. In a patient with existing hypertension, the use of an oral decongestant can result in increased blood pressure. The patient being treated for hypertension should be instructed to consult the prescriber for advice on the use of decongestants.

149. Correct Answer: **2**

Rationale: Alteplase is a thrombolytic drug that acts by converting plasminogen to plasmin. Plasmin is an enzyme that acts to promote the degradation of the fibrin matrix of a clot. The result is the destruction of an existing thrombus. An adverse effect of the action of the drug is bleeding at sites of recent injury from the breakdown of an existing clot or the interference with new clot formation in response to injury.

150. Correct Answer: 1

Rationale: Metoprolol is a cardioselective beta-adrenergic antagonist that blocks the action of $beta_1$ receptors in the heart. Blockade of the $beta_1$ receptors results in decreased heart rate, contractility, and velocity of impulse conduction in the atrioventricular node. In a patient with a myocardial infarction, there is a decrease in the strength of myocardial contractility. Thus the medication controls heart rate and contractility so as to reduce the cardiac workload. The reduction of workload helps to promote a balance between myocardial tissue oxygen demand and supply.

151. Correct Answer: 4

Rationale: The administration route for thrombolytics is intravenous or intracoronary. For maximum therapeutic effect, the drug should be administered within 4 to 6 hours of the onset of symptoms. Early administration acts to limit the size of infarction, improve ventricular function, and reduce mortality.

152. Correct Answer: 4

Rationale: The renin–angiotensin–aldosterone system plays a role in the regulation of blood pressure, blood volume, and fluids and electrolyte balance. An angiotensin-converting enzyme (ACE) inhibitor acts to prevent ACE from acting on angiotensin I. The result is the prevention of the conversion of angiotensin I to angiotensin II. The presence of angiotensin II causes vasoconstriction and the release of aldosterone, which causes the kidneys to reabsorb sodium and water. The action of angiotensin II produces an increased blood volume and vasoconstriction, which in turn contributes to hypertension. Blocking the conversion of angiotensin I to angiotensin II can result in decreased blood pressure.

153. Correct Answer: 4

Rationale: The patient has a low heart rate with symptoms that indicate inadequate cardiac output. Atropine is the drug of choice in this situation. Atropine blocks the cardiac muscarinic receptors and inhibits the parasympathetic nervous system. The blockage of parasympathetic activity results in an increased heart rate. With the increased heart rate, cardiac output will also increase. Cardiac output = stroke volume/beat × heart rate.

154. Correct Answer: 3

Rationale: Alteplase is a thrombolytic drug that acts by converting plasminogen to plasmin. Plasmin dissolves the fibrin matrix of a clot, thereby destroying an existing thrombus. An adverse effect of this medication is bleeding. Alteplase is contraindicated in a patient with a history of bleeding, such as a bleeding gastric ulcer. Severe bleeding or hemorrhage could result from its use in such case.

155. Correct Answer: 1

Rationale: Garlic has antiplatelet effects that can result in bleeding. When coupled with the use of an anticoagulant such as warfarin, the risk of bleeding is enhanced. Nurses should be aware of the potential for such drug–drug interactions between herbal supplements and prescribed drugs and obtain a history including the use of both herbal and prescribed medications.

156. Correct Answer: 1

Rationale: Calcium channels in the arteries and arterioles are involved in the contraction of smooth muscle. Movement of calcium into the smooth muscle cells results in contraction and corresponding vessel constriction. Blocking the movement of calcium into the cell prevents vasoconstriction.

157. Correct Answer: 1

Rationale: Carvedilol is a nonselective beta-adrenergic antagonist that blocks the action of $beta_1$ receptors in the heart and the action of $beta_2$ receptors in the lung, smooth muscles, and skeletal muscles. Blocking the $beta_1$ receptors leads to decreased heart rate, contractility, and velocity of impulse conduction in the atrioventricular node. $Beta_2$-receptor blockade can result in bronchoconstriction, vasoconstriction, and inhibition of glycogenolysis. Because of this drug's effects on the heart, the nurse should assess the patient's current pulse and blood pressure before administering carvedilol. The prescriber should be contacted if bradycardia or hypotension is identified prior to the administration of the drug. Carvedilol is administered orally.

158. Correct Answer: 4

Rationale: The normal therapeutic range for digoxin is 0.5 to 0.8 ng/mL. A digoxin level of 2.9 ng/mL is considered toxic. The nurse

SECTION I

SECTION II

SECTION III

SECTION IV

SECTION V

SECTION VI

SECTION VII

SECTION VIII

SECTION IX

SECTION X

should hold the medication and contact the prescriber. Patients should be instructed in the clinical manifestations of digoxin toxicity, which may include fatigue, nausea, vomiting, diarrhea, visual disturbances (blurred or yellow vision), and dysrhythmias.

159. Correct Answer: 11 mL/h

Rationale: The heparin concentration for the infusion is 100 units/mL (25,000 units/1000 mL = 100 units/mL). The desired dose is 1,100 units/h. The nurse needs to determine the desired rate of infusion in cubic centimeters per hour (mL/h) and can do so by setting up a cross multiplication problem: 1100 units/x mL/hr = 100 units/1 mL/hr x = 11 mL/h.

REDUCTION OF RISK POTENTIAL

160. Correct Answer: 45% risk for developing coronary disease over the next 10 years

Rationale: Based on the data the patient received the following points:

Age: 62 (5 points)

Total cholesterol: 230 mg/dL (1 point)

Smoker (2 points)

Diabetes (2 points)

HDL: 42 mg/dL (1 point)

Blood pressure with treatment: 148/92 mm Hg (2 points)

Total points = 5 + 1 + 2 + 2 + 1 + 2 = 13 points

Coronary heart disease risk = 45% risk for the client in the scenario

A man the same age, with a normal blood pressure, a total cholesterol of 160–199 mg/dL, an HDL of 45 mg/dL who is a non-smoker and has no diabetic history, has an average 10 year risk for coronary heart disease of 21%. Therefore the patient in the scenario is at increased risk for the development of coronary disease over the next 10 years.

The Framingham risk prediction scores place patients in 10-year risk groups. The patient described in this scenario is at high risk for developing coronary heart disease. The average 10-year coronary heart disease risk for an individual who is the same age as this patient is 21%. The low-risk comparison for an individual who is the same age as this patient is 11%. Given that the patient in this scenario (45%) clearly has an increased risk for coronary heart disease, this risk prediction

should be used to establish treatment goals, such as therapeutic lifestyle changes, LDL goals, and the need for medications.

161. Correct Answer: 2

Rationale: The two factors are required for infective endocarditis to develop: a damaged endocardial tissue (thin membrane that lines the heart chambers and valves) and a portal of entry for an infectious organism to gain circulatory access. Infective endocarditis can occur in people with existing heart lesions such as those associated with valvular disease, prosthetic valves, congenital heart defects, and intravenous drug abuse. *Staphylococcus aureus* and *Streptococcus viridans* are often the infecting organisms.

162. Correct Answer: 1

Rationale: Anemia is an abnormally low hemoglobin level and/or circulating number of red blood cells. The result is a decrease in the blood's oxygen-carrying capacity. Symptoms associated with chronic anemia, which are caused by the lack of oxygen reaching the cells, include fatigue, dyspnea at rest, and tachycardia. The lack of hemoglobin results in pallor. The dyspnea and tachycardia are attempts by the body to compensate for the tissue hypoxia by increasing oxygen delivery.

163. Correct Answer: 2

Rationale: Prolonged, uncontrolled hypertension causes the heart to work harder because of the increased peripheral vascular resistance that it is required to pump against. A cardiac complication that develops when hypertension is not treated is left ventricular hypertrophy. Hypertrophy is caused by the increased work of the left ventricular heart muscle when it pumps against increased peripheral vascular resistance. Over a period of time, the increased muscle size decreases the filling capacity of the ventricles and can result in decreased cardiac output.

164. Correct Answer: 3

Rationale: The mean arterial pressure is a representation of the average pressure in the arterial system during ventricular contraction and relaxation. It is an indicator of tissue perfusion. The following formula is used to calculate mean arterial pressure: diastolic pressure + (pulse pressure/3). The pulse pressure is = systolic B/P – diastolic B/P.

165. Correct Answer: 2

Rationale: Morphine is an opioid agonist that mimics the action of endogenous opioid peptides at mu and kappa receptors so as to produce analgesia. Respiratory depression—caused by depression of the central nervous system—is the most serious adverse effect associated with this drug. In the scenario described, the medication produced a serious decrease in respiratory effort. The nurse should stimulate the patient and prepare to administer an opioid antagonist such as naloxone (Narcan). Naloxone competes with morphine for receptor sites and works to block the action of morphine.

166. Correct Answer: 2

Rationale: Fluid retention and pulmonary congestion resulting in dyspnea on exertion and fatigue are clinical manifestations of congestive heart failure. The treatment goals are to relieve the patient's symptoms and enhance the patient's quality of life by optimizing the underlying cardiac dysfunction. Patients are taught to monitor their daily weight and to note any associated changes (such as weight gain and decrease in activity level with dyspnea) that could be indicative of failure.

167. Correct Answer: 3

Rationale: Sequential compression devices are used to prevent the development of deep vein thrombosis. This kind of device consists of a small air compressor that is attached to knee-high or thigh-high sleeves. Air is pumped into the sleeves, which sequentially fill and apply pressure to the ankle, calf, and/or thigh. A sequential compression device helps to increase blood velocity and decrease venous stasis, which is a factor associated with the development of deep vein thrombosis.

168. Correct Answer: 4

Rationale: Pre-renal failure is often caused by hypovolemia, which results in both decreased cardiac output and decreased renal perfusion. One way to increase cardiac output and renal perfusion is to increase vascular volume through the administration of a fluid bolus. The goal of this treatment is to restore vascular volume, increase cardiac output, and improve renal blood flow, thereby preventing further renal damage. If caught early, pre-renal failure can be treated and kidney function preserved.

169. Correct Answer: 1

Rationale: The clinical manifestation of a swollen, reddened area that is cool and painful to palpation is associated with the infiltration of an intravenous access device. Infiltration occurs when fluids or medications infuse into the surrounding tissue. Infiltration is caused by dislodgement of an intravenous catheter from the vein. After finding clinical evidence of infiltration, the first thing the nurse should do is to discontinue any fluids infusing into the device.

170. Correct Answer: 4

Rationale: One function of the skin is to protect the body against invading organisms. When the natural protection of the skin is compromised, such as by a surgical incision, the nurse must observe the wound for any clinical manifestations of infection. The presence of redness, swelling, and cloudy, foul-smelling drainage would indicate inflammation and possibly infection.

171. Correct Answer: 4

Rationale: The increased temperature and respirations are signs of a transfusion reaction. The first action by the nurse when a transfusion reaction is suspected is to stop the transfusion. It is most important that the patient not receive any additional blood, as it is the source of the reaction.

172. Correct Answer: 3

Rationale: Chest pain and shortness of breath on exertion are both symptoms of an imbalance in cardiac oxygen supply and demand. A patient who presents with these symptoms should rest to improve his or her myocardial oxygen supply.

173. Correct Answer: 2

Rationale: Rheumatic fever is an acute, immune-mediated inflammatory disease that follows a throat infection with group A beta-hemolytic streptococci. A complication of the acute phase of rheumatic fever is a carditis of the pericardium, myocardium, and endocardium. The involvement of the endocardium can cause cardiac valvular complications.

174. Correct Answer: 1

Rationale: Immobility is associated with venous stasis, pooling, and increased coagulability of the blood, all of which increase the potential for the development of thrombophlebitis. Thrombophlebitis is the presence of a thrombus in the venous system and the associated inflammatory response in the vessel wall.

175. Correct Answer: 3

Rationale: The computer programmer is at increased risk for the development of thrombophlebitis due to the sedentary lifestyle associated with the job which can lead to venous stasis.

176. Correct Answer: 1

Rationale: One of the most serious adverse effects of excessive levels of potassium is a disturbance in the electrical impulse generation and conduction in the heart, which can lead to lethal cardiac dysrhythmias. ECG changes are often an early sign of elevation. The nurse should observe the ECG for tall-peaked T waves, small P waves, a prolonged QT interval, and ventricular tachycardia, fibrillation, or asystole.

177. Correct Answer: 2

Rationale: Raynaud's disease is an arterial disease of the extremities (commonly the fingers, but occasionally the toes) caused by an excessive vasospasm of the arteries and arterioles. This disease is often triggered by extreme cold or strong emotions. The fingers and toes are innervated only by the sympathetic nervous system fibers. The digits rely on withdrawal of the stimulus to slow or stop the vasoconstrictive response.

178. Correct Answer: 1

Rationale: Cardiac enzyme analysis is used in conjunction with patient history, presentation, and ECG exam to diagnose myocardial injury. In response to cellular injury and damage, certain enzymes are released from the cells; however, most of these enzymes are not specific to a particular cell or organ. By contrast, myocardial contractile cells release a specific enzyme, troponin. Troponin is the most specific cardiac marker for myocardial cell damage.

179. Correct Answer: 2

Rationale: Normal urine output is 30 to 60 mL/h. A urinary output of 20 cc for a 2-hour period indicates a decreased glomerular filtration rate, which might be caused by any of several factors that result in fluid volume deficit. This finding should be reported to the physician for further assessment and intervention.

180. Correct Answers: 2, 4

Rationale: An ECG is a display of the electrical activity of the heart. A normal ECG tracing has the following characteristics:
- An upright P wave
- One P wave before each QRS complex
- A PR interval of 0.12 to 0.20 second
- A QRS interval that is 0.12 second or less
- A positive R wave (first positive deflection after the P wave)
- A regular R-to-R interval
- An isoelectric ST segment (the segment that connects the QRS complex to the T wave—the line is straight and not elevated or depressed)

181. Correct Answer: 4

Rationale: To perform a transesophageal echocardiogram, a transducer is passed into the esophagus by having the patient swallow it. Topical anesthesia and sedation are often used to facilitate conduction of the probe and completion of the procedure. Ultrasound images of the cardiac structures are then obtained. After the procedure and prior to resuming a normal diet, the nurse should ensure that the patient has recovered from the sedation or topical anesthesia and is able to swallow adequately.

182. Correct Answer: 2

Rationale: A pulmonary embolus is a venous thrombus that has dislodged, entered the circulation of the right side of the heart, and become lodged in the pulmonary vasculature. An embolism can be lethal. Its effects ultimately depend on its size and the location where the clot lodges within the pulmonary vasculature.

183. Correct Answer: 4

Rationale: Secondary hypertension is hypertension that is caused by another disease. It can be corrected or cured. A tumor of the adrenal gland, such as a pheochromocytoma, is associated with the development of secondary hypertension. In such a case, surgical removal of the tumor is used to treat the tumor and its associated hypertension.

184. Correct Answer: 2

Rationale: Ideally, the total cholesterol level should be less than 200 mg/dL. The LDL level should be less than 100 mg/dL. Both of the values reported for this patient are high, so the patient should be evaluated for a treatment plan that would seek to reduce these levels and lower his or her coronary heart disease risk.

185. Correct Answer: 3

Rationale: The ECG shows atrial fibrillation. This rhythm is characterized by chaotic impulse formation within the atria at a rate that often exceeds 400/min. Because of the rapid rate of discharge, the atria are unable to fully depolarize and conduction of impulses through the atrioventricular node is sporadic. Blood pools in the atria, and normal clotting can be accelerated. The result is small blood clots (thrombi) that accumulate on the wall of the atria. If the thrombi break away from the atrial wall, they become emboli that can lodge in the lungs, heart, or brain.

186. Correct Answer: 3

Rationale: Orthostatic hypotension is an abnormal drop in blood pressure that occurs upon standing. The 68-year-old patient taking a loop diuretic is at higher risk for the development of orthostatic hypotension. A loop diuretic results in loss of blood volume through diuresis and relaxation of venous smooth muscle, both of which can decrease preload (i.e., the amount of blood returning to the heart). Decreased preload coupled with a patient quickly moving from a recumbent position, where venous blood can pool in the extremities, to a standing position can result in decreased cardiac output and hypotension. The patient should be counseled to report symptoms of hypotension such as dizziness, lightheadedness, and syncope and should get up slowly from recumbent positions.

187. Correct Answer: 4

Rationale: Bibasilar rales are associated with left-sided congestive heart failure. It is caused by pulmonary congestion that occurs from the inability of the left side of the heart to pump adequately, which causes blood to back up and results in pulmonary congestion.

188. Correct Answer: 1

Rationale: Hematocrit is the measurement of the percentage of red blood cell mass in plasma. Dehydration decreases the amount of plasma, resulting in an increased concentration of red blood cells. The greater concentration of red blood cells results in an increased hematocrit finding.

189. Correct Answer: 2

Rationale: In acute coronary syndrome, a thrombus forms within the coronary arterial circulation, impeding or blocking the flow of blood to the myocardial tissues. The inability to deliver an adequate oxygen supply to meet the myocardial tissue's demands results in tissue ischemia. In association with the ischemia, the patient experiences an increase in the irritability of myocardial cells, which can in turn result in dysrhythmias.

190. Correct Answer: 2

Rationale: A stage II pressure ulcer is characterized by skin breaks into the epidermis or dermis. An abrasion, blister, or a shallow crater is often seen in such a case. Edema, drainage, and necrosis can also be found.

191. Correct Answer: 2

Rationale: A myocardial contusion is an area of injury to the heart and the most common result of blunt chest trauma. This injury is characterized by ecchymosis, swelling, and pain. Diagnostic procedures to assess for myocardial contusion include a 12-lead ECG and cardiac enzymes. An ECG is done because approximately one-half of patients with such a contusion develop injury-associated dysrhythmias. Cardiac enzyme tests assess for myocardial injury.

192. Correct Answer: 1

Rationale: The MIDCABG is a cardiac surgical procedure that is designed to reduce the cost, length of hospital stay, and morbidity and to provide an alternative to coronary artery bypass surgery for patients who meet the criteria for this procedure. Patients with left anterior descending lesions or single-vessel lesions for which medical management is not effective are candidates for the procedure.

PHYSIOLOGICAL ADAPTATION

193. Correct Answer: 1

Rationale: Paroxysmal nocturnal dyspnea is a sudden attack of shortness of breath that abruptly awakes someone during sleep. This finding is associated with heart failure.

194. Correct Answer: **3**

Rationale: Cardiogenic shock is the failure of the heart to adequately pump blood. Causes may include myocardial infarction, dysrhythmias, ventricular aneurysm, and acute valvular dysfunction. Treatment includes measures to improve cardiac output and balance myocardial oxygen supply and demand. Interventions administered to accomplish these goals include the use of nitroglycerin to reduce arterial resistance and preload, diuretics to reduce preload, and insertion of an intra-aortic balloon pump to promote coronary and peripheral blood flow.

195. Correct Answer: **3**

Rationale: Fever, chills, back pain, chest tightness, dyspnea, hematuria, and anxiety are all associated with a hemolytic transfusion reaction. Hypotension and vascular collapse can result from the hemolytic reaction. The priority nursing intervention in such a case is to stop the transfusion immediately upon recognition of a potential reaction.

196. Correct Answers: **2, 4, 5, 6**

Rationale: Right-sided heart failure results in the inability to move blood from the venous circulation into the pulmonary circulation. The result is accumulation of blood in the systemic venous circulation. Clinical manifestations of this problem include abdominal discomfort, hepatomegaly, splenomegaly, swollen ankles, and ascites.

197. Correct Answer: **4**

Rationale: Cardiac tamponade is a life-threatening condition that is caused by the accumulation of fluid, pus, or blood in the pericardial sac. The buildup causes an increase in pericardial pressure that does not allow for adequate ventricular filling time, which in turn results in decreased cardiac output. The severity of the condition depends on the amount of fluid present and the rate of its accumulation. Treatment includes relief of the pressure. Pericardiocentesis (i.e., removal of the fluid, blood, or pus accumulation via needle aspiration of the pericardium) is one means of improving cardiac output and reducing intracardiac pressure.

198. Correct Answer: **3**

Rationale: In cardiogenic shock, the heart fails to adequately pump blood. Causes may include myocardial infarction, dysrhythmias, ventricular aneurysm, and acute valvular dysfunction.

199. Correct Answer: **3**

Rationale: The EMT has reported findings from the scene of the accident that are consistent with a myocardial injury. Beck's triad—hypotension, muffled heart tones, and distended neck veins—are classic signs of cardiac tamponade. Hypotension is associated with decreased cardiac output. Muffled heart tones are found due to the fluid or blood accumulation around the heart. Distended neck veins occur because of the heart's decreased ability to accommodate the blood flow and the back up of blood into the vena cava.

200. Correct Answer: **3**

Rationale: Polycystic disease is a condition characterized by dilatation of the tubular structures and cyst formation within the kidneys. Secondary hypertension, a symptom of the disease, results from the compression of intrarenal blood vessels and the activation of the renin–angiotensin–aldosterone system.

201. Correct Answer: **3**

Rationale: The renin–angiotensin–aldosterone mechanism plays a role in blood pressure regulation. The enzyme renin is released by the kidneys in response to stimuli such as decreased blood pressure, decreased blood volume, or decreased sodium concentration. Renin is released into the bloodstream and acts to convert the plasma protein angiotensinogen to angiotensin I.

202. Correct Answer: **3**

Rationale: The cardiac output is the product of the stroke volume times the heart rate. The stroke volume is the amount of blood ejected from the heart with each beat. Given the clinical information in this question, cardiac output = 70 (stroke volume) × 85 (heart rate/min) = 5,950 mL.

203. Correct Answer: **4**

Rationale: A weak, thready pulse is associated with decreased cardiac output. A pulse results from contraction of the left ventricle and ejection of blood into the arterial circulation. A decrease in cardiac output is associated with a thready pulse—that is, a pulse that is not easily palpated.

204. Correct Answer: **2**

Rationale: Variant (Prinzmetal) angina is caused by coronary artery spasm. Prinzmetal and associates first described the condition. Variant angina differs from stable angina in that it can occur during rest and in the absence of coronary atherosclerotic disease.

205. Correct Answer: **4**

Rationale: Atherosclerosis is characterized by the formation of fibro-fatty lesions in the intimal lining of the large and medium arteries. These atherosclerotic lesions reduce arterial elasticity and vessel diameter. Systolic pressure is the peak pressure that occurs during ventricular contraction. As vessel diameter and elasticity decrease, an increased pressure develops in the arteries because they are no longer able to accommodate all of the blood being ejected from the left ventricle. Ultimately, this cascade of events leads to hypertension.

206. Correct Answer: **3**

Rationale: Capillaries are the vessels that connect the arterial and venous segments of the circulatory system. Gases, wastes, and nutrients leave and enter the capillaries through capillary pores found in the basement membranes of the endothelial cells that line these vessels.

207. Correct Answer: **1**

Rationale: The vagus nerve is a part of the parasympathetic nervous system. Stimulation of this nerve results in a decreased heart rate.

208. Correct Answer: **2**

Rationale: Pressure-sensitive baroreceptors are located in the blood vessel and heart walls. Baroreceptors respond to changes in blood pressure and stretch of the vessel walls by stimulating the autonomic nervous system.

209. Correct Answer: **1**

Rationale: The P wave on the electrocardiogram represents atrial depolarization and conduction of the impulse through the atria.

210. Correct Answer: **2**

Rationale: Cool, pale skin is caused by stimulation of the sympathetic nervous system, which results in vasoconstriction and shunting of blood away from the skin.

211. Correct Answer: **3**

Rationale: Metabolic acidosis develops from the lack of tissue perfusion and the conversion from aerobic to anaerobic metabolism. The respiratory system attempts to compensate for the acidosis by increasing the rate and depth of respirations to blow off carbon dioxide.

212. Correct Answer: **1**

Rationale: Fluids are conserved through the stimulation of osmoreceptors which identify an increased osmolality of the blood and act to stimulate the release of anti-diuretic hormone. Anti-diuretic hormone signals the kidneys to reabsorb fluids into the vasculature to maintain intravascular volume and improve preload and cardiac output. Reabsorption of fluid volume into the vasculature results in a more concentrated urine and an increased urine specific gravity.

213. Correct Answer: **4**

Rationale: In order to improve cardiac output, the heart rate increases as a result of sympathetic stimulation of beta$_1$ receptors.

214. Correct Answer: **2**

Rationale: The central venous pressure (CVP) is measured via a catheter placed in the superior or inferior vena cava. The measurement is a reflection of right atrial pressures and, if there is no tricuspid valve obstruction, right ventricular end-diastolic filling pressures. The normal CVP is 2–6 mmHg. In the scenario, the patient is in hypovolemic shock, a condition where preload and right ventricular end diastolic pressure would be reduced. A CVP of 0 mmHg would support a reduction in right ventricular end diastolic filling pressures.

215. Correct Answer: **1**

Rationale: A bruit is an abnormal swishing or blowing sound heard upon auscultation of the carotid arteries. This sound arises as a result of blood flow through a narrow or partially occluded vessel. Arterial occlusive disease is associated with the narrowing of arterial vessels and, therefore, with the development of a carotid bruit.

216. Correct Answer: **2**

Rationale: The mitral valve is located between the left atrium and the left ventricle. The

SECTION I

SECTION II

SECTION III

SECTION IV

SECTION V

SECTION VI

SECTION VII

SECTION VIII

SECTION IX

SECTION X

presence of a stenotic mitral valve hinders the ability of blood to move into the left ventricle, resulting in an increased workload for the left atrium as it works harder to force blood through the diseased valve. Left atrial hypertrophy can develop in association with this disorder.

217. Correct Answer: **3**

Rationale: Angina is a clinical manifestation of ischemic heart disease. Its symptoms include chest pain or a pressure sensation associated with myocardial ischemia. Angina arises when myocardial oxygen demand exceeds supply.

218. Correct Answer: **1**

Rationale: Venous insufficiency results in tissue congestion, edema, and (over time) impairment of tissue nutrition. The brown pigmentation is caused by hemosiderin, an iron-rich pigment that is deposited by the breakdown of red blood cells.

219. Correct Answer: **3**

Rationale: The depth of chest compressions for cardiopulmonary resuscitation efforts on an adult is $1\frac{1}{2}$ to 2 inches. This depth allows for compression of the heart between the sternum and the spinal column when the patient is placed on a hard surface.

220. Correct Answer: **4**

Rationale: In an emergency situation, the delivery and absorption of medications are critical. Ensuring the patency of an intravenous line prior to the administration of medications will prevent medication extravasation into the tissues and promote safe care.

221. Correct Answer: **2**

Rationale: Ischemia entails a decreased supply of blood to myocardial cells. It can be caused by conditions such as arteriosclerosis and acute coronary syndrome. The lack of blood flow to the cells causes the cells to convert to anaerobic metabolism as a result, the body produces lactic acid. Irritation of nerves from lactic acid accumulation results in pain.

222. Correct Answer: **3**

Rationale: The assessment of a carotid pulse is one way to determine the effectiveness of chest compressions. The person performing chest compressions should be asked to reposition and ensure that he or she is delivering compressions at a depth of $1\frac{1}{2}$ to 2 inches over the lower half of the sternum.